£1.99

15

CANCER: CAUSES AND PREVENTION

Swedish Cancer Committee

CANCER: CAUSES AND PREVENTION

Swedish Cancer Committee

Taylor & Francis
London • Washington, DC

UK	Taylor & Francis Ltd, 4 John St., London WC1N 2ET
USA	Taylor & Francis Inc., 1900 Frost Rd., Suite 101, Bristol, PA 19007

Copyright © Taylor and Francis Ltd. 1992

All right reserved. No part of this publication may be reproduced, stored in a retrieval system, or transmitted, in any form or by any means, electronic, electrostatic, magnetic tape, mechanical, photocopying, recording or otherwise, without the prior permission of the copyright owner.

British Library Cataloguing in Publication Data
A catalogue record for this book is available from the British Library

ISBN: 85066-344-X

Printed in Great Britain by Burgess Science Press, Basingstoke on paper which has a specified pH value on final paper manufacture of not less than 7.5 and is therefore 'acid-free'.
Typeset by Ponting-Green Publishing Services,
Sunninghill, Berks.

Contents

Acknowledgements			xiii
Preface			1
Chapter	1.	**Introduction**	3
	1.1	The Swedish 'scene'	3
	1.2	Terms of reference for the Cancer Committee	8
	1.3	Scope of the study	11
	1.4	Working methods	14
	1.5	Arrangement of the report	14
Chapter	2.	**Cancer—a general background**	16
	2.1	Introduction	16
	2.2	What is cancer?	19
	2.3	The distribution of cancer diseases	24
	2.3.1	How common is cancer?	24
	2.3.2	Geographical and temporal differences in the occurrence of different cancers	32
	2.4	Causes of cancer	42
	2.4.1	Examples of causal factors	43
	2.4.2	The overall picture of cancer causes	51
	2.5	The treatment of cancer	57
	2.6	Economic aspects of cancer	62
Part	**I**	**Cancer diseases: considerations of their induction causes and distribution**	67

Chapter	3.	**Mechanisms involved in the induction of neoplasms: fundamental theories and hypotheses**	69
	3.1	Introduction	69
	3.2	Environmental carcinogenic factors: definitions and basic problems	70
	3.3	The mutation hypothesis	71
	3.3.1	General aspects	71
	3.3.2	Repair of DNA damage	73
	3.3.3	What factors are mutagenic and cancer initiating?	74
	3.4	Cancer induction: a process in several steps	76
	3.5	Dose-response relationships	83
Chapter	4.	**Different types of cancer**	90
	4.1	Introduction	90
	4.2	Tobacco	91
	4.2.1	Introduction	91
	4.2.2	Tobacco consumption—survey	92
	4.2.3	Chemical content of tobacco smoke	96
	4.2.4	Smoking habits and risks to the smoker	100
	4.2.5	Risks for non-smokers (effects of passive smoking and effects of smoking on offspring)	121
	4.3	Diet	131
	4.3.1	General aspects	131
	4.3.2	Natural components of the diet that may cause cancer	132
	4.3.3	Components added to the diet in connection with production, storage and preparation that may cause cancer	136
	4.3.4	Components of the diet that may protect against induction of cancer	140
	4.3.5	Alcohol (ethanol)	142
	4.3.6	Drinking water	144
	4.4	Specific chemicals and exposure environments	147
	4.4.1	Introduction	147
	4.4.2	Routes of dispersion and exposure to chemical substances in the environment	149
	4.4.3	Uptake and metabolism in the

vii

	body: chemical dosimetry	154
4.4.4	Exposure to certain substances in Sweden: information obtained from regulatory agencies	160
4.4.5	Examples of exposure to chemical substances associated with cancer induction in humans	187
4.4.6	Concluding evaluations	211
4.5	Physical factors	220
4.5.1	Physical carcinogens—background	220
4.5.2	Ionizing radiation	222
4.5.3	UV light	235
4.6	Interaction effects	243

Chapter 5.	**Studies of variations in cancer mortality and incidence in Sweden**	256
5.1	Introduction	256
5.1.1	Background	256
5.1.2	Information sources	257
5.1.3	Objectives, related investigations, etc.	257
5.2	Demonstrated relationships between incidence of mortality and certain environmental variables	262
5.2.1	Diagnostic routines	262
5.2.2	Socio-economic factors and lifestyle	265
5.3	Estimates of the magnitude of demonstrated correlations	270
5.3.1	Diagnostic intensity	262
5.3.2	Total 'explainable' proportions of incidences	273
5.3.3	Proportions of incidences attributable to urbanization factors and tobacco smoking	275
5.4	Working conditions and occupational exposure	277
5.5	Cancer in relation to other diseases and causes of death—population group correlations	278
5.6	Trends in cancer incidence and mortality	
5.7	Attempts to forecast future lung cancer incidence	285
5.7.1	Men	286
5.7.2	Women	287
5.8	General experience from the data-base analyses described	289

Chapter	6.	**Attempts to quantify the importance of different causes of the number of cancer cases in Sweden**	293
	6.1	Introduction	293
	6.2	Tobacco smoking	295
	6.3	Dietary factors	296
	6.4	Other lifestyle factors, especially sexual habits and fertility pattern	300
	6.5	Infections, inflammations etc.	302
	6.6	General air pollution in urban areas	303
	6.7	Factors in the working environment	306
	6.8	Consumer products	308
	6.9	Physical factors	309
	6.9.1	Ionizing radiation	309
	6.9.2	Ultraviolet light	310
	6.10	Iatrogenic factors	311
	6.11	Conclusions	311
	PART II	**Prerequisites and measures for reducing the harmful effects of cancer diseases**	317
Chapter	7.	**Strategy of cancer prevention—possibilities and aims**	319
	7.1	General prerequisites	319
	7.2	The concept of cancer prevention. Main aims of the strategy	320
	7.3	A special strategy for cancer only?	322
	7.4	Components of the strategy	323
	7.4.1	Extent—general viewpoints	323
	7.4.2	Risk areas and quantitatively important causal factors	327
	7.5	Special policy issues	332
	7.5.1	Importance of a risk policy	332
	7.5.2	Components of a risk policy	334
Chapter	8.	**Information systems relating to cancer and cancer risks**	345
	8.1	Different information systems and their utilization	345
	8.1.1	Published literature	345

	8.1.2	Population-based information systems	345
	8.2	Prerequisites for population-based studies	346
	8.2.1	General remarks about registers ('files')	346
	8.2.2	Cancer registration	352
	8.2.3	Registration of causes of death	354
	8.3	Epidemiological monitoring	357
	8.4	International cooperation	365
	8.5	The Committee's summarized assessments	366
Chapter	9.	**Health education as a component of disease prevention**	372
	9.1	Introduction	372
	9.1.1	Some starting points and delimitations	372
	9.1.2	Health education aimed at preventing cancer—a part of general health education	374
	9.2	Some future aspects of general health education	376
	9.3	Distribution of responsibility and resources among bodies with present health education duties	377
	9.3.1	Role of authorities	377
	9.3.2	Cooperating parties at the local, regional or other levels	380
	9.4	County Councils' health education at present—an activity in the making	383
	9.5	Strategic questions for health education—limitations and possibilities	385
	9.5.1	Can we count on health education to have effects?	385
	9.5.2	Some factors which limit the effects of information	387
	9.5.3	Some factors which contribute to the effectiveness of information	387
	9.5.4	Some ethical questions	388
	9.6	Summary assessment of the Cancer Committee	391
Chapter	10.	**Special measures in certain risk areas**	398
	10.1	Tobacco use and tobacco products	398
	10.1.1	General background	398
	10.1.2	Tobacco smoking must decrease	398
	10.1.3	Legal control of tobacco products	401

	10.1.4	Monitoring the effects of anti-smoking programmes and other studies	412
	10.1.5	Future development	414
	10.2	Diet and dietary habits	414
	10.2.1	Points of departure	414
	10.2.2	The importance of research on diet for cancer prevention	418
	10.2.3	Control of hazardous substances in food	419
	10.2.4	Alcohol habits and alcohol policy	421
	10.2.5	Dietary habits and diet recommendations	421
	10.2.6	Prerequisites for changes of dietary habits	425
	10.2.7	Effects of changing diet	427
	10.3	General air pollution	428
	10.3.1	Background and general considerations	428
	10.3.2	Car exhausts	431
	10.4	Radon in houses	438
	10.4.1	Uncertainty in the risk assessment	438
	10.4.2	Epidemiological study of the association between lung cancer and radon	440
	10.4.3	The proposals for measures given by the Radon Committee	445
	10.5	Indoor air pollution	449
	10.5.1	Background	449
	10.5.2	Considerations by the Cancer Committee	452
Chapter	11.	**Risk management in the legal context**	456
	11.1	Introduction	456
	11.2	Classification of carcinogens	463
	11.3	Certain priorities. Resources for testing	467
	11.4	The availability of exposure data	471
	11.5	Risk evaluation and risk control measures	475
	11.6	Organizational aspects	480
	11.7	Overall conclusions	482
Chapter	12.	**Cooperation and mutual trust in risk control—the role of information**	487
	12.1	Introduction	487
	12.2	Information—openness and secrecy	488
	12.3	Information supply	494
	12.4	Quality of information	498

			xi
Chapter	*13.*	**Health screening for cancer prevention and detection**	502
	13.1	Health screening—background	502
	13.1.1	Some general comments	502
	13.1.2	Screening for the detection of cancer and precancerous conditions	503
	13.1.3	Definition of populations suitable for screening	506
	13.1.4	Screening problems—theoretical aspects	506
	13.1.5	Organization of health screening	512
	13.2	Issues relating to cancer screening in Sweden	513
	13.2.1	Discussion of various cancer types	513
	13.2.2	Gynaecological screening (vaginal cytology)	514
	13.2.3	Screening for breast cancer	520
	13.2.4	Screening for colo-rectal cancer	526
	13.2.5	Screening for lung cancer	529
	13.3	Psychological aspects of screening for cancer	530
	13.4	Overall evaluation	532
Chapter	*14.*	**Review of the organisation of cancer care in Sweden**	535
	14.1	Current situation	535
	14.2	General guidelines for the future	536
	14.3	Coordination by interdisciplinary collaboration, cancer management programmes, counselling and information within the health service region	537
	14.4	Organization within the county health-care framework	538
	14.5	Training	539
	14.6	Psychological, psychiatric and sociomedical aspects of cancer care	539
	14.7	Prevention of cancer, screening programmes and collaboration between basic and clinical research	540
	14.8	Multi-regional collaboration	541
Chapter	*15.*	**Research into cancer and preventive measures**	542
	15.1	Starting points	542
	15.2	The organization and financing of Swedish cancer research	543
	15.2.1	Introduction	543

	15.2.2	The total resources available to cancer research	545
	15.3	Swedish cancer research—types and directions	547
	15.4	Some organizational issues	553
Chapter	16.	**Some general conclusions**	556
	16.1	Introduction	556
	16.2	Starting points, preconditions for ordering of priorities etc.	557
	16.3	Survey of more important proposals and overall cost aspects	562
	16.4	Setting up an advisory health council at the national level	568
Appendix 1:		Summary	572
Appendix 2:		References	594
Appendix 3:		Background documents	619
Appendix 4:		Committee members and experts	624

Acknowledgements

Acknowledgements

The Cancer Committee and the publishers are grateful to the Swedish National Board of Health and Welfare for administration of this project and to the Swedish Government and the Swedish Cancer Society for financial support for the publication of this English edition. Thanks are also due to the National Environmental Protection Board, the National Energy Administration, the Work Environment Fund and the National Institute of Radiation Protection in Sweden for further financial assistance. Without this support, the project could not have been undertaken.

Preface

In 1979 the Swedish Government appointed a special committee to study the question of cancer prevention with reference to the feeling that many cancer cases were caused by environmental factors (in a broad sense, including life-style). Such feelings were at that time beginning to gain strong support among the scientific community.

The Committee was to assess current knowledge concerning factors entailing a risk of cancer and then to recommend a strategy for cancer prevention in Sweden. It was also to pay attention to certain other questions in connection with cancer disease, such as the value of existing programmes of mass health examinations.

This book is based on the report of the Cancer Committee, which was published in Swedish in October 1984, as No. 67 of the *National Official Investigation Series (SOU)* under the title *Cancer—Orsaker, forebyggande m.m. (Cancer—Causes, prevention, etc.)*. The English version presented here has been edited in collarboration with Dr Ulla Swaren, who was a member of the Cancer Committee and also its chief secretary during the final stages of its work.

When the Committee's report was published, it attracted wide attention both in Sweden and elsewhere. However, with the exception of an authorized summary in English included in the report itself, its contents were in Swedish only. The Committee, although now formally dissolved, has been eager to make the full report available to an international audience so as to promote and perhaps provoke more comments, discussion, research and policy making for reducing cancer risks. The original English summary of the Committee's recommendations is included here as Appendix 1.

After two 'scene-setting' chapters, Part I of this book contains the scientific background regarding the causes of cancer and how the risks can be assessed, and also presents new data and assessments for Sweden. Part II contains the Cancer Committee's recommendations which aimed at improving cancer prevention in both the short and long term, and on policies to promote earlier diagnosis of these diseases. Especially important is the Committee's view that cancer care and prevention should not be carried on in isolation, but should be integrated into the general systems for health care and risk control.

The fact that the Cancer Committee reported to the Swedish Government on a matter of interest to many parties, including politicians and other non-scientists as well as the scientific community, meant that different styles were adopted between various parts of the report, and that it was found desirable to include repetitions and summaries of certain sections in other chapters, so that such chapters could be read in isolation.

The original Cancer Committee report was supported by a quantity of detailed background documents from various authors, initiated or otherwise used by the Committee. These are still available only in Swedish, although some may in due course appear in the international scientific literature. In this book, these documents are often cited as a formal literature reference, being the only source of the supporting information, even if they are not easily accessible or comprehensible to most readers. Of these documents, those published in the *Swedish Departmental 'Ds' Series* are now out of print, but should be available through normal inter-library loan facilities. Unpublished documents are part of the Committee archives to be transferred to the Swedish National Archives (Riksarkivet) which operates a certain service for researchers, e.g. after requests via scientific libraries. In these cases, and for other references to Swedish-language publications, a translation of the title into English has been added.

In certain chapters, the relevant 'background documents' contain most of the detailed citations to the original literature upon which the text is based, which have not been repeated in this volume. It is hoped that readers will not find this too great an inconvenience.

In this edition, account has not been taken of developments or subsequent scientific literature since the original report was published, as this would have entailed an impossible amount of extra work. On the whole, it does not appear that anything has happened that would fundamentally alter the Committee's assessments or recommendations. However, a brief summary of some political developments in Sweden that relate to proposals in the report has been added to Appendix I. The only other addition here to the content of the original report is a brief outline of the organization of Sweden's national and local government and of its health care and risk management systems, at the end of Chapter 1, to help readers to understand the structures mentioned throughout the book.

Information on committee members and associated experts is given in Appendix IV.

1
Introduction

1.1 The Swedish 'scene'

To the reader: Section 1.1 is editorial information not included in the original report by the Swedish Cancer Committee.

Some general information

Sweden occupies a large part of the Scandinavian peninsula, with a maximum distance of about 1600 km from south to north. The country's large area, 450 000 km^2, and small population, 8.4 million (1989), means a low average population density, about 20 inhabitants per square kilometre. However, since about 85 per cent live in urban areas, concentrated to the southern part of the country and along the coasts, the population density in rural areas—including forests and the mountainous parts of northern Sweden—is considerably lower. The three largest conurbations, of the Stockholm, Gothenburg and Malmö regions comprise well over 2 million people.

Historically, demographically, religiously and linguistically, Sweden is a relatively homogeneous country. It is only in recent decades that a process of internationalization and growing immigration has become apparent.

Sweden is a highly industrialized country with a diverse range of production, its traditional strongholds being forest industry, steelworks and, during more recent times, metal industry such as car manufacturing. It may be noted that the country generally lacks the large-area concentrations of heavy industry which are to be found in many other countries, for instance the Ruhr district in Europe.

The Gross domestic product (GDP) per capita in Sweden corresponds to about US$ 19 000 (1987). The rate of employment among women is very high, 80 per cent. Unemployment for men and women taken together was less than 2 per cent (in 1989), but is now increasing.

The social security system is well developed; since the mid-1950s this has included automatic health insurance for all citizens.

Health and medical care in Sweden is to a great extent a public responsibility (see below). The same goes for control of factors that imply risks to human health or to the environment as such, with the important addition that the 'producer' of a risk in principle always has the primary responsibility for reducing or eliminating unacceptable risks. Non-governmental organizations including those on the labour market, both employers and employees, play a great role in the Swedish scene and often supplement public efforts.

National and local government

Sweden is a nation state in contrast to a federal state. Her national parliament, chosen after free elections, is the sole maker of laws. Parliament also decides on national taxes and, in broad terms, on allocating funds to ministries and governmental agencies.

According to conditions laid down in each specific law, the Government may issue more detailed legislation for implementation or, as the case may be, delegate such powers to a suitable governmental agency.

With few exceptions the Swedish Government in the sense of ministers and their chancery has no excecutive or operational tasks, and the ministries are smaller than in many other comparable countries. This work is instead carried out by some 100 major central governmental agencies, under the respective ministries. The agencies are compelled to follow directives issued by the Government but are otherwise in many ways independent. A minister cannot interfere in an agency's application of the law in an individual case; appeals against certain types of agency decision are to go to the Government, however, while others go to a special administrative high court. The Government has also other means to exert an influence over its agencies, not least through the resources made available to each one of them.

A central governmental agency with key functions in planning and supervision in the field of health care in Sweden is the National Board of Health and Welfare. This Board will be referred to in several of the following chapters. Control of health risks in other specific fields are exercised by agencies such as the National Board of Occupational Safety and Health, the National Food Administration, the National Institute of Radiation Protection and the National Environmental Protection Board. The tasks of these agencies are dealt with more specifically in Section 1.2 and in Chapter 11.

Parallel to agencies at the national level—and independent of these—there are the governmental county administrations. A county usually has 200 000–300 000 inhabitants, some being bigger such as the county of Stockholm with a population of 1.6 million. These administrations have a wide range of duties, several of which have a bearing on environmental protection. Protection in the working environment, on the other hand, is an example where the regional/local part of governmental responsibility is carried out beside the county administrations, through the Labour Inspectorate.

Local self-government has a long tradition in Sweden, but the laws underlying the current system go back only somewhat more than 100 years. The first such legislation established rural municipal districts on the basis of medieval parish boundaries. It also introduced a regional unit of self-government, the county councils. These are now 26 in number, and their territory normally coincides with the national goverment's regional administration unit, the county.

Municipalities, the term nowadays covering urban areas as well, are around 280 in number since their reduction from about 2500 in the middle of this century, through changes decided by Parliament. There is still quite a span in size, though, from over 600 000 inhabitants (the city of Stockholm) to some with less than 5000.

County councillors and members of the local decision-making body, the municipal council, are directly elected by the people at general elections every 3 years, on the same day as the parliamentary election.

The division of labour between the municipal and county council administrations has so far been based essentially on the principle that tasks requiring a large population base should properly be handled by the county councils.

According to a number of decisions by Parliament over the years, the county councils have been given a wide range of rights and responsibilities, that of answering for the health and medical care of the population in the respective areas being the oldest and still the major task. The county councils will be referred to in several chapters in the following, especially Chapters 8, 9, 13 and 14.

The municipalities provide a wide range of services: housing, roads, sewerage, water supply, education and social services. Local authorities can issue certain supplementary rules to parliamentary laws, applicable within their jurisdiction. With regard to health risk management they play an important role especially as supervisory bodies at the local level.

Both county councils and municipalities have a right to tax their respective populations. Especially for people in the lower income classes, these taxes taken together constitute the predominant part of the direct taxes they have to pay. Besides through taxation, county councils and the municipalities can partly finance some of their activities through national subsidies according to rules by Parliament/Government.

County councils and municipalities are both strong forces in Swedish society. They have also formed their respective association at the national level, for example for lobbying and for direct negotiations with the Government.

The relative independence of the county councils as well as local government through municipal authorities is one of the reasons why investigators like the Cancer Committee, reporting to the Government, usually refrain from elaborating recommendations with a bearing on these organs.

Organization of health and medical services

Health standards in Sweden are relatively high. The average life expectancy at birth is 74 years for men and 80 years for women (1986). Infant mortality is around six per 1 000 live births. There are, however, inequalities in health between different sectors of the population, occupational categories, etc. Expenditure on health care and medical services equals around 9 per cent of the GDP.

It has already been indicated that health and medical services are by tradition a public concern. They are the responsibility of the regional county councils with their rather unique self-government and taxation powers. Private health care exists only on a limited scale. Parliament and Government have the general duty, at the national level, of safeguarding the equal entitlement of all citizens in the country to good health and medical care, of supervising the quality of health and medical services in medical and legal terms, and of ensuring that activities are adapted to national and economic conditions in general.

Below Parliament, the Ministry of Health and Social Affairs and certain administrative agencies, primarily the National Board of Health and Welfare, answer for central governmental tasks in this context.

Legislation passed in the early 1980s lays down that health care and medical services are to be regarded as a single entity; this piece of legislation, when referred to in later chapters, is therefore presented under the translation of the Health Care Act, 1982. County council responsibilities include not only the provision of medical care, as traditionally represented by examination, treatment and rehabilitation, but also health care, including health promotion and disease prevention. Prevention has to be both individualized and addressed to the population as a whole.

Preventive activities in Sweden include maternity care, child health care and school health services. Organized industrial health schemes cover roughly 70 per cent of all employees. Preventive activities have been introduced for other target groups as well, e.g. for the elderly.

There is mass screening for certain cancer forms, discussed by the Cancer Committee in detail in Chapter 13. An infant vaccination programme has been in operation for many years. Dental care is well developed.

As will be seen in the following, the main task of the Cancer Committee has been to investigate matters concerning cancer prevention. However, a brief outline of the medical care system in a stricter sense seems indicated here, especially with regard to the Committee's discussion in Chapter 14.

The number of hospital beds in Sweden is relatively high, about 14 per 1000 inhabitants. In contrast, the number of out-patient visits to physicians is comparatively low—about 2.5 medical treatment visits per year. Hospitals are nowadays fewer but bigger than they used to be and very well equipped. The staff's professional standard can likewise be said to be very high. However, as in so many other industrialized countries, the late 1980s has shown what the public in general regards as an increasing shortage of personnel resources in health and medical care.

Out-patient care is organized into fairly small primary care areas, with one or more health centres where medical treatment, advisory services and preventive care is provided. When these resources are insufficient with regard to a patient's need for diagnosis and treatment, responsibility may be transferred to the hospital system. This operates at three levels:

(a) District county hospitals for 60 000–90 000 inhabitants with at least four specialities (internal medicine, surgery, diagnostic radiology and anaesthesiology).
(b) Central county hospitals for 200 000–300 000 inhabitants (ordinarily one hospital for each county council area) with 15–20 specialities, one of which can be oncology.
(c) Regional hospitals of which there is at least one in each of the six 'health regions' into which the country is divided. Among other things, one such hospital in each region has an oncological centre, which coordinates relevant clinical and other activities in the region, such as the reporting of new cancer cases.

The health regions are an expression of the need for co-operation between county councils, primarily with regard to highly specialized medical care. The regional hospitals are responsible for patients who present especially formidable problems, requiring collaboration between a large number of highly trained specialists and perhaps also special equipment. Their activities are regulated by agreements between county councils included in each of the respective regions.

1.2 Terms of reference for the Cancer Committee[1]

Cancer is a comprehensive term for a number of different diseases characterized by cells in the body changing their normal pattern of growth. In recent years, the number of cancer cases has markedly increased. According to the Swedish Cancer Registry, set up in 1958 at the National Board of Health and Welfare, about 19 000 new cases of cancer were diagnosed that year. In 1972 about 31 000 new cases were recorded. This is a very alarming development.

Cancer is more common in older people than in younger. Around half of the steady 4 per cent per year increase between 1958 and 1972[2] can be explained by increased average life-span. For the remaining increase, i.e. about 2 per cent per year, reliable and unambiguous explanations are still lacking. Furthermore, it is not known why different forms of cancer increase at different rates. The cancer diseases show great geographic variations. A form of cancer common for one country could be rare in another country.

The cancer diseases and their continuous increase pose a very serious problem. As mentioned above, cancer is more common in older people but it also occurs in younger people. Cancer is the most common cause of death in people aged between 40 and 55 years. It is reckoned that one in every five deaths today is caused by cancer. According to medical science a further increase of cancer is probably to be expected.

Intensive research efforts are continuing worldwide in order to gain a better knowledge of how cancer develops, but the causes and induction mechanisms of these diseases are in most cases still unknown. However, much evidence favours the belief that several interacting causes or risk factors are required in order to bring about a cancer disease.

This of course makes the identification of such factors more difficult. The cancer diseases also have a long so-called latency period, i.e. it usually takes several years until a contact with a risk factor leads to a cancer disease. This delay varies, but 15–20 years is common in this context.

Against the background of the large geographic variations of cancer, an expert groups from the International Agency for Research on Cancer in Lyons as well as other researchers have judged that more than 70 per cent of all cancer cases are caused by environmental factors. The term 'environmental factor' here includes not only substances identified as definite or potential carcinogens, but also factors such as the work environment, social milieu and personal life-style, which subsumes smoking habits, drinking habits, etc.

X-rays, radioactivity and solar ultraviolet rays may be mentioned as other examples of factors which can have a triggering effect in cancer induction. A number of substances, such as certain metals, poisons and chemicals, are also able to induce cancer; such substances are released in, for example, the combustion of coal and oil. There is a continuous increase both in the number and quantity of substances in our environment suspected of contributing to cancer induction. There are fears that the incidence of cancer might increase even faster in future than before, especially in view of the latency period mentioned above.

The risk factor perhaps best known is smoking. The connection between smoking, particularly cigarette smoking, and lung cancer has been shown more and more clearly during recent years. The latest report in this field (Smoking and Health, US Department of Health, Education and Welfare, January 1979) has presented further evidence for such a connection. The report has also pointed to a causal relationship between smoking and cancer in other organs such as the kidneys, the bladder and the pancreas. Furthermore, contact with other cancer-causing factors give a considerably enhanced effect when combined with smoking. Thus smoking increases the morbidity and mortality rates of several forms of cancer far above the numbers following from other risk factors alone. This is the case for the combination of asbestos exposure and smoking.

Since it is likely that a major proportion of cancer diseases is environmentally conditioned, disease prevention should be feasible by different measures. The first major requirement will be that the various cancer-causing factors in different environments should be identified with certainty. Today, two methods are used to map out correlations between different environmental factors and the induction of cancer diseases. One method is experimental research based on animal tests and studies of cells and tissues in the test tube. The other method is epidemiological research based on observations of humans through register analyses, studies of specific populations such as certain groups of employees or residents, retrospective studies of persons with a cancer disease and of their environment, and so on. It is mainly through epidemiological studies that it has been possible to demonstrate a causal relationship between tobacco and lung cancer and between vinyl chloride and a certain type of liver cancer.

Cancer research is well developed in Sweden with extensive research in this field being carried out mainly at institutes within the university sector. The research is financed mainly by the Swedish Cancer Society which has a general economic responsibility for cancer research.[3] At the National Bacteriological Laboratory, research is pursued in virology and immunology, both fields being of importance for cancer research. At occupational health clinics and institutes for hygiene there is research into, for example, chemical health risks.

Several governmental agencies are actively concerned with the impact of environmental factors on the state of public health. For example, pharmaceutical products and their effects are monitored by the National Board of Health and Welfare[4], which also maintains a Cancer Registry of all persons with a tumour. The National Food Administration carries out analytical controls of substances in foods which might have cancer-causing properties. The National Environmental Protection Board monitors pollutants of the air and water. The Department of Environmental Hygiene within this Board[5] has studied the effects of radon, heavy metals and arsenic. The Board's products control division investigates substances hazardous to health and to the environment.[6] The National Board of Occupational Safety and Health has overall responsibility for control of the work environment. Its tasks include mapping of risks for occupational injuries, drawing up standards and methods for control and analysis, and research into occupational cancer. This Board also issues guidelines for exposure limits for many substances, including a classification of cancer-causing substances. The National Institute of Radiation Protection is also authorized to act within this field.

From the above, it should be clear that extensive work is being done in Sweden which has a bearing on the connection between environmental factors and cancer. On the international front, co-operation in this field is well developed and is of great importance for Swedish research. However, taking into consideration the strong impact on the state of health of the population from risk factors associated with cancer diseases, further measures need to be taken in order to prevent, as far as possible, the problems and the individual suffering which these diseases entail. For this purpose a special committee ought to be appointed.

The first task of the Committee should be to compile information available from various sources and assess the state of knowledge about factors entailing a risk of cancer. Such a summary of present knowledge is necessary as a basis for further deliberations. In this context it is desirable that the Committee should consider the effects when different cancer-causing factors interact. The Committee ought also to pay attention to how far difference in lifestyle and in the work environment between men and women give rise to different cancer disease patterns.

Against the background of information gathered and the comprehensive knowledge thus obtained by the Committee, it should suggest a realistic strategy for measures to be taken against cancer. In doing so, the Committee should illuminate to what extent more far-reaching changes in life-style, technology, industrial production, etc., would be needed to considerably reduce cancer risks. Here it might be necessary to weigh the goal of good health against other desired objectives such as a person's right to individual freedom. The Committee should also look into what effects such changes could have on societal economy, employment and material welfare. The Committee should evaluate the costs and sacrifices involved.

Based on its recommended strategy for strengthening measures to prevent cancer, the Committee ought also to consider an appropriate resource distribution between the different measures. The Committee should investigate the practicability of coordinating research activities concerning correlations between environmental factors and cancer diseases. The Standing Committee on Social Welfare in Parliament has stressed the desirability of such a coordination (in its memorandum 1977/78, No. 2).

The major task of the Committee should thus be to recommend measures that can prevent induction of cancer diseases. However, the Committee should also pay attention to problems related to the diagnosis and therapy of these diseases.

Once a cancer disease is established in a patient, the prognosis of a successful treatment is better the earlier the disease is discovered. This is the reason for mass health examinations aiming at early discovery of cancer cases. The value of such screening programmes, however, has not been clearly demonstrated, according to some medical experts.

The Committee should examine current work on evaluating mass health examinations for diagnosis of, for example, cancer of the cervix and of the breast. The Committee ought thus to be able to present a basis for decisions on continued use in Sweden of such health programmes.

An organization for the care of cancer patients is now being built by the various county councils. This is being done according to guidelines issued by the National Board of Health and Welfare in its publication (1974, No. 32) on Planning of Oncological Health Care. It should be part of the Committee's task to follow up developments in this field.

1.3 Scope of the study

According to its directive, the Cancer Committee's principal task was to propose *measures which could prevent the occurrence of cancer diseases*. The first stage was to carry out a survey of all the information available on factors which contribute towards the risk of cancer. The next step was to draw up proposals for a realistic strategy regarding measures to prevent cancer against the background of the information collected.

The basis for the Cancer Committee's compilation of information and assessment of the present state of knowledge has of course been the international scientific literature. In addition, the Committee has in different ways sought to gain a picture of the relevant Swedish situation. It was, however, necessary to limit the investigative work to some extent, firstly to keep the outlay of time and resources reasonable, and secondly to avoid overlap with other governmental investigative work in specific related fields.

The starting points for the assessment of cancer cases caused by living habits and other environmental factors are observations of differences between population groups with different living conditions, as well as differences in the trends in incidence of many forms of cancer. With the aid of the international scientific literature, which is now relatively comprehensive, it is possible to identify certain fairly broad causal areas as regards the occurrence of cancer. When trying to pick out individual causal factors, such as specific chemical substances, knowledge is more fragmentary, although the relevant literature on epidemiological and experimental studies, and research on mechanisms of carcinogenesis has yielded a great deal of detailed information. It would not have been a reasonable objective for the Cancer Committee to attempt to make an independent survey, with its own scientific assessments of all the original literature available. Scientific evaluation of research with possible relevance to cancer risks, regarding both fairly large causal spheres as well as specific agents, have been made and published over a long period both nationally in several countries and on an international basis, often by large, well-qualified research groups. Such work goes on within the International Agency for Research on Cancer (IARC), linked to the World Health Organization. The Committee has to a large extent made use of such existing compilations of information and assessments.

Nor was complete coverage of the scientific literature attempted even within the subsections which the Cancer Committee covered in greater detail. Here the Committee tried to work as pragmatically as possible, in view of the aim of the investigation, to produce an *adequate basis for a strategy for the future prevention of cancer*, rather than to produce complete data and assessments in every respect, as is normal in a scientific context. It must be stressed that the selection of literature quoted is therefore uneven. Furthermore, updating of the investigative material while the work was in progress is not necessarily the same within all spheres.

With regard to causal factors arising within particular risk areas, the Committee considered that it did not lie within the mandate of the investigation to deal with all theoretically conceivable components in different environments or products. This is primarily the responsibility of specific governmental agencies. Instead the Cancer Committee chose to illustrate related problems by means of examples and otherwise to discuss policy questions together with principles and priorities for preventive measures.

Introduction

To make a more specific discussion possible, information from the international scientific literature must be matched to Swedish conditions. The Committee therefore sought in two ways to produce a broad picture of the links in Sweden between different cancer diseases and environmental factors, *firstly* from descriptions of the cancer pattern in the country with time, age, geographical changes and other factors and *secondly* from specific exposure data.

The descriptions of the 'disease panorama' include certain of the so-called macroepidemiological studies of statistical correlations with the incidence of cancer diseases of different 'environment-defining' variables, initiated wholly or partially by the Cancer Committee. It was considered important within the Committee to check the value of existing Swedish registers for population-related details, e.g. to indicate which factors must be taken into consideration in future scientific efforts towards identifying the actual causes of disease. Some of these results have subsequently also been used for checking the plausibility of assumptions made about the importance of certain causal factors for the total incidence of cancer in Sweden.

As far as the exposure data were concerned, the Committee considered it desirable, *firstly* to seek to clarify the actual exposure situation in Sweden with regard to a number of known or suspected cancer-inducing chemical and physical agents, and *secondly* to study separately the data access in this sphere. The Committee therefore approached a number of central authorities with responsibility for control and inspection of such agents to obtain a comprehensive basis of relevant data.

Attempts were made subsequently to estimate quantitatively, from these data about conditions in Sweden, or in certain cases by analogies with conditions in other countries, the importance of different causes for cancer in Sweden. This applies to fairly large spheres of risk or causal factors. Specific agents which might be seen to contribute to the occurrence of some of the annually occurring cancer cases have been examplified.

Even though the investigation does not expressly concern itself with cancer research as such, it was clear from the start that, firstly, the specific measures proposed by the Cancer Committee to try to increase the provisions for cancer prevention would in certain cases become recommendations for specific research or development work and, secondly, that continued intensive national cancer research is, generally speaking, of the greatest importance both for the future prevention of cancer and for the development and improvement of methods of diagnosis and therapy. Apart from the fact that the research questions are thus integrated into different sections from the actual investigation work, the Committee also discussed cancer research separately— but within those limits of breadth and depth which can nevertheless be considered to lie within its terms of reference.

With regard to *medical treatment* and *care*, the Committee decided to concentrate on the two tasks specifically quoted in the terms of reference, namely the question of mass health examinations for early diagnosis of cancer, and the organization of the care of cancer patients.

1.4 Working methods

The complex nature of the cancer question and its breadth had to be especially borne in mind with regard to methodology and possible resources. The investigative work within the Cancer Committee was, to a large degree, based on the active participation of members and experts, several of whom made their knowledge available by writing the basic material for chapter drafts. This applies particularly to Professors Lars Ehrenberg and Lars-Gunnar Larsson, but others in the Committee made specific and time-consuming contributions.

To supplement the specialist knowledge represented within the Cancer Committee, external scientific experts and consultants were co-opted by the Committee in a number of different specialist fields, to provide suitable basic material, or otherwise to give advice and opinions. Furthermore, of great importance for the Committee's work have been the contacts which most of the members have in connection with their own scientific work, not least internationally.

The Committee had both written and verbal contact with a large number of national authorities with responsibilities relating to health promotion or risk control, and also received valuable investigative data from the latter. Consultation or informal contacts also took place with certain other governmental committees.

The Committee also had hearings, firstly with representatives of a number of voluntary organizations within the health and environmental sphere, and secondly with some foreign cancer researchers visiting Sweden. A separate hearing was held with external experts on questions of risk–benefit balancing.

In a few cases the Cancer Committee made use of the fact that scientific conferences on relevant risk areas were to be arranged in Sweden under other auspices, which could to some extent save unnecessary work.

1.5 Arrangement of the report

There was unanimous approval of the report, and its conclusions and recommendations, by the Cancer Committee. This report is introduced by a summary chapter (Chapter 2) about cancer diseases, which firstly constitutes a general background to the whole of the following report, and secondly constitutes a point of departure for certain in-depth analyses presented within subsequent chapters.

The report continues in two main parts. Part I (Chapters 3–6) examines the scientific basis of cancer induction, causes and occurrence in the population as it relates to possibilities for prevention. This part contains a number of sections which may be difficult for a non-scientist to follow. Part II (Chapters 7–16) deals with both measures for cancer prevention and certain other questions of importance for reducing the harmful effects of cancer diseases.

A 'special statement' by Committee Member Dr Peter Soderbaum was published as part of the original report. It dealt with the general approach to the investigation, and more particularly with the issue of non-secrecy for toxicological information submitted to governmental agencies. This statement has been condensed and appears here within Chapter 12, to which the remarks contained are most relevant. [*Ed. note.*]

The main part of the original English summary included with the Swedish edition of the report is included here as Appendix 1, along with some brief comments on developments within Sweden that have taken place since the publication of that edition.

Literature references to each chapter or section are compiled separately in Appendix 2.

Notes

1   These terms of reference were expressed in terms of a statement by the Prime Minister to the Swedish Cabinet (on 3 May 1979). [*Ed. note.*]
2   When the terms of reference were given, available Swedish data did not go beyond 1972 [*Ed. note.*]
3   In recent years there has been a considerable increase in the financing of cancer research from the national budget (see Chapter 15) [*Ed. note.*]
4   As from 1990, control of pharmaceutical products is the responsibility of a new government agency, the Medical Products Agency.
5   Since 1980 this department has formed the nucleus of the new National Institute of Environmental Medicine. [*Ed. note.*]
6   As from 1986, most of these matters are handled by a new government agency, the National Chemicals Inspectorate. [*Ed. note.*]

2
Cancer—a general background

2.1 Introduction

In all the developed countries, cancer is responsible for an ever greater share of the overall sickness spectrum. One important reason for this is the increase in average longevity (Figures 2.1 and 2.2), since the risk of cancer increases with age. Since many diseases which were previously common (for example, infectious diseases, malnutrition and infant mortality) have decreased in importance in socially and medically advanced countries, cancer has assumed the role of a common

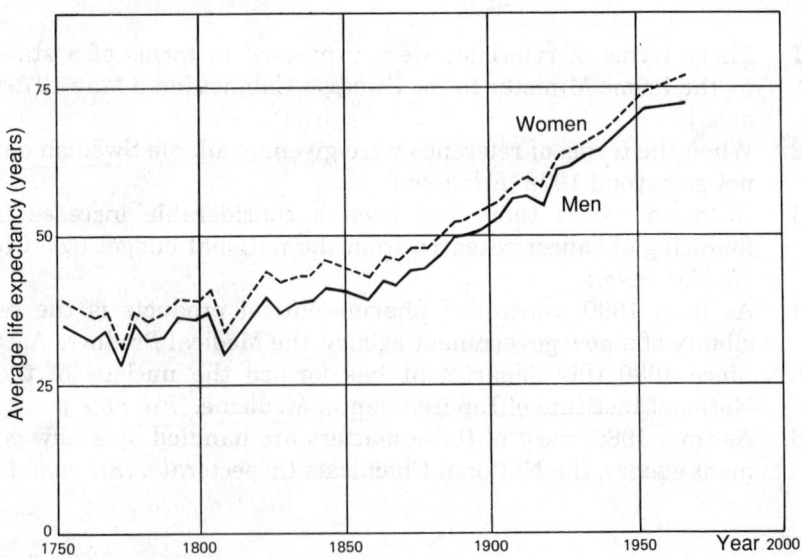

Figure 2.1 Average life expectancy in Sweden since the 18th century. Adapted and updated from Hofsten and Lundstrom (1976).

cause of sickness or death. Another reason for the increase in the number of registered cancer cases is certainly diagnostic. Recent decades have seen improvements in the diagnosis of many cancer diseases—for example, through advances in X-ray diagnostics, cytology and endoscopy—at the same time as greater efforts are put into investigating the nature of the diseases and the causes of deaths particularly among the elderly. Given the current disease spectrum, it is natural that such investigations should today be more concentrated on cancer than previously.

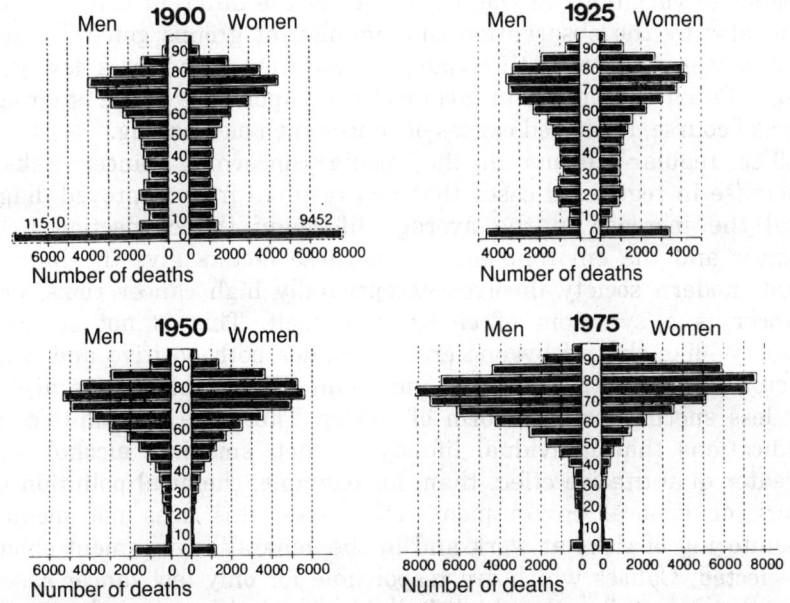

Figure 2.2 Number of deaths in different age groups in Sweden in 1900, 1925, 1950 and 1975. From Bolander and Lindgren, (1981).

The question of whether cancer has become more common in recent decades, after allowing for the changes in the age distribution, is a subject of debate. In the cancer registers of many industrialized countries—that is, in the registers to which new cancer cases are reported—a considerable increase in the age-standardized incidence rate has been noted, but it is likely that this depends, at least partly, on diagnostic factors. If we look instead at the age-standardized cancer mortality rate, which is probably less affected by diagnostic routines, we find that this has altered very little in recent decades. However, considerable alterations which cannot be explained by changes in diagnostic or reporting routines can be observed in the cases of some individual cancer diseases. Common to the countries of the industrialized West, for example, is an increase in the incidence of lung cancer and a decrease in the incidence of cancer of the stomach.

There are many indications that the majority of cancer cases are instigated by the environment. By this is meant the total human environment in the broadest sense, including dietary habits, infectious diseases, sexual habits, the pattern of reproduction, drugs such as tobacco and alcohol, sunlight and ionizing radiation, pharmaceuticals and carcinogenic agents in the general environment and the work place. The importance of the environment is borne out by the geographical variations in the occurrence of the different cancer diseases, and also by the observation that immigrant groups generally acquire the cancer pattern of their adopted country after just a few generations. Other arguments in favour of the importance of the environment are, of course, identified causes of cancer such as smoking.

The regular alarms in the media concerning cancer risks; the increase in registered cases that has resulted from improved diagnosis and the increase in the average life-span; the connection between cancer and the environment; all of these factors give the impression that modern society involves exceptionally high cancer risks, or that cancer is a symptom of civilization itself. This is not so. Modern society—like that of bygone eras—includes both positive and negative factors, from the carcinogenic viewpoint. The problems are also more or less specific for each form of cancer. There are, in addition, many indications that individual life-styles (diet, smoking, alcohol) have a greater quantitative effect than, for example, chemical pollution in the work or general environment. Of course, this does not mean that monitoring of risks at work and in the general environment should be neglected. Causes which are responsible for only few cancer cases can sometimes entail rather high individual risks (for example, in certain work environments), and this makes the checking of potential risk areas worthwhile. Even if the total incidence and mortality of cancer were constant, or only showed small variations, this would not mean that we can assume that the environmental conditions, or the carcinogenic, risks were also constant. Different environmental factors can be of varying importance to different forms of cancer, and our observations reflect the sum of the changes in life-style and other environmental factors.

Reduction of the effects of cancer in society is an important matter, and one that in principle can be achieved in three ways: prevention, improved diagnosis and improved treatment. All three methods must be used in the fight against cancer. The knowledge that the majority of cancer cases are provoked by life-style and other environmental factors probably means that prevention will occupy a more dominant role.

2.2 What is cancer?

Cancer is not a new phenomenon, and does not occur only in man. Cancer diseases have been observed in nearly all vertebrates. The oldest observation has been made in the skeleton of a dinosaur that lived hundreds of millions of years ago. In humans, there are descriptions of obvious cancer tumours, particularly in visible organs such as the breasts and skin, going back thousands of years.

Cancer—that is, malignant tumours—is a collective term for at least a hundred different diseases. These can be quite unlike each other from the point of view of cause, symptoms and prognosis. However, a number of common factors can be defined:

(a) the cancer cells derive from one of the body's own cells,
(b) malignant tumours generally continue to grow in an unlimited fashion, at least when they have reached a size that leads to their being diagnosed,
(c) they often infiltrate, that is, they grow into and destroy normal tissue,
(d) they can spread and cause secondary growths—known as metastasis—in other organs.

The latter three factors—together with the fact that the tumours often produce substances that are toxic to the body, for example, leading to blood deficiency and wasting away—are the reason why a malignant tumour that is not successfully treated will often sooner or later cause the death of the patient.

We can say that cancer cells and malignant tumours are 'antisocial', unlike the other cells and tissues of the body, which develop 'socially' and fulfil their functions according to the body's needs. In fact, from the biological point of view, this 'social' growth is as remarkable as the growth of 'antisocial' structures, that is, cancer.

The normal growth of cells is regulated by complicated biochemical mechanisms. There is minute control of growth and specialization: processes that are still only partially understood. Vital concepts in this area are the genetic code, differentiation and control mechanisms.

THE GENETIC CODE

Cells reproduce themselves through division, where the basic principle is that one cell gives rise to two identical cells with the same genetic code as the original. The code is stored in the chromosomes of the cell's nucleus. The human cell has 46 chromosomes. The genetic code consists of genes, that is, large molecules of deoxyribonucleic acid (DNA). Each chromosome contains a large number of genes. It is estimated that each human cell contains several tens of thousands, perhaps several hundreds of thousands, of genes.

The genetic information is stored in the DNA. By processes that are becoming quite well understood, this information controls the formation of all the proteins which the organism requires in order to function.

Certain cells in the organism constitute tissues which are formed continuously throughout life, through cell division. This is, for instance, the case for skin, mucous membrane, bone marrow and connective tissue. In these tissues there are stem cells which continuously generate new cells at the same speed as the old cells die and disappear.

Other body cells do not, in normal circumstances, reproduce at all, but have a latent reproductive capacity if this is required. The liver cells behave like this. If a part of the liver is destroyed or removed, the tissue loss can be replaced by cell division.

A third type of cell has no reproductive capacity at all. This type represents the highly specialized, final stage of cell development. These are either cells that remain throughout life, for example, certain nerve cells, or cells that have a limited life-cycle and are replaced from a store of stem cells, for example, blood or glandular cells.

Cancer can only develop from cells that are able to undergo cell division. There are many indications that the majority of cancers stem from cells with a disturbed genetic code.

DIFFERENTIATION

All the cells of an individual's body have an identical DNA structure, that is, they have the same basic genetic information. Despite this, both at the fetal stage and later on in life, cells and tissues are developed which have completely different appearances and functions, such as cells of the skin, the nerves, connective tissue and the blood. The process that leads to the specialization of these cells is called differentiation. The biochemical control of these processes is still incompletely understood.

The reason for cells developing in different directions is thought to be that different parts of the genetic information are expressed. The complete genetic information is found first in the fertilized egg cell, and is then transferred to all the cells of the body. In the various cells, only a part of this information is used at each point in time. A thyroid cell and a white blood cell in an individual thus have the same genetic code, but it is a different part of that information in each case that is in operation.

In cancer cells too, only a part of the total genetic information is in operation. But cancer cells are characterized by the fact that the differentiation is disturbed, and is generally less complete than in normal cells. The degree of differentiation in cancer cells varies from one type of cancer to another. We generally refer to poorly differentiated cancer, where the cells appear to be immature, and well-differentiated cancer, where the cells appear to be almost normal. Generally, poorly differentiated tumours are more malignant, that is, they grow and spread more quickly.

The reason for the cancer cell's differentiation shortcomings is probably to be found in deviations in the genetic code. However, there are examples of malignant tumours in which the cells appear to have a normal genetic code, and where it is a disturbance in the differentiation process itself that is responsible for the cancerous nature of the cell.

Recently, some genes have been identified, called oncogenes, which are normally found in all cells, and which, when activated, can initiate cancer. The activation of these genes can be provoked in different ways by carcinogenic viruses, and probably also by physical and chemical agents. One mechanism for activation seems to be a relocation of genes. Even if the oncogenes' part in causing cancer in humans has not yet been fully investigated, this research may lead to the discovery of a common link in the action of different carcinogenic agents.

CONTROL MECHANISMS

During a normal human life-span, about 10 000 million million (10^{16}) new cells are produced. This constitutes approximately 10 tonnes of tissue. Given this tremendous degree of production, it is inevitable that some cells will always be produced with incorrect genetic codes. This can occur by chance, or through the outside influence of, for example, viruses, chemical substances, ultraviolet light or ionizing radiation. The majority of these damaged cells die, but some can survive and, through division, pass on their shortcomings to new generations of cells. Changes in the genetic code in the body cells of a person affect only that person, but changes in the germ cells will, after conception, often lead to an early abortion but may also lead to hereditary diseases in the offspring.

In order to protect the body from such deviant cells, there are control mechanisms. These are basically of two types:

(a) *DNA repair*, for example after damage to the genetic code as a result of chemicals, ultraviolet light or ionizing radiation;
(b) *elimination* of cells with 'incorrect' DNA.

Elimination is probably undertaken in different ways. There are indications that the immune defence system plays a part here. According to one theory, the immune defence system is vital to the prevention of cancer development in cells with a damaged DNA in the same way that we know that immunological phenomena protect organisms from foreign cell material. However, this is a complex matter and has by no means been fully proven. It nevertheless seems

clear that immunological and other control mechanisms play an
important part in the prevention of cancer within the body.

TUMOUR DEVELOPMENT

Figure 2.3 illustrates how a malignant tumour can develop. The steps
in this development are explained as follows:

1. The normal cells reproduce by division.
2. A number of cells are produced that have damaged DNA. These are
   called mutations.
3. Some of the DNA damage is repaired, other damaged cells are
   destroyed. However, some of the damaged cells remain as potential
   ancestors to cancer cells. From some of these pre-cancer cells, a
   true cancer cell can develop, probably through a series of changes.
4. This cell has the ability through division to form a co-ordinated group of cancer cells, a minute cancer core, which can
   be seen only through the microscope.
5. From this minute cancer core, a cancer can develop which is
   clinically noticeable, and which continues to grow.
6. This can in turn lead to spreading and daughter tumours in
   other organs, and finally lead to the death of the patient.

None of the steps in this development is automatically followed
by the next. The appearance of mutated cells need not lead to
the development of a minute cancer core. Not all minute cancer
cores lead to progressively developing cancer tumours. Neither
do all untreated cancers cause death. There are certain types of
cancer which do not usually affect the life-span of the patient.
An example of this is the most common type of skin cancer—
basal cell carcinoma—which grows slowly and which hardly
ever leads to metastasis or to the patient's death. There are
other types of cancer which, while they do spread, grow so
slowly and are so non-toxic that they appear to affect neither
the patient's general health nor his lifespan. In very rare cases,
there can even be a spontaneous regression of a cancer tumour.

DIFFERENT TYPES OF CANCER

As mentioned earlier, cancer is a collective term for a large number of
diseases. Although these have some common characteristics, there are
also great differences. Preventive measures, methods of detecting the
diseases, and means of treatment can differ widely from type to type.
The following major groups can be defined:

(a) epithelial malignant tumours (carcinoma), which are found in skin,
    mucous membrane or glands. Here we find the most common forms

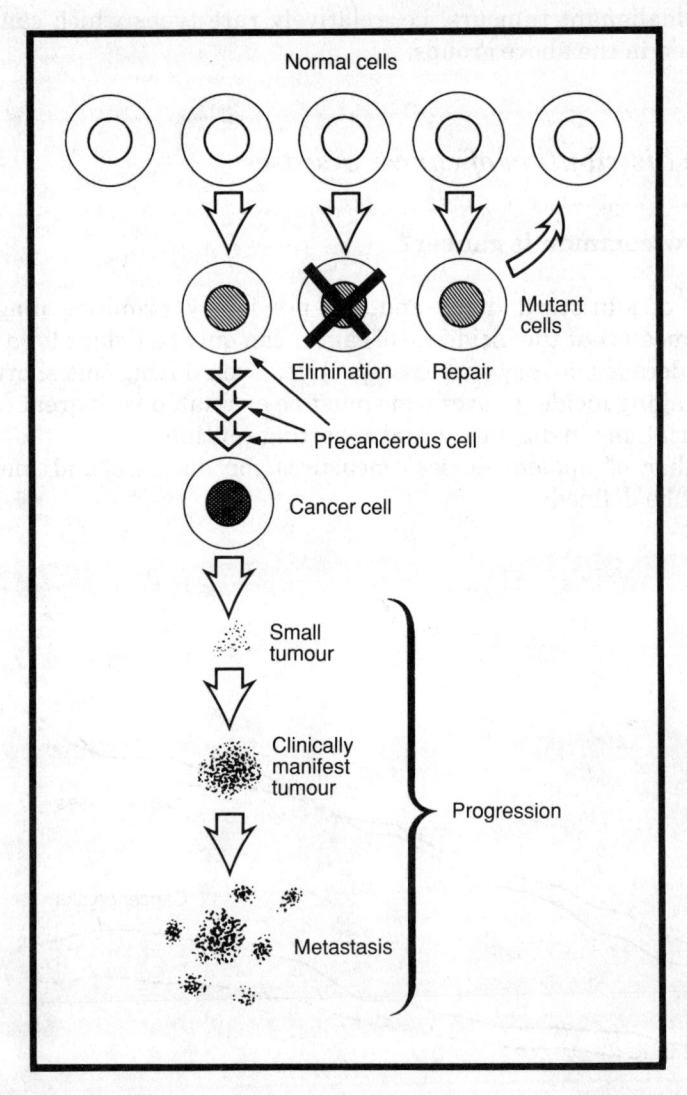

Figure 2.3 Schematic illustration of the development from normal cell to cancer.

of cancer: lung cancer, cancer of the breast, intestinal cancer;
(b) neuro-ectodermal malignant tumours, which are found in the central nervous system;
(c) mesenchymal malignant tumours (sarcoma), which originate in supportive tissues such as connective tissue, fatty tissue, muscles, bones and cartilage;
(d) tumours from the blood-generating organs, i.e. leukaemia and malignant lymphoma;

(e) other malignant tumours, i.e. relatively rare types which cannot be included in the above groups.

2.3 The distribution of cancer diseases

2.3.1 How common is cancer?

The lack of statistical data[1] and the previously primitive diagnostic methods mean that the incidence of cancer can only be judged for a recent period of decades: a very short perspective. Even during this short time-span, changing incidence over time must be evaluated with great caution due to variations in diagnostic and reporting routines.

A number of epidemiological measures for diseases and mortality must first be defined:

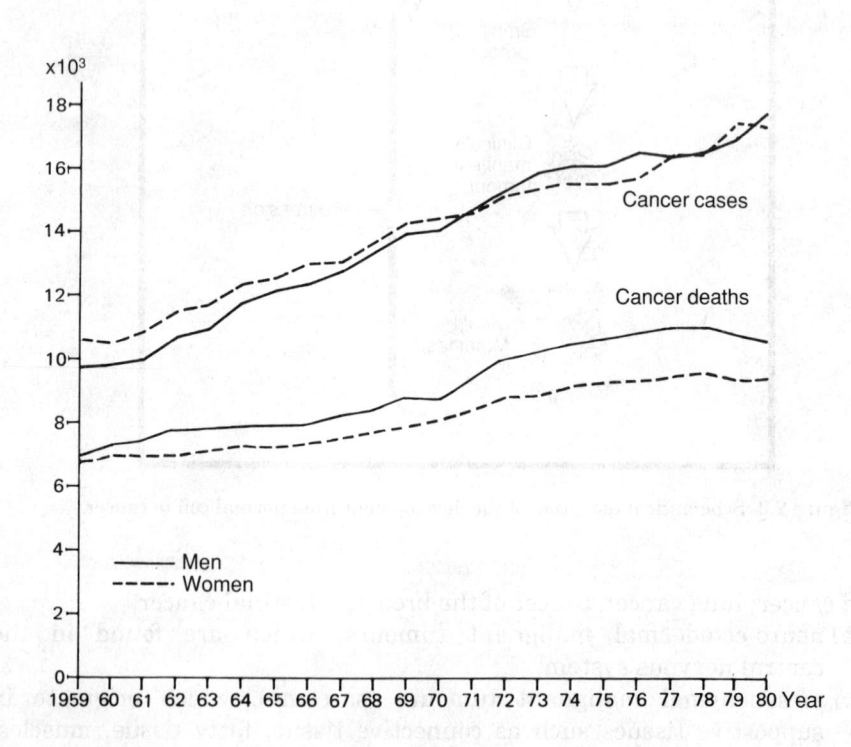

Figure 2.4a The number of annually registered cancer deaths and new cancer cases in Sweden during two decades. From *Cause of Death* (Statistics Sweden) and *Cancer Incidence in Sweden* (National Board of Health and Welfare).

(a) *Incidence rate.* The number of new cases per number of individuals (e.g. 100 000) and period, usually 1 year
(b) *Mortality rate.* The number of deaths per number of individuals and period
(c) *Age-specific incidence rate and mortality rate.* The incidence and mortality rate respectively within a certain age group (e.g. 50–59 years). Given these age-specific data, one can calculate the *age-standardized incidence rate* and the *age-standardized mortality rate*, the incidence and mortality rates which one would expect to find in a study population if this had the same age distribution as a standard population (here usually the 1970 Swedish population).

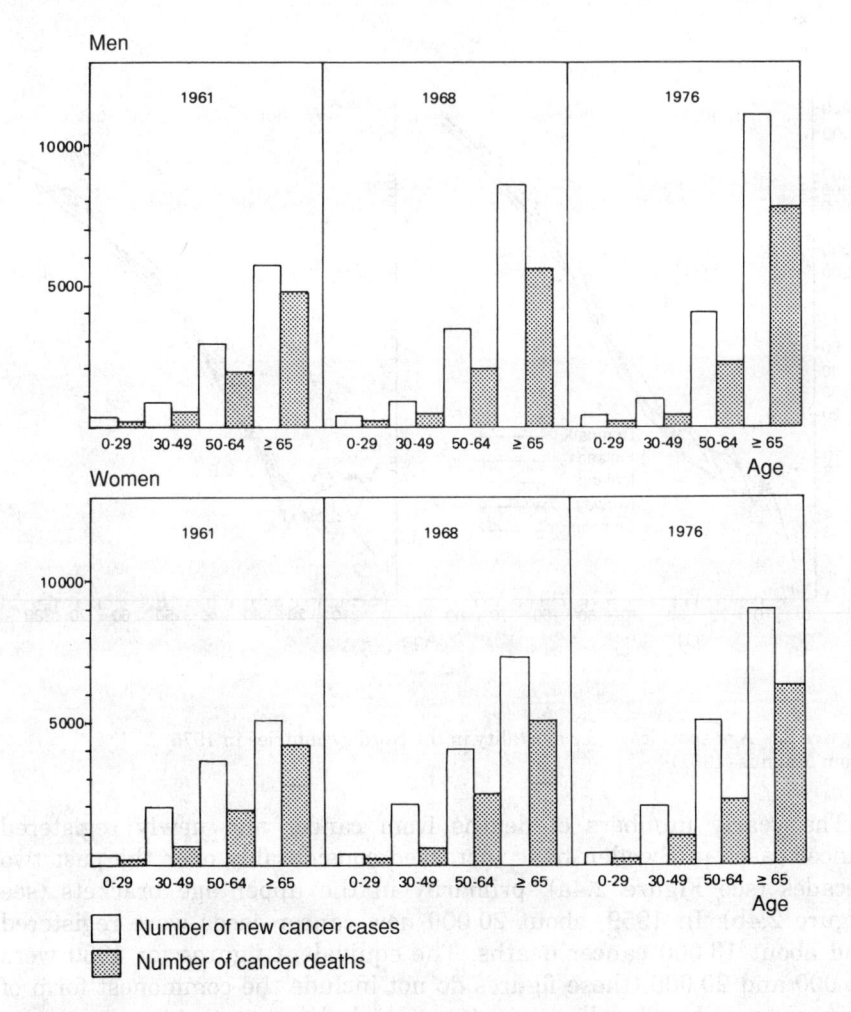

Figure 2.4b Comparison between the years 1961, 1968 and 1976 with cancer deaths and new cancer cases divided into four age groups.

The terms *incidence* and *mortality* are usually used in the text to express the *rates* as defined above (rather than absolute numbers).

In comparing populations with different age profiles, for example when describing changes from one period to another, or between different geographical areas, the age-specific or age-standardized incidence and mortality should always be used, since most diseases, including cancer, have different frequencies in different age groups.

The *prevalence* of a disease indicates the proportion of a population which at a certain point in time has the disease in question. This figure is of interest in connection with mass screening, for example, since the number of cases which may be found depends on the prevalence.

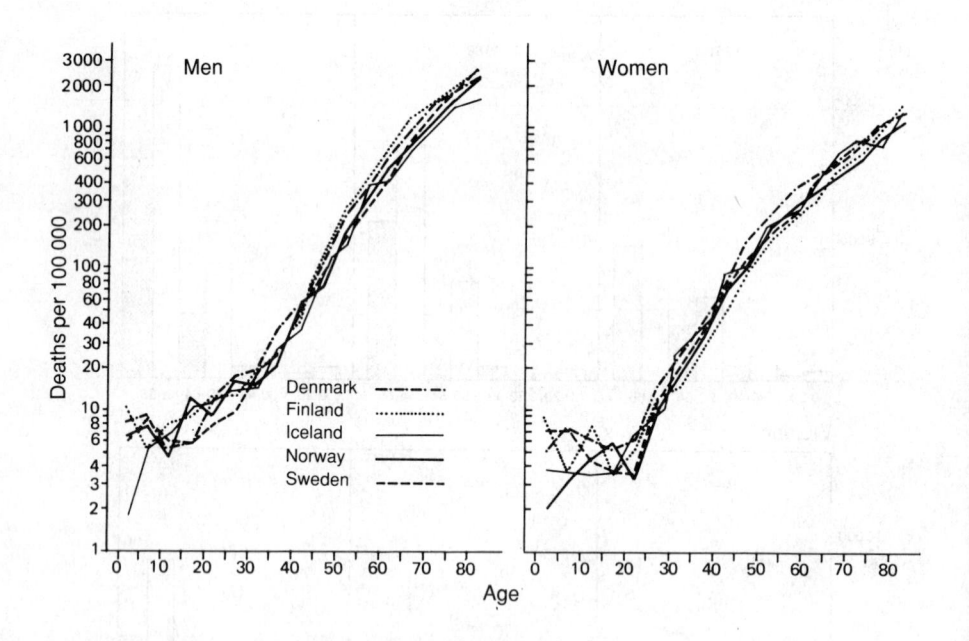

Figure 2.5 Age-specific cancer mortality in the Nordic countries in 1975. From Magnus (1981).

The yearly numbers of deaths from cancer and newly registered cancer cases in Sweden have increased considerably over the past two decades (see Figure 2.4a), primarily in the upper age brackets (see Figure 2.4b). In 1959, about 20 000 new cancer cases were registered and about 13 000 cancer deaths. The equivalent figures for 1980 were 35 000 and 20 000 (these figures do not include the commonest form of skin cancer—basal cell carcinoma—which is very rarely a cause of death). The main reason for these increases is the change in the age profile of the population, since the risk of cancer increases with age. Figure 2.5 shows the age-specific cancer mortality rate in the Nordic countries, and shows how rapidly the rate increases with age, and also how great the similarity is between the different countries.

The age-standardized cancer mortality rate in Sweden has shown little change (+ 0.9 per cent per year for men, ±0 per cent per year for women) during the past two decades (see Figure 2.6). In men, however, we can see

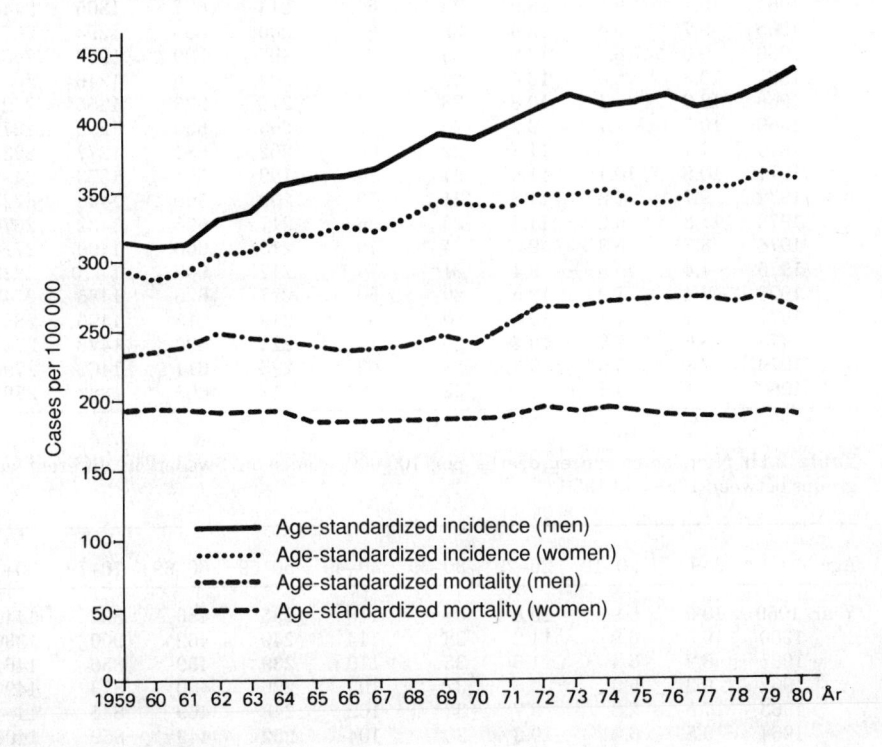

Figure 2.6 Age-standardized cancer incidence rate and mortality in Sweden between 1959 and 80.

an increase in the upper age groups (70 years and over), and especially in the highest age group (80 years and over). (See Table 2.1.)

The age-standardized incidence for the same period showed greater changes. The increase in men was on average 1.5 per cent per year, and in women 0.8 per cent per year (see Figure 2.6). The increase was most obvious in the oldest age groups, although a certain increase could also be seen in the group aged 50–79 years for both sexes (Table 2.2). As already mentioned, these changes must be interpreted with great caution, since improved diagnostic techniques and changes in reporting routines, particularly for the upper age groups, might have

Table 2.1a Number of cancer deaths per 100 000 men in Sweden in different age groups between 1959 and 1980.

Age	0–9	10–19	20–29	30–39	40–49	50–59	60–69	70–79	80+
Year 1959	11.9	8.8	13.1	26	67	201	545	1271	1974
1960	9.9	9.2	12.8	24	73	211	588	1262	1955
1961	10.9	10.8	12.0	28	68	210	591	1240	2018
1962	10.9	7.1	13.3	23	69	211	614	1286	2217
1963	9.1	8.3	13.2	26	65	204	587	1257	2318
1964	10.1	9.2	13.9	23	65	213	577	1305	2140
1965	9.7	9.4	12.8	29	64	200	566	1294	2075
1966	9.0	8.7	12.8	23	65	197	589	1237	2035
1967	10.3	5.4	12.5	22	73	204	585	1246	2041
1968	12.3	8.1	10.8	28	60	215	570	1255	2121
1969	10.7	7.7	12.1	20	71	203	606	1299	2277
1970	7.7	8.5	11.1	22	66	202	581	1277	2238
1971	10.8	10.1	11.5	21	74	199	591	1373	2490
1972	9.7	7.8	11.8	21	70	209	599	1445	2725
1973	11.3	9.2	11.2	23	66	217	606	1432	2676
1974	8.7	6.3	9.8	24	70	213	606	1490	2718
1975	7.4	5.9	9.1	21	79	212	609	1 470	2829
1976	7.4	7.9	12.5	20	60	227	626	1485	2745
1977	8.4	4.7	10.4	20	65	219	615	1496	2863
1978	6.6	7.9	10.4	20	70	221	600	1478	2763
1979	7.8	5.6	9.3	19	63	225	611	1462	2790
1980	7.1	5.6	8.4	22	62	217	601	1383	2791

Table 2.1b Number of cancer deaths per 100 000 women in Sweden in different age groups between 1959 and 1980.

Age	0–9	10–19	20–29	30–39	40–49	50–59	60–69	70–79	80+
Year 1959	10.9	5.9	10.8	38	110	235	480	832	1446
1960	10.5	6.9	11.2	38	114	249	462	900	1336
1961	8.2	6.4	11.8	35	110	239	459	856	1461
1962	9.2	5.9	9.6	32	103	226	450	873	1499
1963	7.5	7.8	9.7	33	102	243	469	845	1434
1964	9.5	6.0	10.3	33	104	252	449	859	1406
1965	9.7	4.4	9.6	28	108	231	441	835	1332
1966	10.7	6.8	7.5	33	105	234	438	831	1361
1967	8.3	4.4	9.9	33	103	228	440	848	1333
1968	8.4	4.5	12.0	37	100	235	433	848	1409
1969	8.3	4.7	9.2	29	116	232	436	844	1446
1970	7.7	4.2	8.4	30	107	236	444	834	1494
1971	6.4	7.6	7.8	30	99	238	420	857	1621
1972	8.9	6.5	10.0	27	97	237	451	935	1562
1973	7.6	2.9	9.5	29	97	221	457	883	1649
1974	8.4	5.7	7.4	26	99	235	457	910	1610
1975	7.4	4.1	7.7	28	96	233	462	879	1627
1976	6.3	4.2	8.8	28	84	230	455	862	1645
1977	6.8	4.2	9.8	26	94	234	456	837	1632
1978	5.4	5.0	7.2	25	94	224	454	849	1619
1979	6.2	4.6	4.1	25	86	237	467	835	1592
1980	5.1	5.2	6.1	27	93	229	458	838	1589

Cancer—a general background

Table 2.2a Number of new cancer cases per 100 000 men in Sweden in different age groups between 1959 and 1980.

Age	0–9	10–19	20–29	30–39	40–49	50–59	60–69	70–79	80+
Year 1959	13.8	14.4	27.3	50	113	317	825	1629	2014
1960	15.3	13.3	22.1	51	118	319	857	1528	1859
1961	12.2	15.2	28.3	52	116	328	837	1504	2039
1962	11.9	11.9	25.2	47	123	328	886	1694	1817
1963	12.4	11.8	26.7	49	106	330	863	1747	1860
1964	11.9	15.0	23.4	53	116	352	901	1914	2484
1965	15.9	14.2	24.5	52	131	346	931	1906	2532
1966	16.2	14.0	25.7	53	121	350	907	1935	2686
1967	16.9	11.8	28.4	51	125	368	927	1856	2790
1968	18.3	14.5	26.8	49	121	357	962	2008	2794
1969	17.2	14.5	26.7	53	143	366	874	2046	3091
1970	16.8	15.5	29.9	52	131	365	965	2019	3006
1971	14.3	17.5	28.6	53	138	364	986	2041	3239
1972	12.9	16.2	30.2	55	135	383	1015	2182	3342
1973	16.7	17.5	29.4	61	139	398	1021	2187	3259
1974	16.3	16.6	27.8	56	141	385	1019	2236	3310
1975	15.2	14.6	28.4	50	143	402	995	2219	3235
1976	14.5	14.5	30.7	54	136	408	1061	2241	3096
1977	14.8	12.6	30.5	41	134	401	1009	2139	3247
1978	18.2	12.3	26.4	48	136	404	1049	2180	3106
1979	17.0	15.3	24.8	51	128	416	1029	2218	3282
1980	17.2	14.9	31.1	53	142	419	1089	2228	3236

Table 2.2b Number of new cancer cases per 100 000 women in Sweden in different age groups between 1959 and 1980.

Age	0–9	10–19	20–29	30–39	40–49	50–59	60–69	70–79	80+
Year 1959	12.7	12.4	29.1	63	256	461	751	1087	1303
1960	12.1	11.3	31.7	102	275	438	712	1060	1118
1961	11.5	12.0	30.3	99	275	454	721	1107	1226
1962	13.0	12.8	31.2	115	287	469	734	1153	1652
1963	12.7	13.6	30.0	100	281	475	745	1142	1489
1964	11.8	14.3	32.7	104	302	474	746	1263	1566
1965	15.4	11.8	31.5	118	311	464	738	1227	1632
1966	11.7	13.4	28.3	116	309	479	762	1281	1704
1967	15.1	12.0	32.7	112	297	480	724	1243	1736
1968	13.3	11.7	33.9	122	305	497	753	1276	1794
1969	13.2	13.2	29.5	111	327	501	801	1304	1941
1970	14.7	10.3	39.0	111	310	503	771	1280	1977
1971	10.3	10.7	36.3	100	303	520	782	1287	1898
1972	12.9	15.3	37.2	102	338	516	821	1351	1938
1973	12.4	10.5	40.2	98	303	510	830	1311	1965
1974	15.4	12.5	36.6	103	294	522	811	1334	1960
1975	14.9	12.1	37.1	95	286	534	819	1279	1885
1976	13.3	12.5	38.5	101	313	522	819	1272	1845
1977	11.3	13.6	40.3	102	306	559	809	1280	1920
1978	13.8	14.7	36.4	99	290	544	877	1305	1828
1979	13.2	12.5	40.3	112	289	566	880	1355	1967
1980	17.9	13.3	36.6	110	293	549	863	1317	1937

affected these figures. One influence of these factors may be seen in the considerably greater increase from 1961 to 1970 than from 1971 to 1980 (see Table 2.6). The rapid changes in the age profile during the 1960s, and the appearance of new therapeutic and diagnostic tools may have led to a gradual increase in the number of reported cases, especially in older patients.

The difficulty of discerning real changes in the incidence and mortality rates from the effects of diagnostic and reporting routines has also been noted in other countries. This is enlarged upon in Chapter 5.

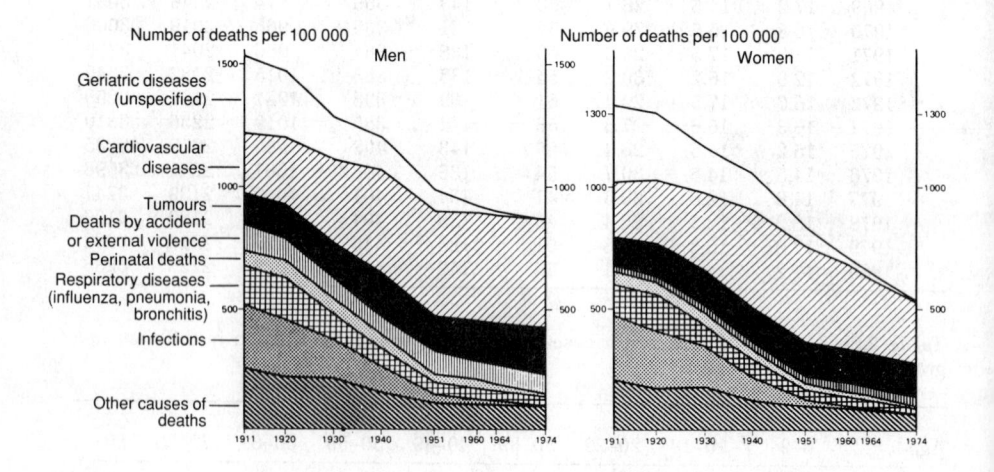

Figure 2.7 Age-standardized mortality in Sweden 1911–1974 divided into some main causes of death. From Carlsson *et al.* (1979).

In recent decades, great changes have taken place in the disease spectrum in Sweden. These changes are clearly reflected in the statistics concerning causes of death. In Figure 2.7, the age-standardized mortality rates for different causes of death are shown for the period 1911–1974. The mortality rate as a whole decreased considerably, largely due to sharp reduction in the infant mortality rate and in deaths from infectious diseases. The diagram also shows changes in the classification of causes of death. The unspecified cause of death 'old-age diseases' was gradually phased out and replaced by more specific causes of death (probably primarily cardiovascular diseases and tumours). Despite this, the registered deaths from tumours have remained at a surprisingly constant level for this period of six or seven decades. Statistics from the other Nordic countries,

Cancer—a general background 31

England, the USA, Canada and others show similar patterns. However, it should be noted that from a preventive viewpoint, it is not sufficient merely to know what changes there are in the total cancer incidence or mortality rates, since these are the sum of individual

Table 2.3a Number of deaths (all causes) per 100 000 men in Sweden in different age groups between 1959 and 1980.

Age	0–9	10–19	20–29	30–39	40–49	50–59	60–69	70–79	80+
Year 1959	257	66	122	151	321	825	2187	6018	16 298
1960	246	62	111	154	326	863	2390	6356	16 791
1961	238	63	107	156	301	848	2327	6076	16 261
1962	239	63	111	147	322	854	2404	6407	17 022
1963	245	69	114	150	311	840	2341	6200	16 997
1964	235	75	115	158	323	867	2333	6150	16 276
1965	223	68	110	169	311	852	2335	6239	16 487
1966	217	67	108	159	336	842	2356	6116	15 944
1967	200	55	114	169	353	865	2357	6142	15 805
1968	197	63	118	181	341	864	2296	6230	16 558
1969	182	63	112	162	357	871	2380	6290	16 263
1970	170	65	110	156	350	854	2273	5862	15 254
1971	163	69	112	164	371	862	2320	6070	15 750
1972	164	64	116	160	375	875	2277	6094	15 601
1973	138	60	111	160	359	877	2345	6117	16 119
1974	136	58	105	160	370	889	2313	6102	15 990
1975	128	58	120	160	376	876	2351	6088	16 094
1976	115	56	115	158	358	919	2375	6226	16 427
1977	113	48	116	159	372	902	2336	5940	15 742
1978	108	54	118	157	359	907	2330	5986	15 649
1979	110	49	110	164	354	925	2292	6033	15 736
1980	103	43	112	153	354	887	2291	5847	15 803

tumour diseases which themselves demonstrate considerable variability.

As a result of the changes in the mortality spectrum, longevity has steadily increased in Sweden (Figure 2.1). This has continued to be the case for the past two decades, although more slowly than over the previous hundred years. The average life-span in 1978 was about 72 years for men, and about 78 years for women. The increase for men in recent years has been entirely the result of the decrease in the infant mortality rate. On the other hand, for women, even the age groups of 40 years and above have shown a decrease in the mortality rate (Table 2.3). The average life-span for those who died of cancer in 1978 was about 71 years both for men and women. If we were to assume that cancer did not exist as a cause of death, and that the cancer victims instead had run the same risk as others in their age group who later died of other causes, then we find that cancer shortened the average life-span by 2–3 years, for both men and women. The loss of years of life for the individuals who die of cancer is nonetheless considerable: about 11 years for men, and about 16 years for women, based on the entire population. The greater loss of years of life in women arises from the fact that certain female cancer forms (cancer of the breast, ovaries and cervix) are quite common among middle-aged or even somewhat younger women. This is also reflected in the average age at which cancer has been diagnosed. This increased between 1959 and 1980 from 65.6 to 68.7 years in men, and from 61.2 to 66.3 years in women, and was always lower for women. The reason for the increased average age at diagnosis is certainly chiefly the result of changes in the age profile in the population.

Table 2.3b Number of deaths (all causes) per 100 000 women in Sweden in different age groups between 1959 and 1980.

Age	0–9	10–19	20–29	30–39	40–49	50–59	60–69	70–79	80+
Year 1959	179	30	53	99	232	557	1571	4905	14 844
1960	185	33	55	101	245	571	1569	5127	15 367
1961	182	31	55	87	226	549	1489	4890	14 895
1962	181	33	48	92	216	536	1487	4904	15 421
1963	179	38	52	92	226	539	1482	4700	14 735
1964	182	33	54	99	218	534	1459	4584	14 073
1965	173	35	47	97	225	525	1416	4505	14 188
1966	155	32	50	94	211	503	1355	4460	13 799
1967	155	28	53	94	219	496	1335	4425	13 617
1968	147	32	51	95	220	513	1339	4471	14 227
1969	120	32	48	94	234	512	1341	4381	13 714
1970	125	34	49	88	220	498	1281	3978	12 707
1971	120	36	43	94	217	492	1244	3939	12 585
1972	116	29	51	87	205	487	1239	3959	12 543
1973	111	31	47	89	202	467	1221	3837	12 628
1974	110	30	44	82	204	476	1208	3782	12 670
1975	96	35	44	84	216	475	1204	3768	12 415
1976	90	32	53	89	201	466	1192	3715	12 826
1977	81	28	45	77	207	467	1143	3489	11 944
1978	81	27	45	77	194	448	1124	3528	11 963
1979	78	27	45	79	190	481	1126	3415	11 951
1980	74	24	43	79	199	464	1129	3388	11 995

2.3.2 Geographical and temporal differences in the occurrence of different cancers

The majority of cancer diseases show considerable differences in incidence from one part of the world to another. These differences are often very great. For example, cancer of the oesophagus and of the nasopharynx and primary liver cancer are all rather rare in the West, but in some parts of the world are among the most common forms.

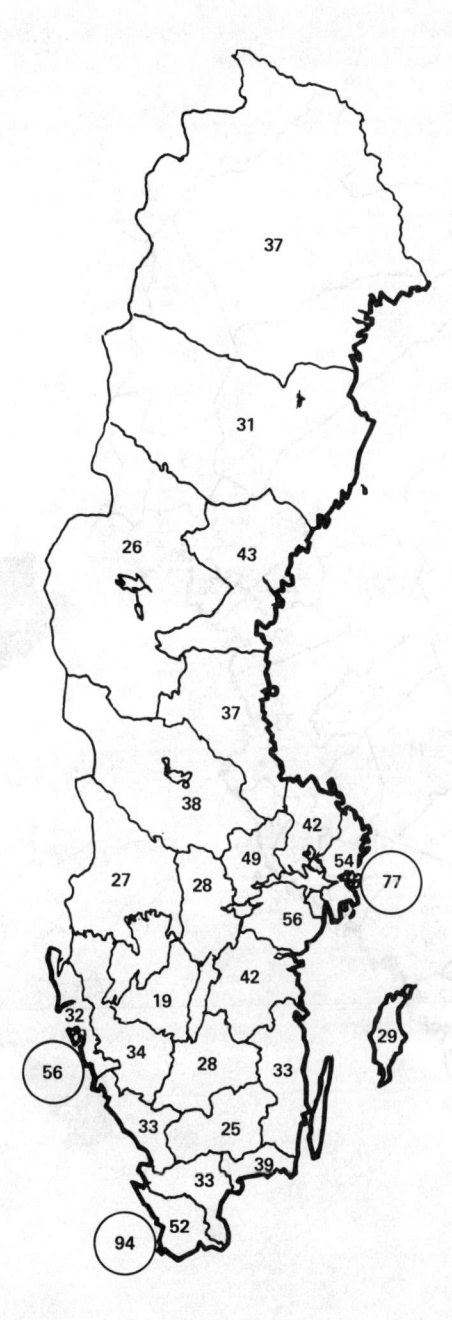

Figure 2.8 Age-standardized incidence of male lung cancer for the period 1977–79 (per 100 000 and year) in the different counties and in the municipalities of Stockholm, Gothenburg and Malmo. (In the figures for Stockholm County, Gothenburg and Bohus County, and Malmohus County, the three mentioned municipalities are excluded. Figures for these municipalities are given within circles.)

34   *Cancer: causes and prevention*

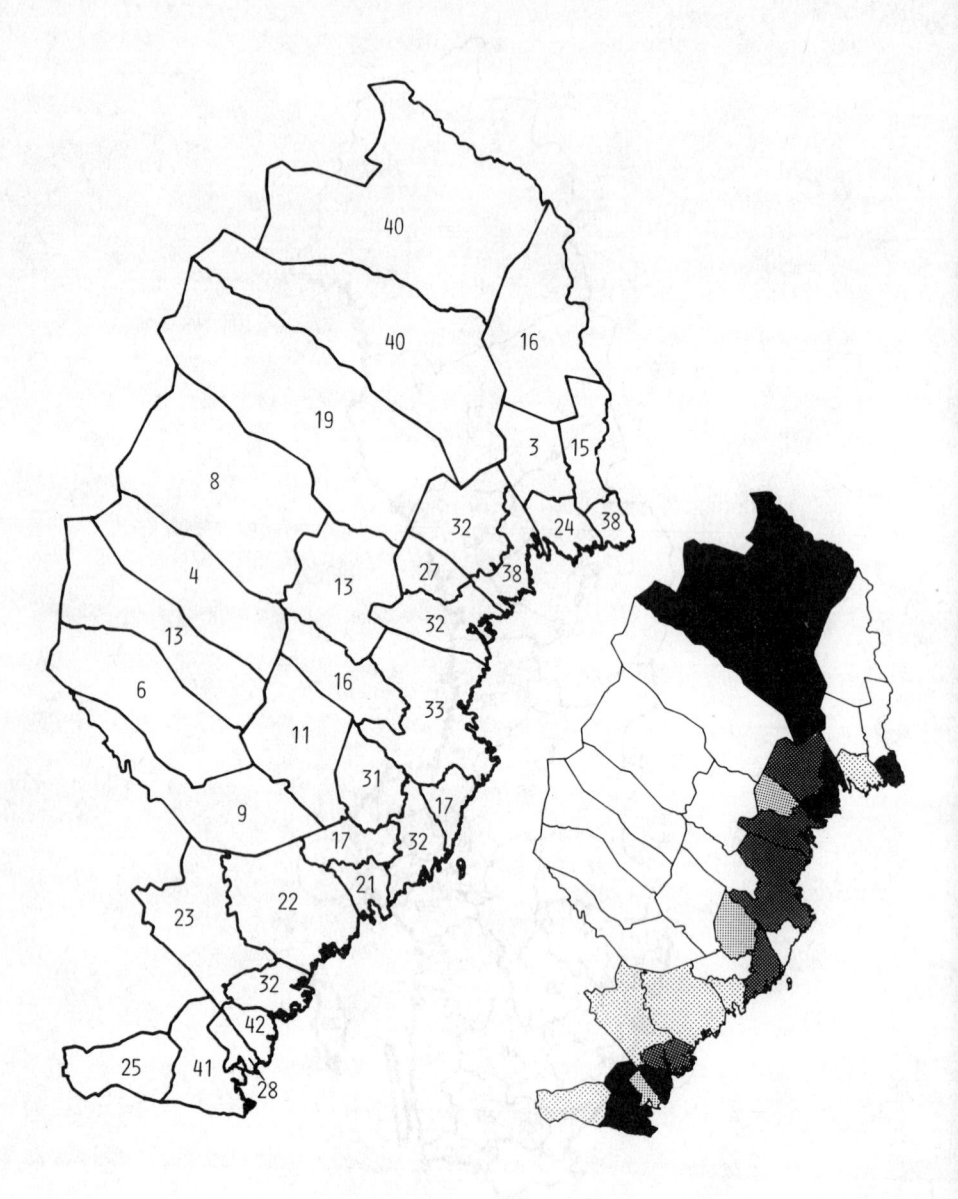

Figure 2.9 Age-standardized incidence of male lung cancer in the different municipalities in the counties of Norrbotten, Vasterbotten and Vasternorrland. Average for the period 1959–78 (per 100 000 and year). Numbers on the left-hand map are represented graphically on the smaller right-hand map.
From Larsson *et al.* (1982).

Another example, an extreme case, is Burkitt's lymphoma, a special form of cancer which occurs in certain parts of Africa, South America and New Guinea, but which is very rare in other parts of the world.

Furthermore, several of the forms of cancer that are common in the West demonstrate remarkable geographical differences in incidence, for example lung cancer and cancers of the colon, stomach, breast and cervix. Differences can be shown not only between countries with widely differing socio-economic and cultural structures, but also between different areas within the same country. Examples of this phenomenon are found in a large US mortality rate study (*Atlas of Cancer Mortality for US Counties 1950–1969* (Fraumeni et al., 1975)), and also in studies from the Nordic cancer registers. For example, male lung cancer in Sweden, as in many other countries, has a higher incidence in urban areas than in rural areas (Figure 2.8). Great

Table 2.4 Age-standardized incidence rates in 1978 for some cancer types in the whole of Sweden, the municipalities of Stockholm, Gothenburg and Malmö, and the county of Örebro.

Cancer site	Sex	Sweden	Stockholm	Gothenburg	Malmö	Örebro county
Total	M	413.2	525.0	431.8	797.8	330.0
	F	350.1	388.5	379.5	492.8	284.6
Oesophagus	M	5.2	11.6	7.8	8.9	4.6
	F	1.6	2.1	1.3	2.0	0.6
Stomach	M	28.6	27.9	32.0	36.6	20.8
	F	15.2	11.6	14.6	15.6	13.1
Colon	M	29.7	36.7	32.5	51.6	27.3
	F	27.0	26.6	30.6	47.2	29.9
Rectum	M	20.1	20.8	21.2	29.7	18.4
	F	12.5	14.2	12.0	18.1	9.3
Lung	M	34.8	76.7	51.5	96.3	25.5
	F	10.7	18.1	14.7	16.3	8.5
Breast	F	91.9	107.3	96.1	153.6	77.7
Cervix	F	14.1	19.7	21.3	16.9	8.8
Uterus	F	20.6	26.2	24.3	21.2	23.3
Prostate	M	89.7	97.4	64.0	174.2	86.1
Kidney	M	17.4	21.7	22.6	25.7	15.2
	F	9.7	10.9	10.4	14.5	3.5
Urinary tract (excl. kidney)	M	27.3	39.6	36.1	4.3	20.2
	F	8.1	10.3	8.8	12.4	7.0

differences in the incidence rate can also occur within a limited geographical area. Many inland municipalities in the northern part of the country, for example, have a very low incidence of male lung cancer compared with the more urbanized coastal municipalities and the two mining municipalities of Kiruna and Gällivare in the far north (see Figure 2.9).

Table 2.4 shows that the total incidence rate was about twice as great in Malmö (the highest incidence in Sweden) as in the county of Örebro (the lowest), and that great differences existed between the rates of, for example, lung cancer, cancer of the prostate, cervix, breast, stomach, colon and urinary tract. Probably, some of these apparent differences reflect real variations, but some differences also seem due to diagnostic factors. In Malmö, the proximity of a highly specialized hospital, a high rate of autopsies, and autopsy methods that include systematic searching for latent cancer may explain, for example, the high incidence of prostate cancer.

Allowing for misleading differences caused by random deviations, diagnostic intensity and reporting routines, the geographic incidence and mortality variations can help to indicate the risk factors involved in different life-styles and other environmental conditions. The same is true of differences between various occupational and ethnic groups. However, such differences cannot alone serve as proof of assumed risk factors. They can only serve as a warning, justifying a more thorough study of the underlying causes, for example in the form of analytical epidemiological studies of cohort or case-control type.

Table 2.5 shows the distribution of cancer cases and cancer deaths registered in 1959 and in 1980 in Sweden with regard to cancer type. Both for men and for women, the five or six most common cancer forms covered 50–60 per cent of all cancer cases. The table also shows that there has been a considerable change in the pattern of cancer over the past two decades. The most striking things are the relative decrease in cancers of the stomach and of the cervix, and the increase in lung cancer. Statistics from many other developed countries show similar changes. Figure 2.10 shows the development of the age-standardized mortality rate in the USA for some of the most common cancers between 1930 and 1973. The total cancer mortality rate was relatively steady, but the mortality rate for cancer of the stomach and uterus decreased, while that of lung cancer increased. In the Swedish registers of deaths and of cancer cases, developments over the past two decades can be studied (Figures 2.11 and 2.12, Table 2.6). Both the mortality and incidence statistics show a sharp increase in lung cancer, primary cancer of the liver and malignant melanoma and a sharp decrease in cancer of the stomach. Furthermore, in the incidence statistics, we can see an increase in cancer of the prostate and of the urinary tract, as well as a less rapid increase in cancers of the breast

Cancer—a general background

Table 2.5 Distribution of new cancer cases and cancer deaths in Sweden among different cancer types in 1959 and 1980.

The most frequent cancer types in men	Cancer deaths 1959	Cancer deaths 1980	New cancer cases 1959	New cancer cases 1980
Total number	6 786	10 647	9 671	17 708
Specific cancer types	%	%	%	%
Prostrate	14.2	16.3	16.0	21.7
Colon and rectum	12.3	11.9	13.4	12.2
Lung	8.0	17.2	7.7	10.5
Lymphatic and blood-forming organs	9.3	10.0	6.7	6.4
Stomach	22.5	9.0	16.2	6.5
Urinary tract (excl. kidneys)	2.6	4.0	4.7	6.7
Skin (excl. melanoma)	0.4	0.3	3.3	3.8
Pancreas	5.2	6.8	4.0	3.7
Liver and biliary passages	2.1	4.4	1.8	2.8
Nervous system	2.4	3.0	3.6	3.0
Malignant melanoma of the skin	1.0	1.3	1.0	2.6

The most frequent cancer types in women	Cancer deaths 1959	Cancer deaths 1980	New cancer cases 1959	New cancer cases 1980
Total number	6 642	9 280	10 549	17 178
Specific cancer types	%	%	%	%
Breast	12.5	16.1	23.1	24.9
Colon and rectum	13.2	13.6	11.1	12.7
Ovary	7.8	7.4	7.1	5.9
Lymphatic and blood-forming organs	8.0	9.2	6.1	6.6
Uterus	1.7	2.3	6.0	5.4
Stomach	15.4	7.4	8.4	4.1
Liver and biliary passages	2.7	7.4	2.0	4.0
Nervous system	2.8	2.6	3.1	3.2
Pancreas	4.1	7.1	2.2	3.4
Cervix	4.4	2.6	8.4	3.0
Lung	2.3	6.5	1.9	3.5
Kidney	2.6	3.5	2.3	2.9
Malignant melanoma of the skin	0.5	1.4	1.2	3.0
Urinary tract (excl. kidney)	1.3	1.9	1.6	2.5
Skin (excl. melanoma)	0.3	0.3	1.7	2.2

and colon, and a decrease in cancer of the cervix. In the mortality statistics, these latter changes are all either less apparent, or are absent. A difference in changes over time between incidence and mortality can have several causes. An incidence increase with no corresponding mortality increase can be due to improved treatment, or to earlier diagnosis, allowing more successful treatment. Another reason could be that we are increasingly discovering biologically more benign cases, which do not shorten the patient's life. As in the case of

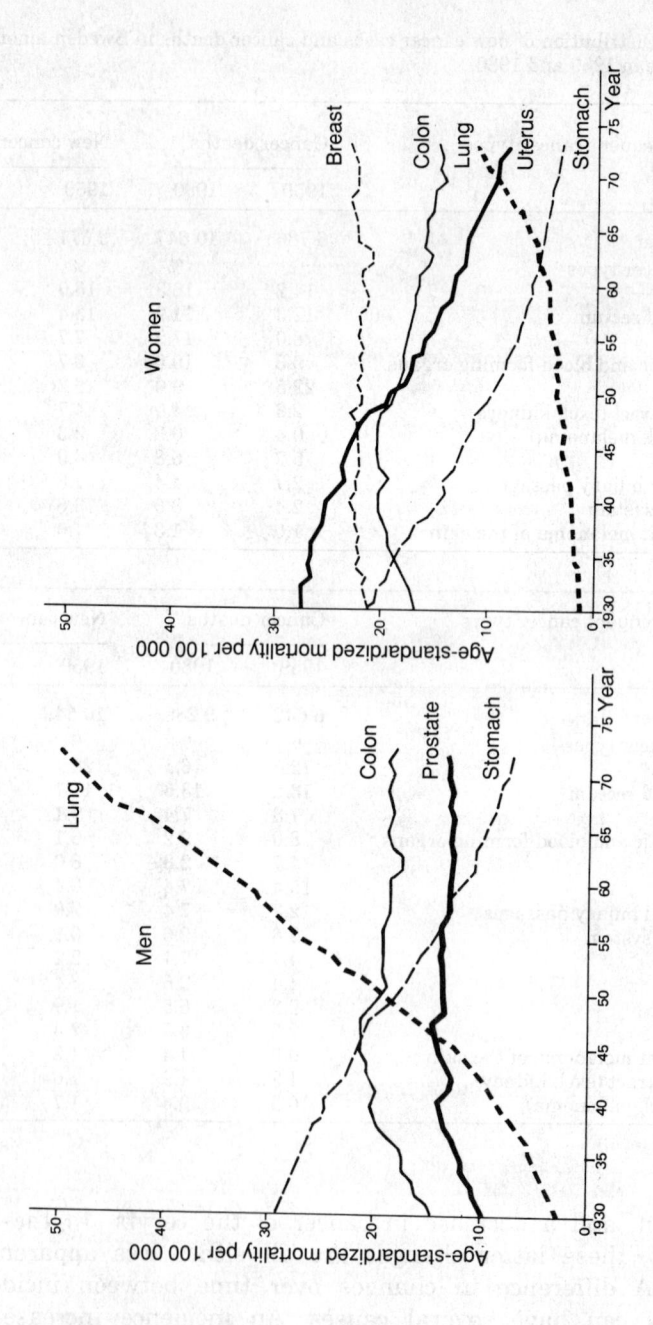

Figure 2.10 Age-standardized mortality for some common cancer types in the USA between 1930 and 1973.
From Weisburger *et al.* (1977).

Table 2.6 Percentage change per year of age-standardized incidence and mortality rates for different cancer types in Sweden during the periods 1961–70 and 1971–80.

		Incidence rate 1961–70	Incidence rate 1971–80	Mortality rate 1961–70	Mortality rate 1971–80
All cancer	M	2.3	0.4	−0.1	0.4
	F	1.5	0.4	−0.5	−0.3
Oesophagus	M	1.1	0.3	0.1	−0.6
	F	−2.7	−3.5	−2.6	−2.8
Stomach	M	−2.7	−2.8	−4.7	−3.7
	F	−2.4	−4.0	−4.3	−3.9
Colon	M	2.1	0.6	0.7	−0.7
	F	2.1	0.5	−0.1	−0.6
Rectum	M	0.6	1.0	−0.8	−0.9
	F	0.9	0.9	−0.6	−1.4
Liver and biliary passages	M	4.8	2.1	4.0	3.7
	F	4.0	1.8	3.7	2.3
Pancreas	M	2.7	−1.4	1.6	−0.7
	F	2.4	0.1	1.8	1.3
Lung	M	3.6	0.8	6.7	2.1
	F	4.3	3.1	6.5	3.3
Breast	F	1.5	1.8	−0.8	−0.8
Cervix	F	−0.1	−4.9	0.3	−3.8
Ovary	F	1.9	−0.6	1.3	0.1
Prostate	M	4.2	0.5	−0.2	0.2
Kidneys	M	3.3	0.7	1.1	1.0
	F	3.1	−0.3	−0.1	−0.2
Urinary bladder	M	4.3	1.4	3.2	0.6
	F	1.8	−0.9	2.7	0.1
Melanoma of the skin	M	5.9	5.4	4.9	2.4
	F	8.2	5.8	3.3	3.3

the total cancer incidence, the increase in many forms was much less apparent between 1971 and 1980 than it was between 1960 and 1970, which may depend on diagnostic and reporting routines.

The question of variations in the incidence of cancer in children is a subject of particular interest, since such variations could indicate the influence of environmental factors at the fetal stage or during the first years of life. The incidence of cancer in children in Sweden, which is very low, has, however, not shown any significant changes over the two last decades (Table 2.2). Nor have any definite geographic variations been shown.

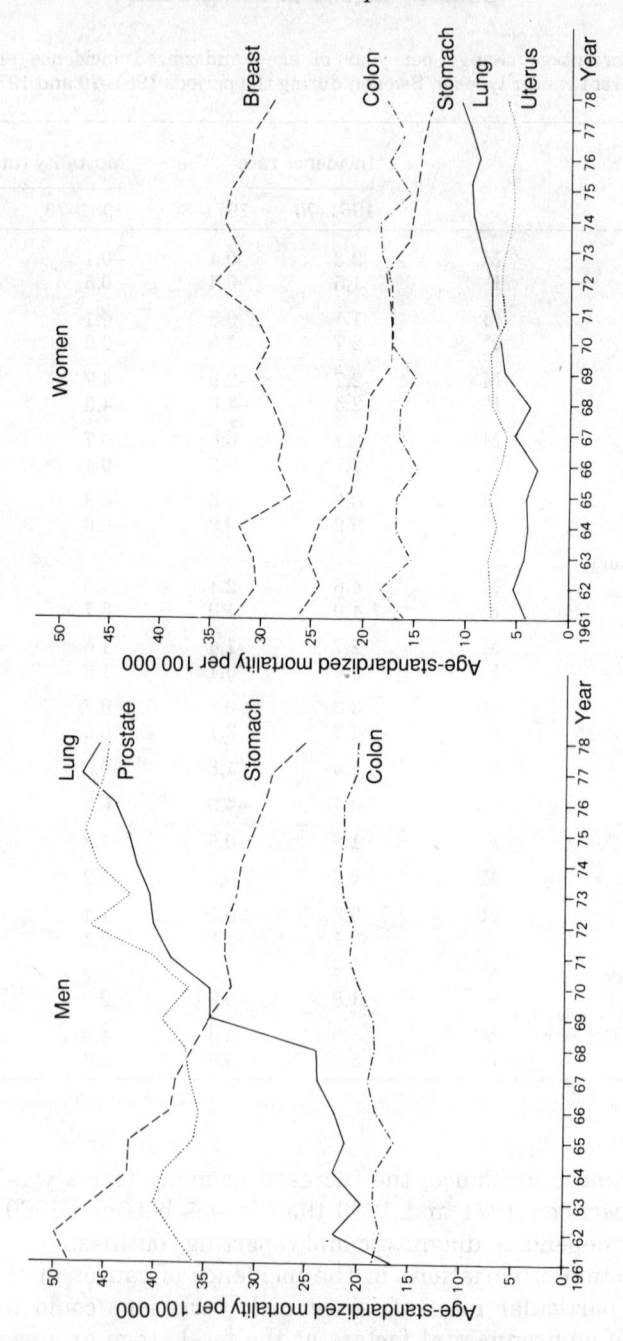

Figure 2.11 Age-standardized mortality in Sweden between 1961 and 1978 for some common cancer types.

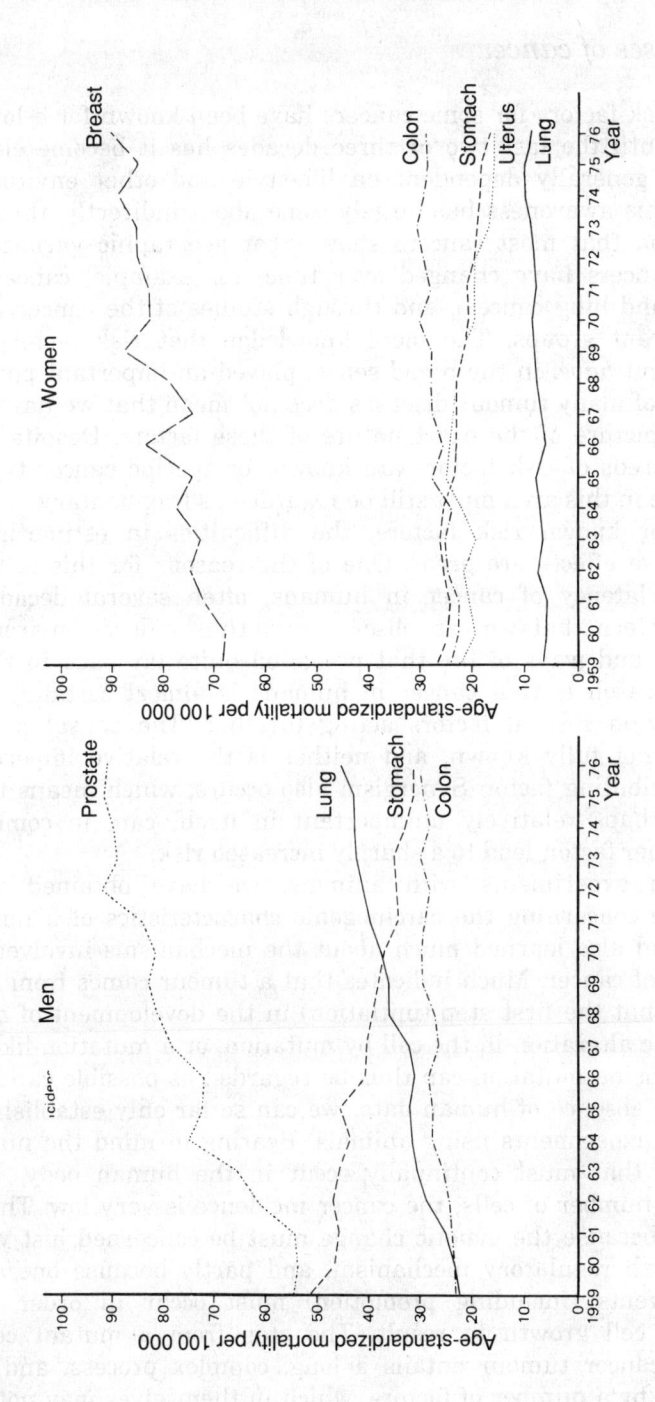

Figure 2.12 Age-standardized incidence in Sweden between 1959 and 1976 for the same cancer types as in Figure 2.11.

2.4 Causes of cancer

Certain risk factors for some cancers have been known for a long time, but not until the last two or three decades has it become clear that cancer is generally dependent on life-style and other environmental factors. This awareness has largely come about indirectly, through the observation that most cancers show great geographic variation, that certain cancers have changed over time (for example, cancer of the stomach and lung cancer), and through studies of the cancer patterns of immigrant groups. The mere knowledge that risk factors in the environment *have*, in the broad sense, played an important part in the incidence of many tumour diseases does not mean that we have a more complete picture of the exact nature of these factors. Despite the fact that hundreds of risk factors are known for specific cancer types, our knowledge in this area must still be regarded as fragmentary.

Even for known risk factors, the difficulties in estimating their quantitative effects are great. One of the reasons for this is the long period of latency of cancer in humans, often several decades. The cancer pattern that we can observe now thus reflects environmental conditions and ways of life that prevailed quite far back in the past. Another reason is that cancer in humans is almost certainly usually dependent on several factors acting together. The causal pattern is generally not fully known, and neither is the relative importance of each contributing factor. Synergism also occurs, which means that one factor, perhaps relatively unimportant in itself, can, in combination with another factor, lead to a sharply increased risk.

Through experiments with animals, we have obtained valuable knowledge concerning the carcinogenic characteristics of a number of agents, and also learned much about the mechanisms involved in the induction of cancer. Much indicates that a tumour comes from a single cell, and that the first step (initiation) in the development of a cancer is a genetic alteration in the cell by mutation, or a mutation-like event. Agents causing mutation can thus be regarded as possible carcinogens, but in the absence of human data, we can so far only establish this in long-term experiments using animals. Bearing in mind the number of mutations that must continually occur in the human body, with its enormous number of cells, the cancer incidence is very low. This could be partly because the genetic change must be concerned just with the cell's growth regulatory mechanism, and partly because one or more further events (including promotion) must occur in order for uncontrolled cell growth to result. The step from a mutant cell to a manifest cancer tumour entails a long, complex process, and can be influenced by a number of factors, which in themselves may not have a mutagenic effect. It is this complexity that partly explains why experimental findings constitute an insufficient basis for a quantitative analysis of the causes of cancer in humans. Some risk factors, even some that have been demonstrated in humans, appear to operate by means other than genetic alteration, and generally at a later stage of the carcinogenic process. It is often difficult to find experimental models for the study of this type of factor. (The mechanisms concerned with the development of cancer are described further in Chapter 3.)

2.4.1 Examples of causal factors

The following are a number of examples of known or suspected causal factors in connection with cancer in human beings. In several cases, the analysis of the causal factors is expanded on and covered in more detail later (see especially Chapter 4 and parts of Chapter 6).

Heredity

In the case of some rare cancer forms, it has been possible to demonstrate a strong hereditary factor. There are also a fairly large number of innate disorders—although these are all rare—which predispose individuals to different forms of cancer. Of greater quantitative importance is the fact that in a number of common cancers (for example breast, stomach, large intestine) a certain hereditary predisposition for the particular cancer form studied has been found. Generally, studies have shown that patients with these cancer forms had close relatives with the same disease more frequently than was expected. Families with a remarkably high cancer frequency have been observed which, combined with the findings that certain individuals can be stricken by more than one cancer form, may indicate a certain hereditary disposition.

It is natural to assume that hereditary factors play a certain part in the induction of most cancer cases, but the quantitative importance of these factors seems still relatively slight when compared to environmental factors. This can be illustrated, for example, by studies of twins where the agreement between single-egg (monozygotic) twins with regard to cancer incidence has generally been slight. For certain cancer forms, however, there are real ethnic differences. One example is malignant melanoma of the skin, which is rare in the dark-skinned races and most common in people with fair or ruddy skin (which is poor in pigmentation).

Tobacco

The carcinogenic effect of smoking tobacco has been well established in a number of epidemiological studies. Tobacco smoking is certainly the main cause of the sharp increase in lung cancer observed in many countries in recent decades. Smoking has also been shown to play a part in the incidence of cancer in other parts of the body, both in direct contact with the inhaled smoke—for example lips, oral cavity, throat and larynx—and in other organs such as the urinary tract and the pancreas, which indicates a spreading of the carcinogenic substance in the body. The question of the cancer risk run by so-called passive smokers (environmental tobacco smoke) is still very much under discussion, particularly with regard to lung cancer, where some epidemiological evidence has appeared. This is discussed in more detail in Section 4.2.5.

Tobacco smoke contains a large number of carcinogenic substances, for example polycyclic aromatic hydrocarbons of the kind found in tar, small amounts of radioactive substances, and nitrosamines. Smoking appears to both initiate and promote the carcinogenic process. This latter point implies that even heavy smokers can reduce the risk of lung cancer by quitting the habit.

Even chewing tobacco and snuff can lead to cancer of the mouth, although the incidence is low. In some countries, for example India, chewing plugs are used consisting of a mixture of betel, tobacco and spices, which explains the high incidence of cancer of the mouth in these parts of the world.

Alcohol (ethanol)

High alcohol consumption raises the risk of cancer in organs that are directly associated with the intake, such as the mouth, throat and oesophagus, and several epidemiological studies have indicated that alcohol and tobacco operate in synergy. Primary liver cancer frequently appears with cirrhosis in alcoholics.

Other chemical factors

Many substances and certain more complex exposure situations have a proven or suspected carcinogenic effect on man on the basis of epidemiological observations. Asbestos is one example (lungs, lung sac, peritoneum). Others are aromatic amines (bladder), vinyl chloride (liver and other sites), the pain-killing drug phenacetin (kidneys, urinary tract), wood dust (nasal cavities), benzene (leukaemia). Carcinogenic polycyclic hydrocarbons such as benzo[a]pyrene are suspected to be a cause of the increased risk of lung cancer which has been observed in workers in coke ovens and gasworks. These substances are formed in oil and petrol combustion, and they also appear in the form of general air pollution. They have been much discussed as a possible contributing factor to the higher cancer incidence (especially lung cancer) found in urban areas. Epidemiologically, this has been difficult to prove because of the simultaneous effects of smoking habits, occupational situations and possibly also other living habits. However, studies have shown it to be probable that some part of the increase in lung cancer in urban areas can be ascribed to general air pollution. A couple of new Swedish studies in this context will be described in Chapter 5. Certain metals, or metal compounds, such as arsenic, nickel and chromium have, in occupational situations, also been shown to have a carcinogenic effect (causing lung cancer).

Nitrosamines and related substances, which can be formed from nitrite and nitrate under certain conditions, are found to be carcinogenic in animal experimental systems, and are highly suspect as human carcinogens. This has led to considerable discussion concerning the use of nitrite as a preservative in beef and pork products. The use of nitrite additives, such as nitrite salting, and even ordinary salting, has become less common in recent years, which may be a cause of the decrease in the incidence of cancer of the stomach. Aflatoxins, which can be formed from vegetable moulds, are highly carcinogenic in experimental conditions (causing liver tumours) and epidemiological studies point to these substances also being carcinogenic in humans. Several cytotoxic drugs which are used in treating cancers are mutagens, and clinical observations have shown that some of them also have a carcinogenic effect.

Internationally, the question of chemical carcinogens is carefully monitored by the International Agency for Research on Cancer (IARC) in Lyons, which publishes collected risk analysis reports based on available experimental and epidemiological observations. Other bodies too, especially the National Cancer Institute (NCI) in the USA, are engaged in this evaluative work. After evaluation of nearly 600 chemicals or exposure situations (covered in the first 29 IARC monographs), the IARC has listed 44 with positive evidence or a suspicion of an association with human cancer, based on epidemiological data. The equivalent list of experimental carcinogens contains between 200 and 300 substances. Bearing in mind the difficulties involved in epidemiologically documenting carcinogenic effects, particularly if they are slight, it can be assumed that the real number of human carcinogens is considerably greater than in the IARC list.

Dietary factors and metabolism

Particularly in the last decade, a lively discussion has been in progress concerning the possible role of the diet in the incidence of certain common cancer diseases, such as cancer of the stomach, large intestine, breast and prostate. Experimental findings and some epidemiological indices make it probable that this role is quite important. Several mechanisms of carcinogenesis are possible. There has been much discussion of the amounts of fat and fibre in food. One possible mechanism promoting cancer of the large intestine is that fats increase the formation of substances such as bile acids in the intestines, which by bacterial conversion may become carcinogenic. A high fibre content reduces the exposure of the intestine's mucous membrane in the bowel to such substances. Experimental and clinical studies have shown that an increase in the fat content of food leads to an increase in prolactin production (a pituitary hormone that stimulates the mammary glands). This could be a mechanism in the development of breast cancer.

Other conceivable dietary risk factors include naturally formed carcinogens such as aflatoxins, food additives such as nitrite, and residues of foreign substances from food production and storage (for example certain pesticides, possible carcinogens in packaging materials, and so on). Substances formed in grilling and frying (polycyclic aromatic hydrocarbons and certain breakdown products from proteins) may also be carcinogenic.

The epidemiological evidence has hitherto consisted of macro-oriented studies (descriptive studies, statistical correlation studies) and to a lesser extent of analyses of individuals, which in this field have considerable difficulties. One example of the broader kind of epidemiological evidence is the correlation observed between fat consumption in different countries and the incidence of cancers of the large intestine and of the breast. Dietary habits in Japan have traditionally been quite unlike those of the West. Japan also has a cancer pattern that differs radically from those of the USA and Europe (more cancer of the stomach and oesophagus, less cancer of the large intestine, breast and prostate). Japanese immigrants in the USA, however, have after two or three generations acquired a cancer pattern similar to the US pattern. The most probable explanation of this is the change in dietary habits.

In this context, it should also be mentioned that certain metabolic dysfunctions promote cancer in the alimentary tract. For example, pernicious anaemia leads to a considerable increase in the risk of cancer of the stomach. Even an operation formerly used for a stomach ulcer (a partial resection) appears to add to the risk. One form of tumour that is interesting in Sweden is cancer of the mouth and throat. Only a few decades ago, this cancer form was not uncommon in women who had previously suffered from iron-deficiency anaemia, which often led to changes in the mucous membrane in the upper alimentary canal. Following the introduction of iron-enriched flour and intensive treatment of this type of anaemia in young women, the incidence of this form of cancer decreased considerably.

In all probability, there are other dietary factors that have a positive effect and that can prevent the development of cancer. This will be discussed later.

Hormonal factors

Giving oestrogen to women, often to alleviate menopausal symptoms, increases the risk of cancer of the corpus uteri, and has also been discussed as a possible risk factor in connection with breast cancer. In the latter case, however, there is a lack of firm evidence. Several epidemiological studies have indicated that women who have not given birth run a higher than average risk of breast cancer, while this risk is lower for women who bore children at a relatively early age. Hormonal imbalance caused by diet has been discussed as a possible cause of cancer of the breast, corpus uteri, ovaries and prostate gland. A very rare form of vaginal cancer can appear in young girls if the mother has taken certain synthetic oestrogen preparations during pregnancy. Cancer of the thyroid appears to be more common in countries with endemic goitre due to a lack of iodine.

Viruses

Viruses cause many tumour diseases in animals. In all probability, there are oncogenic viruses for humans too, although it has been difficult to obtain firm evidence. However, there are strong indications concerning a couple of tumour diseases: Burkitt's lymphoma and nasopharyngeal cancer. In these diseases, one generally finds an increased number of antibodies to a virus (the Epstein–Barr virus) and, in the tumour cells, certain antigens associated with this virus can be found. It has also been demonstrated that viral genetic material is built into the genetic material of the cancer cell in the fashion that one would expect of an oncogenic virus. Since most people are bearers of this virus, it cannot be the sole cause of these cancers. However, it could form a link in a chain of causal events, a chain including certain alterations in chromosomes resulting in the activation of an oncogene.

There are also indications that a virus infection can contribute to cancer of the cervix (the papilloma virus) and primary liver cancer (the hepatitis B virus). With a special type of acute leukaemia (T-cell leukaemia), strong indications have recently been found of a viral aetiology.

Chronic infection and inflammation

Certain chronic infections and inflammations predispose towards cancer. There are well-known correlations between chronic sinusitis and cancer of the paranasal sinuses, between chronic otitis and cancer of the middle ear, between ulcerous colitis and cancer of the large intestine. Skin cancer occasionally appears in old burns, leg sores and fistulas. Some tropical parasite diseases can also lead to cancer, such as bilharzia (bladder) and infections of *Clonorchis sinensis* (liver).

Sexual habits and genital hygiene

In the case of cancer of the cervix, sexual habits play an important part in that the risk increases with the number of sexual partners and with the early commencement of sexual activity. This is borne out both by case control studies and by observations of special ethnic groups. Fimosis predisposes to cancer of the penis, and early circumcision almost entirely removes the risk of this cancer form. There are strong indications that the carcinogenic factor in cancer of the cervix is transmitted by the male, although it is unclear whether this is in the form of a virus or whether it is of a chemical nature. Male circumcision also appears to have prophylactic effect on cancer of the cervix.

Immunological factors

The body has definite defence mechanisms for dealing with deviant, mutant cells, and also with developed cancer cells. Part of this mechanism is probably immunological and, according to one theory, immunological surveillance constitutes an important factor in preventing the development of cancer. Certain innate immunological defects, and also artificial immunosuppression following, for example, a kidney transplant, have been found to lead to an increased incidence of malignant lymphoma (tumours from the body's lymphatic tissue) and even an increase in some other cancer forms. In the case of acquired immunodeficiency syndrome (AIDS) in which a pronounced lowering of the immune defence system is characteristic, an otherwise very rare form of cancer, Kaposi's sarcoma, can appear. The organism's control of cell differentiation and defence against mutant cells is, however, extremely complicated and far from fully understood. No simple connection between, for example, immune defence mechanisms and tumour risks has yet been proven.

Ultraviolet light (sunlight)

Ultraviolet (UV) light causes changes in the DNA of the skin's epithelial cells, which the body generally can repair. Epidemiological studies indicate that, for Caucasian races, excessive exposure to sunlight can increase the risk of cancer of the lip, and of the most common forms of skin cancer (basal cell carcinoma, squamous cell carcinoma and malignant melanoma).

The increase in the incidence of malignant melanoma which has been observed in several countries in recent decades probably depends, at least partly, on the increase in sunbathing. There are indications that intermittent, intensive exposure is especially responsible for the increased risk. In the case of the rare hereditary disease *xeroderma pigmentosum*, the normal DNA repair mechanism is defective and patients with this disease get malignant skin tumours at an early age on skin surfaces exposed to the sun.

Ionizing radiation

Ionizing radiation, for example X-rays and radiation from radioactive substances, may, depending on the type of exposure, lead to different forms of tumour such as leukaemia, cancer of the breast and the thyroid, lung cancer, and cancer of the skin, mucous membranes and supportive tissues.

Together with smoking, ionizing radiation is the best known and studied causal factor in human cancer, and it is also the one for which the dose–response relation in human populations is best known. The reason for this is primarily that we have had access to a large, exposed study population (survivors of the atom bomb explosions in Hiroshima and Nagasaki), and also to some clinical materials. Under more ordinary conditions, ionizing radiation certainly is not one of the major causes of cancer. One exception, however, could be exposure to the radioactive gas radon, which, because of alpha radiation from decay products (known as radon daughters) can give high radiation doses in the lung epithelium. Radon exposure is probably one of the reasons for underground workers in poorly ventilated mines (uranium mines and others) having an increased incidence of lung cancer. Radon exposure is currently under discussion, in many countries, as a risk factor in homes with increased radon content either as a result of the use of building materials containing uranium (especially light concrete), or as a result of radon leaking in from ground containing uranium. Primarily by extrapolating risk data from mineworkers, the Swedish radiation protection authority has calculated that radon in housing in the future may be responsible for roughly 300–3000 cases of lung cancer per year in Sweden. This estimate, however, is very uncertain and it is doubtful whether it is possible to 'translate' (extrapolate) data from mining to housing, which have such different physical and chemical environmental conditions. There is as yet no firm epidemiological evidence of a connection between radon in housing and lung cancer. As radon in dwellings could constitute a serious health problem, this problem is discussed in more detail in Section 10.4.

Difficulties in estimating the risks are also encountered with regard to the low exposures caused by diagnostic radiology, particularly in X-ray diagnostics. Epidemiological data have shown a relationship between exposure of fetuses (during X-rays of the abdomen and pelvic regions of pregnant women) and the development of a cancer in the infant. Epidemiological evidence is also available concerning X-ray examination that has given rise to rather high radiation doses in adults, for example breast cancer in women who have undergone repeated X-ray examinations of the lungs in connection with tuberculosis. For the small doses that usually result from diagnostic radiology, there is no epidemiological evidence of a carcinogenic effect. Using a linear model to extrapolate from observations at high doses to low doses, a small number of cancer cases (roughly the same number that can theoretically be ascribed to natural background radiation) per year could be caused by medical radiology. Chapter 3 addresses the question of extrapolation to small doses in connection with both physical and chemical agents.

The effects of ionizing radiation, at both the experimental and population levels, are being followed with great care by an international committee of experts, the United Nations Scientific Committee on the Effects of Atomic Radiation (UNSCEAR), which publishes regular reports. The American National Academy of Sciences has also appointed committees on Biological Effects of Ionizing Radiation (BEIR) which have played an important role in the field.

Factors in combination

As has been mentioned earlier, cancer in human beings is probably generally the result of a number of factors in combination. Experimental studies have shown that cancer often develops as a result of a series of events in which certain factors may be initiators and others promoters. There are also many substances which are not in themselves carcinogenic, but which can be activated by different enzymes to become carcinogenic. Certain chemical substances can also stimulate the effect or the production of these enzymes and thus function as so-called co-carcinogens. Other co-carcinogenic effects may, for example, be found due to the increased absorption into the body of carcinogenic substances. The chain of events mutant cell–cancer cell–minimal cancer tumour–manifest cancer tumour can also be affected by a number of factors, such as hormone balance, nutrition, stress, immunological factors, and others. It is also of great interest that certain substances which occur naturally in food have been shown in animal experiments to protect against cancer.

In all probability, the situation is at least as complex in man, but our knowledge in this area is as yet slight. The fact that there can be a synergistic effect following exposure to two known carcinogens is, however, quite well established (for example, smoking and asbestos).

The question of whether we can find substances that prevent tumours in humans is of great interest, since this would lead to the possibility of taking general preventive measures. Substances that have been discussed in this context include fibre in food, selenium and vitamin A, where certain indications of a preventive effect even for humans does exist, although firm proof is not yet available.

2.4.2 The overall picture of cancer causes

General aspects

Several attempts have been made in the past to present a quantitative picture of the relative importance of different groups of causal factors (tobacco, diet, other habits, occupational exposures, exposure in the general environment, sunlight, ionizing radiation, and so on) to the total cancer incidence and mortality rates. Table 2.7 shows estimates concerning incidence, one made by a US team (Wynder and Gori, 1977) and one by a European team (Higginson and Muir, 1979). In a more comprehensive analysis of US mortality statistics, and using available epidemiological data, Doll and Peto (1981) attempted to distribute cancer deaths in the USA between different groups of risk factors (Table 2.8).

In these assessments, some of the authors have tried to split up cancer cases according to the most common known or suspected risk factors in such a way that the sum of the various risk columns is 100 per cent. In actual fact, the majority of cancer cases are caused by more than one factor. From an epidemiological viewpoint, a more correct method of expressing the importance of a risk factor would be in terms of the 'aetiological fraction', in other words, the proportion of cancer cases that would not have occurred if the risk factor in question had not existed. With sufficient knowledge of the causes of cancer, the sum of aetiological factors would naturally be much greater than 100 per cent, regardless of whether we are looking at one particular form of cancer, or at cancer as a whole. Tables 2.7 and 2.8 must therefore be seen as highly pragmatic attempts to sort cancer cases into the most important known or suspected cause categories.

Common to these assessments is the fact that tobacco is found to be responsible for a considerable proportion of the total. In Sweden, this proportion is probably somewhat lower because of the relatively lower incidence and mortality rates of tobacco-related cancer forms compared with the USA and UK. Another common feature is that occupational exposure and man-made chemicals in the environment are allocated a relatively minor role. In the studies of Wynder and Gori and of Doll and Peto, diet has considerable importance. This same is true of Higginson and Muir, although here diet is relegated to a heading 'life-

Table 2.7 Attempts to distribute the cancer cases (I) in the USA between different causes according to Wynder and Gori (1977) and (II) in Birmingham, UK, according to Higginson and Muir (1979).

Factor or class of factors	Percentage of all cancer cases			
	I Men	I Women	II[a] Men	II[a] Women
Tobacco	28	8	30	7
Tobacco/alcohol	4	1	5	3
Diet	40	57	–[b]	–[b]
Life-style	–	–	30[b]	63[b]
Occupation	4	2	6	2
Sunlight	} 8	} 8	10 }	10 }
Ionizing radiations			1	1
Iatrogenic factors[c]	–	–	1	1
Exogenous hormones	–	4	–	–
Congenital	} 16	} 20	2 }	2 }
Unknown			15	11

[a] Deduced from histograms. Non-environmental factors equated with congenital and unknown.
[b] Dietary factors have been included in life-style.
[c] Treatment with pharmaceuticals and other measures (diagnostic and therapeutic).
From Doll and Peto (1981).

Table 2.8 Attempt to distribute the cancer deaths in the USA between different causes according to Doll and Peto (1981).

Factor or class of factors	Percentage of all cancer deaths[a]	
	Best estimate	Range of acceptable estimates
Tobacco	30	20 – 40
Alcohol	3	2 – 4
Diet	35	10 – 70
Food additives	<1	–5[b] – 2
Reproductive and sexual behaviour	7	1 – 13
Occupation	4	2 – 8
Pollution (general environment)	2	<1 – 5
Industrial products[c]	<1	<1 – 2
Medicines and medical procedures	1	0.5 – 3
Geophysical factors[d]	3	2 – 4
Infection	10?	1 – ?
Unknown	?	?

[a] Observe that the table refers to cancer deaths and not to cancer cases as in Table 2.7. Males and females are in one group. Doll and Peto stress that the sum of cancer deaths should be considerably higher than 100 per cent due to interactions, if all causative factors had been known.
[b] Allowing for a possibly protective effect of antioxidants and other preservatives.
[c] About the same as consumer products.
[d] Also includes sunlight. The incidence of skin cancer caused by sunlight is considerably higher than the mortality.

style' as a result of the authors' view that causality is difficult to pinpoint. These estimates are concerned with current cancer incidence and death figures, and thus pertain to yesterday's environmental conditions, including life-style. The authors also offer some cautious comments concerning future developments in cancer diseases, and underline the difficulty of making such prognoses.

Viewpoints that deviate widely from the above studies have also been presented. In the unofficial publication, the so-called 'Califano Report', from a number of US federal institutes (Bridbord et al., 1978), an attempt was made to calculate the number of expected cancer cases as a result of a number of known occupational exposure situations (asbestos, arsenic, chromium, benzene, nickel, petroleum products and polycyclic aromatic hydrocarbons). At the same time, sharp criticism was aimed at the 'one effect–one cause' methodology which was said to underlie the models of Higginson and Muir and of Wynder and Gori. According to the authors' calculations, up to 2 million extra cancer cases would occur in the USA in the coming 30-year period as a result of asbestos alone (13–18 per cent of all cancer cases), and the total number of occupationally related cancers would amount to 20 per cent or more of the total for the USA. There are also groups who claim that industrial carcinogenic agents in the general environment (in the air, water and foodstuffs), pharmaceuticals, food additives and the like, together with occupational exposure and smoking are responsible for the majority of cancer cases, thus in general rejecting the life-style theory. One typical representative of this school can be found in Samuel Epstein, whose publication *The Politics of Cancer* (1979) has been much discussed.

Both of these schools have been criticized in a number of works (for example Doll and Peto, 1981). The 'Califano Report' has been criticized for, among other things, not having taken proper account of the degree of exposure, and for itself having used the 'one effect–one cause' method without paying sufficient attention to combined factors (such as asbestos and smoking). Concerning the 'Califano Report' and Epstein's work, it has been claimed that the calculations do not agree with available epidemiological data. For example, the age-standardized cancer mortality rate in the USA has been practically unchanged for the last few decades, while, according to Doll and Peto, a sharp increase would have been the result if industrial occupational exposure and general pollution were to have had such a dominant causal (aetiological) effect. This line of reasoning is correct, provided that no other changes of the same degree took place to affect the cancer death rate in the opposite direction.

All attempts to date to quantify the relative importance of different factors must be regarded as hypothetical because of our limited knowledge of the causes of cancer, and also because of the fact that in individual cases there is almost always a combination of several factors. It is also natural that in this situation many interpretations will be influenced by subjective considerations.

However, with regard to the practical possibilities of cancer prevention speaking broadly, it is valuable that such estimates are made and are being discussed from a scientific viewpoint. In Chapter 6 the Cancer Committee has summarized its own assessments of conditions that have influenced the spectrum of cancer diseases in Sweden. As expected, this picture is largely consistent with results from other Western countries such as Doll and Peto's. Their work has also been of great value to this report.

The possibilities of epidemiological studies

As has already been stressed, the majority of cancer forms demonstrate very great geographical variations in incidence, and the relationship between the highest and the lowest age-standardized incidence, in an international context, can be as high as 10–20, and in extreme cases 100–200. The age-standardized total incidence of cancer, however, shows much less variation, with a relative spread from highest to lowest noted incidence of a factor of around 2–3, based on countries with reasonably reliable cancer registration. A difference of this magnitude can be seen, for example, if we compare the city of New York with a rural population in Norway, or the metropolitan areas of Sweden with some rural communities. That the variation is not greater can be due to a number of reasons. One may be that, in the areas under comparison, there are different environmental factors influencing the development of different tumour forms, and that there is thus an evening out of the total cancer incidence. Another reason may have to do with the principle of competing causes of death, where the various cancer diseases can be regarded as competing with each other. If mortality from one form of cancer is reduced, it obviously does not mean that other cancers will increase, but that the likelihood of one of these occurring in the individual during his or her lifetime increases. A third explanation could be that hereditary factors exert a greater influence on the total cancer incidence than we have assumed, while environmental factors to a great extent govern the cancer pattern.

Population studies involving groups with widely differing lifestyles are of great interest, since these allow us to assess the extent to which cancer diseases should be preventable. (This was the subject of a conference on 'Cancer Incidence in Defined Populations'; Cairns *et al.*, 1980.) Seventh Day Adventists in California have been the subject of one such study. This group does not smoke, they are absolutists and often vegetarians, have restrictive sexual mores, and do not normally engage in industrial work involving high exposures. The study showed that this group not only had a low mortality rate for cervical cancer and for tobacco and alcohol-related cancers (respiratory system, mouth, throat, oesophagus, bladder), but they also had a remarkably low mortality for some other cancer forms (for example large intestine, stomach, breast, corpus uteri, leukaemia). The total age-standardized cancer mortality rate was approximately 60 per cent for men and 70 per cent for women of the general rate for California as a whole. For lung cancer, the difference was considerably greater. Similar results have been found in Mormons in the USA, another group that has strict life-style norms. It is of particular interest that the higher incidence of for example lung cancer in urban areas is not found among Mormons in Utah. This suggests that, if factors other than smoking have an influence, then their effects manifest themselves in combination with smoking. Among Mormon women, but not among men, a higher incidence was noted in urban areas than in rural areas, both for smoking-associated and other types of cancer, an observation that could indicate the influence of factors other than smoking and general air pollution.

One interesting though theoretical question is how large the 'spontaneous' cancer incidence is, that is the incidence that would apply in a population living in an environment that was ideal from a cancer-risk point of view. That such a basal cancer incidence exists is probable for a number of reasons. There are, for example, cancer forms, like infant tumours, which show little geographical or temporal variation in incidence. There is probably a certain risk of cancer in all organs, even under ideal environmental conditions. The risk usually increases with age, but in most cases does not manifest itself because of competing causes of death. Of course, it is not possible with our present knowledge to estimate this theoretical basal cancer incidence. On the other hand, it should be possible, using data from different populations, to calculate a 'minimum' cancer incidence. In the above-mentioned study by Doll and Peto (1981), the authors calculated the cancer incidence that would have existed in Connecticut if every form of cancer had the lowest incidence reported from any country (published in *Cancer Incidence in Five Continents* Vol. II (International Union Against Cancer, 1970)). This calculated incidence constituted only 20–25 per cent of the actual incidence, and the conclusion was thus drawn that 75–80 per cent of all cancer in Connecticut could be 'avoidable'. The view that cancer is avoidable to this extent is naturally only correct if there is no hereditary predisposition to cancer which would assert itself even if the cancer pattern were changed.

As indicated above, even in Sweden there are considerable geographic variations in the incidence of certain cancers. In some studies in conjunction with the work of the Cancer Committee (see Chapter 5) the authors have examined the extent to which incidence data can be linked to available environmental factors (such as degree of urbanization, smoking habits, socio-economic factors), and tried to draw conclusions concerning the statistically 'explainable' proportion of cancers in Sweden. The results of these analyses indicate that more than half of all cancers, and for several individual tumour diseases a major part, is 'explainable' in this sense. It must be pointed out here that the 'explainable variables' that are currently available for such studies are only indirect measures of variations in life-style, occupational pattern, and other factors and they thus cannot indicate the exact causes of diseases (see Chapter 5). That such a large proportion of the incidence rate, like its variation, is 'explainable' in this way, however, shows that further studies of this type aimed at identifying aetiological factors would be meaningful.

Summary

There are many indications that factors in personal life-style are important—perhaps dominant—as causes of the cancer forms that are common in industrialized countries, that is lung, bowel, stomach, breast, prostate and cervical cancers. Some of these factors have been well documented epidemiologically, for example smoking for lung cancer and sexual habits for cervical cancer. In other cases, it is more a question of indirect indices, for example the influence of diet on cancers of the stomach, large intestine and mammary glands.

Another group of aetiological factors may, for restricted groups in society, be of great importance, for example radon in mines, arsenic in smelters, and asbestos. These factors are often well verified epidemiologically, but their total quantitative significance is probably slight.

A third group consists of risk factors that concern many people, but where the risk for each individual is practically negligible. Despite the low individual risk, such factors, by affecting a large group of individuals, could nevertheless provide a considerable contribution to the incidence of cancer, particularly if synergistic effects occur. Factors of this kind include pollution of the air, water and foodstuffs. This group also includes exposure to ionizing radiation via natural background radiation, diagnostic radiology, radon in homes, and perhaps too a number of widespread pharmaceuticals, such as hormones for the relief of climacteric distress and for contraception. Epidemiological verification of these factors is difficult and sometimes impossible to obtain. The risks are therefore often calculated by extrapolation, the justification of which is much debated. Available epidemiological data, for example the detailed analyses by Doll and Peto (1981), indicate that these factors exert a relatively slight influence on the cancer incidence rate. But this does not remove the need for effective monitoring and control systems, since it must be assumed that new substances will sometimes constitute a cancer risk which if possible should be countered at an early stage.

2.5 The treatment of cancer

The treatment of cancer can be specific or unspecific. The former is treatment that eliminates or reduces cancer tissue; the latter is concerned with measures to minimize concern, anxiety, pain and other symptoms, to improve nutritional status and the balance of liquid, to fight infection, or to restore passage in the intestine, respiratory system, and so on.

Specific treatment of cancer can have a curative aim (the complete eradication of the disease), or a palliative aim (to ease or prevent symptoms).

The specific treatment of cancer has developed considerably in this century. Surgical techniques have improved, making more extensive operations possible in some cases. Developments in anaesthetics, artificial feeding, the prevention of infections and thrombosis have led to a sharp reduction in the number of complications and deaths in connection with operations. Plastic surgery and prosthetic techniques have improved the possibilities of reconstruction and rehabilitation following surgery.

Treatment using ionizing radiation, which was made possible by the discovery of natural radioactivity and X-rays in the late nineteenth century, has also developed rapidly. Using radium preparations and what is now conventional X-ray therapy, it was already possible in the early decades of this century to cure cancer forms that were accessible by these methods, for example skin, mouth, throat and cervical cancers. Since the 1940s and 1950s, the physical and technical conditions surrounding radiation treatment have greatly improved and, for example, provided artificial radioactive preparations (such as cobalt-60) and high-energy electron and X-ray radiations from accelerators. All of this, together with improvements in dosimetry and dosage planning, as well as the ability to map the extent of tumours (e.g. using computer tomography), has greatly improved the precision of radiation treatment. Today, it is possible to treat tumours, regardless of their location, with more effective radiation doses and with less risk to surrounding organs than ever before.

Until the 1940s, surgery and radiation treatment (local treatment) were the main specific methods available. Since the 1940s and 1950s, hormone and cytostatic methods have been introduced, with the possibility of treating cancer that has already spread in the body.

Hormone treatment can provide temporary improvement, and sometimes complete freedom from symptoms, but never complete cure.

Hormone treatment is effective in certain cancers of the prostate, breast, thyroid and corpus uteri, and in malignant lymphoma and leukaemias.

Since the first cytotoxic drug (nitrogen mustard) for clinical use was discovered in the USA in the mid-1940s, intensive research into cytotoxic agents has been undertaken. This has involved testing hundreds of thousands of chemical preparations in experimental systems. It is one of the largest efforts in medical history. This has to date produced about 30 clinical drugs with different effects and applications. Even cytotoxic methods have so far been used primarily as palliatives, providing improvement but no cure. However, some rather rare cancers appear to be curable by cytostatic means. Among these are cancers of the testes and the placenta (chorionepithelioma), acute leukaemia (particularly in children) and some forms of malignant lymphoma. There are also indications that cytotoxic methods in combination with surgery and radiation treatment have contributed to the recent improvements in results of treating certain malignant tumours in children.

Quantitatively, the greatest progress in recent decades has been made in the area of palliative treatment. Surgery, radiation, cytotoxic and hormone treatment, together with improvements in unspecific treatment, have all contributed to a more effective alleviation of the symptoms of many cancer patients, and have often led to periods of complete or almost complete freedom from symptoms. This has also led to a radical change in the attitude towards chronic cancer, both on the part of the general public and within the medical profession. It is nowadays self-evident that cancer patients should be looked after and treated in the same manner as patients with other chronic diseases, such as cardiovascular or chronic kidney diseases. This, together with the increased number of cancer cases (a 70 per cent increase in Sweden between 1959 and 1979), primarily as a result of changes in the general age pattern of the population, has resulted in a greatly increased demand for cancer treatment.

It has been calculated that 30–40 per cent of all cancer patients can now be completely cured. However, this differs greatly from one cancer type to another. In certain cancers, the majority of patients can be cured, for example the most common form of skin cancer (basal cell cancer), cancer of the lip, corpus uteri and the testes, and Hodgkin's disease (a kind of malignant lymphoma). In another group, about half of the patients can be cured, for example cancer of the breast, large intestine, mouth, larynx, cervix, malignant melanomas in the skin, acute childhood leukaemia, and certain other children's cancers. There are also types of cancer where the frequency of cure is low, for example cancer of the stomach, lung, pancreas, liver, prostate and oesophagus, chronic leukaemias, acute leukaemias in adults, and malignant brain tumours.

For individual types of cancer, the frequency of cure is often highly dependent on the stage of the disease. Patients with cancer of the breast, large intestine, larynx or cervix at an early stage of development can thus often be cured.

One question often posed is whether the progress in cancer treatment in recent decades has led to a marked increase in the proportion of patients cured. For some cancer types, this certainly is the case. Examples of this are cancer of the bladder (surgery and radiation treatment), Hodgkin's disease (radiation and cytotoxic treatment), cancer of the testes (cytotoxic drug treatment), acute childhood leukaemia (cytotoxic and hormone treatment), certain other malignant children's tumours (surgery, radiation and cytotoxic treatment), and chorionepithelioma (cytotoxic treatment). However, the numbers of patients are fairly small, and cannot be expected greatly to affect the mortality statistics in general. In other cases, earlier diagnosis may have increased the proportion of patients cured without this being ascribed to improvements in treatment. Examples of this are cancer of the breast and the cervix. This is enlarged upon in Chapter 13.

It is possible to obtain a picture of the curability of cancer diseases by comparing the incidence and mortality rates in the Swedish Cancer and Cause-of-Death Registeries. Table 2.9 shows the age-specific incidence and mortality rates for all cancers in men and in women for the periods 1960–4 and 1975–9. The ratio of the mortality rate to the incidence rate, which gives a rough indication of the proportion of patients who die of their disease, was lower in the latter period for all age groups, and the difference was particularly great in the younger age groups. The difference between the incidence and mortality rates also suggests that 25–35 per cent of the men and 35–45 per cent of the women with cancer were cured.

One objective method of studying the prognoses of different cancer diseases is to look at survival rates for cohorts from a cancer register. Such a study has been conducted using Norwegian material from different periods between 1953 and 1975. Table 2.10 shows a comparison of cases registered in the periods 1953–7 and 1972–5. For many types of cancer, the proportion of patients surviving after 5 years was greater in the later period, while for other types of cancer, the figure was practically unchanged. Of course, it is not possible to establish the extent to which the improved mortality–incidence ratio in Table 2.9 and the higher survival rate for many forms of cancer in Table 2.10 depend on diagnosis at an earlier stage, more diagnosis of non-fatal cancer forms, or improved treatment. In all probability, what we see is a combination of these factors.

Much research is currently in progress to find new methods of treatment. Active areas of research are, for example, the development of new cytotoxics and cytotoxic drug combinations, the testing of

Table 2.9 Comparison between cancer mortality rate and cancer incidence rate in Sweden in different age groups during the periods 1960–64 and 1975–79 (incidence and mortality rates expressed as cases per 100 000 and year).

Men

	1960–64			1975–79		
Age	Incidence rate (I)	Mortality rate (M)	M/I	Incidence rate	Mortality rate	M/I
0–9	12.7	10.2	0.80	15.9	7.5	0.47
0–19	13.5	8.9	0.66	13.8	6.3	0.46
20–29	25.1	13.1	0.52	28.8	10.3	0.36
30–39	50.2	24.5	0.49	52.2	20.0	0.38
40–49	115.8	68.1	0.59	135.5	67.3	0.50
50–59	331.5	209.9	0.63	406.1	220.1	0.54
60–69	868.9	591.3	0.68	1020.8	612.3	0.60
70–79	1680.5	1270.6	0.76	2199.0	1478.2	0.67
80+	2234.7	2131.8	0.95	3193.8	2797.8	0.88
All ages	280.9	202.9	0.72	402.1	262.3	0.65

Women

	1960–64			1975–79		
Age	Incidence rate (I)	Mortality rate (M)	M/I	Incidence rate	Mortality rate	M/I
0–9	12.2	9.0	0.74	12.3	6.4	0.48
10–19	12.8	6.6	0.52	13.1	4.4	0.34
20–29	31.3	10.5	0.34	37.8	7.5	0.20
30–39	104.1	44.4	0.43	102.3	26.2	0.26
40–49	284.0	106.6	0.38	296.8	90.9	0.31
59–59	462.2	241.8	0.52	544.8	231.6	0.43
60–69	732.0	457.5	0.63	845.2	458.6	0.54
70–79	1147.3	866.0	0.75	1299.2	851.9	0.66
80+	1367.2	1427.7	1.04	1889.6	1622.1	0.86
All ages	299.3	189.2	0.63	392.5	224.6	0.57

adjuvant cytotoxic treatment or hormone treatment after surgery or irradiation, interferon research, the use of tumour-specific monoclonal antibodies, bone marrow transplants, new forms of ionizing radiation, hyperthermia and radio-sensitizing chemical substances. It is clearly impossible to predict the extent to which, or the time when, a radical improvement of treatment could be achieved. In all likelihood, the coming decades will see gradual progress, primarily for specific cancer forms. However, it is entirely possible, not least in light of the rapid progress from molecular biological studies into the nature of cancer, that new methods could emerge which could alter the situation more radically.

Table 2.10 Five-year survival rates (adjusted for general mortality) in the Norwegian Cancer Register. Comparison between cases registered in the periods 1953–57 and 1972–75.

Type of cancer	Men 1953–7	Men 1972–5	Women 1953–7	Women 1972–5
Lip	92	97	80	100
Tongue	27	40	44	46
Salivary gland	50	77	48	85
Floor of the mouth	34	28	13	41
Other parts of oral cavity	35	65	42	70
Nasopharynx	29	26	6	38
Oropharynx	21	22	29	32
Hypopharynx	7	19	10	27
Oesophagus	2	3	5	7
Stomach	10	14	10	14
Small intestine	25	35	19	41
Colon	27	40	28	41
Rectum	25	36	29	40
Liver	0	5	3	9
Biliary passages	2	7	4	9
Pancreas	0	2	1	3
Nasal cavities and paranasal sinuses	26	37	14	43
Larynx	63	75	63	48
Lungs	7	7	8	9
Breast	54	68	59	68
Cervix	–	–	52	73
Uterus	–	–	64	79
Ovaries	–	–	24	37
Vulva	–	–	57	67
Vagina	–	–	27	31
Prostate	39	52	–	–
Testes	55	67	–	–
Other male genital organs	71	81	–	–
Kidneys	25	36	33	41
Renal pelvis, ureter	12	56	27	53
Urinary bladder	34	40	18	32
Malignant melanoma of the skin	49	65	56	82
Eye	76	55	76	76
Central nervous system	22	26	34	36
Thyroid gland	45	77	55	79
Bone system	20	43	17	31
Connective tissue, muscles, etc.	25	45	44	54
Hodgkin's disease	26	56	36	47
Non-Hodgkin lymphoma	26	35	25	39
Myeloma	13	17	10	21
Chronic lymphatic leukaemia	21	34	25	34
Chronic myelomic leukaemia	15	10	12	6
Acute leukaemia	0	10	0	10

2.6 Economic aspects of cancer

Cancer, cardiovascular diseases, damage caused by external violence and poisoning are the most common causes of premature death in Sweden. Based on an average life-span of 75 years, cancer accounts for about a quarter (or 150 000 per year) of all lost years of life.

Efforts to reduce the effects of cancer by prevention, diagnosis and treatment must naturally be seen primarily from a humanitarian perspective. Nevertheless, it is of interest to know how much of the medical resources available and how much of society's finances are accounted for by cancer. For a number of reasons, it is not possible to make exact calculations, and the rough ones that follow are in the nature of minimum estimates. The reasons for this are as follows.

IN-PATIENT CARE

Based on the diagnosis-related statistics for in-patient care, the number of days in hospital as a result of cancer can be calculated. However, these data do not reveal how many days are indirectly the result of cancer, for example examinations caused by suspicion of cancer, operations conducted to eliminate cancer as a diagnosis, or to remove potentially pre-cancerous changes.

OUT-PATIENT CARE

Out-patient statistics related to diagnosis are not currently available in Sweden. However, sample surveys allow fairly accurate calculations to be made of the proportion of primary-care visits that can be attributed directly to cancer. As in the case of in-patient care, the data do not reveal the consumption of resources which are an indirect result of these diseases. For hospital out-patient care, visits to the oncological clinics should be counted as cancer care. However, the majority of visits are to other clinics, and for these, there are no diagnosis-related statistics available.

OTHER MEASURES

Operations conducted in in-patient and out-patient care are registered but, for the latter, there are no diagnosis-related statistics. For radiation treatment, it can be assumed that this is almost always the result of tumour diseases.

CONSUMPTION OF PHARMACEUTICALS

The National Corporation of Swedish Pharmacies keeps statistics on the drug consumption in the country but not related to individual diagnoses. Pharmaceuticals that are specifically for cancer diseases (such as cytotoxics or anti-oestrogens) pose no problems. However, one cannot tell to what extent the consumption of other pharmaceuticals

Table 2.11 The direct costs for cancer care in Sweden in 1977 (adjusted to 1980 values).

In-patient care (number of care days = 2 141 400)	Sw. kr (millions)
Gastro-intestinal cancer	418
Lung cancer	147
Breast cancer	190
Liver cancer	81
Prostate cancer	157
Leukaemia	54
Other cancers	767
Total in-patient care	1814
Out-patient care	
Primary care (according to a sample)	67
Hospital-associated out-patient care (oncology departments)	83
Pharmaceuticals (according to prescriptions)	48
Radiation treatments (number = 350 000)	35
Total out-patient care	233
In-patient and out-patient care	2047

From the SPRI (1981).

Table 2.12 Distribution of direct costs of medical care and 'morbidity' cost among different diseases in Sweden.

Disease category	Direct care costs (%)	Morbidity costs (%)
Tumours	5.3	3.0
Mental disorders	15.7	18.6
Cardiovascular diseases	13.7	12.5
Respiratory diseases	5.1	11.1
Gastro-intestinal diseases	13.7	5.3
Diseases of bone, joints and other supportive tissues	5.3	25.7
Injuries by external violence and poisoning	7.8	7.7
Others	33.4	16.1

From Herzman and Lindgren (1980).

(such as hormones, vitamins and antibiotics) refers to cancer treatment, since these products are also used for other diseases.

CALCULATIONS

Even with these restrictions, rough calculations of the extent and cost of cancer care are of interest. Calculations by the Planning and Rationalization Institute of the Swedish Health and Social Services (SPRI) on behalf of the Cancer Committee indicate the costs shown in Table 2.11. The in-patient costs are for 1977 (adjusted to 1980 values) and the out-patient costs are from 1980. The costs of operations, radiation treatment, pharmaceuticals and so on relating to in-patient care are included in the general cost. The total costs for in- and out-patient care come to about 2000 million Sw.kr.(about US$300 million)[2]. However, as mentioned earlier, certain costs are underestimated. If we assume that about 90 per cent of the hospital out-patient visits are to clinics other than the oncology departments, and that the costs of medication are about twice those given, a total cost is arrived at of about 3000 million Sw.kr (US$450 million). This is about 6 per cent of the total annual cost of medical health care (approximately 45 000 million Sw.kr (US$6800 million).

The Institute of Health and Medical Economics has made calculations taking into account not only the direct costs of care, but also the morbidity costs (loss of production as a result of sick-leave or early retirement). For the largest disease categories, the percentage proportion of costs is shown in Table 2.12. Practical and theoretical objections can be made to all types of calculations of morbidity costs. However, the table should give a fairly good picture of the costs to society of cancer in comparison with other diseases or injuries. As can be seen, the proportion of cancer diseases in the total cost of medical care and morbidity is fairly low (5.3 per cent and 3 per cent respectively). That the direct costs of care are relatively low can be explained by the fact that cancer patients do not often require in-patient care. The low morbidity costs are a result of the facts that (*a*) the average period of sick-leave is short, since the patient either returns to work or dies, and (*b*) more than half of all cancer patients have reached the ordinary age for retirement.

Note

1 Figures and tables in this chapter without a reference are based on data published by Statistics Sweden (*Dödsorsaker 1959–1980 Cause of Death 1959–1980*) and by the National Board of Health and Welfare (*Cancer Incidence in Sweden 1959–1980*), as well as on primary registry data on cancer incidence.

2 The value of the Swedish Crown (Sw.kr.) in relation to the US dollar has varied considerably during the 1980s. In this book, a figure of around 6.5 has been chosen, although, for example, in 1980 the real dollar value was in fact much lower. [*Ed. note*]

Part I
Cancer diseases: considerations of their induction, causes and distribution

Part 1

3
Mechanisms involved in the induction of neoplasms: fundamental theories and hypotheses

3.1 Introduction

Although our understanding of the mechanisms of cancer induction is still incomplete, it can provide an important basis for investigations into factors which influence tumour induction and the magnitude of their effects. The following review is mainly based on work by Holmberg and Ehrenberg (1984), which contains more detailed discussion and bibliography.

Our knowledge about the mechanisms of induction of tumour diseases has grown out of an interplay between clinical and epidemiological observations and laboratory experiments. There is no reason to doubt that general conclusions from laboratory experiments are valid also for humans, provided that due consideration is given to important differences between human populations and groups of experimental animals. In the experimental study of specific carcinogenic agents (chemicals, radiation) these are often administered in doses that are many times higher than those that humans may be exposed to, and in the experimental situation the individuals vary considerably less than humans normally do with regard to genetic and environmental factors (such as diet) which may influence the induction of tumours. In addition, humans are, in different patterns, simultaneously exposed to many carcinogenic agents which may interact in different ways, while experimental studies generally are carried out with one or two agents at a time. Finally, considerable differences may exist between different strains and species of experimental animals and between experimental animals and humans in their sensitivity to carcinogenic compounds. This may be due to species-specific differences in the metabolism of a compound, in particular its uptake, distribution, transformation and excretion.

3.2 Environmental carcinogenic factors: definitions and basic problems

A tumour may be described as a mass of cells which grows autonomously, without obeying the control signals that normally regulate growth and relations between cells and organs of the body.

The induction of a tumour is a *stochastic* ('random') event. This means that the presence of a carcinogenic factor increases the probability that a tumour will occur. The properties of the tumour are not influenced by the size of the dose. In this respect the carcinogenic effects of chemicals are different from toxic action in the general sense, where the severity of poisoning increases with increasing dose. In the latter case, the influence of the size of the dose at the level of the individual is described as a *dose–effect relationship*. For effects at the level of the group, the term *dose–response relationship* is preferred. A positive dose–response relationship hence means that the number of individuals who develop a tumour increases with increasing dose of a carcinogenic agent. From the point of view of the individual, the probability (risk) that he or she will develop a tumour increases with increasing dose.

A multitude of environmental factors influence the probability of induction of a tumour (see also Chapter 2). In its definition of environment (in relation to carcinogenesis), the World Health Organization mentions the following factors: tobacco, alcohol, diet, radiation, occupational factors, reproductive patterns and sexual behaviour, pollution, iatrogenic factors, consumer goods, infections, geophysical factors and 'unknown factors'. (The latter include such internal factors as disturbed hormonal balance, metabolism or nutritional status.)

The following five points are of importance with regard to cancer prevention:

(a) The induction of a tumour is a multistep process, in which at least two necessary phases, initiation and promotion, have been identified. In addition, each of these phases is influenced by a number of modifying factors, which sometimes operate in complicated patterns of interaction.

(b) On the basis of experimental models, where a tumour cannot occur in an organ if the agent studied is not capable of triggering the first step (the initiation), scientists were previously inclined to define carcinogens, in a restricted sense, as initiators. (The majority of initiators have been shown, when administered either as a high acute dose or as repeated exposures to lower doses, to possess promoter activity also.)

(c) Man is different from the experimental models in that a population is exposed to many initiating as well as promoting and modifying agents. All of these agents—as well as a lack of anti-carcinogenic factors in the diet—show up in a population as factors increasing the incidence, and may, in principle, be objects of preventive measures, provided that they can be identified.

For this reason it is important, from a cancer-preventive point of view, to introduce a wider definition of carcinogens which will include all factors increasing the incidence of cancer. Here the concept of 'carcinogens' will be used in this wider sense.

(d) When applying cancer-preventive measures it is important to neither overestimate nor underestimate the risks of individual carcinogens at the low doses often occurring in the environment. Underestimation means that cancer cases that might have been avoided are occurring. Overestimation of the risk may mean that a product beneficial to human health and prosperity is banned—and may even be replaced by something causing greater risks.

(e) An assessment of the dose–response relationships at low doses requires that consideration be given to the mechanisms. It is generally assumed that initiating agents have linear dose–response relationships without any safe threshold (the initiation itself is a stochastic event); see Section 3.5. The same is probably true for certain particulate promoters. The majority of other carcinogens, i.e. mainly promoters and co-carcinogens, are probably inactive below a certain threshold dose.

Because it is not possible to define a dose below which the risk is zero, a type of risk philosophy must be adopted different to that which may be applied when there is a threshold dose below which there are no harmful effects.

3.3 The mutation hypothesis

3.3.1 General aspects

Already at the beginning of this century it was suggested that the triggering event for the induction of a tumour consisted of a change in the genetic material of the cells, the chromosomes. Since that time an overwhelming amount of evidence has been collected in support of this hypothesis. During the 1960s Brookes and Lawley demonstrated a relationship between the carcinogenic activity of a chemical substance and its ability to react with the nucleic acid DNA (the molecule in the chromosomes which contains the genetic information), and E. and J. Miller demonstrated that almost all chemicals with a carcinogenic activity are also mutagenic (a mutation being a change in the genetic material leading to a change in inherited properties). This is presumably true for most carcinogenic agents, and it is highly probable that the converse is also true: that all chemical compounds (and physical agents) that are mutagenic are also to be considered *potentially* carcinogenic. Since it is much easier and less expensive to determine mutagenic activity than to carry out long-term cancer tests on experimental animals, a number of short-term tests, such as the Ames test, have been developed for the demonstration of mutagenic and, hence, potential carcinogenic activity.

In line with the mutation hypothesis and the stochastic character of the induction of tumours, there is strong circumstantial evidence that a tumour arises from a single cell. Furthermore, recent molecular biology research into 'cancer genes' (oncogenes) has demonstrated how a normal cell may be transformed by mutation into a cell with disturbed or impeded regulation of growth, that is, a cancer cell.

All cells in the body have the same genes. What determines the state of differentiation of the cells, that is, their having developed into components of specific organs or tissues, is that genes are 'turned on' or 'turned off' by control mechanisms according to certain patterns or programmes (see Chapter 2). The transformation of a normal cell into a cancer cell, which does not obey the normal growth-regulating control signals, constitutes a reprogramming. This reprogramming means that certain genes, which in the normal cell should be kept silent or almost silent, are activated ('turned on'). The term oncogenes (or cancer genes) for these genes may be misleading as they are normally present in all cells.

Research into cancer genes is at present moving fast, among other things because of the use of DNA hybridization technology. The activation of these genes can be brought about by certain so-called cancer viruses (in some cases the virus has 'borrowed', and built into its own genetic material, a cancer gene from its host organism). Moreover, the principles of control of gene activity and how a gene may be permanently turned on through a mutation in a control gene are known. Specific structural chromosomal aberrations (known as translocations, a kind of change created by mutagenic agents) in certain positions may lead to an increased risk of cancer since a cancer gene may be turned on when it is moved to a very active region of the genetic material.

A change in the control mechanisms of the cell, which may be related to the effects of cancer viruses, is created by mobile genetic elements, for example transposons, that seem to exist in all types of organisms and to play an important role in the differentiation of individuals and the evolution of species. Such mobile elements were discovered at an early stage in corn by McClintock (the Nobel Prize winner for medicine in 1983).

Mechanisms in the induction of neoplasms

The transfer of mobile elements by transposition seems to be a regulated process which is probably only little influenced by chemical and physical carcinogens. This process has been suggested, somewhat provocatively, by Cairns to be an important mechanism for the induction of cancer. At present there is no evidence for this hypothesis, but it indicates a possible pathway for the induction of cancer in the absence of cancer-initiating agents in the environment. Even if such a 'basic' incidence of cancer existed—about which little is known at present (see Chapter 2)—this would not change anything essential in the arguments concerning the action and avoidability of carcinogenic factors in the environment.

In conclusion, these research results indicate that phenomena as different as infection with a cancer virus, induction of mutation and induction of chromosomal aberrations may lead to neoplastic transformation of a cell by the same mechanism, namely by the activation of certain genes (which presumably play an important role in cell differentiation). Recent experiments seem to indicate that the transformation of a normal cell to a cancer cell requires at least two genetic changes (the two-mutation hypothesis of Knudson (1971)).

3.3.2 Repair of DNA damage

Living cells are equipped with many different systems for the repair of DNA damage. These systems are characterized by very high efficiency, so that only a very small proportion of the DNA lesions remain unrepaired or are erroneously repaired. This proportion may be modified by factors such as the rate of cell division and the inhibition of enzymes. For instance, during the repair ('excision repair') of lesions produced by ultraviolet (UV) light (defects mostly made up by so-called pyrimidine dimers) the first step is to locate the lesion. Then the defective DNA segment is removed and DNA is resynthesized in the gap, after which, in the final step, the ends of the newly synthesized segment and the old DNA strand are linked. This type of repair is, under normal conditions, almost error-free. Other lesions such as breaks in both strands of the DNA molecule may be repaired in higher organisms.

Factors which stimulate cell growth increase the number of tumour initiations at a given dose of carcinogen. This is due to the fact that the repair of DNA requires a certain time and that during a period of intense cell division, the defective DNA is duplicated in many cells before there has been time for the lesions to be repaired. In consequence, the number of errors and hence the probability that a tumour will be induced are increased. A rapid enhancement of the tumour frequency will also be the result if the repair system becomes saturated at high doses. In addition, certain carcinogenic metals seem to disturb the enzymes responsible for synthesis and repair of the DNA.

For lesions produced by certain reactive chemical compounds, such as methylating agents, other repair mechanisms exist. For example, there exists a specific enzyme for the removal of methyl groups from certain positions in the DNA which have been alkylated by a methylating agent. If the carcinogenic substance methyl nitrosourea is injected into young rats at low doses for 5 weeks, tumours are produced almost exclusively in the central nervous system (mainly in the brain). If one large dose is given, tumours arise also in the spleen and in the kidneys. Following longer-term administration at high levels, liver tumours are also formed. The locations of the tumours produced by this methylating agent can be correlated with the capacities for repair in different tissues.

3.3.3 What factors are mutagenic and cancer initiating?

As illustrated in Figure 3.1, tumour induction may be described as a sequence of events from the point where the cells are exposed to a dose of a carcinogenic agent to the growing tumour. At least two of these events seem to be necessary for a tumour to arise: initiation (a mutation or a mutation-like change) which causes the reprogramming of the cell, and a subsequent promoter step. Initiators may be of a physical, chemical or biological character.

Physical factors

Ionizing radiation and UV light are carcinogenic. Ionizing radiation is sufficiently energetic to 'knock out' electrons during its passage through matter, so that molecules become electrically charged (ionized); these ions directly or indirectly cause chemical changes leading to gene mutation or chromosomal aberrations (see also Section 4.5.1).

Ultraviolet radiation, which is a component of sunlight, is electromagnetic radiation with lower energy than gamma and X-rays. It causes excitations leading to characteristic chemical changes in the DNA without the molecule initially being ionized (see Section 4.5.3).

Electromagnetic radiation with longer wavelengths (visible and infra-red light, microwaves, radio waves) lack any known carcinogenic activity.

Chemical factors

E. and J. Miller have pointed out that almost all chemical carcinogens (here, strictly speaking initiators) possess so-called electrophilic reactivity or are transformed in the body to compounds with such reactivity. Electrophilically reactive compounds have groups of atoms with a deficit of electrons and therefore react with electron-rich nitrogen and oxygen atoms in the DNA. The chemical changes in the genetic material produced may, if they are not correctly repaired by the repair systems of the cells, lead to mutation and possibly cancer initiation.

All electrophilic substances that are able to reach the DNA—or compounds which may be transformed to such—may produce chemical changes in the DNA and must therefore, according to Ehrenberg and Osterman-Golkar (1980, 1983), in principle be considered as potential carcinogens in the sense that exposure to such compounds may lead to an increased risk. The ability to produce changes in the DNA that may lead to the induction of cancer varies considerably, however, and for certain compounds the risk increment will be negligible under normal conditions of exposure.

Classes of substances with electrophilic reactivity are:

(a) alkylating (e.g. epoxides such as ethylene oxide and mustard gas);
(b) arylating;
(c) acylating;
(d) nitrenium compounds, with a positively charged nitrogen (including nitrite);
(e) carbonyl compounds, particularly certain aldehydes;
(f) certain metals and metal compounds;
(g) free radicals.

The majority of known carcinogens and mutagens are directly *alkylating* (e.g. alkyl chlorides and epoxides) or are transformed ('bioactivated') in the body to such alkylating agents.

Metabolic transformation often involves an oxidation followed by a so-called conjugation. In the latter reaction the intermediate metabolite formed is enzymatically linked to hydrophilic components naturally occurring in the organism, such as sulphate, glucuronic acid (carbohydrate component) or glutathione (with excretion of the respective mercapturic acid).

Reduction may also lead to bioactivation. Thus, aromatic nitro compounds are often reduced to the corresponding amines or hydroxylamines. Metabolic conversion often implies 'detoxification' of the original substance through the formation of a mixture of products. The metabolic decomposition does not, however, always lead to less toxic compounds being formed. In certain cases, decomposition products which are equally or more toxic than the parent substance may be formed.

A large number of compounds which are not themselves carcinogenic may, in this way, be transformed into intermediate products which are active carcinogens ('the ultimate carcinogen'). Thus, polycyclic aromatic hydrocarbons (e.g. benzo[a]pyrene) and unsaturated aliphatic compounds (e.g. vinyl chloride) are converted to reactive epoxides.

The conversion of foreign compounds takes place mainly in the liver but also occurs in other organs. In fact, low conversion activities exist in most tissues of the body.

Many experiments support the notion that carcinogenic metals—which may also react with the DNA—can react with certain enzyme molecules to give rise to errors in the synthesis of DNA during cell division or, as mentioned, counteract the efficiency of DNA repair.

Certain alkylating and other electrophilic compounds are normal components of the biochemical machinery of cells. At present it is not known to what extent these compounds contribute to the incidence of tumour diseases.

Biological factors

Certain viruses (cancer viruses, oncoviruses) cause, in different ways, changes in the cells, which lead to reprogramming and neoplastic transformation. Such viruses have mostly been studied in laboratory animals. Viruses have not with full certainty been proved to induce cancer in human beings, but there are data to support the theory that viruses play a role in the induction of Burkitt's lymphoma (Klein, 1982), which occurs in certain tropical regions. This is probably true also for some other lymphomas (see Section 3.4). Recently the role of viruses in the induction of acute lymphatic leukaemia has been demonstrated. Other viruses, such as jaundice virus (hepatitis B) and herpes virus, also seem, according to epidemiological data, to play an important role in the induction of liver cancer and cervical cancer, respectively. The mechanism is not clear in these cases; it may possibly be a question of promoter activity.

3.4 Cancer induction: a process in several steps

The mutation or mutation-like event which is the first step in the process finally leading to a growing tumour is generally referred to as the *initiation*. In order for the change produced by the *initiator* in the genetic material, DNA, to be manifested, that is, expressed as changed properties of a cell, the cell must go through a number of divisions. If the cell does not happen to be in a tissue undergoing cell division (e.g. fetal tissue) it may remain 'dormant' for a long time without giving rise to a tumour, provided that another event that promotes cell division does not occur. Such an event is usually referred to as *promotion* and the agents giving rise to the effects are called *promoters*.

Describing promoter activity as promotion of growth is an over simplification. Other events may possibly be necessary for a tumour to arise, but it is difficult to study such events since initiators and promoters both give rise to several different effects. At present, a growth-promoting activity seems to be the only known common property of all agents and phenomena with a direct or indirect promoter activity (the latter, for instance, by effects on the hormonal balance of the body). For promoters there does not yet exist any rapid test such as the Ames test. Promoter activity may be highly specific, as is the case for certain hormones. Furthermore, a large number of widely different phenomena may have an unspecific promoter activity by causing cell damage leading to healing and reparative growth. This includes wounds of various types such as burns, surgical operations and infections. It also includes the toxic action of chemicals which may lead to cell damage or cell death. These effects are often organ specific; for example, carbon tetrachloride and many other compounds exhibit promoter activity in the liver, and vinylidene chloride exhibits such activity in the kidney.

Generally, only one factor at a time is studied in cancer experiments. A carcinogenic effect seen when testing a chemical may be the result of an initiator acting as its own promoter, for example by a toxic activity in a tissue. A promotive situation may also exist for reasons unknown to the experimenter, for instance through the diet. Compounds with both initiating and promoting activity are generally referred to as 'complete carcinogens'. Most initiators act as complete carcinogens when administered as repeated exposures to low levels or in a single exposure to a high concentration. Ionizing radiation is also a complete carcinogen. Maybe it would be more appropriate to speak of the initiating and promoting profile of a factor rather than distinctly differentiating between initiators and promoters. The majority of the investigated 'classical' promoters do not, however, possess any initiating activity in the sense that they bind to DNA or are capable of producing point mutations.

That the cancer incidence is lower than would be expected from mutation frequencies in general and the enormous number of cells in the human body (10^{14}, i.e. 100 million million,) is probably explained in part by the fact that tumour induction requires the co-operation of at least two events, each of which is relatively rare. This low probability for the induction of a tumour appears to be even more easily explained if it is considered in the light of recent results indicating that *two* separate genetic changes are required for the induction of a neoplasm (Section 3.5).

The promoter event and the genetic changes leading to malignancy may, in principle, occur at any time after the initiation. The interactive effects of factors from different sources, or repeated exposures to the same factor, lead to an increased probability that a tumour will arise during the lifetime of an individual; this is reflected in the dose–response relationships for specific factors. In general, the latency time for experimental tumours decreases with increasing dose. There is much evidence that this is true for chronic exposure to complete carcinogens at doses so high that the initiator is also acting as a promoter.

Many initiators, such as ethylene oxide, give approximately the same dose in different organs of the body. In contrast, promoter activity is, as mentioned, often markedly organ specific, with the result that animal experiments with specific compounds have produced an exaggerated impression of the organ specificity of chemical carcinogenesis. Tumours may also be localized to specific organs and tissues if the reactive intermediates are very short lived and thus remain in the organ where they are generated, leading to an uneven distribution of the dose. Furthermore, there may be considerable differences between the capacities for repair in different organs and tissues. It is evident from experimental data that exposure to an initiator may give rise to tumours in different organs provided that a promotive situation is created in them. Human populations show a wide spectrum of promoter situations among individuals, due to infections, tissue damage, hormonal imbalance and so on. If a pure initiator, which gives an even distribution of the dose among the different organs of the body, is administered, one would theoretically expect an increase in the incidence in most of the sites where tumours occur in the population. Ionizing radiation acts primarily as an initiator, and for this reason an increase in the incidence of many of the tumour types which are already present in the Japanese population could be observed among the survivors of the atomic bombings of Hiroshima and Nagasaki.

If only agents with initiating activity were defined as carcinogens, promoters would be closest to the category of co-carcinogens (see below). It is, however, apparent that if a promoter is given to a population under conditions otherwise unchanged, this will be noticed as an increased cancer incidence, provided initiations occur in the population. Preventive measures could be directed either against initiators or against promoters, but of course also against co-carcinogens interacting with them.

Epidemiological attempts to identify carcinogenic agents have, to date, been dominated by methods which favour the detection of agents with organ-specific effects. This has probably also contributed to the fact that knowledge about the most important causes of cancer is still very fragmentary, with the exception of tobacco smoking. Tobacco smoke contains many initiators, but it also has a promoter activity, which appears to be the dominant effect. This explains the interactive effects of smoking, both with (presumed) promoters, such as asbestos, and with initiators, such as ionizing radiation.

At the present state of our knowledge it must be assumed that the multiphase principle developed from animal experiments, implying at least initiation and promotion, is valid also for most human cancers. As mentioned, a second genetic change may be required after the promotion.

Factors which increase tumour incidence by mechanisms that do not involve reaction with the DNA are sometimes called *epigenetic factors*. This concept has been used primarily to characterize carcinogenic chemical compounds (e.g. steroid hormones) which seem to lack mutagenic activity in different test systems. For such agents the existence of a threshold dose below which no carcinogenic activity occurs has been proposed (Weisburger and Williams, 1982). In practice, it may, however, be very difficult to establish the mechanism(s) through which a carcinogenic factor acts. To demonstrate a genotoxic effect can, with certain types of compound, involve considerable technical difficulties, and the absence of a response in a test system such as the Ames test must be interpreted cautiously. Neither does an increased incidence of cancer that appears only after massive exposure to a compound provide adequate support for an epigenetic (i.e. non-genotoxic) mechanism, since the effect may depend on the formation of a genotoxic metabolite via a conversion pathway which is responsible for only a small fraction of the total amount of substance metabolized by the organism. There has sometimes been a tendency to classify all agents for which the mechanisms of action are unknown as 'epigenetic'. Here, no classification of carcinogenic factors into the two categories of genotoxic and epigenetic agents will be attempted; nor is a strict classification into initiators and promoters for regulatory purposes feasible at present. It is, however, important to point out genotoxic mechanisms of action and genotoxic agents as such in discussions relating to risk, policy, and so on.

Modifying factors

Many factors, called *co-carcinogens*, may, without themselves being carcinogenic, enhance the effect of carcinogens. (Promoters may be included in this class, even if it is somewhat misleading, since tumours, in the majority of tissues, seem to require promotion to be induced at all.) Other factors, *anti-carcinogens*, inhibit the induction of tumours. Correspondingly, different carcinogens may enhance *(synergism)* or weaken *(antagonism)* the activity of each other. In epidemiological studies the cooperation between initiators and co-carcinogens (promoters included) shows up as effects of interaction (in a statistical sense) or as multiplicative effects, in contrast to purely additive effects of different factors.

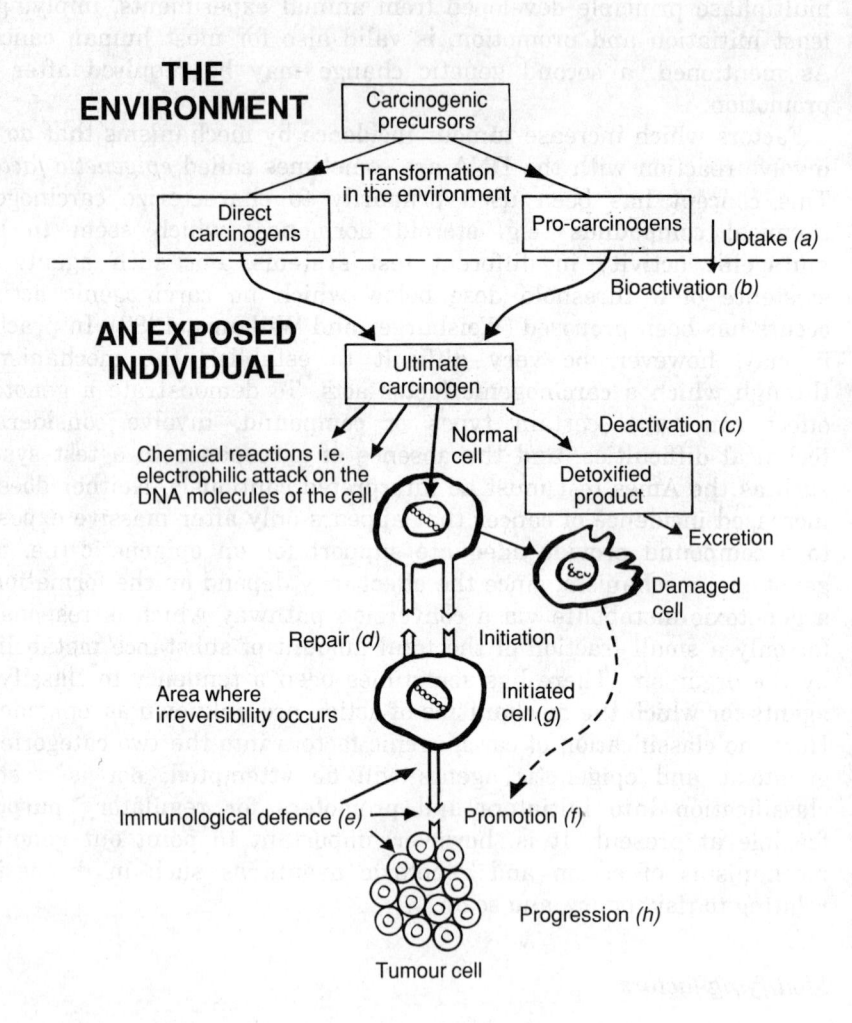

Figure 3.1 Individual steps during the induction of a malignant tumour.
Modified from *Miljöeffekter och risker vid utnyttjande av energi*, Swedish Departmental Series Ds I 1978:27, 1.

In the scheme of chemical carcinogenesis in Figure 3.1 a few ways are shown by which enhancement or weakening of the activity of an initiator can be brought about (reference is made to letters in the figure):

(a) The uptake may be affected in many ways, for instance during inhalation, by damage to lung tissue (e.g. by sulphur dioxide), by the compound being adsorbed to particles, through physical stress causing an increased rate of respiration or through the skin (either directly or by the influence of different solvents). Certain fibres in the diet can probably decrease the uptake through the intestine. One of several ways in which alcohol has been suggested to contribute to cancer risks is by an enhancement of the uptake of carcinogens, in particular those that occur in tobacco smoke, in the pharynx–oesophagus.

(b) and (c) The ultimate carcinogen, which reacts with the DNA, is formed (through bioactivation) as an intermediate in biochemical conversions, which should finally lead to products to be excreted from the body. The ability, particularly of the liver, to give rise to a reactive compound ((b) in Figure 3.1) and to convert this intermediate ((c) in Figure 3.1), may further be enhanced or weakened by pre-treatment with or simultaneous exposure to other compounds. This increases or decreases the dose and thus the effect of the ultimate carcinogen.

(d) Cells have several mechanisms for repairing damage to DNA induced by radiation or reactive chemical compounds. The change(s) in the genetic code which lead to mutation and probably to cancerous transformation arise(s) through erroneous repair or by DNA being synthesized prior to cell division before the repair has had time to take place. The efficiency of repair is influenced in the same way as bioactivation and detoxification ((b) and (c) above), by previous or simultaneous exposure to other agents. In this way sulphur dioxide and arsenic trioxide, for instance, seem to enhance the mutagenic and probably also the carcinogenic action of cancer initiators.

(e) The immunological defence of the body seems to provide efficient protection against types of cancer suspected of being induced by viruses, but it also seems to have a modifying influence on the incidences of other tumours. An impaired capacity for immunological defence, for instance in recipients of transplanted tissue, also favours tumour induction.

(f) The promoter activity of specific agents is certainly modified by many factors, although the mechanisms for this are still unclear. If a certain hormonal balance is regarded as a promoter for breast cancer, the demonstrated connections with fat in the diet and/or obesity may be ascribed to such a modifying activity. The mode of action of dietary fat and obesity is, however, not well understood.

(g) Cell damage, and reparative growth resulting from it, may contribute to promoter activity.
(h) Results from animal experiments suggest that the progression of a tumour sometimes ceases, followed by regression. It is not known what factors may influence such a beneficial process. Animal experiments indicate a possible negative role of stress factors in this context (Weiss et al., 1981). It is also not clear what factors influence the occurrence of metastases. Experimental data indicate, however, that damaged tissue (e.g. lung tissue after exposure to high air concentration of nitrogen oxides (Törnqvist, 1984)), makes the organ more receptive to the growth of metastases. In Figure 3.1 the main emphasis has been put on the initial steps of carcinogenesis. It is conceivable that the progressional phase, which may be seen as an evolution because of changing cell properties, consists of many steps, including genetic changes.

ANTI-CARCINOGENS (not indicated in Figure 3.1)
Many normal components of tissues, such as compounds related to vitamin A, vitamin E and probably vitamin C, as well as the trace element selenium, can, according to experimental studies, counteract the induction of tumours (see Section 4.3). These compounds seem to act as antioxidants, but apart from this their mechanisms of action are still unknown. It is probable that suboptimal levels of these compounds in the diet lead to an increased incidence of cancer. The addition of synthetic antioxidants (e.g. butylated hydroxytoluene) to the diet has also been shown experimentally to decrease the tumour frequency in studies of the effects of chemical carcinogens.

Genetic variation

There seems to be considerable genetic variation in the ability of the body to activate and detoxify carcinogens, to repair DNA damage and to counteract the growth of the transformed cell. Points (b)–(g) in Figure 3.1 provide examples of important mechanisms which may all be subject to such genetic variation. A genetically determined total inability to repair DNA damage gives, for instance, a high susceptibility to skin cancer induced by sunlight. An inherited deficiency in the immunological defence system increases the probability of tumours of types which are probably initiated by viruses. Apart from such drastic abnormalities, genetic variation probably also includes more moderate modifications of physiological and biochemical functions. Mechanisms other than those mentioned here also exist. In case of genetically determined increased susceptibility, tumours arise earlier than otherwise, and in paired sites (e.g. eyes and breasts) often on both sides.

In certain rare forms of strongly family-linked cancers (e.g. retinoblastoma), the genetic changes that otherwise are induced by carcinogens seem to be inherited from the parents.

In some animal experiments it has been shown that exposure to X-rays or chemical cancer initiators leads to a genetically conditioned increase in cancer incidence in later generations, presumably as a result of the mutagenic effects of the initiators on the germ cells. This gives us a hint that our thinking about risk must not be limited to cancer risks in the present generation (including possible effects on the fetus through exposure of the mother) but should also consider the possibility of damage to future generations from smoking habits (Bridges et al., 1979), occupational exposures, and so on. No data are available today which would permit estimation of the extent of such effects.

3.5 Dose–response relationships

Information useful for estimating the magnitude of the risk at a given exposure dose or level of a carcinogenic agent is derived from epidemiological data and laboratory data.

Unfortunately, epidemiological data are at present too uncertain and incomplete to permit an evaluation of dose–response relationships, except mainly for ionizing radiation, tobacco smoking and a few occupational exposures. An estimation of the risk on the basis of experimental data requires a 'translation factor' which takes into account differences between laboratory organisms and humans in their capacities to handle a carcinogenic agent (initiator), that is, data on uptake, distribution, elimination, bioactivation, detoxification, DNA binding and repair of DNA damage (see Figure 3.1). Principles and methods for determining this translation factor, including chemical dosimetry of initiators in blood samples, have been developed by Ehrenberg and co-workers (Osterman-Golkar and Ehrenberg, 1983). Chemical dosimetry of adducts from electrophilic substances to DNA or to a suitable amino acid in a protein is of interest also because it may allow identification of potential carcinogens, for instance in a mixed exposure. The scientific basis for the determination of a corresponding 'translation' factor for promoters is still very uncertain.

Since experimental observations have almost always been made with doses that are considerably higher than those that normally occur in the different environments of human beings, an extrapolation is also required down to current doses (dose defined as exposure level integrated over time) and exposure levels. This, however, confronts us with a considerable difficulty. Existing doses and levels are often in a range where statistically significant observations cannot be made in epidemiological or experimental studies because a population size reasonable from a practical and economic point of view would be too small.

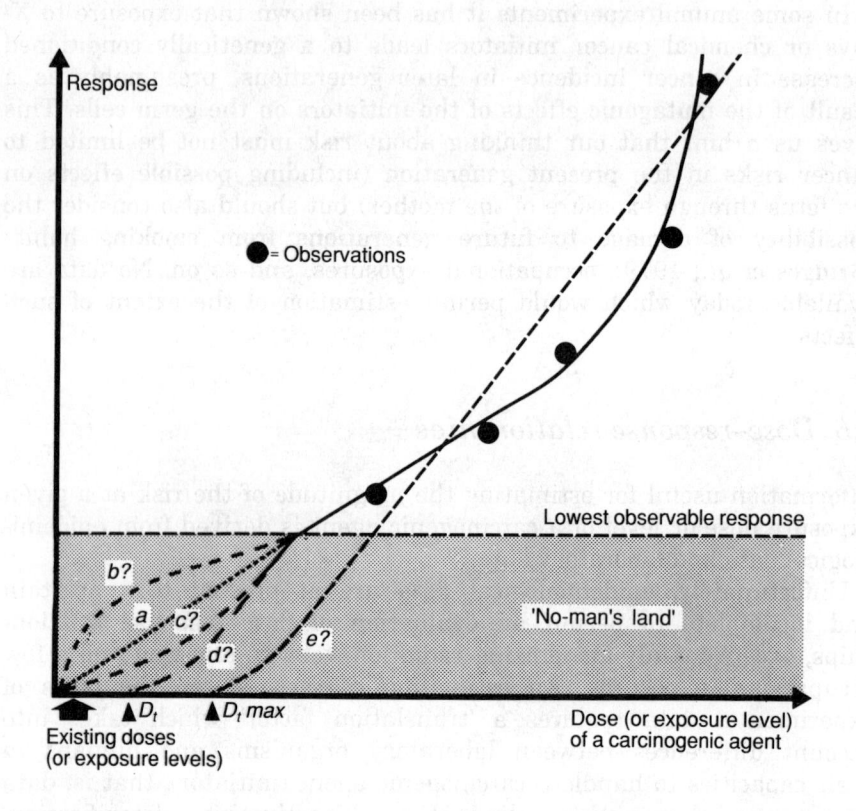

Figure 3.2 The detection limit of epidemiological and experimental observations of cancer incidence or mortality as a function of dose (or exposure level) of a carcinogenic agent. In this context response means the part of the incidence caused by the agent studied, i.e. the differences between incidences in exposed groups and the incidence in the control group. See also the text.

This is illustrated in Figure 3.2. With decreasing dose, the points often seem to approach a straight line, but a linear extrapolation according to curve *a* would lead to an underestimation or overestimation of the risk if curve *b* or *c*, respectively, were true. Exposures in the dose range occurring in the real world would be erroneously judged as 'hazardous' if the true relationship exhibited a threshold dose D_t according to curves *d* or *e*. Against the background of the high efficiency with which DNA damage is often repaired, one could theoretically postulate the existence of a 'safe' threshold below which the risk would be very close to zero. However, as a result of the differences existing in the efficiency of repair in different organs and between different individuals, a threshold dose generally valid for populations cannot be precisely defined.

It is generally assumed that mutations induced by radiation or chemicals display linear dose–response relationships down to the very low doses that occur in different environments. This is in accordance with the plausible assumption that a constant *proportion* of potentially mutagenic DNA lesions are correctly repaired in the low-dose region. To the extent that the mutation hypothesis for cancer initiation is true, it is probable that this holds true also for the *carcinogenic* activity of radiation and chemicals (See Box 1).

It is sometimes claimed that because of statistical uncertainty, it will never be possible to know what the dose–response curve looks like at doses close to zero, and that, consequently, it will never be possible to exclude the existence of a 'safe' dose threshold. Scientific arguments can be raised against this. The lowest possible threshold—if one does exist—can be roughly estimated. Below some very low dose of radiation or chemical an individual cell nucleus will be hit by only *one* ionizing particle or suffer *one* chemical change in the DNA of a type which, if not repaired, can lead to cancer initiation. If a safe threshold exists, it must include this dose. But in certain experiments, radiation-induced mutations in different organisms and cancer transformation in cultured cells have been demonstrated at doses giving less than an average of one 'hit' per cell, which seems to indicate that in these biological systems a dose threshold does not exist. This also seems to be valid for the enhanced incidence of child cancer (in particular leukaemia and central nervous system tumours) following diagnostic examinations of the mothers with X-rays (analyses in UK and the USA by Stewart and MacMahon; see UNSCEAR, 1977). For one chemical substance, ethylene oxide, the same absence of a threshold has been demonstrated for the induction of mutations, and experiments with other compounds point in the same direction. (These data and conclusions have been summarized by Ehrenberg *et al.* (1983).)

Holm *et al.* (1980), in a study of thyroid tumours in patients examined with radioactive iodine (iodine-131) for diagnostic purposes, failed to demonstrate the increase in incidence that would have been expected from a linear extrapolation. This speaks in favour of the conclusion that a carcinogenic effect demonstrated for a certain type of irradiation such as high intensity and a homogeneous dose does not necessarily have to be the same as for another type of irradiation such as low intensity and inhomogeneous dose. This illustrates the difficulties with generalized risk estimations.

The promoter activity of radiation and chemicals which may be attributed to toxic action in some organs is certainly so low at low

Box 1

The substance 2-acetylaminofluorene (2-AAF; *N*–2-fluorenyl-acetamide) produces tumours in the liver and the urinary bladder of mice following administration in food. A conventional cancer test with this compound, including 25–50 animals at each dose and of each sex of a certain strain of mice at three different dose levels, does not permit any conclusions to be made as to the effects of low doses. Such a conventional cancer test costs approximately US$100 000.

In order to study the real appearance of the dose–response curve at low doses, the National Center for Toxicological Research (a laboratory shared by the EPA and the FDA) in the USA completed an extremely expensive experiment with 2-AAF in 1979, using some 24 000 mice at seven dose levels (Staffa and Mehlman, 1979).

For the induction of liver tumours by 2-AAF it was established that the dose–response relationship was in fact linear down to the lowest dose tested.

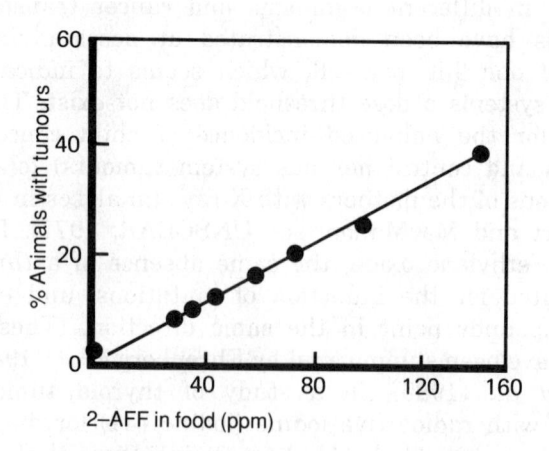

Figure 3.3 The incidence of liver tumours following oral administration of 2-AFF to mice.
From the Office of Technology Assessment (1981) based on a study by Littlefield *et al.* (1979).

doses that a threshold dose may be said to apply. Cancer experiments with individual agents therefore lead—in cases where the same agent is acting as an initiator and a promoter—to the incorrect assessment that the resulting carcinogenic activity generally (at all dose levels) has a threshold dose even if the initiating activity depends linearly on the dose. Since, according to what has been said above, the dose–response relationship at low doses in human populations is primarily determined by the initiating activity (for a given prevailing set of promoter conditions), this erroneous conclusion may lead to an underestimation of the risk.

Various mathematical models have been used for evaluating dose–response relationships and risk estimation at low doses. As far as is known these models have not previously taken into account the fact that the agents studied have both initiating and promoting activity and that these effects may depend differently on the dose. An assessment of different models previously used and of a new biphasic model, for about 150 published experimental investigations of chemicals which have been carried out at four or more dose levels (von Bahr et al., 1984b), indicates that in many cases the existence of a linear component is hidden behind an S-shaped curve for promoter activity. Looking at available epidemiological and experimental data, as well as certain genetic experiments, the provisional conclusion may be drawn that a linear extrapolation to the low doses in 'no-mans-land' (curve a in Figure 3.2) comes closest to the dose–response relationship for the action of initiators. The promoter activity of the same initiators is, however, exceedingly low at low doses. Therefore where there is an even distribution of the dose in the organism, it is conceivable that, for certain compounds, the increase of the tumour incidence and the cancer risk at very low doses concern the tumour types which are already present in a population (i.e. the tumour sites where promoter situations exist for reasons other than the exposure to the compound studied).

Animal experiments, as well as investigations in molecular biology, support the concept that at least two mutational events (or corresponding processes for oncogene activation) are involved in carcinogenesis (the two-mutation hypothesis of Knudson (1971)). This hypothesis has obtained strong support through more recent studies of, for example, retinoblastoma in children (Murphree and Benedict, 1984). From the point of view of cancer prevention does this new hypothesis change the previous views on the relationship between dose and risk, most closely illustrated by a linear relationship, curve a in Figure 3.2?

The two-mutation hypothesis requires a rare coincidence of two, each relatively rare, events and it would therefore give a plausible explanation to the long latency times, to the age dependence of the incidence and to the fact that, at least among younger and middle-aged people, cancer must be considered as a rare disease.

In this context it is important to re-emphasize the difference between experimental animals and humans concerning the requirement that a carcinogen must be complete—something which, if two mutations are required, leads to the incidence being dependent on the square of the dose, with very low risks at low doses as a consequence. For human populations, however, with a complex and variable exposure to both promoters and initiators, it is thus most likely that, at an exposure to an additional initiator, one *or* the other mutational event will be rate limiting for the cancer induction by the factor considered. This implies a linear relationship between risk and dose. The growing support for the mutation hypothesis seems to strengthen this reasoning.

Experimental data indicate that certain deviations may occur upwards or downwards (curve *b* or *c*) from the linear curve. These deviations do not seem to be so large that they can lead to serious over- or underestimation of risks. Certain agents, such as UV-irradiation and methylating agents, exhibit dose–response relationships of types *d* or *e* (Figure 3.2) in mutation experiments, confirmed to a certain extent in cancer experiments (von Bahr *et al.*, 1984b). This speaks in favour of the concept that safe thresholds or 'near thresholds', may exist in certain organisms and organs. These cases mostly concern agents of types that life has always had to protect itself against (methylating agents are normally present in most cells of all species) through the development of highly efficient repair capacity. Also in these cases it would, however, be advisable not to accept safe thresholds which have been demonstrated under special experimental conditions, considering the variation in modifying and genetic factors which exists in a human population.

The importance of not taking the absence of a *demonstrable* effect to mean the absence of any effect can be illustrated by a theoretical example.

A factor, for example a general food additive, is suggested for use at a dose corresponding to a yearly intake which, according to a linear extrapolation, is expected to produce one cancer case in 10 000 persons. An effect of the compound at this dose would, however, not be detected in a conventional cancer test with 100 animals. The number of animals required to detect such a low frequency in an experiment would be 30 000. That individual experiments of this type are likely to give a negative result for statistical reasons is, or course, not a proof that the action of the substance exhibits a threshold dose. Neither can the result be interpreted as if the risk is so low that it may be neglected. If the treated foodstuff is used by a population of 8 million, 800 cancer cases could be initiated per year according to linear extrapolation, a figure which is certainly unacceptable to society.

The increase in the number of experimental animals that would be required to demonstrate a carcinogenic effect with sufficient precision at the concentrations of a food additive or other substance to which humans will be exposed in practice, is, not least for economic reasons, impossible to carry out. Instead, internationally accepted guidelines (among others, OECD (1981)) suggest that the highest level of exposure used in the experiment should be the maximal level that can be tolerated by the experimental animals without seriously affecting their survival. From the cancer incidence observed at such a high dose level, an extrapolation should then be made to a more realistic dose level. The problems with interpreting the shape of the dose–response curve remain, but the use of a linear extrapolation seems to exclude an underestimation of the risk provided that bioactivation is not saturated at high doses. Understanding the mechanisms of action may facilitate the choice of a suitable model for extrapolation. Test substances are nowadays mostly administered orally, irrespectively of the route of administration that may be important for the human case. For many substances oral administration is the most effective route of administration for inducing tumours in experimental animals.

The conclusion that dose–response relationships are to be regarded as linear is not valid for promoters and modifying factors. These agents act in principle by non-genetic mechanisms, and it can be assumed that generally a certain dose or exposure level is required for an effect to be induced. In such cases a linear extrapolation from the high levels where tumours occur in the experiments leads to a considerable overestimation of the risk. This points to the importance of considering the mechanism of action in risk estimation.

4
Different types of exposure

4.1 Introduction

It has been suggested that environmental factors in a wide sense (see Chapters 2 and 3) contribute, to a high degree, to the induction of cancer. It is therefore important to make an inventory of the different kinds of factor in the human environment, including the diet, that involve exposure to factors outside of man himself. These may be subdivided into chemical and/or physical factors. Certain viruses belong here too, although their importance in carcinogenesis is still unclear. Environmental factors which do not entail exposure have been mentioned in Chapter 2. To these belong life-style factors, such as the fertility pattern of women which probably exerts an influence on the hormonal balance.

This chapter deals with the problem of exposure to exogenous chemical and physical factors, alone or together with other factors to which human beings are exposed, and which, often after metabolic change, directly produce damaging effects through chemical reaction in the cells. This also applies to physical factors such as radiation, where the primary effect in cases of hereditary damage or a tumour disease consists of a chemical change in the genetic material of the cells. Other exposure factors act indirectly, for example by influencing the flora of intestinal bacteria or the hormonal balance, with changed chemical reactions in the body as a possible consequence. In certain cases the overall composition of the diet (e.g. the proportions of different nutrients) might act as such an indirect 'chemical factor', while at the same time specific compounds in the diet may be assumed to be of importance and may, through different mechanisms, either promote or counteract the the induction of cancer.

Sections 4.2 and 4.3 deal with exposure sources of a complex nature, namely tobacco and diet, respectively. Tobacco smoking is known to be a strong causal factor in cancers not only of the respiratory tract but also of other organs. There is also growing scientific evidence of the importance of the diet in the context of cancer.

The number of specific chemical compounds to which human beings may be exposed—naturally occurring, for instance in food, as well as synthetic ones—is enormous. To this should be added those compounds which originate in chemical reactions of different kinds: in industrial processes, in combustion and through changes in the environment by the influence of water, light, micro-organisms, and the like. We are probably aware of only a small proportion of these substances at present. Even for those compounds that have been identified, the carcinogenic effects are well understood for only a small number. More or less fragmentary knowledge on a relatively large number of substances is available, however, and the international scientific literature in this field is extensive. This chapter will therefore deal with only a selected sample of substances.

Exposure to chemicals and risks in different environments and from different types of products will be discussed. An essential part of this chapter (Section 4.4) deals with the availability of exposure data, based on an investigation into such data obtained from central control agencies in Sweden.

With physical factors of known, suspected or theoretically possible carcinogenic action, the field is limited (Section 4.5) and therefore more easily described than that of chemical factors. The best known is ionizing radiation, but ultraviolet light is also discussed. Detailed exposure data for ionizing radiation are presented.

Problems regarding 'mixed exposures' and interaction effects are treated separately in Section 4.6.

4.2 Tobacco

4.2.1 Introduction

The damaging effects of tobacco on health were not demonstrated until the 1950s, long after its use had spread over large parts of the world. Since then our knowledge of these effects has continually increased.

In a simplified description of the biological effects of smoking it may be said that the harmful effects are mainly caused by the following factors:

(a) the toxic substance nicotine, which has several effects on the body including a stimulating action which creates a physiological dependence that increases the habit-forming nature of smoking;
(b) carcinogenic and/or irritating components in the smoke associated with several forms of cancer as well as various smoking-induced annoyance reactions and also chronic bronchitis and emphysema;

(c) carbon monoxide, which, as a component of smoke, does not cause cancer but does contribute to the excess mortality rates of smokers from cardiovascular diseases.

In recent decades, tobacco use and especially smoking has been the subject of many studies in several countries. Reliable data on the increased lung cancer risks and excess mortality rates from different diseases among smokers, and data on the consumption of tobacco, have led to wide acceptance of the fact that the use of tobacco constitutes a major general health problem. There is no need to review in detail here the investigations and risk assessments made in other similar contexts, but a selection of data in condensed form is provided. Topics discussed include the mechanisms by which different components in tobacco smoke act with regard to cancer induction, trends in consumption and exposure and, in quantitative terms, the impact of tobacco use on the total cancer incidence in Sweden. For obvious reasons the main subject of discussion and the focus of the available scientific data have long been the risks to smokers themselves. So-called passive or secondary smoking, that is the largely involuntary exposure of everyone who can be reached by the polluted air ('environmental tobacco smoke') in the atmosphere where smoking occurs, has recently been the subject of increasing attention. Since this problem has been less investigated it is treated relatively thoroughly in the following pages. Also, potential health hazards to fetuses and individuals in future generations will be touched upon. In these cases the information is more uncertain, however. The information in this chapter is partly based on a number of reports[1]: from the US Department of Health and Human Services (US Surgeon General, 1979–82); the UK report *Smoking or Health* published in 1977; a report on lung cancer from the International Union Against Cancer (UICC, 1976); and various Swedish studies, especially a report on reduced tobacco use by the Tobacco Committee (TC, 1981). Where no other citation is given, data presented in the following pages were extracted from these reports. Further information has been collected from a number of scientific articles mentioned in the text.

4.2.2 Tobacco consumption—survey

In industrialized countries the greatest increase in cigarette smoking occurred in the first half of the twentieth century. At the same time the consumption of other kinds of tobacco (pipe and chewing tobacco, snuff) decreased. Among males the increase in cigarette smoking in many countries had already begun towards the end of the last century,

25–30 years before women exhibited a similar increase (see Figure 4.1).

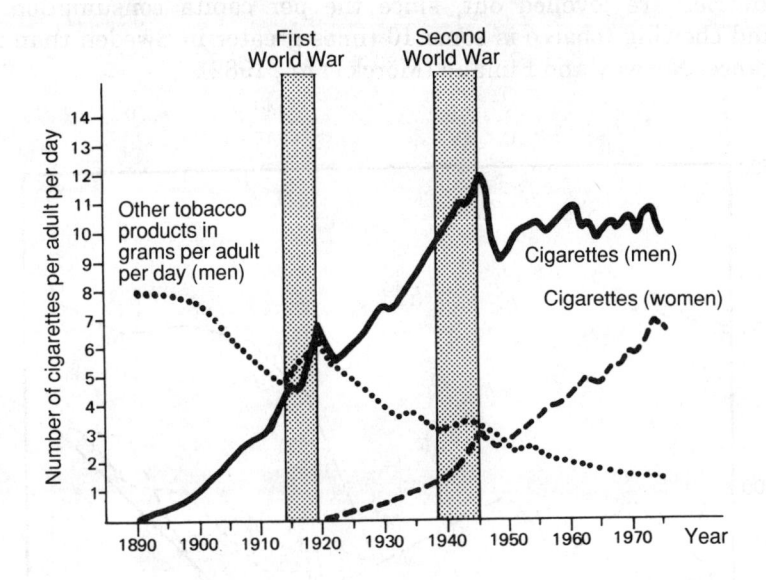

Figure 4.1 Tobacco consumption in Great Britain between 1890 and 1975 (average for all adult men and women). From *Smoking or Health* (1977).

A comparison between the Nordic countries with respect to the annual consumption of cigarettes per person above 15 years of age shows approximately the same increase in Sweden and Norway, from about 270 cigarettes in the mid 1920s to about 1700 in the early 1970s. (See Figure 4.2: in this figure the growing use in Norway of hand-rolled cigarettes, now more than 50 per cent, has been allowed for.) In Finland, where smoking habits developed early, the annual per capita consumption was already high in the 1920s—about 1300 cigarettes per adult—and in the early 1970s it reached about 2000 per person. In Denmark too, smoking habits developed earlier than in Norway and Sweden, with a cigarette consumption of about 500 per year during the period 1920–40. To this can be added the typically Danish habit of smoking cigars, which has certainly been considered less harmful (to the extent that the smoke is not inhaled), but which may nevertheless have implied a considerable contribution to health risks. In the early 1920s this cigar consumption in Denmark, in kilograms per person per year, was greater than the cigarette consumption. In 1980 the consumption of smoking tobacco and factory-made cigarettes in kilograms per person per year) was 2.3 kg in Denmark 2.1 kg in Norway 1.4 kg in Sweden and 1.7 kg in Finland. Included as smoking tobacco were pipe tobacco and finely cut tobacco for rolling cigarettes. If the consumption of chewing tobacco and snuff is also included, the differences between the countries are levelled out, since the per capita consumption of snuff and chewing tobacco is some 10 times greater in Sweden than in, for instance, Norway and Finland (Mörck et al., 1982).

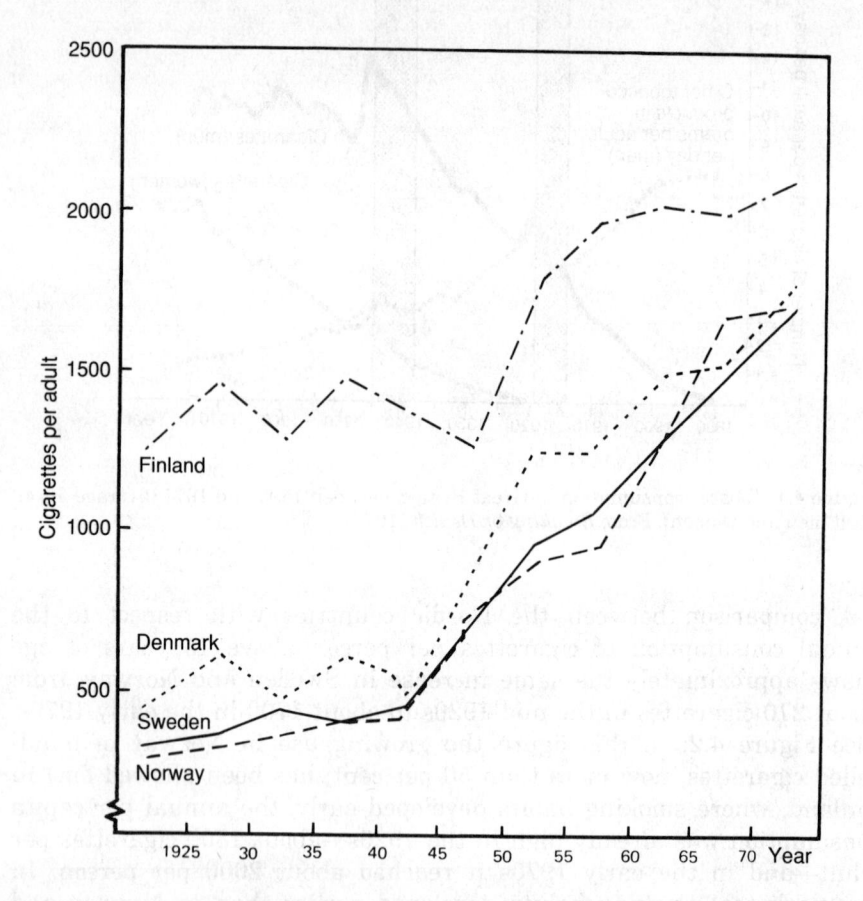

Figure 4.2 Annual consumption of cigarettes per person above 15 in four Nordic countries. Consumption in Denmark, Finland and Sweden comprises only factory-made cigarettes. For Norway, the consumption of hand-rolled cigarettes was calculated and added to that of factory-made cigarettes.
From a report (in Swedish) by a Nordic Tobacco Working Group (NTG, 1975).

The total consumption in Sweden of tobacco (including snuff) has changed little since 1920. It was then 2.2 kg per year per person aged over 15 years. In 1980 the corresponding consumption was about 2.0 kg per per person per year. On the other hand there have been great changes in the pattern of tobacco products consumed, and hence also with regard to the exposure to components in tobacco and tobacco smoke. In 1920 snuff and chewing tobacco constituted three-quarters of the total amount of tobacco consumed, cigarettes being a little less than one-tenth. Sixty years later, in 1980, cigarettes predominated, amounting to two-thirds of the total consumption (by weight). Snuff and chewing tobacco constitute at present one-quarter of the total

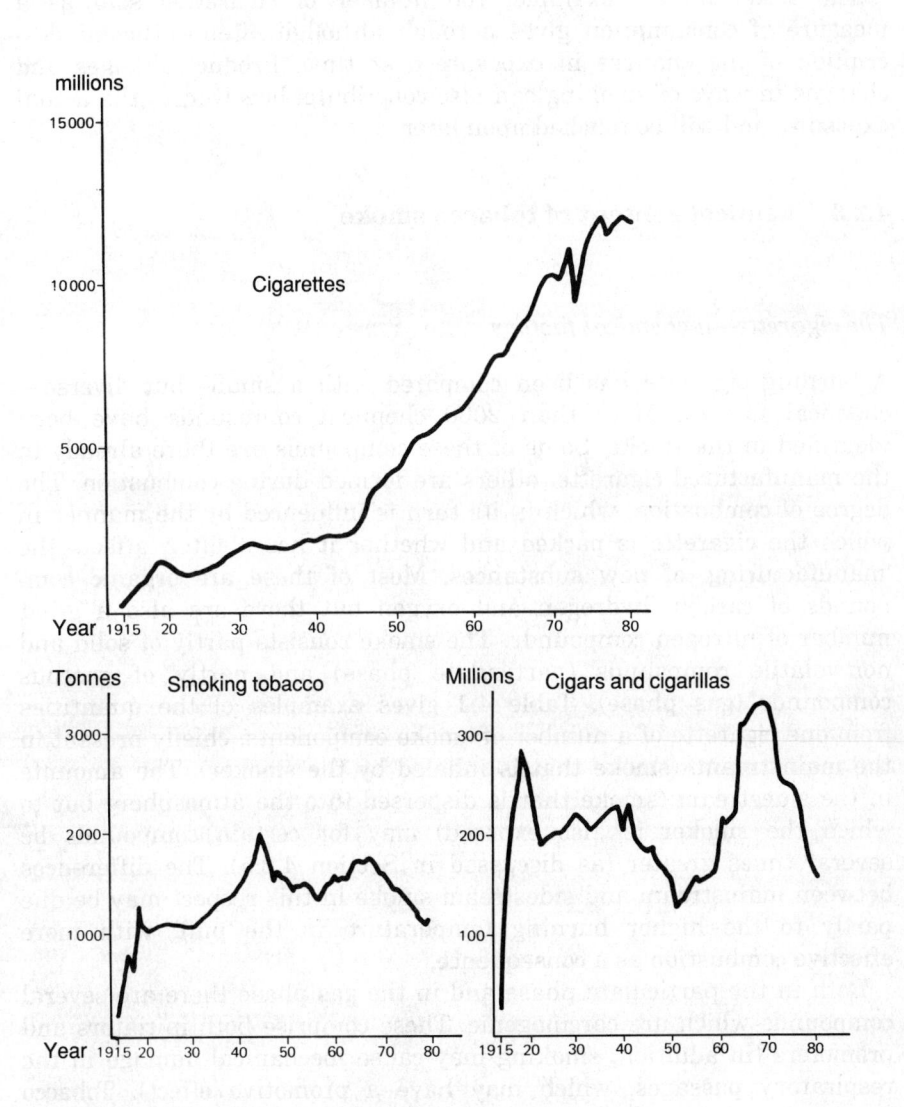

Figure 4.3 Consumption (sales) of cigarette, cigar, cigarillos and smoking tobacco (pipe tobacco and tobacco for hand rolling of cigarettes) in Sweden.
From NTS (1982).

amount of tobacco consumed. Snuff, however, shows an increase of about 50 per cent compared to 1965–70. For the last few years cigarette sales have remained unchanged at 1700–1800 cigarettes per year per person above 15 years in the total population (compared with about 4000 cigarettes per year per person above 18 years in the USA). The sales of cigars and pipe tobacco have started to decline. This development is illustrated in Figure 4.3.

The trend in, for example, the number of cigarettes sold as a measure of consumption gives a rough although often sufficient description of the changes in exposure over time. Product changes and changes in ways of smoking can also contribute, however, to the actual exposure, and will be touched upon later.

4.2.3 Chemical content of tobacco smoke

The cigarette—a chemical factory

A burning cigarette has been compared with a small—but diverse—chemical factory. More than 2000 chemical compounds have been identified in the smoke. Some of these compounds are there already in the manufactured cigarette, others are formed during combustion. The degree of combustion, which in its turn is influenced by the manner in which the cigarette is packed and whether it has a filter, affects the 'manufacturing' of new substances. Most of these are organic compounds of carbon, hydrogen and oxygen but there are also a great number of nitrogen compounds. The smoke consists partly of solid and non-volatile compounds (particulate phase) and partly of gaseous compounds (gas phase). Table 4.1 gives examples of the quantities from one cigarette of a number of smoke components, chiefly present in the mainstream, (smoke that is inhaled by the smoker). The amounts in the sidestream (smoke that is dispersed into the atmosphere but to which the smoker is also exposed) may for certain compounds be several times greater (as discussed in Section 4.2.5). The differences between mainstream and sidestream smoke in this respect may be due partly to the higher burning temperature in the puff, with more effective combustion as a consequence.

Both in the particulate phase and in the gas phase there are several compounds which are carcinogenic. These comprise both initiators and promoters (in addition, smoking may cause mechanical damage in the respiratory passages, which may have a promotive effect). Tobacco smoke therefore may be called a *complete carcinogen*. Besides promoters it also contains co-carcinogens (compounds which amplify the carcinogenic action of other compounds).

Among the most important initiators in the *particulate phase* (here called the condensate) are the polycyclic aromatic hydrocarbons (PAHs) which are contained in the tar. The best known of these, benzo[a]pyrene, has often been used as an indicator substance for

Table 4.1 Amounts of various compounds in the smoke from one cigarette.[a]

	Mainstream range	Mainstream mean value	Sidestream[b]
Particulate phase			
Benzo[a]pyrene	10–50 ng		3.4
Dibenz[a,h]anthracene	40 ng		
2-Naphthylamine	1–2 ng		67 ng
4-Aminobiphenyl	0.8–2.4 ng		140 ng
Arsenic	0.01 µg		
Lead	0.24 µg		
Cadmium	0.12 µg		3.6
Nickel	0.08 µg		
N'-Nitrosonornicotine	0.14–3.70 µg		
Benzene	10–100 µg		
Catechol	60–500 µg		phenols 2.6
Nicotine	0.05–2.5 mg	1.1 mg	2.7
Polonium	1–2×10^{-4} Bq		
Gas phase			
Dimethylnitrosamine	1–200 ng	13 ng	10–40
Hydrazine	24–43 ng	32 ng	3
Vinyl chloride	1–16 ng	12 ng	
Urethane	10–35 ng	30 ng	
Formaldehyde	20–90 µg	30 µg	
Hydrogen cyanide	30–200 µg	110 µg	0.006–0.37
Acrolein	25–140 µg	70 µg	
Acetaldehyde	18–1400 µg	800 µg	
Nitrogen oxides (NO$_x$)	10–600 µg	350 µg	
Ammonia	10–150 µg	60 µg	40–70
Acrylonitrile	3.2–15 µg	10 µg	3.9
Carbon monoxide	2–20 mg	17 mg	4.7

[a] Out of more than 2000 compounds identified in tobacco smoke, analytical data are available for a few hundred. Even for the examples given in this table the data are sometimes very uncertain and may, in some cases, be based on one single determination. In several cases data for content in the sidestream are not available.
[b] Ratio of amounts in sidestream as compared to mainstream.
From US Surgeon General (1979).

PAHs or air pollutants in general. Other important initiators are 2-naphthylamine and 4-aminobiphenyl. There are also small amounts of radioactive materials such as polonium, and small amounts of non-radioactive metals, for instance lead, nickel, arsenic and cadmium. All of these may contribute to the carcinogenic action of tobacco smoke.

The particulate phase also contains nicotine, which is absorbed via the oral cavity and lungs and acts rapidly on the nervous system. It gives rise to several physiological effects; for instance, it acts as a stimulant.

One component of the *gas phase* is carbon monoxide. This compound probably contributes to the excess mortality of smokers from cardiovascular diseases. Other toxic gaseous components are hydrogen cyanide, hydrogen sulphide, nitrogen oxides, formaldehyde, acetaldehyde, acrolein and ammonia. Several gaseous compounds attack mucous membranes and contribute to irritation of the air passages as well as the eyes—a fact well known to those present in rooms where smoking occurs (see Weber *et al.*, 1979). Another contributory factor to this irritation is inhibition of the ciliary activity in the bronchial mucosa. The gas phase contains established cancer initiators such as dimethylnitrosamine. Examples of mutagenic compounds which may act as cancer initiators are alkyl nitrites and alkenes. Other compounds in the gas phase such as oxides of nitrogen (NOx) (Törnqvist, 1984) and aldehydes may also be assumed to contribute to the cancer risk, although in these cases knowledge is still fragmentary.

Tobacco smoke has so far been analysed only to a limited extent with respect to compounds originating from tobacco additives such as flavouring agents.

Composition of tobacco products

During recent decades filter cigarettes and cigarettes with low tar and nicotine contents have been introduced and are now widely available in many countries. For instance, in the USA, the use of filter cigarettes has increased from 1–2 per cent in 1950 to more than 90 per cent in 1979. Furthermore, the average amount of tobacco per cigarette has been reduced considerably in the last few years and the tar content has by and large been halved during the same period. The nicotine content has been cut, too, though the reduction has only been by one-quarter during the last 10 years.

Since the 1950s, filter cigarettes have also come to dominate the Swedish market, and they accounted for 90 per cent of the cigarette sales in 1980 (Svenska Tobaks AB, 1980). The sales of 'light' low-condensate cigarettes (with less tar and nicotine) have increased since the mid-1960s and reached about 40 per cent of the market in the 1970s; among women the proportion who smoke these lighter cigarettes is greater still. In 'old' cigarette brands, too, the condensate content has been reduced. Thus, the most popular cigarette brand in

Sweden, which gave 41 mg condensate per cigarette in 1961, gave half as much 20 years later (Svenska Tobaks AB, 1980).

From 1964 to 1980, the average condensate content in cigarettes sold in Sweden was reduced from 31 mg to 15 mg, and at the same time the nicotine content decreased by one-third, from 1.8 to 1.1 mg per cigarette (Figure 4.4). This implies that the condensate content has also gone down in relation to the nicotine content, from about 17 mg condensate (mg nicotine)$^{-1}$ to about 14 mg condensate (mg nicotine)$^{-1}$.

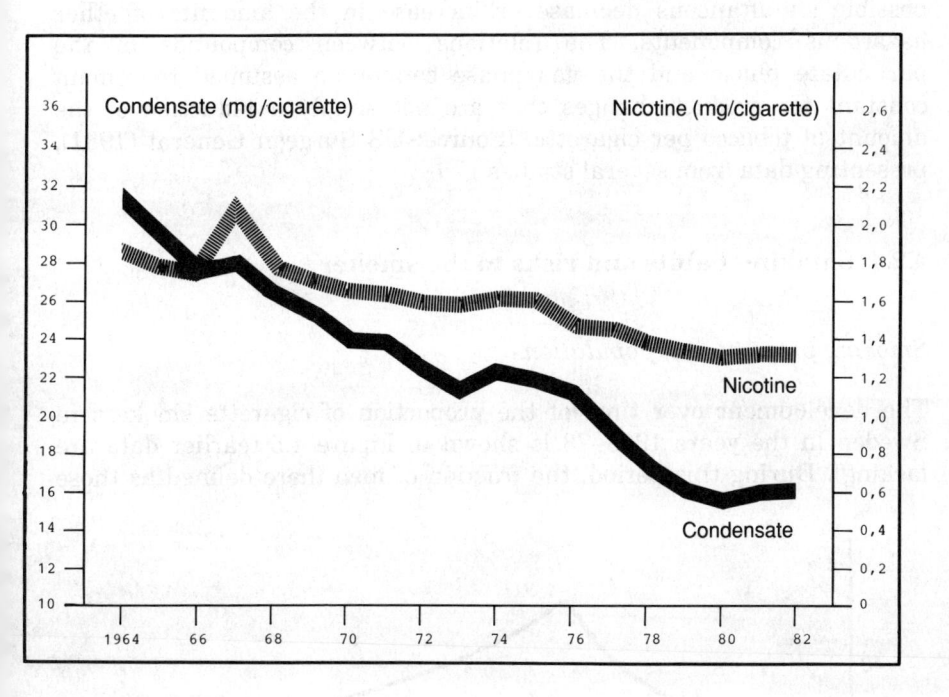

Figure 4.4 Condensate (tar and nicotine) and nicotine, respectively, in Swedish cigarettes for the period 1964–82. Amounts of nicotine and of condensate were determined through analysis of smoke from machine-smoked cigarettes with standardized number of puffs, puff size, etc.
From Svenska Tobaks AB (1983).

In several countries, the product properties mentioned are nowadays analysed and reported regularly for each cigarette type. (This has been a legal requirement in Sweden since 1977.) This makes it possible for the consumer to compare cigarette brands with respect to harmful components in the smoke. Analytical data for the smoke, together with consumption data, also facilitate estimates of exposure changes of different population groups in epidemiological studies. It should be stressed, however, that it is difficult to quantify actual change in health hazards over time, particularly cancer risks. It is thus at present not possible to assess how the risk-decrease (especially for lung cancer) due to a reduced amount of tar per cigarette smoked, has been further enhanced, or on the other hand counteracted, by a possible simultaneous decrease or increase in the amounts of other hazardous components. The relations between compounds in the particulate phase and the gas phase cannot be assumed to remain constant for product changes that are not simply a reduction of the amount of tobacco per cigarette. (Source: US Surgeon General (1981), presenting data from several studies.)

4.2.4 Smoking habits and risks to the smoker

Smoking proportion of populations

The development over time of the proportion of cigarette smokers in Sweden in the years 1963–78 is shown in Figure 4.5 (earlier data are lacking). During this period, the fraction of men (here defined as those

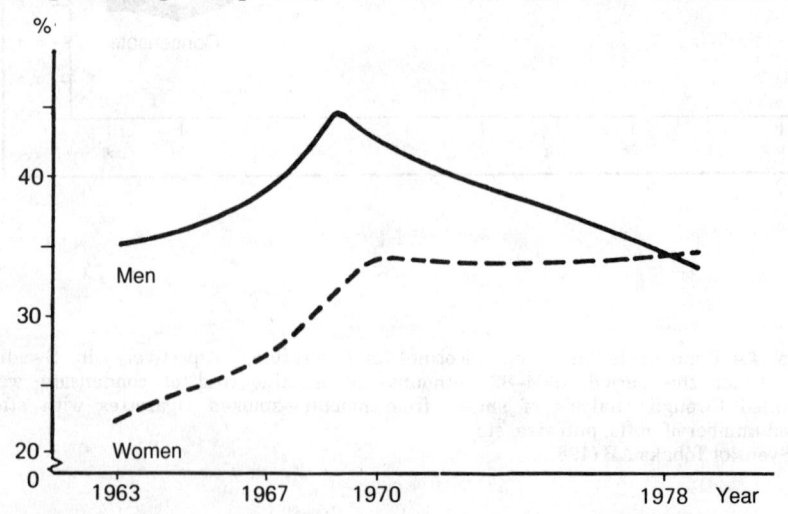

Figure 4.5 Proportion of regular cigarette smokers in the Swedish adult population aged between 18 and 70 years. Regular smokers of pipe or cigars are not included. From TC (1981).

aged between 18 and 70 years) who smoked cigarettes increased continuously up to 1969 but then started to decrease. It is probable that the growing awareness of the danger of smoking has contributed to this decrease. The proportion of regular smokers among women of the same ages increased up to 1970 and has since then remained approximately constant. At the highest level reached (about 1970), every second man and every third woman in Sweden was a smoker. The trends shown in Figure 4.5, indicating that women have overtaken men, have continued, and in 1981 there were 31 per cent regular cigarette smokers among women as against 27 per cent among men. In addition, there were 3 per cent regular smokers of pipes or cigars in the male population. These figures are based on data from the National Smoking and Health Association (NTS).

Among men the proportion of smokers is lowest in the youngest age groups, whereas there is a noticeably high proportion of smokers among younger women (aged between 18 and 24 years; Figure 4.6). A tendency in the opposite direction was evident earlier, the age of starting to smoke of women then being several years later than that of men (SCB, 1965).

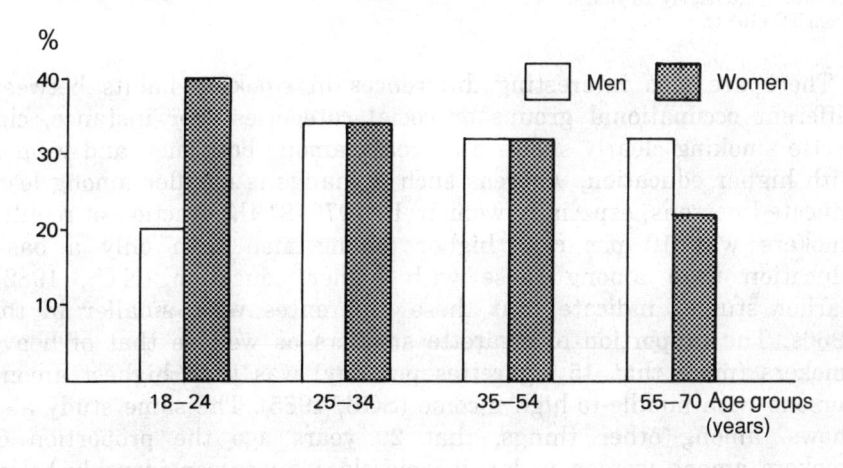

Figure 4.6 Smoking habits in different age groups in Sweden, expressed as a proportion of regular smokers, in 1981.
From NTS (1982).

Since 1975, the Swedish National Board of Education has mapped the smoking habits of pupils in Swedish schools. In the 1970s smoking decreased among both girls and boys in the age groups investigated (Table 4.2). However in 1981, in the sixth school year 6 per cent of the boys and 5 per cent of the girls, and in the ninth school year 23 per cent of the boys and 35 per cent of the girls, were still smokers (NTS,

1982). For the 1980s the trend is thus not unequivocal. The data indicate, among other things, the need for specific information to be given to different groups of adolescents.

Table 4.2 Smokers in primary school in Sweden. Percentage of smokers in respective year's course.

Year	Spring term, year 6[a]		Spring term, year 9[b]	
	Boys	Girls	Boys	Girls
1971	14	16	41	47
1972	10	12	35	47
1973	10	10	31	45
1974	10	12	31	45
1975	12	13	32	45
1976	11	12	27	40
1977	9	11	25	40
1978	10	10	25	38
1979	6	8	21	34

[a] Average age nearly 13 years.
[b] Average age nearly 16 years.
From TC (1981).

There are also interesting differences in smoking habits between different occupational groups or social categories. For instance, cigarette smoking clearly shows a decrease among both men and women with higher education, whereas such a change is smaller among less-educated persons, especially women. In 1976–81 the fraction of regular smokers was 10 per cent higher among men with only a basic education than among those with higher education (NTS, 1982). Earlier studies indicate that these differences were smaller in the 1960s. The proportion of cigarette smokers as well as that of heavy smokers (more that 15 cigarettes per day) was then highest among persons with middle-to-high income (SCB, 1965). The same study also shows, among other things, that 20 years ago the proportion of smokers among women in low-income classes was considerably below the average for all women, especially in age groups above 50 years. The same was true for women in families associated with the occupational category of agriculture, forestry and fishing. The study also showed clear residential differences in smoking habits, with more smokers in densely populated areas and in large cities. As a further example, based on more recent data, it may be noted that labourers as a group smoked more than the average in the middle of the 1970s, and that the unemployed showed still higher figures. The group of single mothers showed an extremely large number of smokers whereas parents of several children were below the average (SCB, 1977).

Actual exposure and uptake

In individual cases, the exposure of a person to the compounds in tobacco smoke from cigarettes depends on the number of cigarettes smoked per day but also on other factors such as the composition of the cigarettes, the size of the smoked part of the cigarette, the number and size of the puffs, and the inhalation depth. Dose–response curves showing the relationship between the number of cigarettes smoked per day and the incidence of lung cancer became available quite early on (see same references given in Figure 4.7). It has been difficult, however, to assess the importance of the other factors just mentioned. A shift to light (low tar, low nicotine) cigarettes may be made up for by 'compensation smoking', through more cigarettes and a changed smoking technique. The importance of differences in the manner of smoking is illustrated by the fact that the absorption of nicotine has been estimated to amount to 5 per cent of the nicotine in the mainstream in the case of mouth smoking compared with 65–95 per cent in the case of inhalation (Greenberg et al., 1952). Certain research is being carried out with the aim of establishing a measure of the actual exposure, for example, through the determination of cotinine (a metabolite of nicotine) or carboxyhaemoglobin in the blood.

Svenska Tobaks AB has estimated that the average exposure to condensate (tar plus nicotine) has decreased according to the following table:

	1964	1974	1979
Condensate	154	116	95
Nicotine	9.0	8.3	7.4

Estimated average annual exposure in grams per cigarette smoker in Sweden.

This calculation was based on data on the proportion of regular smokers, the tar and nicotine contents in the mainstream of cigarette smoke and the total annual cigarette consumption in Sweden. (The latter increased from about 8000 million to about 12 000 million cigarettes in the period 1964–75, since when it has remained relatively constant). However, it is difficult to judge how any changes in the manner of smoking which might have occurred may have influenced the exposure to and uptake of different smoke components that are hazardous to the health. Since the content of tar has decreased faster than the content of nicotine it is reasonable to assume that the actual exposure to tar has decreased, provided that compensation smoking to increase the uptake of nicotine has not occurred. According to a UK review (Stepney, 1980) of various studies of compensation smoking accompanying changes to lighter cigarettes, the number of cigarettes would increase by 9 per cent following a 50 per cent reduction of the nicotine content. Changes in the manner of smoking probably play at least as important a role as the change in number of cigarettes. Fagerström (1981) showed that smokers with heavy nicotine dependence do smoke low-nicotine cigarettes more 'effectively' than they smoke cigarettes with a high nicotine content.

The factors just discussed influencing actual exposure to and uptake from cigarette smoke are probably also valid for other forms of tobacco smoking. In this context available data for Swedish conditions referring to the total consumption (sales) of different product types do not permit further discussion. Certain data on variation in the effects on health between populations indicate, however, that the manner of smoking may be important. (See below for lung cancer and pipe smoking.)

Health effects associated with the use of tobacco

DISEASES, MORTALITY AND LENGTH OF LIFE: GENERAL ASPECTS

The tobacco habit, especially cigarette smoking, has several adverse effects on health, such as impaired physical condition due to decreased oxygenation of the blood and decreased pulmonary capacity, and damage to the mucous membranes of the air passages, often leading to a disturbing bronchitis. Smokers are more susceptible than non-smokers to several diseases, including the more incapacitating ones, and they show higher levels of sick leave from work.

Still more obvious is the increased mortality from various diseases which characterizes smokers, especially cigarette smokers. This relationship may be observed as a shortened mean life-span or as a higher mortality ratio (as an expression of the relative risk (RR)), namely the ratio between the mortality rate for smokers and that for non-smokers. Another way of expressing the individual risk is the difference between mortality rates for smokers and non-smokers. If the figure in the latter case is multiplied by the size of the population, the expected number of deaths due to smoking is obtained. A comparison of this latter number with the actual number of annual deaths indicates the importance of the problem to society.

In a study of British doctors, Doll and Peto (1976) found that the fraction of men aged 35 years who were going to die before retirement (at 65 years) was 15 per cent among non-smokers but 40 per cent among smokers of more than 25 cigarettes per day. In the same study it was shown that those who smoke 20 cigarettes per day shorten their lives by, on average, 5 years.

In comprehensive prospective studies in the USA, Canada and UK the RR of male smokers of cigarettes only was found to be about 1.7 (1.54–1.83). A 10-year epidemiological follow-up (Cederlöf et al., 1975) of participants in a Swedish postal survey study in 1963 (SCB, 1965) of smoking habits of a representative sample of 55 000 persons aged 18–69 years showed a 58 per cent excess mortality for cigarette-smoking men (RR = 1.58) in close agreement with the figure just mentioned. These mortality ratio figures are standardized to the age distributions of the respective populations.

The given excess risks of morbidity and mortality run by smokers, especially cigarette smokers, are statistical relationships which cannot simply be interpreted as causal. Other factors, such as alcohol consumption, stress and malnutrition, which are correlated with tobacco use, may have been direct or contributing causes of the observed morbidity and mortality pattern. Several facts indicate, however, that smoking itself is an important causal factor. (According to what is known as the constitutional hypothesis, certain—partly hereditary—personal characteristics would be the cause of a disposition for disease as well as that of a person acquiring the habit of smoking. This hypothesis seems, however, to lack scientific support.) Unambiguous dose–response relationships are available, showing that the risk increases with the number of cigarettes per day, with inhalation depth, with the tar and nicotine content of the smoke, and so on. It has also been shown that stopping smoking leads to a decrease of the excess risk—15 years after giving up smoking the mortality is nearly the same as that of persons who have never smoked. In addition, the fact that statistical relationships of these kinds between mortality and smoking have been demonstrated in several countries and in populations with different social habits and other life-style factors, indicates strongly that smoking is an essential causal factor.

The higher mortality among smokers applies to various causes of death, but in particular to three disease groups: cardiovascular diseases, cancer (especially of the lungs, other air passages and the oesophagus) and lung injuries (emphysema and bronchitis). In their study of the mortality of British doctors, Doll and Peto (1976) assumed that, for about one-half of the total excess mortality among smokers, the diseases given as cause of death were probably directly due to smoking. The uncertainty of this judgement is mainly due to the fact that the aetiological role of smoking for ischaemic heart disease cannot yet be considered quantifiable.

The excess mortality of smokers in Sweden is illustrated in Table 4.3 with data from the above-mentioned 10-year follow-up of the 1963 postal survey study (Cederlöf et al., 1975). Since this study comprised persons who were 18–69 years old in 1963, the observed mortality may be considered to reflect that of the age interval from about 25 to about

Table 4.3 Mortality in the period 1963–72 among the 55 000 participants, of the ages 18–69 years, in the 1963 postal survey of Statistics Sweden. Standardization has been made to the age distribution in 1970, when about 66 per cent of the Swedish population was in the age interval 18–69 years. The mortality is thus given as number of cases in ages c. 25–c.75 years per 100 000 of the total population. Correction for the decrease of the size of the studied sample was not done.

Causes of death (annual number of cases in Sweden)	Total (smokers and non-smokers)	Non-smokers	All smokers[a] (including ex-smokers)		Smokers of >15 cigarettes/day		Number (%) among smokers and number of cases per year
All causes of death				(RR)		(RR)	
Men	593	491	651	(1.33)	942	(1.92)	102 (=17%) (4 000 cases per year)
Women	372	349	453	(1.30)	616	(1.77)	23 (=6%) (1 000 cases per year)
Cancer of all sites							
Men	140	116	159	(1.37[c])	252	(2.17)	24 (17%) (1 000 cases per year)
Women	112	103	135	(1.31)	192[b]	(1.86)	9(=8%) (400 cases per year)
Cancer of lung and bronchus							
Men	23.0	4.5[b]	37.9	(8.4[b])	79.3	(18[b])	18.5 (≈80%) (750 cases per year)
Women	4.7	2.1[b]	15.5	(7.4[b])	–	–	2.6 (≈50%) (100 cases per year)
Ischaemic heart disease							
Men	206	156	237	(1.52)	256	(1.64)	50 (=25%) (2 000 cases per year)
Women	79	73	108	(1.48)	–	–	6 (=8%) (250 cases per year)

[a] All kinds of tobacco product.
[b] Values uncertain due to small numbers of cases among non-smoking men and smoking women, respectively.
[c] Cigarette smokers only, RR=1.4; smokers of cigarettes and pipe, RR=1.4; pipe smokers only, RR=1.2
From Cederlöf et al. (1975).

75 years, therefore excluding persons in the highest age groups. The mortality seen, 593 and 372 per 100 000 men and women, respectively, thus corresponds to 53 per cent and 40 per cent, respectively, of the total mortality in Sweden. It is estimated that the smoker-related fraction of the total mortality constitutes about 17 per cent and 6 per cent, respectively, in men and women, corresponding to about 4000 and 1000 annual deaths, respectively, in Sweden in the given age interval. Considering that the total mortality is about twice as great in the whole population, it is possible that the total smoker-related mortality may have been some 10 000 cases per year at the most. Because smoking alone cannot be given as the cause of excess deaths

among smokers, the true number with regard to the role of smoking would be lower. This estimate refers to the situation some 15 years ago. A follow-up is therefore called for.

Like studies from other countries this Swedish investigation shows a relatively low smoker-related excess mortality in women. Statistical data of this kind, designating lung cancer, heart attacks and emphysema as typically 'male' diseases, may have lulled women into a false sense of security, into a belief that they constitute a low-risk group, leading to lower motivation to stop smoking. Not least for this reason, it is important to stress that everything argues in favour of there being no difference between the sexes in this respect. The statistical data discussed originate from studies of female populations with small fractions of smokers, where, compared to male smoking habits, the number of cigarettes per day was smaller, the inhalation depth was lower and smoking started later in life. All these differences have thus contributed to a lower dose for female smokers. As for lung cancer (see below and Chapter 5) an increasing number of deaths among women caused by smoking is to be expected when the great number of women who, during the last two decades, took up smoking early in life and who also inhale 'like men', reach higher ages.

MORBIDITY AND MORTALITY: LUNG CANCER

In the case of cancer, scientifically convincing proof is available pointing to tobacco smoking as a dominating causal factor. Tobacco smoking on its own can cause lung cancer because the smoke contains both initiators and promoters of cancer. In addition, substances in the tobacco smoke may produce combined effects with other factors such as occupational exposure to radon daughters, arsenic and asbestos (see Section 4.6).

The lung cancer risk shows a distinct dose dependence, which may be illustrated by the correlation between the relative risk and the number of cigarettes smoked per day (Figure 4.7). The dose dependence shows up also as a decreased risk from smoking filter cigarettes and/or light cigarettes, an increasing risk with increasing depth of inhalation, and a dependence on the 'lifetime dose', that is, the number of years that smoking has been going on (according to compilations by the US Surgeon General (1979)). The last factor is apparently related to the age of taking up smoking (Table 4.4).

A number of investigations outside Sweden indicate that, in general, cigar and pipe smokers run a lower lung cancer risk than cigarette smokers do, evidently due to inhalation of the smoke being relatively rare. The risk to pipe smokers who do inhale, for example cigarette smokers who have switched to a pipe or who sometimes smoke a pipe, is, however, probably similar to the risk run by cigarette smokers. Under Swedish conditions the risk to average pipe and cigar smokers

Table 4.4 Relative risk of mortality from lung cancer (men) as a function of the age of starting to smoke.

Study	Age of starting (years)	Relative risk (RR)
'One million Americans' (Hammond, 1966)	(Non-smokers)	(1)
	25 years and more	4.08
	20–24	10.08
	15–19	19.69
	Below 15	16.77
Japanese study (population census material) (Hirayama, 1975)	(Non-smokers)	(1)
	25 years and more	2.87
	20–24	3.85
	Below 20	4.44
US war veterans (Kahn, 1966)	(Non-smokers)	(1)
	25 years and more	5.20
	20–24	9.50
	15–19	14.40
	Below 15	18.70

From US Surgeon General (1979).

appears to be nearly as high as the risk to cigarette smokers (Cederlöf et al., 1975; Damber and Larsson, 1983).

As to the issue of possible sex differences in lung cancer risks, the same arguments as above concerning mortality in general could be applied. It can therefore be stated that, in all probability, women do not run a lower lung cancer risk than men under similar smoking conditions. The apparently lower lung cancer risk among women compared to men in the same range of cigarettes per day (see Figure 4.7, curve 7, and similar results from other studies) reflects the situation in the 1960s and the 1970s, when women in specific smoking categories ran a lower risk than men because of different smoking habits, especially a late smoking début. To support his assumption that there are probably no sex differences in the smoking-related lung cancer risk, Doll (1978) mentions that Maori women in New Zealand, the female population with the largest number of smokers in the world, exhibit a lung cancer risk that is more than twice as high as anywhere else (it is, for instance, higher than the incidence *among men* in Sweden).

In different populations and countries with 'Western' life-styles, the RR for cigarette smokers compared to non-smokers has been given values in the range 7–14. Part of the variation is due to differences in cigarette type and other dose-determining factors, but the figures are also uncertain because the risk for non-smokers, that is the denominator of the fraction

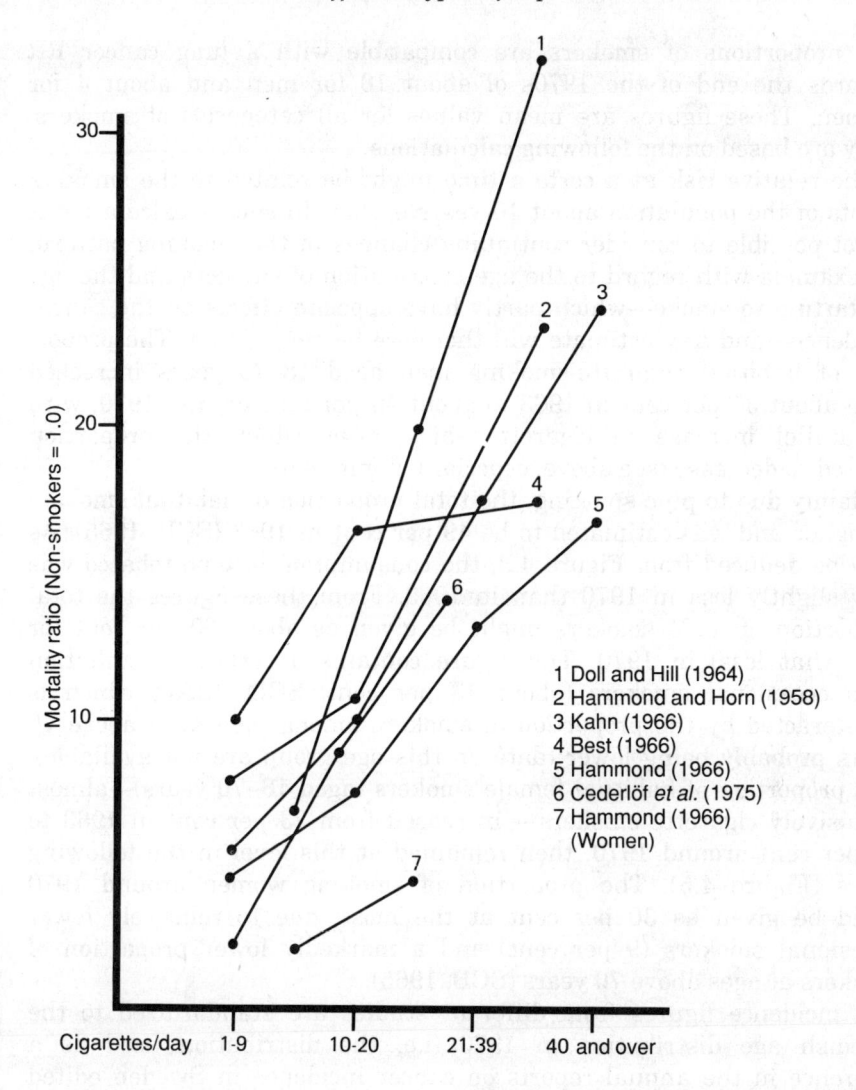

Figure 4.7 Dose–response relationships between number of cigarettes smoked per day and mortality from lung cancer. From Higgins (1976).

1 Doll and Hill (1964)
2 Hammond and Horn (1958)
3 Kahn (1966)
4 Best (1966)
5 Hammond (1966)
6 Cederlöf et al. (1975)
7 Hammond (1966) (Women)

$$RR = \frac{\text{risk for smokers}}{\text{risk for non-smokers}}$$

is uncertain for two reasons: the denominator is often based on small numbers of observations and, in addition, the definition of non-smokers has varied. The only published figure for Sweden (Cederlöf et al., 1975) gives RR = 8 for (average) cigarette smokers. Data for cancer incidences and proportions of smokers are compatible with a lung cancer RR towards the end of the 1970s of about 10 for men and about 4 for women. These figures are mean values for all categories of smokers. They are based on the following calculations.

The relative risk at a certain time might be related to the smoking habits of the population about 10 years earlier. In such a calculation it is not possible to consider continuing changes in the smoking pattern, for example with regard to the age distribution of smokers and the age of starting to smoke—which partly have opposite effects on the cancer incidence—and any estimate will therefore be very rough. The proportion of habitual cigarette-smoking men aged 18–70 years increased from about 35 per cent in 1963 to about 43 per cent around 1970, with a parallel increase in cigarette sales, after which the proportion started to decrease (see above, especially Figure 4.5).

Mainly due to pipe smoking, the total proportion of habitual smokers is higher and was estimated to be 49 per cent in 1963 (SCB, 1965). As may be deduced from Figure 4.3, the consumption of pipe tobacco was only slightly less in 1970 than in 1963. From these figures the total proportion of male smokers might be given as about 60 per cent (or somewhat less) in 1970. This figure contains a certain contribution from occasional smokers (about 13 per cent; SCB, 1965), which is counteracted by the proportion of smokers among men aged above 70 years probably being lower (data on this age group are not available). The proportion of habitual female smokers (aged 18–70 years)—almost exclusively cigarette smokers— increased from 23 per cent in 1963 to 33 per cent around 1970, then remained at this level in the following years (Figure 4.5). The proportion of smoking women around 1970 could be given as 30 per cent at the most, due to relatively fewer occasional smokers (9 per cent) and a markedly lower proportion of smokers at ages above 70 years (SCB, 1965).

If incidence figures from different studies are standardized to the Swedish age distribution in 1970 (i.e. the distribution used as a reference in the annual reports on cancer incidence in Sweden edited by the National Board of Health and Welfare), there is a strong indication that the lung cancer incidence among non-smokers is 5–7 cases per 100 000 per year among men as well as women (Table 4.5). This figure, averaging six per 100 000, may contain a contribution from passive smoking (see Section 4.2.5) and may, in addition, be too high because of uncertainties in the definition of non-smokers which, in some studies, are taken to include occasional smokers and ex-smokers. In 1978 the lung cancer incidence in Sweden was 43.0 per 100 000 for men and 12.2 per 100 000 per women. Thus the respective excess risks are 43 − 6 = 37 per 100 000 for men and 12 − 6 = 6 per 100 000 for women.

If the excess risk among men, is carried by the 60 per cent of the

Different types of exposure

Table 4.5 Lung cancer mortality among non-smokers, standardized to the Swedish age distribution in 1970.

Material	Mortality per 100 000 person-years (with 80% confidence interval)	Source and comments
USA, 10% of deaths in 1948 (men) and in 1958–9 (women)[a]		
Men	7.2 (6.2–8.3)	Haenszel and Taeuber (1964): smoking habits 1–2 years before death
Women	5.4 (5.1–5.8)	
Men + women with permanent residence		
Urban areas	6.1	
Rural areas	2.6	
'One million Americans[b]' ('never smoked regularly')		
8.5 years follow-up Men	7.0 (5.7–8.3)	Hammond (1966)
Women	c. 5 (uncertain)	
12 years follow-up; mean value of sub-periods Men	8.5 (6.6–9.8)[c]	Garfinkel (1981); see also Garfinkel (1980)
Women	5.7 (5.4–6.0)	
American war veterans ('never smoked or smoked occasionally')		
1954–62 Men	6.6 (5.6–7.6)	Kahn (1966)
British doctors		
1951–71 Men	(c. 7)	Doll and Peto (1976) (only 7 cases)
Japanese women	6.4[d]	Hirayama (1981)
husband non-smoker	(4)[d]	(32 cases)
husband smoker	(7)[d]	(142 cases)
Swedish data		
Twin registry		Hrubec (1983)
Men	3.9 (1.9–7.2)	(5 cases)
Women	6.8 (5.4–8.2)	(26 cases)
Postal survey of smoking habits 1963; 10 years follow-up		Cederlöf et al. (1975)[e]
Men	(6.3)(3.5–10.6)	(7 cases)
Women	(5.2)(3.7–6.7)	(19 cases)
Building workers, 1971–8		
Men	7.6 (4.4–12.3)	Schmalensee (1983)[f]
Means of the three studies:		
Men	6.2 (4.5–8.4)	(20 cases)
Women	6.1 (5.0–7.5)	(45 cases)
Men and women	6.15 (5.2–7.3)	(65 cases)

Footnotes on p. 112.

a   The study comprises 10 per cent of all deaths from lung cancer in the USA (except two states), among white men during 12 months and among white women during 24 months, in all c. 2200 men and c. 700 women, respectively, with adequate information of residence(s) and smoking habits. Corresponding information on the population in general was obtained as a supplement to official census data for a sample of about 65 000 of each sex. See also Haenszel et al. (1962).
b   A prospective study, initiated in 1959 by the American Cancer Society (ACS), in which 68 000 voluntary field workers recruited participants in the study among their acquaintances; it is therefore doubtful to what extent the sample is representative.
c   Variation between observation periods (see Garfinkel, 1981)
d   Japanese age distribution from the age groups of 40 years and over standardized (tentatively) to Swedish age distribution in 1970 with c. 45 per cent aged 40 and over.
e   Raw incidences according to Cederlöf et al. (1975), provisionally age standardized with a correction for under-representation of ages around 75 years and upwards.
f   From a health study by the Construction Industry Foundation for Industrial Safety and Health; for study design see Engholm et al. (1982)

population who are smokers, the corresponding RR would be 37/(0.6 × 6) = 10. In the same way the RR to women is estimated at 3–4. The uncertainty of these RR estimates is proportional to the uncertainties of the estimated number of smokers. Relative risk is subject to strong regional variations and shows higher values in large cities and lower values in rural areas, even after allowing for differences in the proportions of smokers. These variations in RR are probably largely due to differences in smoking habits with respect to the starting age and the number of cigarettes per day as well as in the inhalation depth which is correlated with the other parameters.

In their review of cancer in the USA, Doll and Peto (1981) estimated that 85–90 per cent of the approximate 95 000 recorded lung cancer deaths in 1978 could be assumed to be causally related to tobacco smoking. Correspondingly, the above figures imply that, if six cases of lung cancer per 100 000 per year occur among non-smokers, about 85 per cent of the 43 cases per 100 000 in 1978 among men in Sweden are due to tobacco smoking, partly in interaction with other exposures. In a similar way it may be estimated that at present around half the lung cancer cases among women are due to cigarette smoking.

TRENDS IN SWEDEN

From 1960 to 1972 the age-standardized lung cancer incidence in men increased from 24 to 44 per 100 000 per year, nearly a doubling in less than 20 years (Figure 4.8). The real increase may have been somewhat less because of underdiagnosis, particularly among the higher age groups at the beginning of the period; see Chapter 5. The relative rate of increase for women has been the same: from five to 10 per 100 000 per year. In the last few years a decrease in the incidence of lung cancer in men has been observed, especially in large cities, whereas the increase seems to have continued among women. These developments should be compared with the changes in smoking habits; as

Different types of exposure 113

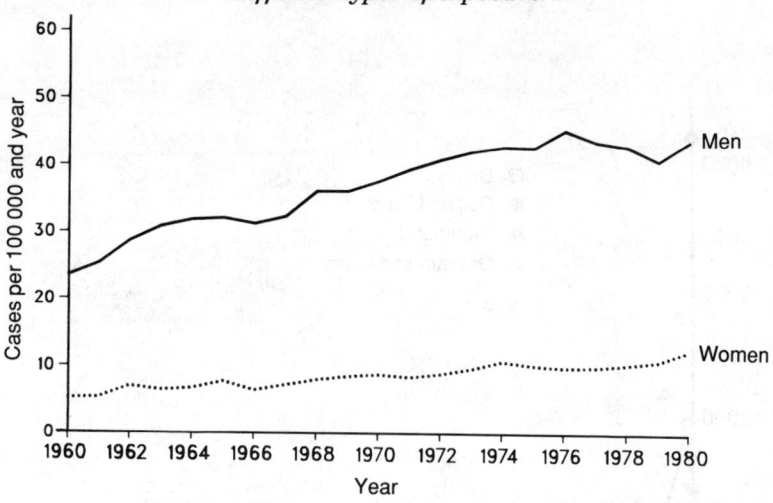

Figure 4.8 Age-standardized lung-cancer incidence for men and women in the years 1960–80 in Sweden. (For the incidence in specific age groups, see Table 5.13.) From NBHW (1980).

illustrated in Figure 4.5, the proportion of regular smokers among men reached a peak in 1969 followed by a decrease. In addition, the tar content of cigarettes was halved between 1964 and 1980 (Figure 4.4).

In women a continuing increase in the incidence of lung cancer is expected because the number of smokers peaked later than for men. In Chapter 5 these changes over time will be discussed more fully. As a consequence of the previous increase in smoking among girls, women aged around 45 years exhibited, in 1980, approximately the same lung cancer incidence as men in the same age group, whereas for those aged around 70 years the incidence was still some five times lower than that of men of equal age (compare Table 5.13).

CHANGES IN LUNG CANCER INCIDENCE AFTER CESSATION OF SMOKING

A couple of years after a previous smoker has stopped smoking, his or her excess lung cancer risk has decreased considerably; and after 10 years it is about one-quarter of what it would have been if smoking had not been given up (Figure 4.9). This rapid decrease in the risk is probably due to the carcinogenic action of tobacco smoke being to large extent a promoter action which, in principle, is reversible. However, the observation that the excess risk to ex-smokers does not decrease to zero, but seems to approach a value some twice that for people who have never smoked, is compatible with the fact that the smoke's components include initiators, the effects of which are, in principle, irreversible (Chapter 3). Section 5.7 discusses the health consequences of a discontinuation of smoking in Sweden.

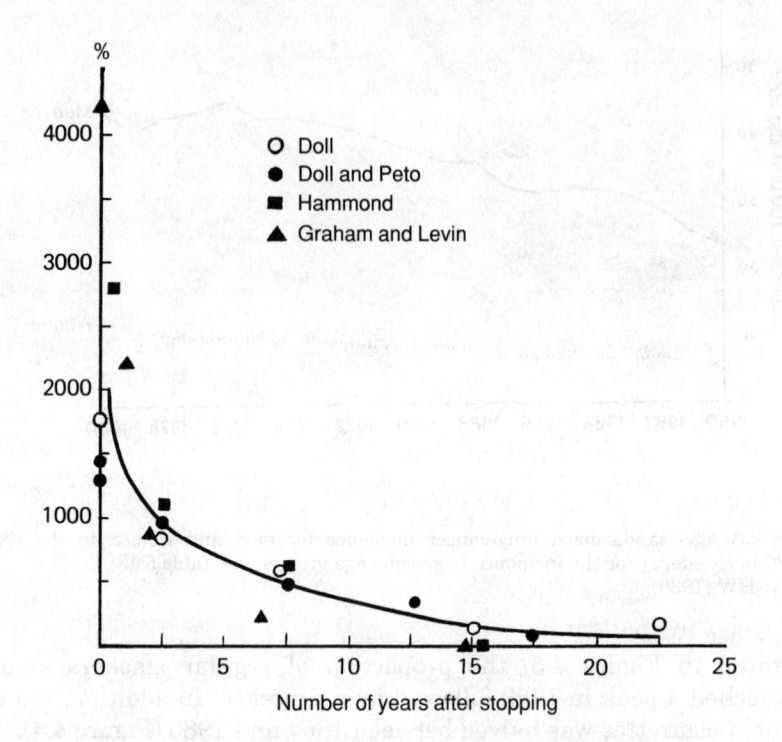

Figure 4.9 Effect of cessation of smoking on the mortality from lung cancer. The curve, which applies to ex-smokers (men) shows how the excess risk, given as the percentage of the risk to non-smokers (= 100 per cent), decreases with time after smoking has been stopped. After a long time a (total) risk about twice as high as that of non-smokers is approached. (This figure is a summary of four studies.)
From Reif (1981).

MORBIDITY AND MORTALITY FROM OTHER CANCER DISEASES: AN ESTIMATE OF THE TOTAL IMPORTANCE OF SMOKING

In several investigations, strong correlations between tobacco smoking and incidence or mortality have been demonstrated for cancer of the upper respiratory tract (oral cavity, larynx and pharynx) and the oesophagus. The risk of cancer of these sites is not dependent on inhalation depth and is therefore not lower among pipe and cigar smokers than among cigarette smokers. The risk of cancer of these sites also shows a correlation with alcohol consumption. A synergism (combined action) between alcohol and tobacco smoking has been demonstrated, in which alcohol has been assumed to act as a promoter or co-carcinogen. Furthermore, cancer in the oral cavity is more common among users of chewing tobacco, and the incidence of lip cancer is strongly associated with pipe smoking in particular.

Cancer initiators absorbed from tobacco smoke are expected, in principle, to act systemically (to spread in the body), with an increased incidence of tumours at sites other than the directly exposed ones. Various studies indicate increased tumour frequencies among smokers especially in the urinary bladder but also in the kidneys and the pancreas. The increased risk of bladder cancer might very well be due to a considerably raised content of mutagens in smokers' urine. Statistical correlations of smoking with an increased risk of cervical cancer might be due mainly to correlations between smoking and living habits that play an aetiological role for this disease, but cigarette smoking has also been pointed to as a causal factor (Buckley et al., 1981).

A certain excess mortality, for smokers, from cancer of other sites too is observed particularly in large investigations, for example the studies of 250 000 war veterans (Kahn, 1966; Rogot and Murray, 1980) and of 1 million US citizens of both sexes (Hammond 1966; Garfinkel, 1980, 1981); see further compilations in the first comprehensive official US report (US Department of Health, Education and Welfare, 1964). However, because of a strong focusing of interest on the above-mentioned 'smoking-related' cancer types, little attention has subsequently been paid to this more general excess tumour incidence among smokers. Because other aetiological factors which are correlated with smoking habits were not taken into account in these studies, causal relationships cannot be considered proven, but they are highly probable for the following reasons.

Smoking entails the uptake into the body of a large number of substances with mutagenic and cancer-initiating properties. According to the general principles for distribution in the body and for dose–response relationships (as discussed for example by Holmberg and Ehrenberg (1984)) in this context smoking is therefore expected to give rise to an increased risk of cancer at most sites (observed examples of systemic effects in smokers are, for instance, enhanced frequencies of cytogenetic disturbances in white blood cells as well as of sperm abnormalities). The observed excess risk at sites not usually associated with smoking, about 30 per cent in male cigarette smokers, is further compatible with other estimates of the cancer initiating action of tobacco smoke in this context (Ehrenberg, 1984a). This excess risk also shows a dose-dependence and is lower among ex-smokers (Kahn 1966).

THE TOTAL NUMBER OF CANCER CASES IN SWEDEN CAUSED BY SMOKING
For calculation of the aetiological fraction (E), due to smoking, of the cancer incidence at sites other than the lung and bronchus, Swedish incidence data for non-smokers are not available.

If the incidence for non-smokers, I_o, is known, E may be calculated from the mean incidence, I, thus:

$$E = 100\frac{I-I_o}{I} \%$$

This expression is independent of the proportion of smokers and their RR and, hence, of uncertainties in the estimates of these values. At present the calculation of E has to be based instead on estimates of the proportion of smokers (P_S) and their RR thus:

$$E = 100\frac{P_S(\text{RR}-1)}{1+P_S(\text{RR}-1)} \%$$

Estimates of E and of the number of cancer cases caused by tobacco smoking are given for men and women in Tables 4.6a and 4.6b respectively. Values for RR were taken from the large US investigations (Kahn, 1966; Hammond, 1966). These studies were not planned to allow for confounding factors. At the same time the excess risks comprise interacting factors as well. Different studies show a certain variation in RR, particularly for the oral cavity and the pharynx (US Surgeon General, 1979); in a Swedish (Cederlöf et al., 1975) and a Norwegian (Lund and Zeiner-Henriksen, 1981) prospective study no significant excess risk of cancer of these sites was demonstrated for either sex; these studies were small, however. Data concerning cancer of the urinary organs also show a variation in RR.

Relative risk of cancer sites other than those which have been associated, with a high degree of certainty, with smoking (i.e. 'Others' in Table 4.6) is about 1.3 for men. Because of uncertainty over contributions from causal factors other than smoking, the calculated E of 15 per cent has been lowered and is here given as about 10 per cent.

The estimate for women of the total number of cancer cases caused by smoking is still more uncertain, except for lung cancer (see Table 4.6a).

According to these estimates about one-quarter of all cancer cases in men should be attributed to tobacco smoking. In women about 7 per cent (5–10 per cent) of cases seem to be caused by tobacco smoking. The uncertainty of the latter figure is due mainly to the relatively large and very uncertain number of cases at sites not usually associated with smoking. Thus, as an average for both sexes, some 15 per cent of the cancer cases in Sweden should be considered to be caused by tobacco smoking, partly in interaction with other factors. The uncertainty interval in this figure may be 12–20 per cent.

It should be emphasized that this estimate concerns cases occurring today (the calculation being based on the disease statistics of 1979) as

Table 4.6a Estimate of number of cancer cases in 1979 among Swedish men with tobacco smoking as causal factor. For lung cancer the aetiological fraction (E) was calculated directly from incidence data, but for other sites it was based on estimates of relative risk (RR) and the proportion of smokers in the population (see text).

Site	RR	E (%)	Total number of cases in 1979	Number of cases due to smoking (rounded)[a]
Lung and bronchus	(c. 10)	85	1710	1450
Other sites associated with smoking, with high degree of certainty				
Lip, oral cavity, pharynx	6.2	75	438	350
Oesophagus	4.6	70	210	150
Larynx	9.0	85	187	150
Pancreas	2.5[b] (1.8–2.5[c])	45	591	300
Urinary organs (except kidney)	2.0[d]	40	1060	400
Kidney	1.5	25	710	150
Sum of 'tobacco smoking associated' sites	3.4[f]	60	4906	3000
Subtotal: 'tobacco smoking associated' except lung and bronchus	2.4[f]	45	3196	1500
Others	1.3	(15)[e] 10[e]	12 048	(1800)[e] 1200[e]
Total: all cancer	(1.6) 1.5[f]	(28) 24	16 954	(4750)[e] 4150

[a] Based on exactly calculated values of E.
[b] Swedish values (mortality) 3.1 for men and 2.5 for women (Cederlöf et al., 1975).
[c] Range of observations made in other countries (US Surgeon General, 1979).
[d] RR for mortality ≈ 2 in several studies (US Surgeon General, 1979); Swedish value for incidence among all smokers 1.9 (Cederlöf et al., 1975). Higher values have been observed in Italy (from a case-control study, Vineis et al., 1983 reported RR = ≈ 8 at 20 cigarettes per day) and in Norway (from a study in 1981, Lund and Zeiner-Henriksen have given RR = 3.1 for men and 3.8 for women).
[e] The calculated value was lowered to 10 per cent because of uncertain aetiology (see text).
[f] Weighted mean values.

Table 4.6b Estimate of number of cancer cases in 1979 among Swedish women with tobacco smoking as a causal factor. For method, see Table 4.6a.

Site	RR	E (%)	Total number of cases in 1979	Number of cases due to smoking (rounded)
Lung and bronchus	(4)	50	525	260
Other sites associated with smoking with a high degree of certainty[a]				
Lip, oral cavity, pharynx	4	50	139	70
Oesophagus	3	40	92	40
Larynx	8	70	16	10
Pancreas	2.5	30	565	170
Urinary organs (except kidney)	2	25	398	100
Kidney	1.5	15	517	80
Cervix uteri	1.5[b]	15	543	80[b]
Sum 'tobacco smoking associated' sites			2795	810
Subtotal; 'tobacco smoking associated' except lung and bronchus			2270	550
Others[c]	1.1	3	14 506	450
Total: all cancer		7	17 301	1250

[a] A lower figure for the average RR compared to male data except for larynx cancer, where the correlation with smoking is strong, has been presumed for cancer in upper respiratory organs and oesophagus because of lower smoking intensity among women and because of influence by other aetiological factors. For pancreas, kidney and other urinary organs, Swedish and other data do not indicate great differences in RR between the sexes (see US Surgeon General, 1979).

[b] An RR of 3.0 was calculated from Swedish data (Cederlöf et al., 1975); in the Norwegian study (Lund and Zeiner-Henriksen, 1981) RR was calculated to be 2.1 It is assumed here that one quarter of the excess risk is due to smoking (see Buckley et al., 1981). The calculated number of aetiological cases will be underestimated because of the greater number of smokers, relatively seen, at lower ages.

[c] Here lies the greatest uncertainty. It is true that some effect has been shown concerning some tumour locations but the interpretation is made more difficult by effects in the opposite direction on mortality in cancer of the breast and colon (Hammond, 1966); an effect in this direction is also seen in Norwegian data, Lund and Zeiner-Henriksen, (1981)), possibly a consequence of differences in dietary habits between smokers and non-smokers. A systemic cancer-initiating effect should, however, be considered as existing, 'stratified' over other effects and thus also including these locations.

a reflection of the smoking patterns of some 10 years earlier. It is probable that changes in smoking habits in the last few years have had the effect that the aetiological *fraction of cases induced today* is somewhat lower for males but the fraction is considerably higher for females, in any case for young women (see Section 5.7).

SNUFF AND CHEWING TOBACCO: CANCER RISKS

As mentioned in Section 4.2.2, the consumption of tobacco products other than for smoking, i.e. snuff and chewing tobacco, is considerable in Sweden. According to a study of smoking habits in 1982 (NTS, 1982), 14 per cent of men were taking snuff regularly, with considerably higher figures among the young. The most important difference concerning exposure, compared to other uses of tobacco, is that no combustion is involved. On the other hand, snuff and chewing tobacco contain compounds known to be carcinogenic. For instance, relatively high concentrations of nitrosamines have been found in snuff, even if the average amount of these compounds appears to have decreased in recent years (Österdhal and Slorach, 1983).

Apart from local effects at directly exposed sites, one should in these cases also expect a possible systemic action in other organs. The total cancer risk cannot be estimated at present. For the cancer type primarily associated with these ways of using tobacco, namely cancer of the oral cavity, there seem however to be no more than a few cases annually in the whole of Sweden. Considering the recent increase in snuff consumption in this country, basic data permitting a complete risk estimate for this factor are nevertheless called for. The International Agency for Research on Cancer (IARC) is working on a monograph on snuff and chewing tobacco which will evaluate the available scientific literature on cancer risks from the use of these products[2].

Summary assessment of risks to smokers

Tobacco use, particularly cigarette smoking, has several adverse effects on health through impaired lung function, damage to the mucous membranes and air passages, etc. Still more obvious is the increased mortality from different diseases that characterizes smokers.

As a result of their smoking pattern in the past, women have contributed considerably less than men to the overall smoker-related mortality in Sweden. However, the proportion of women who are regular cigarette smokers is now, on average, somewhat greater than that of men. Among men, smoking is more prevalent in the higher age groups, whereas among women the smokers are mostly younger or middle-aged. If smoking habits do not change, it is therefore to be expected that the number of cases of illness and deaths due to smoking will increase among women, when these age groups reach those higher ages at which the effects of smoking usually become manifest as diseases. Among men a considerable decline in smoking has occurred since a maximum some 15 years ago.

Scientifically convincing proof is available that tobacco smoking is a major cause of lung cancer in men in Sweden, the aetiological fraction of cases in 1979 being estimated at 85 per cent. There is no reason to assume that the lung cancer risk is smaller in women with the same smoking pattern as men, although in the year investigated the aetiological fraction was estimated at about 50 per cent. In the light of what has been said about changed smoking habits in women, particularly in the lower age groups, a future increase may be expected of the *number* of lung cancer cases in women as well as of the *proportion* of cases caused by smoking—unless a drastic decrease in smoking can be brought about. The same conclusion applies to other cancer diseases as well.

Other tumour diseases that can with great certainty be related to smoking comprise cancer of the lip, oral cavity and pharynx, oesophagus, pancreas, urinary organs and kidney. The aetiological role of tobacco smoking varies for these diseases (see Tables 4.6a and 4.6b), but a high aetiological fraction has been given here in the first instance for sites with direct exposure to smoke. Somewhat lower aetiological fractions were assumed for the three last-mentioned sites. For women, cancer of the cervix should be added, which, at least to some extent, seems to be directly caused by smoking.

For other tumour diseases not usually associated with smoking, it is also assumed that tobacco smoking is responsible to some extent, although causal relationships cannot be considered as proven. Smoking involves the uptake of a large number of substances with mutagenic and cancer-initiating properties. To a variable extent these substances should be presumed to be distributed within the body, an assumption which is supported by certain observed systemic effects (other than cancer) in connection with smoking. It is therefore to be expected that smokers run an enhanced risk of cancer of most sites, and this has been observed in studies of large populations. The uncertainty of the estimates of these excess risks has to be emphasized, however.

About one-quarter of all Swedish cancer cases in men can be attributed to tobacco smoking, and about 7 per cent in women. Thus, as an average for both sexes, some 15 per cent of the cancer cases in Sweden are considered to have tobacco smoking as a causative factor, partly in interaction with other factors.

4.2.5 Risks to non-smokers (effects of passive smoking and effects of smoking on offspring)

Background

As stated above, an assessment of the detrimental effects due to the use of tobacco also must include considerations of health hazards to people other than smokers. In the last few years especially, 'passive smoking' or so-called environmental tobacco smoke, has been discussed from this point of view, particularly with regard to the risks of lung cancer. It has already been mentioned that tobacco smoke contains a large number of carcinogenic substances, initiators as well as promoters. Major proportions of these substances are discharged in the sidestream smoke and therefore pollute homes, work premises, public premises and vehicles, and are inhaled by people present there. It is further possible that a growing fetus might run a risk of ill-health if the mother smokes, or is exposed passively to tobacco smoke, during pregnancy. Unweaned infants may be exposed to harmful compounds via breast milk if the mother smokes (or is exposed indirectly to tobacco smoke).

The question of hereditary injury due to genotoxic agents, including those in tobacco smoke, has been discussed in general terms in Section 3.4.

The lung cancer risk from passive smoking has been studied by epidemiological methods, and has been extensively studied and explicitly questioned. If dose–response relationships for cancer initiation and mutation are assumed to be linear it follows, however, that the risks of such indirect consequences of tobacco smoking are greater than zero. From the point of view of preventive measures it is urgent to clarify whether this excess risk is so high that it should be considered a serious health hazard.

Passive smoking

INVOLUNTARY EXPOSURE TO TOBACCO SMOKE
For most of the many compounds emitted from a burning cigarette, a major proportion enters the sidestream smoke (see Table 4.1 and US Surgeon General (1979)). An inhaling smoker absorbs for instance only 35 per cent of the tar, 20–30 per cent of the benzo[a]pyrene (BaP) formed and about 3 per cent of volatile nitrosamines and 2-naphthylamine. The rest of the products go into the atmosphere, and if the smoker does not inhale—as is often the case with cigar smoking—these fractions are still larger. For this reason the air in indoor environments where smoking occurs will be polluted by components

which in different ways constitute risks to any non-smoker present as well as to the smokers themselves.

The levels of pollution reached in a room depend on the number of cigarettes (or cigars, etc.) smoked per unit of time, the size of the room, ventilation conditions, and so on. Increased, sometimes greatly enhanced, levels of smoke components such as carbon monoxide, nicotine, respirable particles, BaP, oxides of nitrogen, aldehydes and nitrosamines have been observed under experimental as well as field conditions, the latter mainly in public premises such as restaurants and public transport (Repace and Lowrey, 1980; Schmeltz et al., 1975) In addition, metals such as cadmium and radioactive polonium are mostly emitted into the smokers' environment. Increased indoor levels, due to smoking, of mutagenic and therefore potentially carcinogenic compounds were demonstrated in a Norwegian–Swedish study by Löfroth et al. (1983); in this study the mutagenic activity of particles was determined by means of an Ames test in a large office building on a day when no smoking occurred and on a working day with normal smoking (a few thousand cigarettes in the building). The mutagenic activity was considerably higher in the latter case.

The absorption of tobacco smoke components by non-smokers has been demonstrated by findings of carboxyhaemoglobin and of nicotine and its metabolite cotinine (Rylander et al., 1983; Ehrenberg, 1984a). The fact that this uptake also includes mutagenic compounds follows from the raised mutagenic activity in urine from exposed non-smokers.

Air pollutants from cigarette smoking have been shown to cause various health effects among exposed non-smokers. In several studies, children of smoking parents have been shown to run an increased risk of infectious diseases of the air passages. Relationships of this kind were observed particularly in the first year of life (Harlap and Davies, 1974) but also among teenagers (Cameron et al., 1969; Colley, 1974; Holma et al., 1979). The correlations with the parents' smoking habits apply to acute as well as chronic symptoms. As a more objective measure of effects of passive smoking, diminished pulmonary function, established by a physical method, has been demonstrated in children of smoking parents (Tager et al., 1979).

Annoyance reactions of various kinds, such as eye irritations, have been shown in sensitive people subject to moderate concentrations of the components of tobacco smoke (Weber et al., 1979).

It is probable that reactive, and therefore cell-damaging, components in tobacco smoke, such as aldehydes (especially acrolein) and oxides of nitrogen, play a role in the origination of all the effects mentioned.

LUNG CANCER—EPIDEMIOLOGICAL STUDIES

In 1981 three studies, from Japan, Greece and the USA, were published on the lung cancer risks for non-smoking women with husbands of different smoking habits. In all three studies a somewhat higher risk was found when the husbands were smokers, and this increase was statistically significant in two of the studies as shown in the following table:

Source	Observed number of lung cancer cases in non-smoking women with: non-smoking husbands	smoking husbands	Relative risk	95% confidence interval of risk	Significance
Hirayama (1981a)	32	142	1.66	1.02–2.30	$P < 0.05$
Trichopoulos et al. (1981)	11	29	2.40	1.03–5.59	$P < 0.05$
Garfinkel (1981)	65	88	1.17	0.79–1.55	Not significant
Total	108	259	1.49	1.16–1.82	$P < 0.01$

The Japanese investigation (Hirayama, 1981a) was a prospective cohort study and comprised a relatively large number (about 90 000) of non-smoking wives, 40 years and older in 1966, who were observed for 14 years. Both the women and their husbands were interviewed on their smoking habits by postal questionnaires. During the study period, 174 deaths from lung cancer occurred among the non-smoking women. In 32 cases (out of 21 895) the husbands were non-smokers (or smoked occasionally), in 86 cases (out of 44 184) they were ex-or moderate smokers (1–19 cigarettes per day) and in 56 cases (out of 25 146) the husbands consumed 20 cigarettes or more per day. After age standardization within the cohort these figures correspond to mortalities of 8.7, 14.0 and 18.1, respectively, per 100 000 person-years. This trend compared with increasing smoking intensity strongly supports the existence of a causal relationship between risk and the husbands' smoking habits, and this impression is amplified by the appearance of the trend in two age groups (men below 60 years and men aged 60 years or over) and in two occupational categories (the husbands were subdivided into agricultural and other occupations).

The Greek investigation (Trichopoulos et al., 1981) was a case-control study in which 51 female lung cancer cases and about 160 control persons (admitted to hospital for orthopaedic treatment) were interviewed about their own and their husbands' smoking habits. Of the female lung cancer patients, 40 were non-smokers. In this case too there is a significantly increasing trend with an increasing number of cigarettes per day smoked by the husbands.

The US study (Garfinkel, 1981) was a prospective study comprising about 177 000 non-smoking women for whom the smoking habits of the husbands could be certified. The relative risk was estimated at

1.27, established when the husband smoked less than 20 cigarettes per day and 1.10 when he smoked 20 cigarettes or more per day. Neither value is significant (Garfinkel gives confidence intervals of 0.85–1.89 and 0.77–1.61, respectively), nor was any dose dependence shown.

These three studies have been discussed extensively by the scientific community, with arguments for and against their weight as evidence, and for and against the hypothesis that passive smoking entails an enhanced lung cancer risk. For instance, Hammond and Selikoff (1981) have stated that certain additional positive evidence is required in order to convince us that this hypothesis is true. The US Surgeon General in 1982 drew the following conclusion with reference to the studies discussed: 'Although the currently available evidence is not sufficient to conclude that passive or involuntary smoking causes lung cancer in non-smokers, the evidence does raise concern about a possible serious public health problem.'

It has sometimes been argued that the results of the US study were in some way contradictory to those of the other two studies, thereby decreasing their weight as evidence. Such an argument is erroneous. The US study does not contradict the two others in the sense that it could demonstrate the absence of an excess risk among passive smokers (see table above). It simply is not sufficiently informative. It appears from the upper limit of the 95 per cent confidence interval that this study is unable to exclude a 50–60 per cent excess risk due to passive smoking. It is difficult to evaluate the US study because it was a by-product of an investigation with other purposes, within complete presentation of data for non-respondents, follow-up time and age distributions of compared groups.

A statistical analysis of pooled data from these three studies, which were the first investigations of correlations between lung cancer risk and passive smoking and which have been widely debated, shows an amplified significance. This analysis gives the 95 per cent confidence interval 1.49 ± 0.33 and $P<0.01$. One should, however, pay attention to the justified criticism which has been directed towards the studies concerning the validity of data and the possible occurrence of confounding factors. Certain differences between Japan, the USA and Greece in relative risk are to be expected because of social differences with regard to such factors as the occupational situation of women with exposure in the work environment and the smoking habits of husbands in earlier marriages.

From the studies mentioned, the epidemiologically indicated lung cancer risk which may be related to passive smoking amounts to about two cases per 100 000 per year over the whole age distribution. (The figures in the Japanese study correspond to risks of four and seven cases per 10 000 person-years to women whose husbands are non-smokers and smokers, respectively, and the excess risks are approximately the same in the two other studies). This means that the excess risk is small and therefore difficult to demonstrate statistically. In addition, possible effects of several confounding factors contribute to the evidence of a causal relationship between passive smoking and lung cancer being questionable. The statistical correlations between an increased lung cancer risk and passive smoking have, however, become further amplified through more recent data. Thus the Greek investigation has been widened to a subject group twice as large, with an amplified significance ($P<0.01$) for a linear trend (Trichopoulos et al., 1983). Positive correlations have also been obtained in a US (Correa et al., 1983) and a West German (Knoth et al., 1983) investigation. A study in Hong Kong (Chan and Fung, 1982) shows a diminished relative risk of lung cancer (RR = 0.75) for wives of smoking husbands. This study has, however, so large a statistical margin of error (a 95 per cent confidence interval from about 0.4 to about 1.3) that it cannot contradict the studies with positive results. (The fact that a large fraction of the cases belong to a histological type (adenocarcinoma) that is only weakly related to tobacco smoking appears to stretch the margins still more.) In a previous study not discussed so far (Miller, 1978), reduced life expectancy was shown for wives of smoking husbands and also an increased cancer risk (personal communication Miller, 1983). Also Hirayama (1983), in an updating of his material to 1981, has confirmed the previously observed relationships. In this study a significantly increased incidence of cancer of the nasal sinuses for wives of smoking husbands was also discovered.

The fact that positive correlation appears in populations in different parts of the world strengthens the impression that the observed increase in lung cancer incidence does reflect a causal relationship. The statement that exposure to environmental tobacco smoke implies an unacceptable cancer risk would gain further credence if a risk estimate based on exposure dose of smoke components could confirm the epidemiological observations. Such a risk estimate has been calculated by Ehrenberg (1984a) as summarized in the following section.

LUNG CANCER—EXPOSURE DOSE AND RISK

As mentioned in Section 4.2.3, much of the carcinogenic material in smoke is discharged into the smoker's environment. Levels reached in the air have been determined for carbon monoxide, which may be used as an indicator of gaseous components, and for particles as well as nicotine and BaP, which may be taken to indicate levels of particle-bound compounds. Only a few representative measurements have been made in dwellings, and for that reason the exposure levels in homes have to be calculated. Most measurements originate from public premises, public transport and the like, but they are useful for confirmation of the reliability of calculation methods. Since particles precipitate relatively rapidly onto surfaces in a room, the equilibrium concentration of particulate compounds will be lower than the corresponding levels of gaseous compounds, compared to the relative amounts emitted into the air during tobacco smoking.

In a supplementary study to his first investigation, Hirayama (1981b) estimated that, on an average, male smokers spend about 5 hours daily of their time awake in their homes, and that they smoke about seven cigarettes during that time. With certain assumptions concerning reasonable room size (33 m^3) and a low rate of air exchange, Ehrenberg (1984a) applied the model of Repace and Lowrey (1980) and estimated a content of respirable particles of 0.5 mg m^{-3} when smoking was occurring. A recalculation of this figure for the content and uptake of BaP and for the lung cancer risk gives one case per 100 000 person-years as a most likely risk value under the conditions indicated by Hirayama. The risk coefficient used in this context was assumed to have the risk from air pollutants in coke oven and tar work, with BaP as the indicator substance, as a lower limit and the risk from cigarette smoking, also indicated by the BaP uptake, as the upper limit. This means, in principle, that the author assumed the dose–response curve in the case of the low uptakes of carcinogens in passive smoking to have a slope three times lower than the curve extrapolated linearly from the risks at the higher uptakes by active smokers. A lower slope is compatible with the assumption that a great part of the risk run by the smoker is caused by a promotive or co-carcinogenic action that does not appear at low doses.

There are of course great uncertainties in these calculations, partly because several important parameter values could only be roughly estimated. At lower efficiencies of air circulation the risk could be considerably higher than the given value, since pollutant levels in the air may be considerably higher in the immediate surroundings of a smoker. In addition, several smokers often get together in leisure hours with raised exposure levels as a consequence. According to the dose–response model applied by Ehrenberg (from Pike and Henderson 1981), the risk is strongly affected by the number of years of exposure. The risk to persons exposed to tobacco smoke right from childhood might thus be some four times greater than if exposure started at ages of around 20 years.

The overall uncertainty was judged to be a factor of 10 upward and downward. This uncertainty interval includes an overestimate of the possible risks, especially as the major carcinogens in environmental tobacco smoke are bound to particles which may be absorbed to a lesser degree in the case of passive smoking than of active smoking, as indicated in one study (Hiller *et al.* 1982). If, on the other hand, compounds in the gas phase are the essential contributors to risk, a smaller uptake of particles in the case of passive smoking would play a more limited role in the risk; the contents in air of particles and BaP would then only be indicators of the total pollution from tobacco smoke. If gaseous carcinogens, such as certain nitrosamines which appear almost exclusively in the sidestream smoke, are essential risk factors, the estimated risk may be an underestimate. This underlines the importance of identifying the principal carcinogenic components and of clarifying the important relationships between exposure levels and absorbed amounts.

In this debate it has been said that the risk from passive smoking shown epidemiologically, for example in Hirayama's study, would be unreasonably large, considering that it would constitute a considerable part of the risk run by actively smoking women. However, the risk appears realistic if one considers the relatively low risk of lung cancer to smoking women as compared with the risk to smoking men, partly due to the later starting age and the lower degree of inhalation that have characterized women smokers.

To sum up, the attempt referred to above to calculate the lung cancer risk from passive smoking generates a most probable value of the same size as that determined in the epidemiological studies. Although the estimated risk is very uncertain—with an uncertainty interval of about one order of magnitude—this result supports the conclusion that passive smoking constitutes a real risk factor.

OTHER TUMOUR FORMS
Most absorbed carcinogens are distributed systemically in the body and produce a dose contribution and an increased risk in organs other than the lungs. This is probably the main reason for the 40–50 per cent increase in the incidence of cancer at sites other than the air passages and the oesophagus that is shown by medium cigarette smokers (see Tables 4.6a and 4.6b) These risks run by passive smokers, of cancer at sites not directly exposed, were estimated from different determinations of the ratio between the incidences of tumours of these sites and of the lung among active smokers (Ehrenberg, 1984a). The estimation that the incidence of these tumours taken together is at least as high as that of lung cancer could serve, for the time being, as a base to be used in rough estimates of the risks also run by passive smokers.

SUMMARY
Since the epidemiological studies and the estimate based on exposure dose lead to compatible results concerning the lung cancer risk from passive smoking, it appears justifiable for the present to base estimations of *individual risks* in known exposure situations on the calcula-

tion by Ehrenberg (1984a) assuming a linear dose–response relationship and bearing in mind the great uncertainty interval.

Basic data permitting an estimate of the average exposure of the Swedish population to environmental tobacco smoke are not available. The *collective risk*, that is, the total number of cases attributable to this factor, can therefore only be discussed if certain assumptions are made concerning the number of exposed persons and the average exposure to environmental tobacco smoke. As a basis for such an estimate – and mainly in order to give an example of how a calculation might be done – Ehrenberg presumed that half the population at most is exposed under conditions similar to those prevailing in the epidemiological investigations discussed. According to this example about 30 lung cancer cases and of the order of 100 cancer cases altogether might be induced annually because of passive smoking, probably in interaction with other factors.

RELATION TO OTHER AIR POLLUTANTS

Exposure to general air pollutants in urban air implies an increase in cancer risks, roughly estimated at 100–1000 cases annually in Sweden (Section 6.6). The lower limit of this range is thus approximately equal to the estimated corresponding risk from passive smoking. It should be emphasized that these factors may confound each other in epidemiological analyses. Since the proportion of smokers is greatest in urban areas, especially large cities, passive smoking will be most common in these regions. It is in fact possible that environmental tobacco smoke partly explains the urban–rural difference in levels of general pollutants to which part of the corresponding difference in cancer risks has been ascribed.

Passive smoking is related in a different way to radon-daughter exposure. The levels of both environmental tobacco smoke and radon daughters increase with decreased ventilation and, moreover, tobacco smoke leads to increased levels of radon daughters through their adsorption to the smoke particles (Bergman and Axelson, 1983). In studies of relationships between cancer risks and radon daughter levels in dwellings, the effects of passive smoking have therefore to be considered in addition to effects of active smoking (see Section 10.4).

Risks of injury to the growing fetus and the new-born child

Most substances (organic chemicals as well as metal ions) absorbed from tobacco smoke freely pass through the placenta, with the possible consequence that the child will suffer ill-health if the mother smokes or is otherwise exposed to tobacco smoke during pregnancy.

An expected effect of such exposure is an increased cancer risk to the child. According to epidemiological studies the fetus is highly sensitive to the carcinogenic action of ionizing radiation (UNSCEAR, 1972, 1977). Druckrey et al. (1967) in comprehensive experiments, particularly with nitrosamines, demonstrated a similar high sensitivity of fetuses to chemical carcinogens. Several of the compounds in tobacco smoke are likewise effective transplacental carcinogens in animal experiments (Everson, 1980), and in experiments with hamsters, cigarette tar has been shown to lead to cancer in the offspring (Nicolov and Chernosemsky, 1979; see US Surgeon General, 1981). It appears that the exposure of pregnant females gives rise to tumours in the adult offspring animals. Certain data on transplacental carcinogensis in man are available, but they are still scanty and uncertain (concerning tobacco smoking, Hinds and Kolonel 1980; concerning occupational exposures, Hemminki, et al., 1981; concerning diet etc., Preston-Martin et al., 1982)

The possibility of carcinogens occurring in breast milk should also be considered. A sometimes strong mutagenic activity has been demonstrated in aspirate of breast liquid (Petrakis et al., 1982). An association with smoking has so far not been studied but it seems reasonable to assume that breast feeding is a potential indirect exposure route for carcinogens from tobacco smoke. It was shown early on that nicotine may occur in the breast milk of smoking mothers (Emanuel, 1931; Perlman et al., 1942), and the presence of nicotine and its metabolite cotinine has been established in the milk of non-smoking women exposed to environmental tobacco smoke during work (Hardee et al., 1983).

The effects of exposure on the fetus are not limited to an increased cancer risk. Several health effects have been observed to be more or less strongly correlated with the mother's smoking habits. In the report from the US Surgeon General (1982) on the health consequences of smoking for women, these risks are summarized in some 20 points. Among other things it is stated that reduced birth weight, decreased body length and increased risks of spontaneous abortion, fetal death and neonatal death seem to be directly caused by the mother's smoking during pregnancy. According to the report this also holds for other disturbances such as pre-term delivery. Further, an increased risk of malformations is also a probable consequence of maternal or paternal smoking, but has not been shown unambiguously. Congenital heart disease, however, according to Pirani (1978), shows a significant increase among babies of smoking mothers. In the case of an observed increase in ill-health among children, the role of exposure during pregnancy cannot be separated from the effects of passive smoking after birth. According to the US report there are also indications of reduced intellectual capacity in children whose mothers smoked during pregnancy. Some of these effects on the fetus may have genotoxic mechanisms (Pelkonen et al., 1979; Vaught et al.,

1979), but carbon monoxide and nicotine are considered to be important aetiological factors (Pirani, 1978).

A correlation between smoking and reduced fertility has been observed in both women and men, the latter as concluded from physiological and morphological disturbances during spermatogenesis (US Surgeon General, 1980).

Summary assessment of risks to non-smokers

The question of cancer risks from direct exposure through passive smoking has been studied epidemiologically for lung cancer. Although three investigations published in 1981, taken together, indicate an increased lung cancer risk from passive smoking, the organization and conduct of these investigations was such that they cannot be considered to demonstrate unambiguously the existence of such a risk. However, a few later studies and follow-ups amplify the impression that observed increases in incidence reflect a real causal relationship. International scientific activity in this area is at present high, and new epidemiological investigations in the next few years are expected to provide a clearer picture of health effects from passive smoking.

At present it is indisputable that cancer initiators are absorbed upon involuntary exposure to tobacco smoke. Therefore passive smoking must imply a certain increase in cancer risk. Data that could permit an estimate of the *size* of this risk are at present incomplete and imperfect. However, calculations on the basis of exposure dose, although subject to a wide margin of error, yield a (most probable) value for the lung cancer risk which is not incompatible with the results of the epidemiologic investigations. The suspicion that passive smoking does cause lung cancer in man to a non-negligible extent has thus obtained further support.

Considering the cancer risks of smokers, it is also reasonable to assume that cancer initiators in environmental tobacco smoke imply an enhanced risk of cancer of sites other than the lung, the overall cancer risk being approximately twice as great as that of lung cancer.

The individual risk varies, of course with the exposure conditions, and would mostly be low but in extreme cases a substantial risk cannot be excluded. Any estimate of the expected annual number of cancer cases in Sweden due to passive smoking would at present be very uncertain since the average exposure is not known. The importance must be stressed of further epidemiological studies and studies of exposure doses and other factors, which could permit a more reliable risk estimate.

Children are mostly unable to avoid the health hazards from involuntary smoking and therefore constitute a special ethical problem. Children of smoking mothers may be exposed to genotoxic and other compounds which might exert an action either in the fetus during pregnancy or later through inhalation or via breast milk. Nor can it be excluded that injuries may arise to the genetic material of the gonad cells of smoking men or women, leading to hereditary diseases or an increased tendency to the development of certain diseases, including cancer, in later generations. To the extent that such risks exist, passive smoking too should be assumed to exert some action. Certain observed effects have been related to maternal smoking; with regard to cancer risks causal relationships have, however, not yet been proven by epidemiological methods.

4.3 Diet

4.3.1 General aspects

The normal human intake of food and drink (about a couple of kilograms per day) constitutes without doubt our most important confrontation with environmental chemicals. This holds for both the quantity absorbed daily and the chemical diversity of food components.

In experimental studies Tannenbaum demonstrated as early as the 1940s that a reduced total intake of food decreased the incidence of certain spontaneous and chemically induced tumours. The importance of the composition of the diet was also shown in these early studies; for instance a reduced fat intake led to a lower tumour frequency. Earlier still, Watson and Mellanby (1930) had found that adding butter to the diet of animals provoked an increased incidence of skin tumours induced by chemicals. Later observations confirmed that this is valid for several chemical carcinogens and different animal species (Baumann and Rush, 1939; Tannenbaum, 1942; Lavik and Baumann, 1943; Carroll and Khor, 1975).

In the last decade the major role of living habits ('life-style') in cancer risks has become increasingly obvious. Dietary habits are of particular importance in this context—compare the classification by different authors of environmental factors to which variations in cancer incidence or mortality have been related (see Tables 2.7 and 2.8). On the assumption that the major part of all cancer cases are due to environmental factors in a broad sense, it has been said that diet could play an aetiological role in as much as 60 per cent of all cancer cases among women and 40 per cent among men (Gori, 1979). In their extensive review of causes of cancer in the USA, Doll and Peto (1981) suggest that between 10 per cent and 70 per cent of all human cancer may be causally related to dietary factors.

Correlations between cancer incidence and dietary habits have, for example, been observed in population studies of immigrants, whose cancer-incidence pattern changes from that of the home country to one characteristic of the host country (as seen among Japanese immigrants in the USA). Other examples are epidemiological studies of specific populations which live in the same environment but have different dietary habits. Epidemiological studies only rarely permit, however, a clear identification of causal factors in carcinogenesis. By contrast, animal experiments can be conducted with more strict control of different variables such as dietary factors. Results from such studies support the conclusions from epidemiological investigations that the diet and its composition may exert an influence on most cancer diseases, including several of those most common in Sweden.

As implied above, results from animal experiments cannot be directly translated to man. Different species may respond in different ways to exposure to one and the same dietary component, and spontaneous tumours may be affected differently from experimentally induced tumours (Alcantara and Speckmann, 1976). In attempts to demonstrate causal relationships between diet and cancer, one has mostly to rest content with indications, since for natural reasons 'proof' in these cases—like those of other suspected causal factors—can only rarely be obtained. If, however, the results of several experimental studies (if possible in different animal systems) and human epidemiological studies (if possible in different populations) give concordant results, the total impression given by the collected evidence will be that a causal relationship between intake of the dietary component studied and the incidence of a certain tumour disease is likely to exist. Additional support for such a hypothesis may be obtained if one succeeds in clarifying the mechanisms by which the dietary component operates in the body.

In the following pages a general survey is given of our state of understanding with respect to components in the diet that are believed to increase or reduce cancer risk (Sections 4.3.2– 4.3.4). When applicable, these data are discussed in relation to specific cancer types in Sweden. In a couple of separate sections discussions follow on alcohol (Section 4.3.5) and problems pertaining to drinking water (Section 4.3.6).

In a separate section on specific chemicals and exposure environments (Section 4.4), certain data relating to exposure situations in Sweden for specific chemicals, including their occurrence in foods, are presented and commented on.

4.3.2 Natural components of the diet that may cause cancer

Relationships between the composition of foods and cancer risks are complex, and comprise interactions of initiators, promoters and co- and anti-carcinogens. Furthermore, the strong interdependence between amounts of different components in the diet has to be considered: at a constant calorie intake, for instance, a reduction in protein leads to an increased intake of other components. Despite these difficulties certain patterns begin to appear and, when epidemiological observations and experimental data point in the same direction, a reasonable basis for cancer-preventive measures develops.

Concordance of epidemiological and experimental data is available, for example with regard to the relationship between intake of fat and mortality from cancer of the colon and rectum (in both men and women) and breast (in women). For both sites comparisons of statistical data from different countries generate relationships which are nearly linear, starting from mortalities from these diseases which are close to zero at the lowest daily fat intakes (concerning the colon, see Wynder (1975) and Armstrong and Doll (1975); concerning breast cancer, see Carroll (1975)).

In Sweden *colo-rectal cancer* is responsible for some 12 per cent of all cancer cases in both men and women, with altogether about 4200 cases annually. Third-World countries in Africa and Asia show relatively low incidences of colon cancer. Immigrant studies support the assumption of an environmental influence. Among Japanese in Hawaii, the mortality from colon cancer increases in the first immigrant generation (Shils 1979). The increase in colon cancer incidence in Japan has also been related to the growing contribution of Western habits to the Japanese food culture (Wynder and Reddy, 1977). Studies in Israel have revealed a higher incidence of colon cancer among immigrants from Asia and Africa (Modan et al., 1975).

If fat does play a role in the aetiology of colon cancer, questions arise concerning the mechanism behind this relationship. A currently accepted hypothesis is that dietary fat intake (a) increases the secretion of bile acids, cholesterol and related compounds (neutral steroids) into the intestine, and (b) shifts the composition and metabolic activity of the intestinal flora towards an increased number of bacteria that change bile acids and neutral steroids into metabolic products, some of which may act as promoters and others as initiators. A number of animal experiments have given support to the hypothesis concerning the importance of dietary fat in colon carcinogenesis as well as to the assumption that bacterially changed bile acids—for example deoxycholic and lithocholic acids—may play a promoter role in the origin of colon cancer (Wynder and Reddy, 1977).

In the last few years it has turned out that some 20 per cent of all persons excrete mutagenic compounds (positive in the Ames test) in the faeces. Vegetarians seem to produce less mutagens in the faeces than people with mixed diet (Kuhnlein et al., 1981). It seems likely that these compounds are produced metabolically by intestinal bacteria from bile acids, cholesterol and similar endogenous compounds.

The relevance of these findings is still uncertain, but they show that our own body and bacteria in the intestine are able to give rise to genotoxic compounds. (The relation between mutagens and carcinogens was discussed in Chapter 3.) Under these conditions cancer promotive processes become particularly interesting, especially those associated with the diet.

Breast cancer is the most common form of cancer in women and in Sweden is responsible for some 25 per cent of all female cases, or about 4300 cases annually. As with colon cancer, there are indications from epidemiological as well as experimental studies of a dependence on environmental factors (Shils, 1979; Carroll, 1977; MacMahon, 1979). In contrast to colon cancer, no change in breast cancer incidence after emigration from a low-risk country, for example Japan, to a high-risk country, such as the USA, can be observed until the second generation, that is, the children of the migrants (Wynder and Hirayama, 1977).

Both amount and type of dietary fat are of importance for the promotion of mammary tumours in experimental animals (Hopkins and Carroll, 1979), but it is difficult to arrive at definite conclusions as to which type of fat (saturated or unsaturated) is most active in this respect (MacMahon, 1979). A certain amount of polyunsaturated fatty acids in addition to a high total level of dietary fat seems to be necessary for promotion of mammary tumorigenesis after administration to rats of an initiator (Hopkins and Carroll, 1979).

An increased risk of mammary cancer has also been associated with a disturbed hormonal balance, and it has been suggested that part of the effects of the diet in mammary carcinogenesis may have this mechanism (Gray *et al.*, 1979). A high-fat diet increases the prolactin level in the serum, and one theory has been that this could lead to promotion of breast tumours (Chan and Cohen, 1975).

The present state of knowledge in this field was surveyed in 1982 by an expert group in the USA the Committee on Diet, Nutrition and Cancer (cited as US National Research Council (1982); this report includes a large number of references).

The US group drew the conclusion that of all the food components it had studied, the combined epidemiological and experimental evidence was strongest for a causal relationship between fat intake and cancer. Both epidemiological studies and animal experiments provide convincing evidence that an increasing intake of total fat increases the tumour incidence of certain sites, particularly the breast and colon, and—conversely—that the risk is lower with lower fat intakes.

The Cancer Committee expresses a similar opinion. With as much certainty as can be reasonably achieved, the *total* fat intake must be considered to play an essential role in the incidence of cancer both of the breast and of the colon. It is even possible that this factor is the major one for cancer of these sites. The available scientific data do not yet permit conclusions to be drawn as to possible differences between the influence of *specific types* of fat, although it is probable that such differences exist.

Another cancer for which incidence is also positively correlated with fat intake is cancer of the corpus uteri (endometrium). This disease shows a geographic pattern of distribution similar to those of breast cancer and colon cancer. Overweight post-menopausal women are especially prone to this disease (Armstrong, 1977). Other factors, too, have been shown to exert an influence on the incidence of this cancer form (see Chapter 6). In all, some 1100 cases occur annually in Sweden.

Other forms of cancer for which fat intake may be an important factor, but where additional knowledge is required to prove the causal relationships, are cancer of the prostate, ovary, pancreas and kidney (see US National Research Council, 1982). With regard specifically to prostate cancer, case-control studies showed a correlation between high fat consumption and the incidence of this disease (Zaridze, 1983). Prostate cancer has a higher incidence in Sweden than any other male tumour disease.

The total fat consumption in Sweden is close to 40 per cent of the human energy supply, as in the USA and several other countries in Western Europe. The same total intake of fat in various populations may result from diets of different composition. As an example, in Sweden the proportion of the fat that originates from meat consumption is lower than in many other countries whereas the contribution from milk products is correspondingly higher. In 1980, 24 per cent of the fat intake in Sweden derived from meat and fish (the latter being 2 per cent only) and 21 per cent from milk and milk products excluding butter. In the USA the corresponding figures were 36 per cent and 12 per cent, respectively.

As stated above, statistical data from different countries reflect nearly linear relationships between fat intake and mortality from colorectal or mammary cancer. These relationships might be interpreted to mean that these two tumour diseases, the most common ones in Sweden, could be nearly completely eliminated through a drastic reduction in fat intake. This would of course be a misinterpretation; the observed linearity of the relationships between 'dose' (as daily intake of fat per person) and response may be a consequence of the effects of interactions with other factors, operating in different directions. These may also include variations within the countries concerned, as well as uncertainties in the determination of mortality in relation to fat intake. One is certainly entitled, however, to assume that these data at least partly reflect truly existing correlations.

A cancer which is rapidly decreasing in Sweden and in other developed countries, and which has also been associated with nutritional factors, is *stomach cancer* (ventricular cancer). It has been suggested that the decreasing occurrence of this cancer is due to a diminishing consumption of salted foodstuffs (Joossens *et al.*, 1979) and a rise in consumption of fruit and fresh vegetables (Bjelke, 1978; Tulinius 1981). A high intake of nitrate (see Törnqvist, 1984) and an inadequate intake of vitamin C have been particularly pointed out as causal factors of this disease (Miller, 1983).

Although fat is an essential natural food component which is probably of great importance in the origination of cancer, several pieces of evidence indicate that other natural dietary components may also play a role of this kind. Of special interest in this context are common salt (naturally occurring or added to foods) and substances in vegetable materials, often with complicated and peculiar chemical structures. Several components in foodstuffs from the plant kingdom are mutagenic in laboratory tests.

Taken together, the available data suggest that carcinogens occurring naturally in vegetable materials—including relatively rare foods such as certain mushrooms—are probably of little significance to the overall cancer incidence in Sweden. Also the individual risk is probably low except possibly in cases of a very unbalanced diet. There are, however, reservations due to the incompleteness of our present knowledge. Methods applied up to now do not permit us to exclude with certainty the occurrence of natural carcinogens in foods which might contribute considerably to the total cancer incidence, especially if there are carcinogens of a low potency that are difficult to extract and occur in widely used foodstuffs. It is obvious that proof of the existence or non-existence of such carcinogens requires a scientific methodology quite different from those now available (see discussion on early warning systems in Chapter 8 and Ehrenberg (1984c).

4.3.3 Components added to the diet in connection with production, storage and preparation that may cause cancer

Advances in food technology have in various ways led to new chemical substances in foodstuffs, whose relation to the diet–cancer complex has to be discussed.

The earliest example was heating as a means of food preparation, which also causes chemical reactions. An important step in the origin of stable social cultures in different climates was taken with the invention of methods, adapted to the respective type of climate, for the preservation and storage of foods (salting, smoking, drying, etc.). Refrigeration and freezing techniques have recently changed the picture in industrialized countries, with less need for other preservation techniques. At the same time chemical technology has led to profound changes in all the steps of production, storage and preparation of foods, with the consequence that foreign compounds may appear in the food consumed. Since chemical–technical interventions at various stages partly lead to such compounds being in the food, the consequences of these technologies are discussed together.

Synthetic fertilizers nowadays play a major role in agriculture. Nitrate may be taken up into intensely cultivated crops, so much so that some of it remains at consumption; this could be of some, but probably only of minor, importance in the context of cancer risks. Under suboptimal storage conditions nitrite may also be formed. The presence of nitrosamines has been demonstrated in the body after consumption of spinach together with amine-containing food items such as fish (Törnqvist 1984). Uptake of certain metals that contaminate fertilizers (e.g. cadmium) or precipitate from polluted air may also be of importance, although the magnitude of a possible cancer risk is not known.

Chemical pesticides are likewise of importance in food production all over the world, before as well as after harvest or slaughter. Both vegetables and animal foods contain residues of stable compounds (e.g. DDT) or their metabolites (e.g. DDE) or of compounds not completely decomposed into inactive products before consumption. Imported foodstuffs may differ from locally produced ones in composition and levels of residues; DDT for example is no longer used in Sweden. Carcinogenic activity has been ascribed to certain of these pesticides. As far as is known, the levels in Swedish foodstuffs are mostly low (see Section 4.4.4) and individual risks may thus be assumed to be low. However, available data do not permit an estimate of the contribution of pesticide residues to the total cancer incidence.

Synthetic hormones, such as diethylstilboestrol, with known carcinogenic properties, have been used in some countries in animal husbandry, and can lead to residues in the meat. Epidemiological data on the effects are, however, not available.

Fungus attacks on stored vegetable products or even before harvesting, may lead to the occurrence in foods of carcinogenic or otherwise toxic *mycotoxins*, particularly aflatoxin from the mould *Aspergillus flavus*. Aflatoxin is a very potent carcinogen; for instance, the relatively high incidence of liver cancer in Uganda has been ascribed to human consumption of cereals stored under unsatisfactory conditions conducive to mould attacks (Alpert *et al.*, 1971). Aflatoxin has also been found in concentrated fodder in Sweden and can be formed on mouldy bread. In certain cases very high levels of aflatoxin have been encountered. (For references and further discussion, see Section 4.4.) It should also be mentioned that during fermentation common yeast may give rise to urethane, a potent carcinogen occurring at varying levels in bread, wine and beer. This compound cannot be excluded as a cancer initiator of considerable importance (von Bahr *et al.*, 1984b).

Smoke curing leads to the contamination of foodstuffs with certain pyrolysis products such as polycyclic aromatic hydrocarbons. Some scientists have described correlations between the incidence of stomach cancer and the consumption of smoked foods (Dungal, 1961; Haenszel *et al.*, 1976). Research on this aspect of modern smoking methods is in progress.

A large number of compounds occur in the diet as *food additives* applied with the aim of increasing the shelf life (preservatives), or of improving colour, flavour or consistency. The most important of these compounds seem to have been tested for genotoxicity, in certain cases including cancer tests, but certain types of additive, especially several flavouring agents, appear according to internationally available data to have been insufficiently studied (see also Section 4.4.4). Compounds giving positive results in cancer tests are usually not allowed in Sweden; certain colouring agents are banned, for example. This is not the case with the sweeteners saccharin and cyclamate which seem to act as promoters at very high intakes and which, therefore, most probably involve negligible risks at the usual low intakes. Another exception is nitrite, the use of which as an additive is well regulated and limited in Sweden. Its potential risk from the formation of nitrosamines in the body should be balanced, however, against the benefit aimed at, namely prevention of the dangerous disease botulism, caused by the action of a micro-organism, *Clostridium botulinum*, during storage of certain foods. Nitrate, which is partially transformed into nitrite by micro-organisms in the saliva, was previously common in salted products but is now used only to a limited extent in Sweden.

Certain plastic *packing materials* have been shown to give off small amounts of monomers, such as vinyl chloride and acrylonitrile, known to be carcinogenic. The contents of these compounds are now strictly regulated in Sweden and their risk contribution can be considered extremely small. Packing materials for foods may, however, contain several other potentially carcinogenic compounds (plasticizers, benzidine-based colouring agents, etc.) which, by migration into the packed foodstuffs, may give rise to exposures of unknown magnitude (see Section 4.4.4).

The relevance of *food preparation methods* in the generation of carcinogenic compounds constitutes a very interesting question. It has been known for a long time that heating foodstuffs leads to the formation of mutagenic compounds. Several of these have later been shown to be carcinogenic in animal tests. To what extent they also involve a real hazard to humans is less clear.

In the early 1960s it was reported that benzo[*a*]pyrene (BaP), an established experimental carcinogen, and other polycyclic aromatic hydrocarbons (PAHs) appeared in considerable amounts in charcoal-broiled meat (Lijinsky and Shubik, 1964). It was later reported that

PAHs are formed by smoking and frying as well (Engst and Fritz 1977). PAHs, which include several well-known experimental carcinogens, are easily formed during incomplete combustion of organic matter and also occur in tobacco smoke, car exhausts and gaseous emissions from certain industries. These sources of PAHs are discussed in other sections of the book (see for example Section 4.4.5). Although BaP and other PAHs may be formed by the heating of foodstuffs, it is generally thought, that BaP found in food is mainly due to precipitation from polluted air. Some exposure data on BaP are given in Section 4.4.

There are many indications that compounds other than PAHs are the most important genotoxic compounds formed during heating of foodstuffs. It has, for instance, been shown that the mutagenic activity in the surface layer of grilled fish or meat is some 10 000 times greater than could be explained by the content of BaP (Sugimura et al., 1977). This activity is mostly studied by the Ames test, although other short-term tests have also been used. In systematic model studies, Sugimura's research team showed that the amino acid tryptophan is especially liable to give rise to mutagens when heated (Sugimura and Nagao, 1979). Recent results show that mutagenic pyrolysis products of tryptophan can induce liver cancer in mice following administration in food (Matsukura et al., 1981).

The occurrence of mutagenic activity has also been studied in heated foods of other kinds. Thus heating of carbohydrates may likewise lead to the formation of mutagens (Sugimura and Nagao, 1979; Spingarn et al., 1980).

Heating may also provoke chemical changes involving food additives such as nitrite in bacon. Volatile nitrosamines are formed in frying of Swedish bacon (Josefsson and Nygren, 1981). This group of substances includes several potent carcinogens. The nitrosamines appear especially in the frying fumes and in the remaining frying fat.

Westermark (1984a) has discussed, in terms of elementary chemical kinetics, a few models of the influence of temperature, during preparation and preservation of foods, on the formation of mutagenic pyrolysis products and how their concentrations might be restricted. The formation of mutagens appears to increase strongly with increasing temperature over a quite narrow range, and the formation of mutagens might therefore be reduced considerably by avoiding frying temperatures above the lower limit of this range. It is not unlikely that the formation of mutagenic compounds during the heating of foods might constitute a significant risk factor among those specific environmental factors which are responsible for human cancer, particularly with respect to initiating agents. As mentioned, certain such mutagens have been shown to be carcinogenic in animal experiments. It is at present not known to what extent the Swedish population is exposed to mutagenic and cancer-initiating agents through the heating of foods, whether industrially manufactured products or foods which are not heated until their preparation by catering services or in the home. Further research is needed into the mechanisms of generation of mutagens, as well as research on foods. It is important that studies of the latter type be performed nationally because differences between foods, for instance with regard to protein composition and enzymatic reactions before cooking (such as meat tenderized to various degrees), as well as differences in cooking techniques, may make it difficult to 'translate' research data from one country to another.

4.3.4 Components of the diet that may protect against induction of cancer

Sections 4.3.2 and 4.3.3 have focused on factors in foods which can *induce* cancer. Other factors in the diet act to inhibit carcinogenesis. A number of compounds with the ability to prevent tumour induction and/or inhibit tumour growth have been identified in experimental investigations and are also the subject of studies in man. Examples of possible protective mechanisms are: inhibition of the formation of, or inactivation of, reactive metabolic products (e.g. peroxides); inhibition of the action of promoters; inhibition of the uptake of carcinogens into the body; and effects on the bacterial flora of the intestines. Certain studies have indicated that *dietary fibre* may reduce the effects of certain carcinogens (Kritchevsky, 1977). This may be due to adsorption of carcinogenic substances onto the fibre. Fibre has also been shown to reduce the transit time of the intestinal contents through the intestine (Harvey *et al.*, 1973). Both these effects may lead to a reduced uptake of carcinogens from the intestine. Epidemiological studies indicate a correlation between a low fibre content in the diet and an enhanced risk of colon cancer (Cummings, 1981a). It has, for instance, been suggested that the relatively high fibre consumption in Finland might contribute to the incidence of colon cancer being relatively low there, despite a high fat intake (Reddy *et al.*, 1978). As just mentioned, the composition and metabolic activity of the intestinal bacteria is probably of significance in the formation of intestinal tumours. Dietary fibre may have an influence on the composition of the flora and on the bacterial metabolism, resulting in protection against colon cancer (Cummings, 1981a). There is, however, still some uncertainty with regard to the importance of high fibre intake. Certain recent investigations indicate that a protective effect against colon cancer is restricted to certain types of fibre (Cummings, 1981b).

In the international literature it has been suggested that several vitamins act as protectors against cancer. In experimental studies, lack of vitamin A and its 'pro-vitamins', especially β-*carotene*, has been shown to lead to increased numbers of tumours after administration of chemical carcinogens (Cohen et al., 1976) and treatment with vitamin A reduces the number of tumours (Hogan, 1979). Concerning vitamin A, prospective and retrospective epidemiological studies show certain correlations between a low level of retinol (a form of vitamin A) in the blood or a low intake of β-carotene (a factor in various vegetables which is transformed to vitamin A in the body), and an increased cancer risk (Peto et al. 1981). The observed protective action of vitamin A through β-carotene is not strong, which might indicate that the individual risk is affected only to a minor extent by changing the diet. This protective action might, however, be of greater significance to the total cancer incidence, since such action has a bearing on large population groups and a majority of cancer forms.

Ascorbic acid (vitamin C) appears, in animal experiments, to protect against nitrosamine-induced ventricular cancer by destroying nitrite, with reduced nitrosamine formation as a consequence (Mirvish et al., 1972). Certain epidemiological observations indicate that a larger intake of fruit and other vegetables rich in vitamin C reduces the risk of cancer (Bjelke, 1978; Tulinius, 1981). However, it is difficult with data of this kind to draw conclusions as to the identity of the active factor (it is not necessarily vitamin C). Nor do there seem to be any data available which convincingly prove the theory that very large intakes of vitamin C are useful as a preventive measure.

Vitamin E, which counteracts peroxidation of lipids, has been shown to reduce the cancer incidence in certain experimental systems. Epidemiological data supporting this observation are not available.

A protective action of the element *selenium* against cancer of several types is indicated by experimental as well as epidemiological data (Schrauzer, 1976; Willett et al., 1983). Selenium is needed for the normal function of glutathione peroxidase, an enzyme that eliminates hydrogen peroxide and hydroperoxide in cells acting, in principle, as an antioxidant. Selenium is very toxic at high doses, a fact that has to be considered in connection with possible official recommendations on selenium intake. The question of the role of selenium is important in Sweden, because of relatively low levels in the soil and, therefore, also in locally produced foods in large parts of the country.

Butylated hydroxyanisole (BHA) and *butylated hydroxytoluene (BHT)* are used in the food industry to prevent foods turning rancid by autoxidation of fats. Both BHA and BHT have been shown to counteract carcinogenesis in experimental animals. Part of this effect may be related to the ability of these compounds to capture ('scavenge') free radicals (see Holmberg and Ehrenberg, 1984). BHT, however, seems to also act as a promoter of lung cancer in mice.

In the 1960s it was suggested that certain compounds (*indoles*) occurring, for example, in brussels sprouts, could counteract the development of chemically induced cancer. This has since been supported by studies of several forms of cabbage including brussels sprouts. Hypotheses on the possible mechanisms of action of these compounds have been presented (Wattenberg and Loub 1978).

Several diseases are associated with exceptionally low potassium levels in the body. According to certain observations (Jansson 1983) there is a correlation of the *sodium-to-potassium ratio* in the diet and drinking water and in tissues with the incidences of several tumours. This demands further studies.

The above-mentioned US expert group has summarized the present knowledge concerning inhibitors of carcinogenesis as follows:

The group 'believes that there is sufficient epidemiological evidence to suggest that consumption of certain vegetables, especially carotene-rich (i.e. dark green and deep yellow) vegetables and cruciferous vegetables (e.g. cabbage, broccoli, cauliflower and brussels sprouts), is associated with a reduction in the incidence of cancer at several sites in humans. A number of non-nutritive and nutritive compounds that are present in these vegetables also inhibit carcinogenesis in laboratory animals. Investigators have not yet established which, if any, of these compounds may be responsible for the protective effect observed in epidemiological studies' (US National Research Council 1982). The group has made a similar assessment of fruit, particularly citrus fruits.

The general statement by the US group emphasizes the importance of including fruit, vegetables and whole-grain cereal products in the daily diet, since high intakes of these foods have been inversely correlated with the incidence of various cancer diseases; this statement is supported by experimental data, especially with regard to fruit and vegetables.

Such scientific assessments as are feasible at present of possibly protective agents and their efficiency apply to the composition of the *whole* diet, not to *single* components in specific food items. Although certain animal experiments have been conducted with one compound at a time, it is not yet possible to discuss data for separate components. Therefore, while the importance of large groups of foodstuffs, such as fruit, vegetables and whole-grain cereals, must be underlined, the scientific basis is too weak to allow any firm judgements to be drawn on the possible impact on public health from addition of specific protective components to the diet. However, this points to a field of research which could produce results of great practical importance.

4.3.5 Alcohol (ethanol)

Alcoholic beverages and ethanol in other forms have long been supposed to be a contributing cause of cancer of the oral cavity, pharynx, larynx and oesophagus, and seem to produce these effects in multiplicative interaction (see Section 4.6) with tobacco smoking (Tuyns et al., 1977; Tuyns, 1978). The risk of cancer at these sites among persons who smoke and drink regularly may be 100 times higher than that of persons who do neither. In studies of the importance of social factors, a considerable excess risk has been observed among divorced men (see Chapter 5).

In this context it has been suggested that the alcohol acts as a promoter (by causing cell injury) or as a co-carcinogen (by facilitating the absorption of carcinogens in the upper alimentary tract). Injury to the liver through the use of alcohol leads to an increased risk of primary liver cancer, an effect that has been attributed mainly to a promotive action.

Alcohol was shown in the 1950s to cause chromosomal aberrations in leguminous plants (Rieger and Michaelis, 1960) and a similar effect was recently demonstrated also in man (Natarajan, 1980) Alcoholics exhibit higher frequencies of various structural chromosomal aberrations, which appear independently and are added to the corresponding effects due to tobacco smoking. Experimental data indicate that acetaldehyde, the primary metabolic product of alcohol, is probably causing this injury to the chromosomes. Carcinogenic properties of acetaldehyde have also recently been shown in animal experiments (Feron et al., 1982). Ethanol may therefore act not only as a promoter or co-carcinogen but, via this metabolite, also as an initiator, with an increased risk also of types of cancer other than those mentioned above.

The traditionally alcohol-related tumour types, which are at the same time smoking-related, amount in Sweden to around 5 per cent of the total cancer incidence for men and around 1.5 per cent of that for women. Among non-smokers in Western Europe and North America the risk of cancer of those sites, even at a considerable alcohol consumption, is thought to be comparatively low, corresponding to a relative risk of 2–3 (Rothman and Keller, 1972). More than half the cases in Sweden of cancer of the sites in question should be ascribed to the combined action of alcohol and smoking. To this should be added an unknown but limited contribution to other cancer forms which certainly include primary liver cancer. According to a very rough estimate, something of the order of 500 cases annually (and certainly not more than 1000 cases) are caused by alcohol consumption in Sweden. Epidemiologically observed variations in risks between different alcoholic beverages probably depend on other specific components due to raw materials and production processes. Data on human cancer in man so far available point primarily to a correlation of risk with high alcohol consumption. In these studies it has sometimes been considered difficult, however, to establish the total alcohol intake (references in US National Research Council (1982)). The risk run by 'moderate drinkers' thus cannot be assessed with any certainty but appears to be small.

4.3.6 Drinking water

In a discussion of possible exposure to carcinogens via drinking water several different compounds including naturally occurring ones have to be considered.

It is to be expected that bodies of water into which industrial pollutants are deposited will sometimes contain compounds with mutagenic activity, since a large number of chemicals have this property. Biological characterization with short-term tests of industrial emissions (Rannug, 1980) into water has also produced positive results (i.e. mutagenicity) in certain cases in Sweden. This does not mean that mutagenicity was demonstrated in the water itself, since the dilution may have been very great. Several municipalities are wholly or partly dependent on raw-water resources which are to some degree exposed to industrial pollutants, but it is not possible at present to decide if this involves significant risks of cancer. A general aim is to keep total pollutant levels in industrial emissions as low as possible, and the conditions concerning supplies of drinking water seem to be far more favourable in Sweden than for example, in densely populated, highly industrialized areas of Europe.

In several countries directly acting mutagens have been demonstrated in chlorinated drinking water. Such compounds probably originate in the chlorination process (see below). There is also a possibility that mutagenic compounds might be released from materials used for water pipes.

Drinking water may contain compounds originating from purification and disinfection procedures, especially certain halogens and halogenated compounds. If the water contains organic matter such as humic acids, chlorination may lead to the formation of chorinated compounds (especially chloroform) which according to studies in several countries appear in treated drinking water (Victorin 1980). In Sweden the content of these compounds—mainly chloroform—is less than 25 μgl^{-1} in most drinking water (Norin et al., 1981).

Chloroform as an aerosol is not mutagenic in experiments with bacteria (Simmon and Tardiff, 1978) but has shown mutagenic action in yeast (Callen et al., 1980). Metabolites of chloroform can bind covalently to protein, but binding to DNA is very slight (Clemens et al., 1979; Pereira et al., 1982; Reitz et al., 1982). In animal experiments chloroform meets certain criteria for being considered as carcinogenic (National Cancer Institute, 1976; weak significance obtained by Pereira et al., 1982). Calculations of the human cancer risk from results of animal experiments may only be considered as rough estimates. On the basis of such theoretical calculations, Victorin (1980) estimates that a daily consumption of 2 litres of water containing 100 µgl^{-1} chloroform would lead to 0.03 cancer cases per million persons per year. For Sweden, where the average chloroform concentration is well below 100 µgl^{-1}, this might thus mean less than one cancer case every 5 years. The experimental data referred to above indicate that the effect of chloroform should mainly or wholly be ascribed to a promoter action of the kind that appears only at high intake levels (Reitz et al., 1982). Hence, the chloroform risk estimate just mentioned is probably a considerable overestimate. It should be pointed out, however, that the directly mutagenic and cancer-initiating activity demonstrated in chlorinated drinking water (Bull et al., 1982) is not due to chloroform; during chlorination other mutagens too are formed from organic matter in the water.

Certain US and Dutch epidemiological studies indicate statistical correlations between cancer risk and the concentration of chlorination products in water (DeRouen and Diem, 1977; Buncher et al., 1977; Crump and Guess, 1980; Zoeteman et al., 1982). Later studies of the case-control type, in which known confounding factors were allowed for, confirm these results and indicate causal relationships and raised risk of at least certain forms of cancer (Gottlieb and Carr, 1982; Kanarek and Young, 1982). However, considering that the concentrations of chlorinated organic compounds are very low and that these compounds were shown in experiments to be *weak* carcinogens, maybe mainly of a promoter type, it appears unlikely that such compounds at current levels could make more than a negligible contribution to the total cancer risks in Sweden. Doll and Peto (1981) make the same assessment in their study of cancer risks in the USA. One should, however, agree with these authors that the question has to be watched and that it deserves further studies considering that any pollutant levels in drinking water—even if they are low—imply life-long exposure.

One issue concerning the quality of drinking water which has been observed for a long time is the levels of *nitrate* and *nitrite*, especially due to leakage of plant nutrients from the use of nitrogen fertilizers and sludge. Occasional very high levels of nitrate in Swedish water supplies, usually from private wells, have mostly been due to technical defects in the supply, such as contamination by surface water, leaking sewage disposal systems and other problems or point-sources, for instance dunghills. Intensive fertilization of sandy soils has also sometimes led to high levels of nitrate and nitrite (NBHW, 1981). According to a later study (Thoms and Joelsson, 1982), there may be as many as 100 000 people in Sweden using water from private wells with nitrate levels above 50 mgl^{-1} which is a value not to be exceeded for children under 12 months. (The recommendations generally characterize waters with a nitrate level of more than 30 mgl^{-1} as 'noteworthy' from the hygienic point of view'.) Except for locally elevated levels of nitrate, the total exposure in Sweden appears to be low—in the sense that the content in municipality tap water is usually well below the limit. This guiding principle for a maximum nitrate content in drinking water has, however, been set for reasons other than possible cancer risks. It is difficult to assess these risks but they cannot be excluded, particularly with regard to the possibility that nitrate might be reduced to nitrite, which is mutagenic and may lead to the formation of mutagenic and carcinogenic compounds (nitrosamines) in reactions with other substances in the body (Törnqvist, 1984).

Investigations of tap water in Sweden have revealed the presence of nitrite, especially in outlying districts of certain municipalities where the water distribution system requires long pipelines. One explanation may be the production of nitrite via bacteria from ammonium compounds which occur naturally but which are also added at waterworks during purification processes (Victorin and Stenström, 1975). The possible contribution to cancer risks cannot be assessed at present.

The question of *asbestos fibres* in drinking water has recently been the subject of an investigation in Sweden (Guzikowsi, 1980). The source may be asbestos-cement pipes for water distribution, a relatively common system in Sweden. An increase in the water acidity would contribute to a dissolution of the cement, thus releasing asbestos. It is not known for sure if asbestos is carcinogenic when ingested. Epidemiological studies have demonstrated a carcinogenic action of airborne asbestos mainly in the lungs. A weak and less certain effect of this kind has also been observed in the gastrointestinal tract (Selikoff *et al.*, 1973), however, and possible exposure via drinking water therefore needs to be included in a surveillance of asbestos. Basic data for an assessment of the total exposure of the population via drinking water are still scanty, but they are hardly alarming (see also Section 4.4).

The total exposure in Sweden to *radon* via drinking water is probably negligible.

Some *heavy metals* have been shown to be carcinogenic in various studies. It has long been known that pipes used for drinking-water may release metals under certain conditions. Quite a new aspect of possible exposure to heavy metals has, however, appeared through continuous *acidification* in Sweden, not least through the raised levels in atmospheric precipitation of acidic sulphur and nitrogen compounds. Besides increased risk of corrosion of pipes, metals may be mobilized from sediments in surface water supplies as well as from soil and rock to groundwater supplies. In addition, human beings may be exposed indirectly via plants and animals contaminated after uptake of metals. These effects of acidification may become an extraordinarily severe problem of environmental toxicology.

Correlations between the levels of heavy metals in surface water and acidity have been established. In strongly acidic water (pH 4.5), for example, the cadmium content is 10 times higher than in less acidic water (pH 5.5). Sufficient data on the background levels of heavy metals in groundwaters are still lacking for Sweden. It is therefore not possible to tell whether these levels have been influenced by acidification. Those studies available indicate, however, that metal in the upper soil layers (1 m deep) are released and transported down to the groundwater. The levels of heavy metals in water percolating down through acid soils are much higher than those in the surface water. In most areas the deeper soil layers, due to the higher pH value, act as a 'sink' for the transport of metals. Another aspect is that very high levels of heavy metals may be released into water pipe systems from malfunctioning de-acidification filters (NEPB, 1984).

Acidification is continuing in Sweden (Swedish Ministry of Agriculture, 1982), but available analytical data on metal levels in water do not warrant an assumption that cancer risks so far have increased.

4.4 Specific chemicals and exposure environments

4.4.1 Introduction

It is reasonable to assume that the chemical identity of many compounds to which man is exposed—via air pollution, foodstuffs or by other routes—is unknown. Among these substances carcinogens may be present.

Data from epidemiological studies are available for only a few agents. The number of substances investigated by means of animal experiments is considerably larger, but is still very limited in relation to the great variety of compounds with which man may come into contact. In addition, other experimental data besides studies for carcinogenicity in animals—primarily results from mutagenicity tests indicating the general genotoxic potential of a substance—are of interest in this context. An evaluation of the available documentary material can be carried out with reference to one or more of the following areas:

(a) nature and scope of the material (human data, bioassays, mutagenicity studies, etc.);
(b) the carcinogenic potential of the substance;
(c) the carcinogenic potency of the substance (dose–response relationships in bioassays and in epidemiological material);

(d) the scientific quality and usefulness of data from individual studies (their value as 'evidence');
(e) the magnitude of risk to defined individuals or populations under current exposure conditions.

The depth of analysis and the nature of criteria used for evaluating the cancer risks of a substance depend to some extent on the aim of the evaluation. Thus, until quite recently the International Agency for Research on Cancer (IARC) in Lyons, a scientific body, had not considered the degree of risk in its evaluations. This aspect often assumes importance where administrative decisions are concerned, such as those taken within a regulatory agency.

In order to obtain an overview of the exposure situation for individual chemicals within Sweden, various government regulatory agencies were asked for certain information regarding a selection of reasonably well-documented substances. A secondary aim was to investigate the existence and availability of this type of data. A number of substances evaluated by the IARC and by the National Cancer Institute (NCI) in the USA were selected, for which there were well-founded suspicions of carcinogenicity on the basis of specific criteria (see Section 4.4.4). There was no intention to provide an exhaustive list of all possible chemical cancer risks, nor did the Cancer Committee at this stage hold any scientific discussion of the carcinogenicity of these particular substances.

In these lists complete carcinogens predominate, that is, substances which act as both initiators and promoters (see Chapter 3). To ensure that other types of agent were covered to some extent, a number of possible promoters and other agents thought to exert a modifying influence on carcinogenesis were added as a separate list.

This study seems to be the first large-scale attempt to review available exposure data for carcinogens and suspected carcinogens in the entire Swedish environment. The design of the survey also made it possible to consider drawing conclusions on total exposure for particular substances, by a synthesis of information on different kinds of product or from various environments.

Since exposure analysis provides the basis for risk estimation — appraisal of the degree of hazard under prevailing conditions of exposure—this section starts with a general outline of the various routes for dispersion of and exposure to chemical substances in the environment (Section 4.4.2), including various approaches to the estimation of exposure, with different degrees of precision. In order to provide additional guidance in interpreting various exposure data, the concepts of 'exposure' and 'dose' are further clarified in Section 4.4.3.

In connection with the reports on exposure acquired from government agencies (Section 4.4.4), a more detailed account follows (in

Section 4.4.5) for a limited number of compounds, industrial processes, and the like. The conclusions can be found in Section 4.4.6.

4.4.2 Routes of dispersion and exposure to chemical substances in the environment.

The capacity of a chemical compound to cause injury to man is in part a function of the properties of that substance, and in part dependent on the actual exposure to it. For this reason, analysis of exposure is of paramount importance in any risk estimation.

Exposure analyses mainly concern two major issues:

(a) the dispersion of a substance in the environment from a source up to, but not including, the interface between the body and its surroundings where uptake may occur;
(b) the course of events from the uptake at the point of contact (absorption) up to the biological target in the body, where the substance may exert its action.

This section will look at the first of these issues: routes of dispersion and exposure to chemical substances in the environment.

In the complex range of substances with which man is continuously in contact through breathing, eating, drinking and touch, compounds of natural origin cause the highest exposure levels. Such substances, and compounds formed in large volumes by various forms of human activity (carbon dioxide, sulphur dioxide, etc.), are as a rule easily measured, so satisfactory exposure data are in general available.

However, it is well known that out of the approximately 60 000 synthetic compounds in actual or potential industrial use (most of which will sooner or later end up in the external environment) exposure data—derived from direct analysis and expressed as concentrations in samples derived from biota, foodstuffs, soil, air, and so on— exist only for a limited number. Even when such information is available, the quality is uneven with respect to the representativeness of the samples, the sampling methods and extraction procedures employed, and the precision of analysis. Often the results cannot be verified because the concentration of the substance to be analysed varies over time, and because the original sample was disposed of after analysis was completed. This overall picture is substantiated by the exposure data obtained from certain regulatory agencies, which are presented in Section 4.4.4.

On the other hand, the importance of precision in such analytical data should be related to the potential significance of the properties and effects of the chemical under prevailing exposure conditions. In comparison with situations where current exposure levels can only be considered insignificant, an entirely different standard with regard to quality and scope of analyses must obviously be adopted when there is only a small safety margin between daily intake and the level where damage occurs. Thus, in many cases an idea of the order of magnitude of the concentration of a chemical in various media may suffice. However, for known or suspected carcinogens where a linear dose–response relationship cannot be excluded, one has to consider no less than three aspects when working with exposure analysis, namely: exposure level, dose (exposure over time) and the number of exposed individuals. Since a high collective dose is bound to affect appreciably any estimated incidence figures, the last aspect is of interest also at low individual doses. In certain cases knowledge of the composition of the target population can be significant (e.g. pregnant women). The results of the exposure study, with data from the various government agencies covering a multitude of substances of relevance to carcinogenesis, should be assessed against this background.

The first step in characterizing an exposure profile is to estimate the approximate exposure levels under various conditions. If such an appraisal indicates a potential risk to humans, a more thorough analysis will be called for. In the absence of measured concentrations, certain methods are available for judging the degree of exposure based on other kinds of information.

In the simplest case, such an assessment can be derived from basic data on the physico-chemical properties of the substance, its chemical structure, technical function and use, production volumes, means of disposal, and so on. When usage does not involve a way of handling which creates dust or aerosols, information on vapour pressure will indicate the upper limits for the concentration of a chemical in inhaled air, which in turn can be employed as a basis for calculating a maximal inhalation dose. Based on chemical structure and solubility in various solvents, certain assumptions can then be made concerning uptake and distribution in the body—assumptions which improve the basis for a semi-quantitative estimation of dose. A low solubility in aqueous media in a pH range similar to that in the human gastrointestinal tract may point to a low absorption upon oral administration. The range of particle sizes of finely divided materials may furnish evidence of inhalation hazards from handling methods which involve the generation of dust and so forth.

These considerations may in many cases be entirely adequate—at least when appraising whether or not a certain level of exposure, in the context of available toxicological information, is sufficiently high to justify further research.

Determination of exposure: general considerations

For products intended for direct administration to humans (such as foodstuffs or pharmaceuticals) exposure levels and doses are the most readily defined. In other cases of (usually unintentional) exposure, the feasibility of measuring or predicting exposure on the basis of mathematical models is most favourable when the path between source and target population is short, for example with the direct exposure of workers in the workplace or of consumers to household chemicals. Such direct exposure may occur at any stage in the life cycle of an industrial chemical: during production, transport, storage, processing, consumption and disposal (destruction, recovery).

Exposure in the workplace and in the home

In the production of basic chemicals (such as in the petrochemical industry), today's highly automated processing technology uses closed systems to a great extent, so the production phase rarely involves significant worker exposure in the factory itself. Except for accidents, this is also true for the transport and storage phases in a chemical's life-cycle. Although the number of people involved is generally limited, processing and professional use of many substances involves the highest exposure levels, implying potentially high individual risks. Moreover, for the majority of human carcinogens, their carcinogenicity was first revealed in connection with their professional use.

Consumer usage of a product suggests the likelihood of exposure of a large number of individuals. The skin is highly exposed to many household chemicals. The risk of accidental ingestion is obviously also higher in the home than in the workplace. Although the same range of chemicals is often employed for hobbies and other leisure activities (paints, lacquers, solvents, etc.) as for certain professional uses, the exposure characteristics differ profoundly in certain respects. Consumer use is usually of a more or less temporary nature but may occur under rather uncontrolled conditions caused by inadequate protective equipment, poor ventilation, and other factors. However, in comparison with professional usage, consumer exposure as a rule carries a low risk to the individual.

Even in the absence of detailed measurements, exposures can be estimated by using mathematical models based on physico-chemical data, information on function, use, and so on. For direct exposure reasonably precise estimates may be made for the various phases in the life-cycle of a chemical (US EPA, 1979b; OECD, 1983). Accurate information on the production techniques employed (degree of automation, points of release, process temperature, ventilation conditions, the proximity of workers to points of release, protective measures, etc.)

combined with monitoring data from analogous situations (a chemical with similar physico-chemical properties, identical processing equipment), enables an estimate of exposure at the workplace to be obtained. For many purposes this is sufficiently accurate and can be calculated in the absence of specific monitoring data.

Computation models for consumer use have also been developed for a number of categories of household products, which can be utilized as a basis for a crude estimate of the exposure dose.

Exposure via the external environment

In many situations, unintentional human exposure occurs via one of several different environmental routes. The exposure of suckling infants to polychlorinated biphenyls (PCBs) in their mother's milk is an example of a more complex route. Here the exposure results from the mother's consumption of food such as herring, which in turn has been polluted via the aquatic food-chains by PCBs released from capacitors, hydraulic oils, and other areas of industrial use.

The intentional application of certain chemicals in the general environment such as pesticides, accidents resulting in leakage, waste disposal sites, and emissions from industrial plants and incinerators may all release different agents into the human environment. Such releases can indirectly lead to human exposure through pollution of drinking water and inhaled air. Foodstuffs may be contaminated by uptake in crops, aquatic organisms and the like.

The various physical and chemical processes by which chemical substances move from one environmental medium to another, across an interface, are not fully known. In these cases assessing total human exposure is fraught with uncertainty.

By a variety of chemical, biological and physical processes, transformation, degradation and immobilization of emitted compounds occur in the external environment. In many cases this eliminates any harmful effects, but occasionally a transformation may generate compounds which are more toxic to humans. The formation of methylmercury from inorganic mercury by micro-organisms in lake sediments and of ozone and peroxyacetylnitrate (PAN) in photochemical smog are well known examples.

Sediments are the final sink for many persistent substances and factors which influence adsorption of such compounds to sediments are therefore of great importance. However, since the substance exists in equilibrium between sediment and the aqueous phase in contact with sediment, immobilization is not absolute. Several processes can occur which promote active relocation from sediment to water and from water to air. Acidification, for example, can contribute to mobilization of various metals bound to sediments.

The distance travelled by particles in the atmosphere is dependent on their size. Large particles are deposited close to the emission source, while small particles and gaseous substances more readily follow the air currents and may travel long distances—in some cases to other countries, or even other continents.

The release of chemicals into the environment may occur from particular local sources (point sources) such as a specific factory chimney, or by so-called diffuse emission, due to several methods of use of the same chemical or its use affecting wide areas (e.g. motor vehicles, application of fertilizers). This distinction is important in view of the difficulties involved in estimating total exposure doses from emission data for substances with a dispersed and diverse pattern of use. Thus, in an extensive survey of the uses of cadmium in Sweden, only 15–20 per cent of the atmospheric deposition could be accounted for by known emission sources, and similar estimates have been made for substances such as PCBs and lead.

The characteristics of 'recipients' of emissions (the various bodies of water or other environmental media into which the pollutants are deposited), exposure levels for target organisms in the ecosystems as a function of time in the various environmental compartments (air, water, soil, sediment and biota), and the availability of the compound for uptake (bioavailability) are the main parameters that decide the ecotoxicologically relevant exposures to a substance. This may or may not include human exposure.

In most cases insufficient data for estimation of these key parameters are available, so one has to resort to data which are only indirectly linked to final exposure ('surrogate data') but which are more readily available. Based on a description of the uses and functions of an industrial chemical—the characteristics of the recipient, the volume and character of the emissions, the distribution of the compound between the different environmental compartments, type and velocity of transformation, as well as the physico-chemical properties of the substance—at least semi-quantitative estimates of exposures in the external environment may be obtained. However, for many chemical substances adequate information is lacking in these respects too.

By combining the data elements mentioned above, certain predictions can also be made for human exposure through the external environment. Degradability, the tendency to accumulate in living organisms (bioaccumulation) and progressively increasing concentrations as the substance passes from one trophic level in the food-chain to the next (biomagnification) are properties of the substance *per se* which play a decisive role in human exposure, for example through food.

For a long time, quite sophisticated methods have been available for estimating the distribution of a substance in a given situation, for example, for calculating its diffusion and transport of a substance in the air near a point source. Predictions of total exposure where movement between different media is involved are considerably more difficult.

When making predictions of dispersal routes and of final concentrations reached in the various environmental compartments, the parameters 'predicted environmental distribution (PED)' and 'predicted environmental concentration (PEC)' play a central role. Both parameters give an estimate of the exposure level of a substance in different media.

The main difference between the two parameters lies in the fact that while the PEC gives an estimate of *concentrations* of a certain substance emitted by a point source during non-equilibrium (dynamic) conditions in different media, the PED denotes the estimated final *distribution* of substance between different media under equilibrium or non-equilibrium conditions. The PED is easily calculated using fundamental physico-chemical data for the substance. The most commonly employed model uses the thermodynamic parameter *fugacity* and presupposes in its simplest form only knowledge of molecular weight, water solubility, vapour pressure, absorption coefficient to soil particles, and the partition coefficient between octanol and water (Mackay, 1979; Mackay and Paterson, 1981; Wood, 1981). With certain foreseeable exceptions, estimates theoretically derived by this approach correspond well to measured distributions for a number of substances.

The PED has limited usefulness when assessing actual exposure, but provides guidance for more advanced exposure analysis relating to the environmental medium where presence of the chemical concerned is expected to be of greatest importance.

The PEC gives a more specific and accurate basis for risk estimation, but the calculation requires much more information (Wilmot, 1976; Simons, 1973, 1980). Knowledge of for example a number of local geographical conditions which characterize the recipient of the emission (meteorological, hydrological, hydrodynamic data, etc.), emission volumes and variations with time, are essential when calculating this parameter.

4.4.3 Uptake and metabolism in the body: chemical dosimetry

Factors modifying the effects of exposure to chemicals

In the following section (4.4.4), exposure data submitted by various Swedish governmental agencies for a series of chemical substances are presented. However, such data cannot be directly interpreted in terms of degree of cancer risk. In order to deduce correctly the relationship between exposure and effect, a knowledge of factors affecting the pathway of a substance to the critical organ or tissue where it may exert its effect is necessary. In other words, one has to know how uptake, distribution, biotransformation and excretion of a compound modify the exposure dose, in order to facilitate the calculation of a true 'target dose', directly related to the effect.

In addition to its physico-chemical properties, the effects of a substance on the body are governed by a series of other factors. among the most important are:

(a) the *amount* of the chemical to which the body is exposed—the dose;
(b) the *manner* in which the body comes into contact with the chemical (inhalation, dermal contact, ingestion);
(c) the *period of time* during which the body is exposed (acute or chronic exposure);
(d) the manner of *distribution, biotransformation* and *excretion* of the chemical;
(e) the *sensitivity* and *state of health* of the individual;
(f) simultaneous exposure to other agents with which *interaction* may arise.

In order to cause injury, the chemical must be able to penetrate the protective layers which separate the tissue from the environment. Inside the body, barriers exist which prevent the free passage of certain foreign (sometimes toxic) substances between various tissues and organs, for example from the bloodstream to the central nervous system (the blood–brain barrier), or from the circulatory system of the mother to that of the fetus (the placental barrier).

The diverse layers of the *skin* form the body's major protective barrier, where in particular the outer layer, the epidermis, affords the best defence. Since the thickness of the horny layer of the skin varies in different parts of the body, the degree of uptake will vary accordingly. Thus absorption through the skin of the palm is much slower than through the skin of the upper arm. Mechanical trauma or alkalis and acids causing damage to the skin increase penetration drastically, and substances which normally are not absorbed through the skin may then do so. The simultaneous presence of solvents or oils may likewise accelerate penetration.

Absorption via the *gastrointestinal tract* is the main route of entry for many foreign substances. Although the capacity for uptake will depend on the characteristics of the compound, absorption may, in principle, occur along the entire passage from mouth to rectum. To some extent particles and certain types of fibre (for example particles of azo dyes, cellulose and asbestos fibres) may be taken up from the gastrointestinal tract without any previous degradation.

Toxic substances passing through the alimentary tract may be degraded and inactivated by the action of the gastric juices or by diverse enzymes. In other instances the toxic substance may actually be produced in the gastrointestinal tract itself, as with carcinogenic nitrosamines formed from nitrite and naturally occurring amines. Under the influence of the intestinal microflora, aromatic nitro compounds can also be reduced to carcinogenic amines. Finally, the intestinal flora can reduce nitrate to nitrite which is subsequently taken up by the bloodstream.

In the workplace, exposure through ingestion as a rule plays a minor role. Contact with toxic agents by inhalation and dermal contact predominates.

For chemicals that are *inhaled* in the form of dust or aerosols, particle size influences the toxic action. At sizes below 5 µm particles are deposited mainly in the alveoli.

Larger particles over 5 µm, deposited in the upper respiratory tract, are transported to the pharynx by movements of the ciliated epithelium lining the upper air passages (mucociliary transport) and are then either coughed up or swallowed. Transport of foreign particles from the alveoli also occurs via specialized white blood cells, called macrophages, as well as the lymphatic system.

In the lungs absorption of compounds in the gaseous phase, or of liquids in the form of aerosols, often occurs rapidly and efficiently, in part due to the large inner surface area of the lungs (50–100 m^2). As a rule, absorption of volatile substances in the lungs can be directly related to their solubility in the blood.

The body possesses certain mechanisms besides those of repair, which modify the effects of absorbed chemical compounds. The following are of the greatest importance:

(a) distribution of the substance around the body after uptake;
(b) biotransformation (metabolism) of foreign compounds to less toxic products and to products which are excreted more readily;
(c) excretion of the substance and its breakdown products via urine, faeces and exhaled air.

Uptake of a substance in the bloodstream is followed by its distribution to the tissues and organs. Toxic substances then often accumulate in specific organs and tissues. Certain compounds reach their highest concentration at the site of their toxic action. However, for other substances concentration does not necessarily imply damage to the tissue in question. Thus, lead is predominantly accumulated in bone but exerts its toxic action in various soft tissues. DDT is stored in fat where relatively high concentrations can be reached without obvious symptoms of toxicity being observed. However, in the case of starvation the fatty deposits are mobilized, and accumulated DDT is released into the blood during a short period of time, resulting in toxic effects.

Many lipophilic compounds are excreted with great difficulty or hardly at all. As was mentioned in Chapter 3, the human body possesses enzyme systems which do, however, eventually break down and metabolize such substances to more water-soluble products that can be more readily eliminated in the urine.

Foreign compounds are excreted in various ways. Elimination by the *kidneys* constitutes by far the most important route. However, certain substances like lead and DDT are excreted from the liver in *bile* to the small intestine. For gaseous substances like carbon monoxide, and also for volatile solvents like certain alcohols, ketones and ethers, elimination from the lungs in expired air constitutes an important route. Excretion in the milk by a nursing mother can have serious consequences for an infant.

Finally, although exposed to identical levels, *individuals* can differ with respect to sensitivity and state of health, resulting in different target doses, and hence different risks to the individuals. Normal liver and kidney function is, for example, a prerequisite for normal transformation and excretion of a number of drugs and toxic compounds. When such substances are administered to patients suffering from injury of these organs, potentiation or prolongation of pharmacological and toxicological effects may result. Age is another factor which may be of great importance. Thus, in the newborn the mechanisms responsible for transforming toxic substances (e.g. oxidation, conjugation) are not fully developed.

Considering the great differences in individual human sensitivity to various toxic agents, it is easy to understand that the differences in sensitivity between animal species may be even greater. This *species variation* is explained by differences in absorption, in mechanisms of degradation and excretion, in the rates of transformation and by physiological and anatomical differences.

Exposure and target doses—chemical dosimetry

The dose of a certain substance (defined as the concentration of the compound over a period of time in a certain target area) is of crucial importance in determining whether or not injury will occur and also the type of damage arising. As discussed in Chapter 3, the dose relates to the *degree* of injury (the dose–effect relationship) for toxic effects other than neoplasia and mutations. The occurrence of tumours is affected by dose such that the *incidence* of tumours (the dose–response relationship) increases in a population (the number of individuals with tumours; in bioassays also the number of tumours per individual), and the latency period decreases. Here, different concepts are at work which may roughly be classified into the following two categories:

(a) Exposure dose.
(b) Target dose: Total body burden
Tissue and organ doses
Subcellular target doses (true target doses).

The exposure dose is often expressed as milligrams per kilogram of body weight of the substance administered over a certain time by oral intake (peroral), by skin application (dermal) or by injection (parenteral administration). Inhalation exposure doses are usually expressed as milligrams of substance per cubic metre or as parts per million in the inhaled air over a certain time. Thus, exposure dose is equal to exposure level x time. Here the concept of 'dose' will always have this connotation. However, in medical literature the term 'dose' is commonly used in the sense of exposure level (milligrams per kilogram, parts per million, etc.), at a point in time.

Exposure doses are not corrected according to the amount of substance which actually reaches and is taken up by the tissue where it exerts its action (target dose). Despite its inherent limitations, the correlation between exposure dose and effect, as well as the relation between exposure and the incidence of, say, a specific disease, represents the most common way to express dose–effect and dose–response relationships. It should be stressed that the concentration of a substance, for example in inhaled air often fluctuates greatly over time. This implies that measurements of this type provide exposure doses from which it may be extremely difficult to estimate total dose over a more extended time period. In such a case, a series of statistically representative measurements over time is essential.

The relation between exposure dose and target dose will, to a greater or lesser degree, be affected by the factors just mentioned which all modify the effects of chemical exposure. In particular, considerable differences can exist between true target doses and the oral or dermal exposure doses. For this reason, attempts have been made to find ways of correlating target doses with more easily measured exposure doses. However, information on such correlations which might permit a 'translation' of exposure data to target doses exists for only a few substances.

The blood is in permanent contact with the organs and the tissues and is the body's main transport medium for nutrients, dissolved gases, foreign substances, and so on. This fluid, consequently, provides a suitable and, above all, easily accessible medium for estimating dosage. For a long time, the *concentration in blood plasma* has for this reason been employed in pharmacology to derive better estimates of the variations in the concentration of drugs in certain target organs and tissues. By introducing suitable correction factors it is then possible to compensate for differences between plasma levels and the level in the actual target organ or tissue. In certain cases the measurement of the *concentration in urine* of a substance, or of some transformation product derived from it, may be more convenient. However, rapid fluctuations in the levels of many compounds in blood and urine pose a problem with this kind of data. Thus, blood lead concentrations can be used as an indicator of the exposure of an individual over a limited period immediately before the actual sampling, but constitute a poor measure of total *body burden* (body dose), that is, the amount of the chemical accumulated by the organism over a longer period. Body doses or tissue doses can sometimes be determined by direct analysis of samples from different organs where a certain substance has a tendency to accumulate, such as lead in teeth, cadmium in the renal cortex and DDT and PCBs in fatty tissue. For living individuals this approach is feasible only under exceptional circumstances (such as teeth from 7-year-old children) and, apart from biopsies, material from autopsies usually has to be relied upon when estimating a long-term (sometimes lifetime) dose. Finally, this is only possible for compounds with slow excretion such as asbestos, heavy metals (cadmium and lead),and certain organic compounds of low biodegradability like PCBs and DDT.

For substances causing mutation and cancer initiation, the path is long between exposure and the primary changes of cellular DNA which generate these effects. This is particularly true in situations where the active substance ('ultimate carcinogen') is not identical to the compound initially administered, but is a reactive intermediate formed through the organism's own metabolic processes. There is reason to suppose that the fundamental chemical changes resulting in mutation and initiation of neoplasia are basically the same in all living organisms. Nevertheless, when exposure dose is related to cancer incidence or mutation frequency, the complex history of the 'ultimate carcinogen' often means that there is a great difference in sensitivity between diverse organisms—and even between strains belonging to the same species.

Since the critical target molecule here is DNA, the target dose determined in this structure as the amount of active substance bound to DNA (DNA adducts) over a certain period should provide the most relevant basis for determining a dose–response relationship in the context of hazard assessment (Ehrenberg, 1984c).

For some genotoxic compounds such as ethyl methane sulphonate and ethylnitrosourea, it has been possible to determine the true target dose, expressed as the number of alkylations per nucleotide (unit of DNA), and to correlate these doses with measured mutation frequencies. It has thus become evident that the biological efficiency per unit dose shows great similarities in such different systems as mouse sperm, fruit fly and cell cultures of human fibroblasts (Ehrenberg, 1980; Streisinger, 1983). In other words, with information on true target doses it is feasible to extrapolate the results from experiments with lower organisms to man with much higher accuracy than has previously been possible.

However, routine measurements of dose according to the principle above require a highly sensitive and specific method. Certain advances have been made in determining DNA adducts, but the possibilities of directly measuring DNA adducts are limited by the small amounts of DNA which can be obtained from a person without discomfort and risk, as well as by the fact that the DNA adducts exhibit a relatively short lifetime due to chemical instability and biochemical repair. In this context pioneering work on dosimetry and methods for risk assessment based on such data has been carried out by Ehrenberg and his research team at Stockholm University. Osterman-Golkar and Ehrenberg have developed a method based on the use of haemoglobin as a representative and easily accessible tissue standard. A blood sample contains 1000 times more haemoglobin (the red protein of red blood cells) than DNA. Furthermore, haemoglobin is stable throughout the lifetime of the red blood cell—in man about 4 months. It has been shown that basic chemical (reaction kinetics) laws can be employed with an adequate degree of precision for calculating reaction velocities in the various organs of the body. Furthermore, an estimation of the degree of chemical change in DNA based on the concentration of haemoglobin adducts in the 'general' case yields estimates identical to those obtained by direct analysis of the DNA adducts.

Analytical determination of adducts to reactive amino acid residues (cysteine, histidine, N-terminal valine) in haemoglobin has been shown to provide a sufficiently sensitive method for determining tissue dose in man for carcinogens like ethylene oxide, at levels which are currently found in the workplace and in the external environment. However, from the technical point of view, the method is laborious and considerable scientific effort will be required before this approach can be applied to a broader spectrum of chemical substances (Ehrenberg *et al.*, 1983).

4.4.4 Exposure to certain substances in Sweden: information obtained from regulatory agencies

As was mentioned in the introduction to this section (4.4.1), two groups of substances were identified for inclusion in the survey of exposure data:

(a) substances and groups of substances considered as carcinogens or suspected carcinogens (in humans or animals) by the IARC or NCI at the time when supporting data were collected for the survey (1980);
(b) substances and groups of substances characterized as promoters, co-carcinogens or inhibitors in a literature review.

All of these substances were incorporated in three lists (Memorandum, 1980; Säfwenberg, 1980) together with the criteria used in classifying them. In the following summary of the survey results, a few other compounds are included which were judged to be of special interest by the agencies consulted.

The substances evaluated by the IARC were taken from an article published by Tomatis (1979), reviewing 29 substances, groups of substances or types of exposure where the IARC has judged that sufficient evidence is available from studies in humans to support a causal relationship between exposure and human cancer. Also included are substances and types of exposure for which limited evidence of human carcinogenicity exists, which indicates that a causal interpretation is credible, but that alternative explanations, such as chance, bias or confounding factors, could not adequately be excluded. The survey also contains 236 substances for which the IARC considered that either sufficient or limited evidence of a carcinogenic potential existed based on investigations in laboratory animals.

According to the IARC, *sufficient evidence* of carcinogenicity in experimental investigations implies that the substance in question has caused an increased incidence of malignant tumours: (a) in multiple species or strains; or (b) in multiple experiments (preferably with different routes of administration or using different dose levels); or (c) to an unusual degree with regard to incidence, site or type of tumour, or age at onset. Additional evidence may be provided by data on dose–response effects, as well as information from short-term tests or on chemical structure.

The IARC's definition of *limited evidence* implies 'that the data suggest a carcinogenic effect but are limited because: (a) the studies involve a single species, strain or experiment; or (b) the experiments are restricted by inadequate dosage levels, inadequate duration of exposure to the agent, inadequate period of follow-up, poor survival, too few animals, or inadequate reporting; or (c) the neoplasms produced often occur spontaneously and, in the past, have been difficult to classify as malignant by histological criteria alone (e.g. lung and liver tumours in mice)'.

Tomatis's review covers the first 21 volumes of the series of monographs entitled *Evaluation of the Carcinogenic Risk of Chemicals to Humans*, published by the IARC. A more recent summary of the IARC evaluations was published in October 1982 covering volumes 1–29 (IARC, 1982). In this review, certain amendments were introduced. The experimental basis for short-term tests (DNA damage, mutagenicity, chromosomal anomalies, and various other additional endpoints)[3] was appraised with respect to the three levels 'sufficient evidence', 'limited evidence' and 'inadequate evidence'. Furthermore, a classification into four categories (1, 2A, 2B and 3) was added, summarizing the evaluation of carcinogenic risk to humans of 155 substances or exposure environments on the strength of supporting evidence from the three areas of human carcinogenicity, in experimental animals, and short-term tests.

Group 1 includes 30 types of exposure where a causal association between the exposure in question and human cancer must be considered to exist. Group 2 comprises types of exposure which should be regarded as probably carcinogenic to man. These are divided into two sub-groups: in group 2A are placed 14 types for which the evidence for human carcinogenicity is fairly strong, and group 2B includes 47 types where the supporting evidence is weaker. The remaining 64 chemicals and exposure environments, group 3, could not be classified as to their human carcinogenicity, according to the IARC. A number of potent animal carcinogens, such as certain nitrosamines, fall outside this classification scheme. In administrative decision making the finding of carcinogenic activity in an animal study naturally carries considerable weight, as it also does when data on humans are completely lacking.

It should be pointed out that the mere designation of a certain exposure environment as being associated with an increased cancer risk (e.g. isopropyl alcohol manufacture, occupational exposure to pheneoxyacetic acid herbicides, etc.) cannot be taken to imply the identification of the substance(s) responsible for causing cancer. The IARC here clearly makes the distinction: 'The compound(s) responsible for the carcinogenic or probable carcinogenic effect in humans cannot be specified.'

The NCI list, taken from an article by Griesemer and Cueto (1980), is based on a classification system which is specifically adapted to the NCI's own testing programme utilizing mice and rats. The compounds included in the circulated excerpts from this list for the exposure survey are divided into five categories according to the following criteria: very strong evidence for carcinogenicity in two animal species (rat and mouse); very strong evidence in one species and sufficient evidence in another; very strong evidence in one species and none in the other; sufficient evidence in two species; sufficient evidence in one species and none in the other. In all, the NCI list comprises roughly 100 compounds, of which about 20 also have been covered by the IARC.

Both systems of classification are based on the strength of the scientific evidence and are thus not concerned with the magnitude of the hazard (the carcinogenic potency). In comparison with the NCI system, the demands set by the IARC on completeness and quality of the supporting documentary material to establish 'sufficient evidence' are usually the more exacting.

The list containing potential promoters, co-carcinogens and inhibitors is based on a literature survey carried out by the secretariat of the Cancer Committee (Säfwenberg, 1980). For obvious reasons this list cannot be compared with those based on the evaluations made by the IARC and NCI. Furthermore, current knowledge about promoters and similar agents must be described as inadequate. In several instances a substance has been characterized as, for example, a co-carcinogen on the basis of a single report in the literature. As in the cases of PCBs and urethane, a few compounds classified as experimental carcinogens by the IARC (presumably with initiating activity) can also be found under the promoters heading in this literature survey. In all, the list includes 40 substances or groups of substances. Both promotive and inhibitory effects on the formation of tumours have been noted in separate experiments for some of them.

The three lists total more than 400 compounds, groups of compounds or other types of exposure.

In 1980 the Swedish National Board of Occupational Safety and Health, the National Environmental Protection Board, the National Food Administration and the Pharmaceuticals Department of the National Board of Health and Welfare were asked to provide summarized exposure data for substances included in these lists. The point of departure was substances which the agencies judged to be of importance in this particular context, but also others which could be suspected of occurring in an area under their respective jurisdiction. The information requested included occurrence, areas of usage and exposure levels. If possible, the information given was to include collective doses for the more important substances. It was understood that each agency should decide for itself the amount of work to be put in, taking into consideration the accessibility of existing information. In other words, the procurement of entirely new data was not expected.

During 1981 each of the four authorities provided its report. In addition, during 1982 the Products Control Board was approached for similar information.

The accessibility of exposure data is to some extent influenced by the different regulatory systems used by each authority. More information about legislation and such factors can be found in Chapter 11.

Protecting the individual at work is the main concern of the Board of Occupational Safety and Health. In this field the handling of chemicals usually involves relatively few people, and individual doses are of primary concern. On the other hand, occupational exposure to commonly used solvents and such like may involve more people and be important in terms of collective doses. The exposure of large population groups to chemicals in food, drinking water and the air, where the individual dose and risk is in general low, has quite a different significance for the collective dose. For pharmaceuticals too, the collective exposure of a larger population, over and above individual dose, may be of interest depending on the type of drug involved.

For these reasons, exposure via foods is given a prominent role in this section. As for intake of carcinogenic substances by way of air and drinking water, the available information, except for a few compounds, is mostly inadequate for detailed analysis. However, intake of carcinogenic substances by these routes seems to have little effect on the total tumour incidence.

Because no specifications were laid down on format, completeness and other aspects, the reports obtained from the government authorities are rather dissimilar in character and therefore difficult to present in a consistent and uniform manner. The data are summarized in a highly condensed and somewhat edited form in Tables 4.7–4.18.

The Products Control Board

Except for products subject to special legislation (such as pharmaceuticals and foods), the Products Control Board has a central coordinating function controlling all products which may constitute a hazard to human health due to their chemical composition and manner of handling. The Board is endowed with extensive legal powers to control the various ways in which chemicals are handled. As for the regulation of carcinogenic compounds, this was mostly limited to the classification of a series of carcinogens as 'poisons', which automatically resulted in a number of restrictions on the substances themselves and also on products containing them. The classification is based solely on the properties of the substances themselves, regardless of the actual concentration levels to which different populations may be exposed.

Working from the NCI list the Products Control Board carried out searches in the data-base on chemical products which is being built up by the Board—the Products Register. At that time (August 1982) the register contained some descriptive information such as composition and volume on approximately 12 000 products, mainly basic industrial chemicals, derived from a total of about 100 000 products for which the Board had formerly collected information on trade name, name of importer, etc. (Table 4.7).

Table 4.7 Substances from the NIC list covered by the Products Register of the Products Control Board in Sweden until 1982.

Substance	No. of products[a]	Volume per year (tonnes)[b]
2,4-Diaminotoluene	1	<1
1,2-Dibromoethane[c]	1	1–10
N,N'Diethylthiourea[c]	3	1–10
1,2-Dichloroethane	17	>10 000
2,4-Dinitrotoluene	3	100–1000
1,4-Dioxan	9	10–100
Ethyl tellurac[c]	2	1–10
Hexachloroethane	6	100–1000
Chloroform[c]	19	30–300
Chlorothalonil[c]	1	<0.4
Nitrilotriacetic acid	4	10–100
Nitrilotriacetic acid, tri-sodium salt	14	1000–2000
2-Nitro-p-phenylene diamine	1	<1
N-Nitrosodiphenylamine	5	10–100
p-Benzoquinone	1	<1
Selenium sulphide	1	1–10
1,1,2,2,-Tetrachloroethane	3	100–500
Tetrachloroethylene[c]	17	5000–10 000
1,1,2-Trichloroethane[c]	1	100–500
Trichloroethylene[c]	34	10 000–20 000
Trimethylthiourea[c]	1	<1

[a] Number of products containing the substance in question, mainly basic industrial chemicals. The compound may also occur as an impurity in additional products.
[b] Approximate ranges of quantities imported and/or produced per year. The annual volumes have been estimated on the basis of the concentrations present in each product and the range of annual product volumes.
[c] The substance was also evaluated by the IARC.
From NPCB (1982).

Since it had so far not been possible to consider the presence of individual substances in complex products, the picture of their occurrence in products on the Swedish market is necessarily incomplete. Furthermore, it was felt that unless the register information is supplemented by relatively detailed data which will permit estimates of dispersing, modes of use and so on, a complete products register will still be of only limited value as a tool for assessing chemical exposure.

In estimating exposure in Sweden to the various listed substances, the information in many cases has been based on data found in the international literature, which according to the Products Control Board is often adequate provided that methods of handling are relatively well defined.

In addition, exposure data from Sweden and from other countries were presented for di-(2-ethylhexyl) phthalate (DEHP), benzene, lead, cadmium, 1,2-dibromoethane and 1,2-dichloroethane (see Table 4.8).

Cadmium and lead had not been considered by the Board from the viewpoint of carcinogencity, but exposure analyses were carried out for other reasons. For important pesticides, Swedish exposure data were available in the form of analytical data for pesticide residues in foods. For certain products, measurements of occupational exposure had also been carried out earlier in Sweden.

The exposure profile for cadmium seems to have been very thoroughly analysed. Here information is provided on the whole life-cycle of the substance—from its production, release and dispersal in the environment up to its concentration in the target organ in the human body (NEPB 1982).

Among the pesticides in the IARC and NCI lists, captan, daminozide, dicofol, chloramben, chlorothalonil, lindane, tetrachlorvinphos, trifluralin and quintozene are registered for use in Sweden. Information on sales volumes is available for all registered pesticides. Tetrachlorvinphos and chloramben are employed in such small quantities within the country that the total (collective) exposure to these compounds is negligible.

Information on residues in foods was acquired from random sampling of Swedish and imported food products by the National Food Administration. Since the corresponding Swedish data are lacking, estimates of total intakes of certain pesticides via food are based on data from other countries. For this reason these assessments are, of course, uncertain. Swedish occupational exposure data were presented for lindane and captan. Evaluation of occupational exposure to quintozene was based on experience outside Sweden.

For lead, DEHP and a number of pesticides—as with cadmium— the dose contribution from foods appears to make up a relatively large proportion of the collective dose. Since only incomplete data were available on total intake of these substances via food, the total exposure picture remains unclear with respect to man. On the other hand, representative data do exist on tissue levels for lead, especially in blood.

The National Board of Occupational Safety and Health

The National Board of Occupational Safety and Health looked thoroughly at all three lists of substances providing the basis for the investigation, first of all with regard to their known or suspected *occurrence* in the work environment. More detailed information was then presented on the *use of* and *exposure to* substances listed by the IARC and NCI and substances denoted as promoters.

Some compounds were ruled out immediately as for example 14 substances listed by the IARC which were presumed not to be

Table 4.8 Representative concentrations in air of organic lead compounds (tetramethyl-lead and tetraethyl-lead), 1,2-dibromoethane, 1,2-dichloroethane and benzene in some typical exposure situations.

	Organic lead compounds (μgm^{-3})	1,2-Dibromoethane+ 1,2-dichloroethane (μgm^{-3})	Benzene (μgm^{-3})
Urban ambient air (street with heavy traffic)	0.1–0.5	0.35–2.2	84–430
Multistorey carparks	0.6–4.7	1.8–3.7	200–920
Petrol station	0.6–4.7	4.9–7.5	460–1300
Autorepair shop	–	8.7–12.2	720–1000
Loading petrol, bulk terminals (different loading systems); short-exposures (15–20 mins)		–	1800–7300[a]
Cleaning of paint brushes, engine parts, etc. in an enclosed space[b]; maximum short-exposure		about 600–1200 (dichlorethane)	18 000–37 000
average exposure		–	3 700
Hygienic limit values			
(*a*) Full day value	50	4000 (dichloroethane)	16 000
(*b*) Short-term value	–	–	30 000

[a] The exposure conditions may show considerable variation depending on the technical arrangements and the manner of loading.
[b] Petrol containing 0.4–0.8 g organic lead per litre and 3.2 per cent benzene.
[c] A hygienic limit value in the workplace, according to current Swedish legislation, stands for maximal 'acceptable' average exposure concentration, measured (*a*) during a full day's work (usually 8 hours) or (*b*) during each period of 15 minutes or less. The latter applies to some substances, the effects of which usually have a rapid onset. Another type of short-term value, usually also measured during 15 minutes, serves as an approximate guideline for protective measures.
Data from the Products Control Board to the Cancer Committee in 1983.

produced commercially in Sweden. Of those listed by the IARC and NCI, the Board identified 105 of interest only in connection with the production and use of pharmaceuticals, pesticides, and as laboratory chemicals.

A special source of information used by the Board comprises surveys made within certain branches of Swedish industry (by the printing, textile and paint industries).

When there were no reliable Swedish data on the use of a chemical, the Board resorted to international sources, for example, the documentary material from the IARC. For obvious reasons, this often lists a considerably broader scope of use/occurrence than is applicable under Swedish conditions.

Substances found to be present in the workplace in Sweden in this investigation were checked against existing rules. The National Board of Occupational Safety and Health controls carcinogens by means of a special regulatory system involving the use of three separate lists of substances (A, B and C) which, on the basis of epidemiological and experimental data, have been judged to carry cancer risks. Category A includes substances which may, under no circumstances, be produced or used in the workplace. Carcinogens belonging to category B may be produced or used by permit from the Labour Inspectorate. Substances belonging to categories A and B are considered to potentially increase the cancer risks even at low exposure levels. Category C contains substances which have been assigned hygienic limit values (the highest concentration of an air pollutant to which a worker may be exposed to without suffering adverse health effects). Consequently, substances included in this category may be used in the workplace provided that the regulations on hygienic limit values are followed.

List A of prohibited carcinogens included 13 substances in 1981. Certain of the compounds are, nevertheless, described as existing in Sweden. This can be explained by the fact that the Board has issued exemptions in a few cases (mostly for use in research laboratories, etc.) when adequate conditions for their safe use appear to be fulfilled. Another reason is that low levels of these carcinogens may occur as impurities in certain products.

Generally speaking, several compounds that were known to occur in Sweden, such as polycyclic hydrocarbons and nitrosamines, are not intentional components of products, but appear as impurities or are generated during certain processes (combustion, etc.) and may thus give rise to an exposure entailing a cancer risk. Such exposures may also occur at some workplaces where raw materials for food production or animal feed, containing naturally occurring carcinogenic agents such as mycotoxins are being processed.

In Table 4.9 information is given on the occurrence and use of individual substances classified as carcinogens or probable carcinogens for humans by the IARC (groups 1 and 2 according to the 1982 review) as well as regulatory classification in Sweden (categories A, B or C). Compounds which are used as active ingredients in drugs, or which may not be employed in the workplace at all (category A), have not been included, nor have complex mixtures or combined exposures where the carcinogenic agent(s) have not been identified.

Four substances, of greater industrial importance, which are being produced in Sweden, were the subject of a wider presentation by the Board, who gave an account of their historical development, including

Table 4.9 Substances in the work environment, classified as carcinogenic or probable human carcinogens by the IARC (1982).

Substance	Regulatory classification category (in Sweden)[a]	Area of use[b]
Acrylonitrile	C, 1978	Production of polymers, coatings, (no production in Sweden at the present time)
Arsenic, certain arsenic compounds	C, 1974	Smelters (Rönnskär), wood preservation, glass industry
Asbestos	C, 1974 (except for Crocidolite which belongs to cat. A)	Production of brake-linings, service stations, demolition of buildings, etc.
Benzene	C, 1974	Coking plants; in gasoline
Benzo[a]pyrene	C, 1981	Formed upon pyrolysis of coal in gas and coking plants; in coal tar
Beryllium and beryllium compounds	C, 1974	Production of beryllium ceramics, alloying metal, fluorescent tubes, electronics
Diethyl sulphate	B, 1974	Chemical industry (certain branches)
Dimethyl sulphate	B, 1974	Chemical industry (certain branches)
Chromium and/or certain chromium compounds	C, 1974 1978 (chromic acid and chromates)	Spraypainting, chromium plating, production of industrial paints
Nickel and/or nickel compounds	C, 1974	Production of electric accumulators steel industry
o-Tolidine (3,3'dimethylbenzidine)	B, 1974	laboratory chemical
Mustard gas (bis-(2-chloroethyl)sulphide)	B, 1978	No known use in Sweden
Vinyl chloride	C, 1974	Production and processing of PVC

[a] According to the current list of hygienic limit values in 1981 from the National Board of Occupational Safety and Health. In the workplace the use of substances belonging to category A is prohibited; compounds belonging to category B require permission from the Labour Inspectorate, and category C-substances are carcinogens given a hygienic limit.
[b] According to the National Board of Occupational Safety and Health.

information on production volumes. These are benzene, ethylene oxide, formaldehyde and vinyl chloride.

Formaldehyde was not included on any of the lists submitted but this compound was later classified as an animal carcinogen by the IARC (1982). The compound is in widespread use in the production of phenolic and urea–formaldehyde resins, in the paint and adhesive industries and others, and may also be present in products like chipboard.

In Sweden the extraction of benzene from coke-oven gas began in 1915, and during World War II several plants were constructed for this purpose. Then the production of benzene derivatives from crude oil was introduced, a process which nowadays predominates. The production of ethylene oxide started just before World War II. At present only one such plant exists, at Stenungsund, with a capacity of 40 000 tonnes year^{-1}. The production of formaldehyde has steadily increased since World War II and now amounts to about 220 000 tonnes year^{-1}. The production of vinyl chloride in the plants of Stockvik and Stenungsund amounted to a total of 105 000 tonnes in 1974.

For 16 of the substances evaluated by the IARC and for one compound on the NCI list, data on exposure levels were available. In general, this information relies on measurements reported by the Labour Inspectorate. From this source, it is clear that the material is extensive for some chemicals but more limited in other cases.

When calculating collective doses, it is necessary to know the size of the populations exposed within various industrial sectors. However, this information is difficult to acquire.

The number of employees in different sectors is recorded in official statistical material obtained through population and domicile censuses. (The Swedish classification standard is based on the international industry classification, issued by the United Nations.) In order to define the subject population more narrowly, a description of the occupations would be required, and especially the number of workers engaged in a particular operation or process. However, there are not enough available statistics of this nature. Additional information can be obtained from the membership records of trade unions. A reasonably exact description of the population exposed can therefore be obtained only in cases where specialized studies of a particular substance or work population have been carried out.

Estimates, presented as collective exposure doses (Table 4.10), have been calculated for arsenic, asbestos, benzene, ethylene oxide, vinyl chloride and formaldehyde. Because there are only crude estimates of the number of workers exposed, the collective doses are correspondingly imprecise. This is particularly true for large population groups exposed to low or moderate levels. For small, heavily exposed populations estimates of collective dose are likely to be more accurate.

Table 4.10 Summary of annual collective doses[a] for some substances in the work environment.

Substance	Current situation	Situation in the past (before about 1970)[b]
Arsenic	4×10^3 mg	About 5 times higher
Asbestos	3×10^{11} fibres	About 150 times higher
Benzene	8×10^6 mg	No information given
Ethylene oxide	5×10^6 mg	2–20 times higher
Vinyl chloride	4×10^6 mg	25–75 times higher (1945–74)
Formaldehyde	12×10^6 mg	No information given

[a] In estimating, the Board has considered the quantities inhaled.
[b] Number of times by which the collective dose was higher in comparison with the current situation.

Information from the National Board of Occupational Safety and Health (1981).

The National Food Administration

The main report of the National Food Administration includes information on concentrations of approximately 20 substances occurring in foods. This survey covers substances evaluated by the IARC as well as compounds included in the list of promoters and other modifying agents. These concentrations, combined with known consumption volumes of different foodstuffs, yielded estimates of the average intake of the substances in question (in individually related doses). Subsequently, extensive additional information was supplied on pesticide residues, nitrosamines, polycyclic hydrocarbons, heavy metals, as well as substances capable of migrating from packaging materials, and so on.

In Table 4.11 the concentrations are given for some of these substances, mainly related to foods containing particularly high levels, or those which account for a major proportion of the total intake of that chemical. Human carcinogens (groups 1 and 2A of the IARC classification) have been grouped together, along with compounds for which human data are lacking but where the evidence available (e.g. very potent experimental carcinogens inducing tumours in multiple locations and in several animal species) justifies considering them as human carcinogens. Certain nitrosamines belong in this group. Exposure data for some other substances of interest in this context are also given.

The intake is given here as the average burden per person per year in Sweden, obtained by multiplying the consumption of different foods per person by the sum of the concentrations found. The fact that only

Table 4.11 Concentration levels of some substances in foods.

Substance	Foodstuff	Concentration in mg kg^{-1} or mg l^{-1}	Approximate intake (mg person^{-1} year^{-1})
Human carcinogens or substances which when ingested in food may constitute a high cancer risk (see text).			
Aflatoxin[a]	Peanuts	0–0.005	Low
Acrylonitrile[b]	Beer, soft drinks	<0.005	0.018
Arsenic[a]	Fish	1–5	30
	Shellfish	5	10
	Total	–	55
Asbestos[a]	Wine	A few fibres per litre	–
	Drinking water	<0.03– –3 × 10^6 fibres per litre	–
Benzo[*a*]pyrene[c]	Smoked fish	0.001	0.003
	Grilled sausages (open fire)	0.054	–
	Green-leaf vegetables	0.0001	0.01
	Margarine	0.0005	0.01
	Total	–	0.03
N-Nitroso-dimethylamine[d]	Smoked fish	0.0005–0.0035	–
	Fried bacon	0.0014	–
	Beer	<0.0001–0.0065	0.011[e]
N-Nitroso-pyrrolidine[d]	Fried bacon	0.011	–
	Salted pork	0.003	–
Volatile N-nitrosamines, taken together[d]	Fried bacon	0.013	–
	Salted pork	0.004	–
	Cocoa	0.002	–
	All food stuffs	–	0.04–0.4[f]
Vinyl chloride[b]	Margarine, etc.	<0.002	<0.04
Substances for which carcinogenic activity in man is not proven			
Cyclamate[a]	Sweetener	–	700
Saccharin[a]	Sweetener	–	1800
Diethylhexyl-phthalate (DEPH)[b]	Plastic sealing for bottle caps	<0.01 mg/l	–
PCBs[a]	Salt-water fish	0.1	0.8
	Baltic herring, herring	0.3–0.6	1.6
	Butter	0.03	0.2
	Human milk	0.02	–
	Total	–	6
Toxaphene[a]	Baltic herring, herring	0.4	0.8

[a] Report from the National Food Administration to the Cancer Committee, 3 April 1981.
[b] Memo from the National Food Administration on substances in packaging materials, 20 October 1983.
[c] Memo on PAHs in foods from the National Food Administration, 19 October 1983.
[d] Memo from the National Food Administration (B.-G. Österdahl) on N-nitroso compounds in foods, 25 October 1983.
[e] Österdahl (1983).
[f] Slorach (1981).
Data from the National Food Administration (1981).

part of the total range of foods has been analysed may be a limitation, and in some cases may have resulted in an underestimation of the intake. However, according to the National Food Administration, the analysed samples should be large enough to give an estimate of the average intake of a given substance which is correct within a factor of 10. On the other hand, population groups may exist which exhibit divergent patterns of consumption, resulting in a higher intake of chemicals.

Among the *mycotoxins,* data are given for *aflatoxin* and *sterigmatocystin.* Aflatoxin has previously (early 1970s) been found in relatively high concentrations in shipments of nuts, primarily intended for marketing during the Christmas season, and was earlier also identified in milk in Sweden. It would seem that no detectable quantities can now be found in milk and only negligible concentrations in foods such as peanuts or flour. In some products (e.g. pistachio) used by bakeries, aflatoxins have also been identified in recent years. Recently, aflatoxin has been found too in mouldy soft bread and other foods (Dich et al., 1979). On the other hand, the mycotoxin sterigmatocystin has not been found in spite of analyses of a large number of bread products and cereals. Nevertheless, certain data indicate that the problem with mycotoxins may be greater than appears from the analytical results presented by the National Food Administration in connection with the exposure survey.

The levels of aflatoxin in some of the bread samples investigated were surprisingly high (greater than> 15 000 µg kg^{-1} in the zone closest to the mould colony in one sample). In addition, diffusion of considerable quantities to non-infested regions was also demonstrated. This implies that the risk of aflatoxin exposure from eating visibly mouldy bread will not be eliminated by cutting out the infested regions. Preservatives have only a limited inhibiting effect on mould growth and on toxin production. Experiments with bread artificially inoculated with *Aspergillus flavus* (stored at 22°C) demonstrated that even after 48 hours, when the mould colony had a diameter of only about 0.5 cm, aflatoxin in a concentration of 30 000 µg kg^{-1} (the highest permissible level in foods is 5 µg kg^{-1}) was present in the zone closest to the colony. In Sweden about 200 million kg of bread is eaten annually. Even infestation of a small percentage with occasional toxin-producing colonies may result in considerable collective doses. Information about aflatoxin formation in foods other than bread attacked by moulds is very scanty. Furthermore, nuts are not the only food items imported into Sweden where contamination by aflatoxin has been found.

Although sterigmatocystin has not been demonstrated in foods in Sweden, experience in the USA has shown that zearalenone and sterigmatocystin may be present in beans and peas. A limited Swedish investigation covered 73 samples of dried brown and white beans as well as yellow and green peas. In addition to the sporadic occurrence of *Aspergillus flavus* and *A. versicolor*, a number of other toxin-producing fungi were found (the brown beans especially exhibited a high degree of infestation: 23–43 per cent of the samples were infected by *Aspergillus* species, 22–25 per cent by *Alternaria* species and high levels of ochratoxin). *Aspergillus versicolor* can produce sterigmatocystin. In a series of 194 samples of beans and peas, zearalenone—but not sterigmatocystin—was directly identified in one sample. This investigation covered samples taken during the period 1976–1978 (Åkerstrand and Josefsson 1979).

Arsenic occurs mainly in fish and shellfish. In Sweden an extensive series of analyses of the total content of arsenic in food has been made in more than 800 food samples. The arsenic in fish is mainly present in an organic form, while inorganic arsenic may be found in considerable quantities in wine due to the use of arsenic-containing pesticides in vineyards (Pershagen and Vahter, 1979).

Asbestos may also be found in wine, and in low quantities in drinking water (see Section 4.3.6). Wine can be contaminated by asbestos when older filtration techniques have been employed. However, such methods are used only in the production of certain brands.

Benzidine-based dyes are or have been used to a certain extent for dyeing materials which come into contact with foodstuffs. The migration of carcinogenic amines such as 3,3¹-dichlorobenzidine can occur from these materials. However, no comprehensive information exists on the types of colouring agents used in food-packaging materials in Sweden, and analytical data are not available.

BaP and other *(PAHs)* are found predominantly in smoked and grilled fish and meat products, but also in leafy vegetables, margarine and cooking oils. The total intake of nine different PAHs has been estimated to be on average 1.2 mg person^{-1} year^{-1}.

Pesticide residues included in the IARC and NCI lists of experimental carcinogens which are routinely analysed for in foods (captan, chlordane, chlorothalonil, DDD + DDE + DDT, dicofol, dieldrin, heptachlor, hexachlorobenzene, lindane, quintozene and toxaphene) are identified on a more or less regular basis especially in imported foods. Analytical data for 1976–80 have been given by the National

Food Administration (NFA, 1982) in a special report ('pesticide residues in fruits and vegetables on the Swedish market 1976–1980',) The results—which are not claimed to be representative of all Swedish consumption—are presented as a distribution of the number of various product samples with residue levels within given ranges, normalized with respect to maximum acceptable levels as prescribed by the agency.

The *plasticizers DEHP and DEHA* (di-(2-ethylhexyl) phthalate and adipate) are present in packaging materials made of PVC (polyvinyl chloride). According to the National Food Administration, low levels of DEHP (below the detection limit of 0.01 mg l^{-1}) are thought to occur in soft drinks, etc., originating from the plastic seals of bottle caps, and a higher exposure to DEHA may possibly be obtained from cheese (7–20 mg person^{-1} day^{-1}).

Since the wrapping foils in question are also used for the packaging of other types of fatty foodstuffs (minced meat, etc.), the average total individually related dose should also include contributions from such sources. The presence of DEHP in bottle caps may cause a negligible contamination of soft drinks and similar products, and DEHP has been detected in certain other countries. However, the experiments with migration of DEHA may be taken as also representative of DEHP. To the extent that foil containing DEHP is employed, this implies that a correspondingly high contamination of foods by this plasticizer may occur, but it has not been possible to assess the scope of present use of this type of foil. The extent of utilization of DEHP in other types of packaging materials is not clear, but is thought to be very limited.

Among the *heavy metals*, the National Food Administration presented data on cadmium, chromium, lead and nickel, while pointing out that scientific evidence has not yet proved these agents to be carcinogens when administered via food. Since the total loads of cadmium and lead are of toxicological interest in other respects, the agency has made estimates of total intakes of these metals in food (Slorach, *et al.* 1983).

Problems associated with the presence of *nitrosamines* in food have been the subject of a special report ('Nitrates, nitrites and *N*-nitroso compounds; studies on their chemistry, occurrence and toxicology with special reference to Swedish food', published in 1981 in *Vår Föda 33* (Suppl. 2)).

Volatile nitrosamines are found in a number of foods, especially in nitrite-cured meats and smoked products but also in spices, cocoa, whisky, beer, chewing tobacco and snuff. In Sweden the highest levels have been identified in snuff, chewing tobacco, and fried bacon. In addition, snuff and chewing tobacco contain high concentrations (up to 80 mg kg dry weight^{-1}) of non-volatile nitrosamines such as N'-nitrosonornicotine (the same nitrosated agent found in tobacco smoke that has been demonstrated to be an experimental carcinogen).

The formation of nitrosamines from nitrite and amines is a universal process which may occur during the preparation and storage of food products, but also in the alimentary tract of humans. Appreciable quantities (about 10 µg kg^{-1}) of dimethylnitrosamine can be formed in tuna-fish salad kept a few hours at room temperature in vinegar-based salad dressing (Josefsson and Nygren, 1981). In the acid environment, dimethylnitrosamine is formed from dimethylamine in the tuna and nitrite generated by bacterial reduction of nitrate present in the salad.

There is every reason to believe that many of the identified nitrosamines are human carcinogens, but it is impossible at present to quantify the risk associated with their presence in foods. In spite of the current uncertainty as to the level of risk caused by nitrosamines in the diet, a series of measures to reduce exposure have, nevertheless, been proposed in the report on nitrates, nitrites and *N*-nitroso compounds mentioned above. Examples of such measures which, according to the National Food Administration, are regularly applied include the addition of ascorbate together with nitrite upon preservation in order to reduce the formation of nitrosamines. Other recommended measures are a reduction of the consumption of vegetables with very high levels of nitrate (e.g. red beetroot), and avoiding over-fertilization with nitrogen-based fertilizers in agriculture, etc. Regulatory action to reduce the levels of nitrosamines in certain products has been taken in the USA.

Vinyl chloride can migrate from packaging materials made of synthetic polymers and has previously been found in concentrations up to 0.6 mg kg^{-1} in the actual food. However, the quality of packaging materials has improved to such an extent that nowadays hardly any detectable quantities of vinyl chloride can be found. Sweden was the first country in the world to introduce a highest acceptable level for vinyl chloride in foods (0.05 mg kg^{-1}) in 1975. Improvements in analytical methods allowed this level to be reduced to 0.01 mg kg^{-1} in 1978.

The Pharmaceuticals Department of the National Board of Health and Welfare.

Information on the active constituents of pharmaceuticals registered in Sweden is recorded in the pharmaceuticals information data-base of the National Board of Health and Welfare.[4] For each substance the following exposure-related information is available:

(*a*) number of packages sold, in thousands;
(*b*) number of doses sold, in thousands (e.g. number of millilitres of solution, number of tablets, grams of ointment, etc.);

(c) number of defined daily doses per thousand inhabitants per day;
(d) number of defined daily doses in thousands, expressed as total consumption during 12 months.

The figures recorded refer to sales in the wholesale trade of pharmaceutical products to the pharmacies. However, stock levels in pharmacies are kept so low that the statistics may be regarded as a measure of the sales from the pharmacies. The fact that prescribed drugs are not always completely consumed, so that the actual consumption volume in general is lower, has not been taken into account.

The data-base also covers information on pharmacologically inactive constituents, that is, those added to products for technical reasons, for example colouring agents, fillers, stabilizers and similar agents. Data are also recorded concerning the use of certain substances in manufacturing processes which are eliminated from the formulation and, consequently, do not occur in the finished product to any appreciable extent (solvents, etc.).

The Board provided data on approximately 40 active substances in various defined pharmaceutical products, as well as their pharmacological classification. Inactive constituents from the exposure survey lists were also reported, but little quantitative information was available. Some drugs for which registration had been cancelled were also mentioned in the Board's report. One such example is the drugs containing arsenic trioxide, of which the last registrations were withdrawn in 1971. A review of the consumption of certain substances during the period 1972–1980 was also given.

On the basis of this documentation it is not possible to form an opinion in each individual case as to the justification in allowing the use of these substances. However, the Committee has drafted a brief overview dealing with some of the substances which have been the focus of international attention (see Section 4.4.5).

Among the compounds that are possibly carcinogenic in man are a number of active constituents of drugs for cancer therapy, as well as certain hormones used in gynaecological practice in Sweden. One substance, metronidazole (see Table 4.12), is present in some common preparations employed in the treatment of large groups of patients for certain infections (e.g. colpitis caused by *Trichomonas vaginitis*). However, they are only intended for short-term treatment (7–14 days), according to conditions stipulated in the product registration.

A couple of other substances, phenytoin and phenobarbital, are classified as 'drugs for use in psychiatric disturbances, organic neuropathies, etc.,' and are used mainly in treatment of epilepsy.

There is considerable exposure to oestrogenic and progestogenic steroid hormones; oral contraceptives, in particular, account for a large part of the total consumption.

In Table 4.12 exposure data (relating to 1980) are given for a number of carcinogenic, or suspected carcinogenic, active agents in pharmaceutical products, expressed as the number of defined daily doses and the total amount sold. Some pharmacologically inactive ingredients are also included.

The problems associated with the use of carcinogenic drugs (or those suspected of being carcinogenic) are discussed in general terms in Sections 4.4.5 and 4.4.6.

The National Environmental Protection Board

The report from the National Environmental Protection Board contained exposure measurements carried out in Sweden of the concentrations in air, soil, water and some indicator plants (mosses, lichens) of some of the substances included on the lists circulated by the Cancer Committee. Further, certain data were presented on volumes of various substances emitted into air and water from stationary sources and from motor vehicles, together with an adaptation to Swedish conditions of exposure and emission data taken from a report prepared for the US Environmental Protection Agency. In the report from the National Environmental Protection Board, estimates of the total exposure to seven compounds were included. Finally, an account of the historical trends for emissions from motor vehicles and energy production was given.

There is also a separate review, in Swedish, by the Institute for Water and Air Pollution Research, of the literature on environmental measurements from Sweden and other countries (IVL, 1980).

In Table 4.13 selected data on air exposure measurements from Sweden are given. The period during which samples were taken varied from 24 hours to 1 year. Some random samples were also included. The maximal concentrations of some of the compounds are sometimes far above the reported averages. Within certain industrial communities, for example, there are measurements of chromium and lead showing maximal levels 10–25 times higher than the average. High concentrations of metals in soil, water and certain plants have most often been found in the vicinity of industrial complexes emitting such a chemical. Besides substances listed for the exposure survey, the Board also reported on the occurrence of some agents such as ethylene, formaldehyde, methylene chloride and perchloroethylene.

Table 4.14 gives data on emissions into air and water from the burning of fossil fuels, from waste incineration and other kinds of combustion (heating of homes, etc.), gasoline-and diesel-powered vehicles, and different types of industrial plants.

In addition, the National Environmental Protection Board has estimated doses on the basis of exposure measurements in ambient air

Table 4.12 Exposure data for certain carcinogenic (or suspected carcinogenic) substances in pharmaceuticals.

Substance	Quantity sold (kg)	Daily doses (thousands)
Cardiovascular preparations		
Acetamide[a,b]	0.3	17
Reserpine	0.1	321[c]
Preparations for blood disorders and malignant tumours		
Cyclophosphamide	24	313
Dactinomycin	–	3
Chlorambucil	0.5	48
Melphalan	0.8	83
Thiotepa	–	23
Chemotherapeutics and antifungal preparations		
Griseofulvin	544	1089
Metronidazole	461	901
Antiparasitic agents		
DDT[d]	89	–
Agents for psychiatric disturbances, organic neurological diseases, etc.		
Phenobarbital	833	9624
Phenytoin	2174	7245
Antipyretics and analgesics		
Phenacetin[e]	1458	2472
Preparations used in gynaecology and obstetrics–oestrogens		
Ethinyloestradiol	6	146 578
Mestranol	0.3	7 317
Oestradiol	29	22 000
Oestriol	6	6428
Preparations used in gynaecology and obstetrics–progestogens		
Ethynodiol[g]	–	–
Medroxyprogesterone	82	14 699
Megestrol	0.03	7
Norethisterone	8	13 451
Norethisterone acetate	13	1549
Antiseborrhoeic agents		
Selenium disulphide	979	27 279
Pharmacologically inactive ingredients		
Brilliant blue FCF	–	–
CI 42090 (colouring agent, used in one medical shampoo and in a preparation against Parkinson's Disease)	–	–
Captan (preservative[b])	5	–
Thiourea[a,b] (in two sedatives, one intended for children)	–	–

[a] The substance was present in pharmaceuticals in 1981, but has since been removed.
[b] Classified as an active ingredient in the report from National Board of Health and Welfare.
[c] Consumption has drastically decreased since 1980. The number of defined daily doses for the 12-month period preceding the last quarter of 1983 was 135 000.

d Includes some uses in veterinary medicine.
e The registrations of all preparations containing phenacetin were cancelled in 1982.
f Does not include conjugated oestrogens, which are present in one product.
g Present in one product in 1980 and 1981. Information on used quantities not available.
Information from the NBHW (1981).

for arsenic, benzene, BaP, ethylene oxide, formaldehyde and vinyl chloride in Sweden. Whilst taking into account seasonal and geographical (such as urban, suburban or sparsely populated areas) variations in the different places, the agency has also calculated yearly average values for pollutants in the air inhaled by inhabitants of small communities and residential areas of various sizes (Table 4.15).

It is emphasized by the Board that data for emissions and the presence of carcinogens in the external environment are scarce, and that improvements in the analysis of exposures are urgently needed. The supporting documentation for the dose calculations is considered very unreliable with respect to the occurrence of these substances in diverse locations (e.g. in homes, vehicles, and different urban areas) and also concerning the length of time spent by individuals in different environments. Therefore the dose estimates should be regarded merely as a preliminary attempt to acquire data applicable to Swedish conditions, with the overall aim of assessing the order of magnitude of the doses involved.

Many carcinogens or suspected carcinogens, to which widespread exposure occurs and which are thought to increase the cancer incidence in urban environments, originate from the combustion of fossil fuels. This type of pollutant has been the subject of extensive analysis.

With the exception of communities near heavy chemical plants, domestic heating, energy production and motor vehicles account for most of the carcinogens found in the external environment. The volume of motor vehicle traffic was very small before 1950 and domestic heating at that time was mainly by means of separate small stoves usually burning wood or coal. The period 1950–1960 was characterized by a switch to oil. Central district heating plants became increasingly important in the heating systems of the central urban areas. In the early 1980s oil accounted for 90 per cent of the total consumption of fossil fuels. The number of cars increased dramatically from approximately 0.3 million in 1950 to 3.0 million in 1980. During this period the number of inhabitants residing in urban areas increased from about 4 million to 6.6 million. (In section 6.6 it is estimated that approximately one-fifth of the Swedish population, or just under 2 million, is prone to the exposure characteristic for European urban area conditions.)

Different types of exposure

Table 4.13 Examples of concentrations of various substances in air measured in Sweden.

Substance	Measurement conditions	Air concentrations[a]
Benzene	Urban area: street (min.–max.)	26–110 µg m^{-3}
	Urban area: street (random sampling, average)	45–450 µg m^{-3}
Benz[a]anthracene	Background ambient air (21 days)	0.8 ng m^{-3}
	Urban area: street (average: 14 days)	0.9 ng m^{-3}
Benzo[b]fluoranthene	Background ambient air (average: 21 days	0.8 ng m^{-3}
	Urban area: street (average: 14 days)	3.2 ng m^{-3}
Benzo[a]pyrene	Background ambient air (21 days)	0.2 ng m^{-3}
	Urban area: street (average: 1 year)	6 ng m^{-3}
Cadmium	Urban area: street (monthly, min.–max.)	2–3 ng m^{-3}
Chromium	Urban area, roof level (10 days, average–max.)	8–20 ng m^{-3}
	Different industrial communities (monthly values, average)	40–240 ng m^{-3}
1,2-Dibromoethane	Urban area: street (average: 4 days)	0.1–0.8 µg m^{-3}
1,2-Dichloroethane	Urban area; street (average:4 days)	0.25–1.4 µg m^{-3}
Formaldehyde	Indoor air, child day care centres (min.–max.)	100–300 µg m^{-3}
Hexachlorobenzene	Background ambient air	0.006 ng m^{-3}
	Urban area	0.3 ng m^{-3}
Nickel	Different industrial communities (monthly values, average)	60 ng m^{-3}
PAHs, total	Urban area: street (average: 24 hours) (19 compounds)	50 ng m^{-3}
PCBs,	Background ambient air (average: 23 days)	0.2–0.3 ng m^{-3}
	Urban area (average: 23 days)	0.05–2.6 ng m^{-3}
Sulphur dioxide	Urban area (maximal daily averages)	400–600 µg m^{-3}
	Urban area (Oct.–March, average)	40–140 µg m^{-3}

[a] Note that two different concentration scales are used.
Data from the NEPB (1981).

Table 4.14 Total emissions into air and water of various substances (tonnes year^{-3}, 1978) in Sweden.

Substance	Emissions into air (tonnes year^{-1})	Emissions into water (tonnes year^{-1})
Acrylonitrile	0.5	
Arsenic	125	760
(Asbestos	4000[a])	
Benzene	3800[a]	
Benzo[a]anthracene	0.5[a]	
Benzo[a]pyrene	5	
Beryllium	0.5	
Cadmium	10	4 (6)[b]
Carbon tetrachloride	25	
Chromium	150	260 (280)[b]
1,2-Dichloroethane	400	0.5
Ethylene	14 000[a]	
Formaldehyde	2300[a]	
Ethylene oxide	35	
Nickel	200	90 (120)[b]
PAHs, total (15 substances)	200	
Vinyl chloride	800	4
Sulphur dioxide	690 000	

[a] Emission mainly from motor vehicles (the asbestos data do not refer to quantities emitted but to volumes used for brake linings in motor vehicles).
[b] Includes municipal sewage plants. Since many smaller industries are connected to municipal sewage plants, there is a risk of double recording here.
Data from the NEPB (1981).

The situation regarding emission of pollutants from domestic heating has improved in Swedish urban areas, although the compensatory increase in traffic volume means that the overall pollution situation has not significantly changed. The variations in emissions of BaP[5] are evident from Figure 4.10. Since motor vehicle exhausts are much more poorly dispersed than emissions from domestic heating systems, the situation has, in fact, deteriorated more than is evident in this figure (with regard to oxides of nitrogen, see also Törnqvist (1984)).

Different types of exposure

Table 4.15 Exposures for all or part of the Swedish population, expressed as concentrations per cubic meter of inhaled air multiplied by the number of exposed persons.

Substance	g m^{-3} × number of individuals exposed
Arsenic (total population)	0.016
Benzene (urban population)	31
Benzene (customers filling cars at service stations)	0.8
Benzo[a]pyrene (total population)	0.004
Ethylene (total population)	45
Ethylene oxide (population of Stenungsund)	0.000 08
Formaldehyde (exhausts from motor vehicles: total population)	10
Vinyl chloride (populations of Stenungsund, Stockvik, and Sundsvall)	0.35

To obtain the annual absorbed collective doses, the values should be multiplied by the average volume of air (about 7000 m^3) inhaled per person per year, then by a conversion factor giving the fraction of the substance present in the inhaled air which is absorbed by the body.
Data from the NEPB (1981).

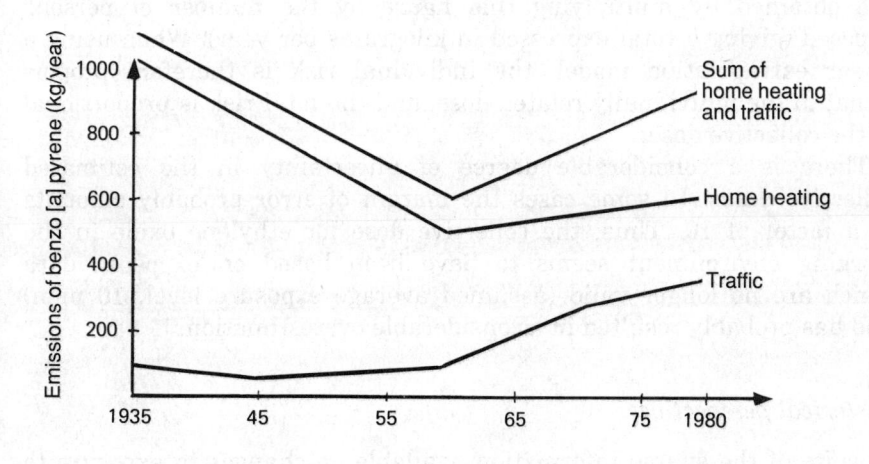

Figure 4.10 Emissions of benzo(a)pyrene in urban areas in Sweden originating from the heating of homes and urban traffic.
From NEPB, 1981

To illustrate the changes in the levels of air pollutants from motor vehicles, the emissions of various substances are shown in Table 4.16.

Table 4.16 Emissions of various substances[a] from gasoline and diesel-powered vehicles (tonnes per year).

Year	Particulates (soot)	Nitrogen oxides	Hydrocarbons (total)	Carbon monoxide	Lead[b]	Benzo[a]-pyrene
1960	13 000	55 000	73 000	460 000	–	0.15
1970	17 000	118 000	140 000	870 000	1800	0.28
1980	20 000	164 000	175 000	1 100 000	1100	0.35

[a] Suspected carcinogens and others.
[b] 705 tonnes in 1982. The information refers to the total volumes of lead in gasoline sold annually.
Data from the NEPB (1981).

The annual *individually related doses* in Table 4.17 have been quantified as milligrams per person. As a rule, this refers to the quantity which, on average, is ingested or inhaled by the population or a group of individuals in question (the degree of absorption will of course vary). The corresponding annual *collective doses* in Table 4.18 are obtained by multiplying this figure by the number of persons exposed (giving a total expressed in kilograms per year). When using a linear extrapolation model, the individual risk is therefore proportional to the individually related dose, and the total risk is proportional to the collective dose.

There is a considerable degree of uncertainty in the estimated collective doses. In some cases the margin of error probably amounts to a factor of 10. Thus, the collective dose for ethylene oxide in the working environment seems to have been based on exposure data which are no longer valid (assumed average exposure level, 10 ppm) and has probably resulted in a considerable overestimation.

Historical perspectives

In spite of the sparse information available on changes in exposure to carcinogenic substances, certain conclusions can be drawn looking from a historical perspective.

For compounds where the Board of Occupational Safety and Health has presented collective doses for different times, there has clearly been a drastic reduction in the exposure levels. The general improvements in occupational safety introduced during recent decades, such

Table 4.17 Individually related doses for various substances.

Substance	Doses in mg person^{-1} year^{-1} for 1981 (for asbestos in fibres person^{-1} year^{-1})				
Arsenic	80	Metal works	0.011	(0.004–0.018)[c]	55[a]
			0.042	Skellefteå	
			0.249	Skelleftehamn	
Asbestos	1×10^9	Production of brake linings (100)[b]		?	?
	0.2×10^9	Service stations			
	0.1×10^9	Demolition, etc			
Benzene	20	Service stations (10 000)[b]	29	(10.5–42)[c]	
	100	Taxi drivers (2000)[b]			
	200	Car repair garages (30 000)[b]			
	2000	Gas truck drivers (500)[b]			
	4000	Coking plant (50)[b]			
Benzo[a]pyrene	?		0.004	(0.001–0.006)[c]	about 0.03
			0.0245	Sundsvall	
Ethylene oxide	20×10^3	e.g. at Berol Kemi (250)[b]	0.07	Stenungsund (8000)[b]	–
Vinyl chloride	about 700	Processing (3000)[b]	10.8	Stockvik and Sundsvall (94 500)[b]	<0.4
			183	Stenungsund (8000)[b]	
Formaldehyde	1300	Different industries (7000)[b]	8.8[d]		
	2 600	Laminates and other industries (1000)[b]			

[a] Mainly as inorganic arsenic.
[b] Figures in parentheses refer to the number of exposed induviduals in cases where the doses do not cover the whole population of Sweden.
[c] Figures in parentheses refer to variations betweem different parts of the country.
[d] Values based on data from other countries
Based on information from the Board of Occupational Safety and Health, the National Environmental Protection Board, and from the National Food Administration (NBOSH, 1981; NEPB, 1981; NFA, 1981).

as protective equipment for workers, switching over to closed systems and improved ventilation, have meant that as a rule exposure to chemicals in the workplace has been substantially reduced.

Exposure of the general population to a number of carcinogens and to substances suspected of being carcinogenic has also been eliminated, or at least drastically reduced, in the case of pharmaceuticals

Table 4.18 Approximate collective doses for various substances.

Substance	Doses[a] in Kg/year (1981)		
	OSH	NEPB	NFA
Arsenic	0.004	0.09	440
Asbestos	3×10^{11}(fibres)	?	?
Benzene	8	230	–
Benzo[a]pyrene	?	0.03	0.2
Ethylene	?	300	–
Ethylene oxide	5	0.0006	–
Formaldyhde	12	70	
Vinyl chloride	4 (1975–80)	2.5	?

[a] Some of the collective doses refer to a limited population group, others to the entire population. Table 4.17, which lists individually related doses, provides the relevant details.

Based on information from the Board of Occupational Safety and Health (NBOSH, 1981), the National Environmental Protection Board (NEPB, 1981), and from the National Food Administration (NFA, 1981).

and foods. A number of potentially carcinogenic food additives—especially colouring agents—have been banned, and even though some problems remain, modern agriculture and food-processing technology here contributed to a striking reduction in the infestation of crops and other staples by mycotoxin-producing fungi. However, not all the implications of these developments can be easily assessed. Although detailed information is hard to come by, it seems that a corresponding change has also occurred regarding the elimination of carcinogens from other types of consumer product.

While certain chemicals capable of causing cancer have been reduced or eliminated from products, new substances have been introduced which may or may not have been well tested. It can be taken for granted that certain of these will be found to be carcinogenic. Although their effects on the *total* cancer incidence may be very limited, their use by particularly exposed smaller population groups, for example in the workplace, may imply an increased risk to the individual (see Chapters 2 and 6). With the introduction in a number of countries of such measures as notification procedures requiring certain minimum testing of new chemical substances before their commercial release, the chemicals introduced in the future will, as a rule, be more fully investigated than in the past (EEC, 1979; OECD, 1981/2).

4.4.5 Examples of exposure to chemical substances associated with cancer-induction in humans

As a supplement to the data described earlier in this chapter, this section will summarize the current understanding regarding carcinogenicity of a selection of substances, industrial processes and occupational exposures, where a cause-and-effect relationship between exposure and neoplasia in man has been demonstrated with varying degrees of certainty. Individual substances, mixtures of chemical substances, and exposure environments are discussed, for which there is considered to exist sufficient evidence for a causal relationship, based on epidemiological studies. In addition, examples are provided where although human data are inadequate, experimental results and/ or other factors strongly suggest that a chemical should be regarded as carcinogenic in man. Using Swedish exposure data the Cancer Committee has also attempted to make a rough estimate of the level of risk for some of these agents. However, in the majority of cases data are lacking for carrying out such a quantification of risk. Finally, consideration has been given to a few substances where the causal relationship between exposure to these compounds and neoplasia in humans cannot be considered as proven, but where the Cancer Committee finds it justified to give a comprehensive evaluation due to public debate involving these agents or due to other circumstances.

This brief survey is based to a considerable extent on a report by Holmberg and Säfwenberg (1984)—a review on occupational carcinogens—as well as on the revised and amended treatise on carcinogens published by the IARC (1982). It should again be emphasized that the assessments of the IARC do not concern the *size* of the risk involved, but the completeness and strength of *proof* of carcinogenicity.

For most identified chemical human carcinogens these characteristics have come to light in the context of *occupational exposure*. For this reason, cancer hazards in the work environment form a major part of this section.

In many instances a significantly increased risk associated with a certain activity has been noted, without the causative agent being obvious. In such cases the results from animal experiments can be used as supporting evidence when evaluating a suspected human carcinogen. In recent years experimental investigations indicating a carcinogenic potential of a certain substance have in some cases preceded the discovery of such a risk for man by use of epidemiological methods.

The latency period for occupationally induced cancer is often several decades. On the other hand, occupational cancer is often diagnosed at a considerably lower age than would normally be expected, considering the average age when cancers due to other causes make their first appearance. It should also be taken into account that the observed risk is associated with a 'historical' exposure (perhaps decades before), while measures introduced in the area of occupational hygiene, changed production procedures and so on may have already changed previous exposure patterns considerably.

Although *agents present in food* are probably decisive factors in the induction of some cancers, only with certain mycotoxins has it been possible to relate the appearance of cancer with any high degree of probability to specific chemical compounds. Even here, the epidemiological evidence is ambiguous. Hazards associated with mycotoxins have been discussed in Sections 4.3 and 4.4.4.

In comparison with the situation regarding carcinogens in foods, the conditions for successfully establishing a causal relationship between *exposure to pharmaceuticals* and neoplasia by epidemiological methods tend to be considerably more favourable. There is convincing proof of carcinogenic activity in man for several active pharmaceutical constituents. At the same time, the special problems associated with drug therapy should be emphasized, where risk of exposure to known or suspected carcinogens must be balanced against the benefits obtained. This situation may be exemplified by some types of cancer treatment.

The examples below are listed in alphabetical order, except for industrial processes, occupational exposures and pharmaceuticals which have been placed at the end of this section.

Some specific chemical substances

AFLATOXINS
Aflatoxins (B_1, B_2, G_1, G_2, M_1) constitute a group of chemically closely related, extremely toxic mycotoxins, which under certain conditions are produced by the common moulds *Aspergillus flavus* and *A. parasiticus* that infest grain, nuts and other basic commodities and foods. The risks of infection and toxin production are greatest under warm, humid conditions, so the situation is most serious in tropical and subtropical regions (WHO, 1979). In Sweden, high concentrations have been found in imported products like peanuts, Brazil nuts, bitter almonds, apricot kernels and in animal feed such as peanut flour. The

formation of aflatoxin in, for example, mouldy bread may be a potential problem also in Sweden. Cattle given toxin-containing fodder excrete aflatoxin in their milk, mainly as breakdown products (aflatoxin M_1), but detectable quantities are no longer found in Swedish milk.

The IARC has judged aflatoxins to be substances which are probably carcinogenic to man (group 2A of its list of carcinogens).

The extremely potent carcinogenic action of aflatoxins has been demonstrated in at least eight animal species, including the rhesus monkey. Liver tumours are consistently induced, but tumours also appear at other sites. Concentrations as low as 1 µg/kg in the feed (aflatoxin B_1) have been reported to produce a tumour incidence of 10 per cent in rats. A concentration of 0.3 mg kg^{-1} in the feed induces acute liver damage in pigs after 3–4 months. The high incidence of primary liver cancer among populations in Africa and Asia has been connected with the high levels of aflatoxin identified in foods from these regions. The simultaneous presence of infection by the hepatitis B virus, which probably contributes to an increased risk, makes it more difficult to establish a causal relationship here. One risk assessment based on exposure data from North America (a linear extrapolation model at low doses) indicated that a considerable number of primary liver cancers in the USA could, theoretically, be explained by the presence of aflatoxin in food (Crouch and Wilson, 1981).

Aromatic Amines

The possibility of a causal relationship between occupational exposure to certain aromatic amines and bladder cancer was being discussed even at the end of the last century. A number of epidemiological studies have linked the appearance of bladder cancer to exposure to the aromatic amines 4-aminobiphenyl, benzidine and 2-naphthylamine. These compounds have been evaluated by the IARC and there is sufficient evidence to prove a cause-and-effect relationship. 2-Naphthylamine is a potent carcinogen. For certain heavily exposed categories (distillation workers) it has formerly been reported that bladder cancer was induced in 100 per cent of the workers after a long period of exposure to this compound.

In Sweden the use of these amines in the workplace has been completely banned for several years.

The production of the dye auramine, involving simultaneous exposure to other compounds as well, has been considered to be clearly associated with bladder cancer in man. Oral administration of technical-grade auramine in high doses has induced liver tumours in rodents, and subcutaneous injection has been found to produce local sarcoma in rats. Although the bioassays therefore provide certain supporting evidence ('limited evidence' according to the IARC) that auramine itself is the aetiological factor associated with the production of this dye, other carcinogenic agents may have been involved. In Sweden auramine has certain uses, but since it can only be employed with permission from the Labour Inspectorate, exposure is obviously limited.

ARSENIC

According to the IARC, inorganic arsenic may induce cancer of the lung as well as of the skin in exposed individuals. An increased incidence of lung cancer has been found in workers employed in smelters and gold mines, in vineyards where they have been using arsenic-containing pesticides, and in certain sectors of the chemical industry. In addition, there are indications that other types of tumour such as lymphoma and haemangiosarcoma of the liver may be induced by inorganic arsenic compounds in the workplace. In Sweden an increased mortality from lung cancer has also been observed in workers employed in smelters (see Box 1).

Arsenic exposure in Sweden has been reduced to an appreciable extent in the workplace by the introduction of a low hygienic limit value (0.05 mg m^{-3} in inhaled air) and by other protective measures. The annual dose from arsenic in urban air has been estimated to be about 0.01 mg person^{-1} year^{-1}, corresponding to an average concentration of 1.5 ng m^{-3} including elevated levels in the vicinity of Rönnskärsverken (see Table 4.13). Using linear extrapolation it can be deduced that this level may give rise to about one case of lung cancer per year. Insofar as arsenic acts as a co-carcinogenic factor, this may be an overestimate.

Exposure to inorganic arsenic in drugs and drinking water containing high concentrations (0.5–1 mg l^{-1}) has been shown to produce in humans certain diseases of the skin (multiple basal cell carcinoma, squamous cell carcinoma and Bowen's disease). No evidence is available to support the view that organic arsenic compounds of the types present in foods (Table 4.11)—shellfish in particular—can cause neoplasia in man. On the other hand, thorough studies have not been conducted.

Investigations in experimental animals indicate that inorganic trivalent arsenic may induce lung cancer (Ishinishi *et al.*, 1980; Rudnay and Borzongi, 1981; Pershagen *et al.*, 1983). On the other hand, inorganic arsenic does not seem to be mutagenic (Löfroth and Ames, 1978; Rossman *et al.*, 1980). In bacteria and in human cells arsenic can interfere with repair of DNA (Jung 1971, Rossman *et al.*, 1977) which could indicate a co-carcinogenic effect. Indications of interactive effects between exposure to arsenic trioxide and BaP and the induction of pulmonary tumours in experimental animals support this hypothesis (Pershagen *et al.*, 1983). In this respect, the interaction

Box 1

A case study of occupational arsenic exposure

Wall and Taube (1983) have carried out a detailed study of the occupational environment at Rönnskärsverken, a large metalworks in northern Sweden. They analysed the increased mortality from lung cancer among the workers, and proved a link with work at the roasting kilns, as well as with certain other activities where exposure to arsenic occurs. Among a total of about 4000 employees with approximately 55 000 man-years of employment at the smelter, 76 deaths from lung cancer occurred during the period 1928–76. Of these cases 30 may be ascribed to the effects of arsenic, possibly in combination with other air pollutants. The relative risk for lung cancer associated with work at the roasting kilns (corresponding to the 30 cases) has been estimated to be 2.46 for non-smokers and 3.63 for smokers, giving an average value of about 3 for the whole group. Interaction between exposure to arsenic and smoking is discussed in Section 4.6.

On the basis of previous epidemiological studies (see US EPA 1978), a three fold increase in risk as a result of exposure to 0.05 mg arsenic m^{-3} air^{-1} during at least 25 years can be calculated. The present arsenic level (since 1970) during work at the roasting kilns in Rönnskärsverken is estimated to be 0.04 mg m$_3$. This value corresponds to an increase in the risk of lung cancer due to 1 year's exposure of (0.04/0.05×25) × 200 per cent = 6.5 per cent. Furthermore, since the number of individuals exposed has decreased from 100 to 50, it can be estimated that this value corresponds to 0.03 induced cases per year. The collective dose was about five times higher before 1970 (100 individuals × 0.1 mg m^{-3}), inducing about 0.15 cases per year. Exposure levels during the 1930s and 1940s were probably another 5–10 times higher, corresponding to approximately one case per year per 100 exposed workers. It appears that the risk contribution from exposure to arsenic in the glass industry and in connection with wood preservation, which are the other major areas of use of arsenic compounds (see Table 4.9), are considerably lower.

between arsenic and smoking in workers employed in smelters is also of interest (see Section 4.6).

Asbestos

The name 'asbestos' is applied to a group of naturally occurring silicate minerals. Exposure occurs through inhalation—and to some extent by swallowing—of airborne fibres. Asbestos is widely used, and potential risk groups can be found in several occupational categories. Cancers which have been primarily implicated in asbestos exposure are lung cancer, mesothelioma of the pleura as well as of the peritoneum and possibly also neoplasia of the larynx and the digestive tract. The mechanism for the carcinogenic action of asbestos is not yet known. Asbestos is not mutagenic and evidence suggests a promoter-like or other co-carcinogenic action, although exhibiting a linear dose–response relationship (see von Bahr et al., 1984b; review by Nicholson et al. 1981). The latency periods are remarkably long. It has been assumed that lung cancer may be induced by all commercially important asbestos varieties, i.e. chrysotile, amosite, anthophyllite and crocidolite, or by mixtures of them. Single cases of mesothelioma have occurred in individuals not occupationally exposed but living in the vicinity of asbestos plants or crocidolite mines and in persons who have come into contact with asbestos-exposed persons in their homes. The various types of asbestos probably differ in their carcinogenic activity in man. The amphibole group, in particular crocidolite (of which occupational use is prohibited in Sweden), has been considered to be more potent than the chrysotile type of fibres. However, comparable dose–response data for different types of fibres are not available. Clarification of this issue is complicated by the fact that mixed exposures are usually involved (at least in industry).

The estimates reported for the risk of lung cancer due to asbestos exposure vary greatly. Based on the higher values published, exposure for 1 year to 1 fibre ml^{-1} [6] corresponds to a risk increment of 4–9 per cent. This would produce about 40 cases per year in Sweden for exposures before 1970 and approximately 0.3 cases per year for present conditions. However, the true values may be considerably lower.

Asbestos and tobacco smoking act synergistically in induction of lung cancer (see Section 4.6). Data presented by Hammond et al. (1979) indicate a purely multiplicative interaction between the two factors, yielding a very great increase in risk for the combination of asbestos and smoking.

In Sweden the occupational use of asbestos is now extremely limited. However, occasional exposure will continue for quite some time, especially in the repair or demolition of existing buildings or piping systems insulated with asbestos, and in repair and servicing of brake systems in motor vehicles. Industrially produced goods, which have contributed to some increase in the natural levels in air and water, are responsible for some exposure of the general population to asbestos, but nevertheless, this is low in comparison with occupational exposure conditions.

BENZENE

This organic compound, which is metabolized to a reactive epoxide, is carcinogenic to humans. The different types of leukaemia (non-lymphatic) induced by occupational exposure to benzene or by mixtures containing it, are well known and in Sweden benzene has been classified as a cancer-inducing substance (category C). The largest number of workers nowadays exposed to benzene are employed at petrol stations and service garages. Since benzene is present in petrol, most of the population will be exposed to it to some degree. Typical air concentrations in Swedish urban areas (streets with heavy traffic) are 0.08–0.45 mg m^{-3} (Johnsson and Berg 1978). These may be compared with the current hygienic limit value in the workplace of 16 mg m^{-3}.

The fact that a total of about 120 million litres of benzene in petrol are distributed annually throughout Sweden may give a misleading impression of the size of the actual exposure to this carcinogen and the resulting risk. Several epidemiological studies have permitted a quantitative assessment of the absolute risk of leukaemias due to exposure to benzene. These show that benzene has a relatively low carcinogenic potency. A US expert group has estimated that some 60 cases of leukaemia per year could be ascribed to *all* sources of exposure in the USA (US EPA, 1979a). For Sweden this would correspond to about 1.9 cases. Based on the collective doses derived for Sweden the following (crude) risk estimates[7] are obtained:

Occupationally exposed
(about 42 500 persons;   0.3 cases of leukaemia per year.
see Table 4.17)

The general population   3 cases of leukaemia per year
(8 million, but mainly the
metropolitan population of
about 2 million)

The cancer risks associated with benzene in petrol have been much debated. Isolated cases of toxic effects on the bone marrow associated with unprotected handling (cleaning, etc.) of petrol containing exceptionally high levels of benzene (over 15 per cent) have been reported from other countries. In several extensive cohort studies of workers handling petrol, no increase in the leukaemia rate has been noted. However, the possibility of detecting a small increase in these investigations was limited. On the other hand, an increased incidence of leukaemia has been observed in a Swedish case-control study involving certain professions (chauffeurs, truck drivers, employees at petrol stations, chain-saw operators, drivers of excavators) where workers are exposed to engine fuels and/or combustion products (Brandt et al., 1978). However, the cause of this increase may in part be ascribed to other common external factors. Another study (Berlin et al., 1977) of the frequencies of chromosome aberrations in white blood cells (a sensitive index for exposure to benzene) covering drivers of diesel trucks, crews of tankers, workers in coke oven plants, and employees at petrol stations is of interest in this context. The results demonstrate that the frequency of chromosomal aberrations in the various occupational categories could not be linked to exposure to benzene, but that some other agent—probably related to the combustion of diesel fuels— had caused or had contributed to the chromosomal anomalies observed in the truck drivers. Furthermore, several investigations have demonstrated the genotoxic properties of diesel exhausts (for references, see for example Albert et al., (1983)).

BERYLLIUM AND BERYLLIUM COMPOUNDS
Beryllium and its compounds have been proven carcinogenic in rats, rabbits, and monkeys. In rats and monkeys pulmonary tumours are induced upon inhalation, intra-tracheal administration or intra-bronchial implantation. Intravenous injection of beryllium and its compounds produces osteosarcoma in rabbits.

Certain epidemiological investigations indicate that beryllium induces lung tumours in humans when inhaled. According to the IARC there is sufficient evidence of carcinogenicity of this substance in animals and limited evidence of its carcinogenicity in man.

In Sweden these compounds are classified as carcinogens, with a hygienic limit value in the workplace (category C).

CADMIUM
Intramuscular injection of metallic cadmium and cadmium sulphide induces sarcoma at the site of injection. In rats and mice subcutaneous administration of soluble cadmium compounds, for example the sulphate or chloride, elicits testicular atrophy followed by testicular tumours. On the other hand, no increase in cancer incidence was detected when rats were administered cadmium chloride in their food at a concentration of 50 ppm. for 2 years. After continuous exposure to an aerosol of cadmium chloride, lung tumours could be induced in rats at very low concentrations (down to 13 μgm^{-3}). There was an almost linear correlation between the incidence and the dose inhaled (Takanaka et al., 1983). Even before this last study, the IARC considered that sufficient evidence for the carcinogenicity of cadmium in animals existed.

An increased incidence of cancers of the prostate and lung has been reported in workers exposed to high levels of cadmium. However, available epidemiological data are ambiguous, and there is only limited evidence of the carcinogenicity of cadmium in man.

The Board of Occupational Safety and Health in Sweden has classified cadmium as a carcinogen, with a hygienic limit value (category C).

CHLORINATED ETHERS

Bis-(chloromethyl) ether has been shown to be a potent human carcinogen. Epidemiological studies of occupationally exposed workers have demonstrated a causal association between lung cancer and exposure to bis-(chloromethyl) ether as well as to technical-grade chloromethyl methyl ether. The assessment of the chloromethyl methyl ether has been complicated by the fact that it contained 1–8 per cent of bis-(chloromethyl) ether as an impurity.

In Sweden the production and use of bis-(chloromethyl) ether and chloromethyl methyl ether in the workplace is prohibited (category A according to the Board of Occupational Safety and Health).

CHROMIUM COMPOUNDS

An increased risk of lung cancer has been demonstrated in workers employed in the production of chromates, although the identity of the chromium compound(s) responsible for this effect has not been established. The experimental evidence is strongest for calcium chromate. However, when administered orally, chromium compounds are not considered to be carcinogenic. Chromic acid and chromates have been classified as carcinogens with established hygienic limit values (category C) by the Board of Occupational Safety and Health.

ETHYLENE OXIDE (OXIRANE, 1,2-EPOXYETHENE)

This gaseous compound is an important basic material for the chemical industry and is used in the production of surfactants, glycols, glycol ethers, plasticizers, etc. It is also used for the sterilization of medical equipment and as a pesticide. In Sweden its use as a pesticide is, however, limited to the preservation of museum specimens and for the treatment of spices. This latter application produces residues of ethylene chlorohydrin (2-chloroethanol), another substance possessing genotoxic properties (Gustafsson, 1981).

In rodents, inhaled ethylene oxide induces leukaemia, mesothelioma and brain tumours (Snellings et al., 1981; Lynch et al., 1982). In the same animals the compound also produces stomach tumours on intragastric intubation (Dunkelberg, 1982). Furthermore, the substance has been proven to be genotoxic in a number of systems. In view of these most recent findings, there can be no doubt whatsoever that ethylene oxide should be considered as an animal carcinogen.

In two Swedish investigations of limited groups of workers exposed to ethylene oxide, an increase in the incidence of leukaemia and tumours of the stomach was found (Hogstedt *et al.*, 1979a,b). However, three other studies have been carried out in other countries where no increase in cancer incidence could be detected (Joyner 1964; Thiess *et al.*, 1981; Morgan *et al.*, 1981).

With regard to the limited size of the Swedish epidemiological studies as well as the factor of simultaneous exposure to other carcinogens in one of them, the IARC, in 1979, considered the available evidence insufficient to prove a causal association.

It should be emphasized that the three negative epidemiological studies referred to above suffer from such methodological deficiencies as to preclude their being relied on as evidence *against* the existence of an increased risk of the magnitude indicated in the Swedish studies. In view of the reaction pattern of ethylene oxide, characteristic of a directly alkylating agent, which readily penetrates to the different target organs in the body, and its established genotoxic action, as well as the convincing results from the bioassays it seems prudent to await the results of future analyses of exposed populations before ruling this substance out as a human carcinogen. The estimated yearly collective dose in the Swedish working environment (5 kg, see Table 4.18) corresponds to the quantity inhaled during work for 2000 hours per year at the present hygienic limit value of 5 ppm. The air concentrations are probably lower now and the estimated exposure dose is, if anything, too high. A few cases of cancer could possibly be induced at this dosage level.

The Board of Occupational Safety and Health has classified ethylene oxide as a carcinogen and lowered the previous hygienic limit value as a consequence.

Ethene (ethylene) is transformed to ethylene oxide in the body. At low levels about 8 per cent of the quantity inhaled by rats and mice is transformed to this reactive agent (Ehrenberg *et al.*, 1977). Ethylene is an important basic chemical in the petrochemical industry. It is found together with other alkenes in exhaust from motor vehicles and is consequently present in ambient air in urban areas. Ethylene is also produced endogenously in the human body. These substances also occur in tobacco smoke (Osborne *et al.*, 1956). The estimated yearly collective dose in Sweden (300 kg) would correspond to about 25 kg of ethylene oxide, which could, theoretically, induce a few cases of cancer each year. The fact that formation of ethylene oxide has been demonstrated only in animal experiments leaves the effects of ethylene in man uncertain.

FORMALDEHYDE

This is a basic chemical with numerous applications in the chemical industry. Half of the volume of formaldehyde produced is used in the production of synthetic polymers such as urea and phenol–

formaldehyde resins. These are used mainly in adhesives for the production of chipboard, board and plywood. Urea–formaldehyde concentrates are also employed in various processes for surface treatment, in paper products and insulating foams. In the latter case the increased levels of formaldehyde measured in indoor air in certain environments have been the subject of particular attention. In the textile industry formaldehyde is used in the production of creaseproof, flame-resistant and non-shrinkable cloth. In addition, acetal resins are synthesized from formaldehyde. The substance is formed during various combustion processes and is therefore present as an air pollutant in, for example, urban air and tobacco smoke. Formaldehyde is also formed naturally in the human body by various metabolic processes.

Inhaled formaldehyde induces neoplasia in the nasal cavities of rats and mice. According to the IARC, there is sufficient evidence both of animal carcinogenicity and of genotoxicity.

In three epidemiological investigations including occupational categories subject to long-term exposure to high concentrations of formaldehyde—embalmers, pathologists, and workers employed in the production of formaldehyde—no increase in risk has been found for neoplastic disease of the respiratory tract. On the basis of these results the IARC considers that there is no evidence for human carcinogenicity of formaldehyde. However, these investigations are limited in scope and extensive epidemiological studies are being conducted in the USA and the UK. Recently published results have indicated an increased mortality due to tumours of the brain and kidney in groups occupationally exposed to formaldehyde. However, the cause–effect relationship must still be considered uncertain, taking into account simultaneous exposure to other substances (Swenberg et al., 1983).

Because of its reactivity, formaldehyde has an extremely short lifespan in the body. In view of this and its high aqueous solubility, it can be assumed that the action of formaldehyde in the rat and mouse is restricted to the contact surfaces of the upper respiratory tract. At the concentrations in inhaled air that produced tumours in the animal experiments, extreme irritation of the mucous membranes occurs, resulting in tissue damage after a time. Under such conditions formaldehyde may exert a definite promotive action, implying that linear extrapolation of the results from the animal experiments to the low dose range where man is exposed in different situations results in an appreciable overestimation of risk. However, the facts that formaldehyde is an electrophilic agent, that its genotoxic activity has been demonstrated in several systems, and that it induces oncogenic transformation, lend support to the view that it should not be merely regarded as a promoter.

Phenoxyacetic Acids and Chlorophenols

The possibility of an association between human neoplasia and phenoxyacetic acids, chlorophenols or the impurities present in them has been the subject of considerable attention during recent years, particularly in the light of certain Swedish epidemiological studies. In two case-control studies dealing with soft-tissue sarcoma and in one analogous study on malignant lymphoma, Hardell (1981) and co-workers found that occupational exposure to preparations containing phenoxyacetic acids or chlorophenols was considerably more frequent in people with such cancers than in the controls. In these investigations exposure to phenoxyacetic acids was associated with a 5–8-fold increase in risk for these types of neoplasia and exposure to chlorophenols was associated with a 3–8-fold increase. In a later similar study related to cancers in the nasal cavities and in the nasal and laryngeal region, a corresponding risk associated with exposure to chlorophenols—but not to exposure to phenoxyacetic acids—was observed. In two case-control studies on colon cancer and primary liver cancer, no significant increase of risk associated with phenoxyacetic acids or chlorophenols was found.

Cases of soft-tissue sarcoma, appreciably more than expected, have also been reported in some US cohorts of workers employed in the production of trichlorophenols (mainly 2,4,5-trichlorophenol). However, negative results have also been found in some cohort and case-control studies. In a report by a Swedish Special Panel (1982) given the task, *inter alia*, of evaluating available documentary materials on more important pesticides from the aspect of health hazards, the Panel presented a detailed discussion on the phenoxyacetic acids, using the products most commonly employed in Sweden as the point of reference. In an analysis of health registers, no adequate evidence was found of an association between these neoplasias and occupations involving frequent handling of phenoxyacetic acids. However, bearing in mind the macroanalytical design of this study, its results are not statistically incompatible with the results presented by Hardell (1981) and co-workers provided, among other things, that the lower limit of Hardell's confidence interval (about a three-fold increase in risk) is taken into account. A large cohort study involving workers carrying permits for spray application has been initiated but in 1984 was not yet complete.

In short-term tests phenoxyacetic acids and chlorophenols do not appear to possess mutagenic properties. Neither have extensive animal experiments provided any clear-cut evidence of their carcinogenic effects. However, for two substances of interest here, namely

2,4,6-trichlorophenol and tetrachlorodibenzo-*p*-dioxin (TCDD, present as an impurity in 2,3,5-T), apparent carcinogenic properties have been revealed in animal experiments.

On the basis of the investigations by Hardell and co-workers, the US cohort studies, and the findings from the animal experiments mentioned, occupational exposure to phenoxyacetic acid herbicides and to chlorophenols was classified in group 2B by the IARC in 1982, meaning that such an exposure is probably carcinogenic to humans but that in this case is limited. According to the IARC, the available documentary evidence will not, on the other hand, permit the classification of individual phenoxyacetic acids or chlorophenols as human carcinogens.

In summing up, the Cancer Committee concludes that it is possible that occupational exposure to phenoxyacetic acids and chlorophenols—in particular to the often highly contaminated products previously available on the market in Sweden—has resulted in a certain increase in the total cancer risk. If so, the health register studies presented by the Special Panel provide proof that the risk increase must have been very low. However, the studies of Hardell and co-workers indicate that for certain specific types of neoplasia the relative risk increase may have been considerable. The risk increases observed so far have been for occupationally exposed individuals. Whatever exposure of the general public may occur, the doses are bound to be small and the resulting individual risk in such cases negligible. Since this issue concerns chemicals that are widely used, involving the potential exposure of many individuals, this is a field that needs further epidemiological and experimental studies.

PLASTICIZERS FOR PVC

According to the IARC the documentary evidence for the plasticizer di-(2-ethylhexyl) phthalate (DEHP) permits classification of this compound as an animal carcinogen. For di-(2-ethylhexyl) adipate (DEHA) the evidence available is limited. The substances do not seem to possess any genotoxic properties. Adequate epidemiological data are also lacking. Exposure to DEHP and DEHA in Sweden and their toxicological properties have been analysed in detail by a group of experts appointed by the Products Control Board. Direct exposure in Sweden of humans in connection with the end use of these plasticizers present in plasticized PVC has been expected, as a rule, to be extremely low according to the Products Control Board, in the exposure survey. Considerably higher exposure has been found in certain categories of processing industries, and is also associated with dialysis of patients suffering from kidney disease, with the use of blood products, and with the use of plasticized PVC as packaging material for foods (see Section 4.4.4).

SOOTS, TARS, MINERAL OILS AND POLYCYCLIC AROMATIC HYDROCARBONS (PAHs)

Under this heading are included several products derived from various fuels, in particular fossil fuels, including certain constituents which can be characterized chemically—including polycyclic hydrocarbons (e.g. BaP). These substances have long been present in the human work environment, and neoplasia of the scrotum was described as an occupational disease in chimney-sweeps by Percival Potts as early as 1775.

Soots, coal tar and distillation products derived from them, such as creosote oil, anthracene oil and pitch, have been demonstrated to induce skin cancer in humans. Furthermore, a causal association exists between skin cancer (including that of the scrotum), and exposure to mineral oil. There are certain indications that oil mist may cause other types of cancer, for example in the lungs, nasal cavities and gastrointestinal tract. According to the IARC there is sufficient evidence to show that these products are carcinogenic in man.

The change-over to the modern solvent-refined oils—involving the elimination of a number of carcinogenic impurities from these products—as well as the introduction of protective measures in the field of occupational safety, have resulted in a drastic reduction in the number of cases of malignant disease which may be ascribed to oil exposure in recent years. To all appearances, skin cancer caused by mineral oils is nowadays rare.

The carcinogenic activity of the combustion products of different fossil fuels has been associated, among other things, with polycyclic hydrocarbons such as BaP. According to the IARC there is sufficient evidence of the carcinogenicity of BaP in several animal species. In addition, there is sufficient evidence to demonstrate a causal connection between cancer in humans and certain types of occupational mixed exposures where BaP appears as *one* of the components involved.

Exposure to BaP as such will occur solely in scientific laboratories. In the workplace and in the general environment, BaP occurs together with other PAHs. As a rule BaP in these circumstances only accounts for few per cent of the total PAHs. Where the air is polluted by exhaust products (including tobacco smoke) from the combustion of oil, coal or other types of organic matter, a number of other substances also appear. BaP and several other PAHs are mutagenic as well as carcinogenic. This is also true for several compounds of structurally diverse types formed by combustion. Exposure to PAHs occurs in the working environment, especially in coal-gas plants and coke oven plants, in aluminium factories and in the production of carbon electrodes, in the handling of pitch and asphalt, as well as in chimney-sweeping.

It is important to realize that, depending on the context, risk estimates based on BaP may have different meanings:

(a) the substance BaP itself (particularly in risk estimates based on animal experiments);
(b) BaP as an indicator substance for the whole category of PAHs or POM (polycyclic organic matter; also including compounds with other atoms, in particular nitrogen and sulphur);
(c) BaP as an indicator substance for all carcinogens involved.

The reason why BaP has been so frequently used as an indicator substance for air pollutants is apparently historical; it was identified quite early on as an active component in the classical complex of mixed occupational carcinogens represented by soot and pitch. Because of its instability it is in fact not suitable as an indicator substance (see Ehrenberg, 1984a).

Because of the great variations occurring during different combustion cycles—even in the same source—and because BaP only represents a small part of the total genotoxic activity of the pollutants in air, this substance is a poor indicator of the carcinogenic effects of air pollution (Holmberg and Ahlborg, 1983; Lundberg et al., 1983). The risks associated with the relatively high concentrations of BaP in an aluminium plant, for example, can therefore not be assessed by the same procedure of extrapolation as used for air pollutants in an urban area, since the levels of BaP and PAHs here are mixed with lower levels of other mutagens/carcinogens.

In the body BaP and other PAHs are transformed to mutagenic and carcinogenic epoxides. Due to initiation caused by alkylation of DNA, a linear dose–response relationship can be expected. In epidemiological investigations an increased incidence of neoplasias of the lung, bladder and skin has been demonstrated in workers exposed to PAHs at work (Lundberg et al., 1983).

Within an uncertainty factor of 2, inhalation of air containing 1 ng BaP m^{-3} (used as an indicator substance for all combustion pollutants) leads, according to Pike, to a risk of lung cancer of 10^{-5} per year (Pike et al., 1975). The calculated collective dose in Sweden (see Table 4.18) corresponds to an average air concentration of 0.5 ng m^{-3}. Using Pike's risk coefficient this would correspond to about 40 cases of lung cancer in the whole of Sweden per year, mainly confined to densely populated urban areas, which contain about 2 million inhabitants. This estimate is not significantly different from the risk of lung cancer associated with air pollution in urban areas calculated by Cederlöf et al. (1978)— 5–10 cases per 100 000 persons per year—and is of the same magnitude as the 'urban factor' which appears in different contexts in epidemiological investigations (see Chapter 5). When used as a point of reference for the calculation of expected cancer risk induced by general air pollutants, it should be realized that BaP, other PAHs and the majority of initiators also contribute doses and therefore cancer risks to other organs than the lung (Ehrenberg and Törnqvist 1984). In comparison with exposure via inhaled air, the largest intake of BaP is from consumption of foodstuffs (see Section 4.4.4).

In experiments with mice and cell cultures the cancer risk associated with absorption of BaP as such has been tentatively compared to the corresponding risk associated with gamma radiation (Forsberg-Karlsson et al., 1983). The uptake of 1 mg BaP (kg body weight^1 was considered to give effects of the same magnitude as 7 rad (0.07 Gy) of gamma radiation (i.e. 1 mg BaP kg^{-1} corresponds to 7 rad-equivalents). The relation between man and mouse as to the dose of carcinogenic metabolite(s) has not yet been determined, and the risk estimate given above should therefore only be used in risk calculation with great caution. With an average intake through inhalation of 4 µg BaP per person per year, and using a risk coefficient for cancer induction of 2×10^{-4} per man-rad (2×10^{-2} per man-Sv), 0.5 cases of cancer (total) would be expected to occur annually in a population of 8 million people. As explained in more detail in Section 6.6, 'the urban effect' may contribute about 100 cases of lung cancer with a margin of error of at least a factor of 2. The total number of cases of cancer per year may lie within the range 100–1000. The contribution of BaP here appears to be less than 0.3 per cent of the cases, and total PAHs—having an effect approximately five times greater—could be responsible for a few per cent of the total risk. These figures are probably representative for smoking too, and are also in accordance with the relatively low excess risks found in aluminium plants in comparison with the high exposures to PAHs.

SYNTHETIC SWEETENERS

The IARC has expressed the opinion that certain evidence exists of carcinogenic activity (bladder cancer) for cyclamate and saccharin administered orally at high doses to experimental animals. Sufficient evidence of genotoxicity is not available for these compounds.

No increased risk of neoplasia has been found in consumers of artificial sweeteners, in spite of extensive epidemiological studies. However, it cannot be entirely excluded, on the basis of these investigations, that these substances may act as weak promotive carcinogens, having no or insignificant effects at low intakes.

VINYL CHLORIDE

In 1974, more than 40 years after vinyl chloride was first used in the chemical industry, the first cases of angiosarcoma of the liver were reported in workers employed in the production of PVC (polyvinyl chloride). The first report was rapidly followed by others from various parts of the industrialized world, each independently demonstrating that exposure to vinyl chloride is associated with an increased risk of cancer in man. Besides the liver, tumours were also found in the brain, lung and lymphatic system. Vinyl chloride is carcinogenic in the mouse, rat and hamster as well.

In Sweden two cases of haemangiosarcoma have been reported to be associated with the production of PVC (Byrèn and Holmberg, 1974). An additional three cases have been found in a population of 700 workers at risk (unpublished study). A cohort study from plants producing PVC confirmed this observation, in that a 4–5-fold increase in the risk of liver and pancreatic tumours was found. However, no increased cancer risk could be demonstrated for any part of the body in a cohort study of workers employed in the PVC-processing industry (Holmberg et al., 1979).

The IARC considers that there is sufficient evidence of the carcinogenicity of vinyl chloride in humans. In Sweden exposure to this substance has been limited by the introduction of a low hygienic limit value in the workplace: 3 mg m^{-3}.[8]

Certain industrial processes and occupational exposures

THE CONSTRUCTION INDUSTRY
In Sweden a significant excess risk of neoplasia of the respiratory organs has been noted in tube fitters, workers employed in insulating work and painters (Englund 1980). In addition, increased incidences of cancer of the stomach and larynx were observed among the tube fitters, and of the larynx, oesophagus and liver in painters. The aetiology here is obscure. For the tube fitters and workers employed in insulating work, asbestos has probably played a role in neoplasia of the respiratory tract.

THE RUBBER INDUSTRY
In the rubber industry a large number of chemicals are handled, several of which are suspected carcinogens. Types of cancer noted in epidemiological studies outside Sweden include leukaemia, neoplasia of the bladder, stomach, lungs, and possibly also of the skin, duodenum and prostate as well as lymphoma. According to the IARC, sufficient evidence exists here to establish a causal association. In a recently published study (Holmberg et al., 1982) of the Swedish rubber industry, an increased mortality from neoplasms of the digestive and respiratory systems was observed in certain production workers. Furthermore, an increase in morbidity from tumours of the liver and pancreas as well as malignant melanomas was noted.

Work in Chemical Laboratories

In a study of Swedish chemical engineers who graduated from the Royal Institute of Technology in Stockholm during the years 1930–1959, a significant excess mortality has been demonstrated in comparison with architects who graduated during the same period (Olin and Ahlbom, 1980). The relative mortality increase in neoplasia among the chemists can mostly be classified in two categories: leukaemia/lymphoma and brain tumours (gliomas). The aetiology is not clear, but certain studies indicate that chemical exposure during training and subsequent professional activity is of major importance. This type of exposure has not been evaluated by the IARC.

The Leather Industry

Elevated incidences of nasal cancer (adenocarcinoma) have been noted in workers employed in shoe manufacture. Here leather dust has been held responsible. In addition to adenocarcinoma, other types of nasal neoplasia were also found. A few studies indicate an association between neoplasia of the bladder and work in the leather industry. Benzene, which was formerly used as a solvent by shoemakers, also led to the appearance of leukaemias among these workers.

According to the IARC there is sufficient evidence to prove that cancer results from certain exposures among such workers.

Nickel Production

High excess incidences of cancer of the lungs and nasal cavities have been reported in investigations outside Sweden among workers in older smelters. Occupational safety precautions introduced appear to have reduced the risk greatly and, according to the IARC, no increase in risk has been noted in a series of recent investigations. The observed carcinogenic action has been attributed to nickel sulphides and/or nickel oxides and possibly nickel carbonyl. In experimental animals nickel subsulphide and nickel carbonyl have both been shown to induce pulmonary tumours when inhaled.

Nickel and its compounds have been classified as carcinogens with hygienic limit values by the Board of Occupational Safety and Health.

Wood Products Industry (Excluding Pulp and Paper)

Studies from Sweden and other countries have demonstrated excess neoplasia of the nasal sinuses (adenocarcinoma) in workers employed in the furniture-making industry. Wood dust is considered the causative agent in this case. Relative risks in the order of 10–100 have been reported for this comparatively rare type of tumour. In a few studies an association between nasal cancer and work in the lumber and sawmill industries has been suggested.

Wood dust has been classified as a carcinogenic agent with a hygienic limit value by the Board of Occupational Safety and Health.

Pharmaceuticals

All drugs may cause side-effects, and their use presupposes that a balance is struck between the benefits of the preparation and the risk of side-effects. The risk of neoplasia induced by drug therapy is one of the side-effects which must be taken into consideration. The clinical status of the patient and the degree of risk determine whether or not a risk of this nature is acceptable. In diseases characterized by short survival, and in grave illnesses where no adequate therapeutic alternatives are available, the risk of cancer may be ignored. In more benign conditions with a favourable prognosis even a small cancer risk can be unacceptable. Since even a small individual risk may involve a considerable number of induced cases of cancer, particular vigilance is required in the case of preparations widely used for treating groups of patients with expected long survival (e.g. analgesics, sedatives, hypotensives, antibiotics and oral contraceptives).

Table 4.12 presented sales volumes in Sweden of carcinogenic drugs, or drugs suspected of being carcinogenic, for the year 1980. Below, two areas covering specific problems are discussed: therapy using cytostatics, and hormone therapy. In addition, comments are given on certain other constituents of pharmaceuticals.

CYTOSTATICS ('CELL-POISONS')

These agents kill cells, or inhibit their replication by interfering with the synthesis of DNA, RNA and proteins. Most of these compounds have genotoxic properties in short-term tests and several have also proved carcinogenic in animal experiments. The demonstration of carcinogenic effects in man has, for several reasons, been surrounded with considerable difficulties. One problem has been that these drugs have been used to a great extent for the treatment of patients who by the nature of their illness have a short life expectancy. Another reason is that a combination of several cytostatic agents or a combination of cytostatics and radiotherapy has often been used, making it difficult to clarify which agent(s) was responsible for the carcinogenic effect. The different cytostatic agents have produced a variable carcinogenic response in experimental animals. Alkylating agents such as nitrogen mustard, cyclophosphamide, and similar compounds have as a rule shown a carcinogenic effect, while the so-called antimetabolites (5-fluorouracil, methotrexate, 6-mercaptopurine, cytosine arabinoside, etc.) and the mitotic poisons (vinca alkaloids, podophyllin derivatives) have usually produced a negative or questionable carcinogenic response. For some cytostatic preparations exhibiting complex effects on

DNA and RNA and on cell division (adriamycin, dacarbazine and the nitrosoureas BCNU and CCNU), sufficient or limited evidence of carcinogenicity in animals is available.

According to the IARC there is sufficient evidence of carcinogenicity in humans for the following alkylating agents: cyclophosphamide, chlorambucil, Myleran R (busulphan; 1,4-butanediol dimethane-sulphonate) azathioprine R, melphalan and the combination MOPP (which contains nitrogen mustard, vincristine, procarbazine and prednisone); the last is used mainly for the therapeutic treatment of Hodgkin's disease. Other alkylating compounds which appear as active constituents in cytostatics like lomustine (CCNU, 1-(2-chloroethyl) - 3 - cyclohexyl - 1 - nitrosourea), BCNU and dacarbazine should for practical purposes also be considered as carcinogenic to humans on the basis of experiments in animals and other evidence.

Consequently, it must be assumed that several cytostatics possess a certain carcinogenic action, even though this has been demonstrated by epidemiological methods for only a few compounds. At the same time it should be emphasized that the incidence of malignant tumours induced by chemotherapy—as in the case of radiation therapy—appears to be low.

The treatment of incurable cancer remains the major indication for the use of cytostatics, that is the therapy of patients with a relatively short expected survival, where a carcinogenic effect may be ignored. For small groups of patients cytostatics may have a curative effect (certain tumours in children, malignant lymphoma, malignant tumours of the placenta). The serious nature of the illness and the lack of equally effective therapeutic alternatives make it necessary and acceptable to disregard the risks of inducing a new cancer. Whenever possible, more carcinogenic combinations of cytostatics are replaced by other preparations believed to possess a lower carcinogenic activity.

The risk of carcinogenic effects with adjuvant therapy must be considered a much more serious problem. Such chemotherapeutic treatment is given to patients who are free of symptoms after radical surgery and/or radiotherapy, with the intention of obliterating remaining but undetectable tumour cells, in order to prevent tumour recurrence. In such a situation it is not possible to judge on a case-by-case basis which patients can really benefit from the therapy, and the effects can be evaluated only by statistical studies on the frequency of recidivation and on survival. If a large proportion of the patients were to remain free of symptoms even without adjuvant treatment (as is the case in mammary and intestinal neoplasias), the possible benefits must be balanced carefully against the risks of serious side-effects (including cancer induction). It is important that benefits in the form of reduced tumour recurrence and improved survival should be unambiguously documented. Adjuvant therapy using cytostatics is therefore often tested by controlled prospective studies in order to facilitate future evaluation of the results and the side-effects.

Cytostatics are also used to induce immunosuppression in patients suffering from auto-immunological disorders or in patients who have undergone transplant surgery (e.g. a kidney transplant). The most commonly used preparation here is the alkylating substance azathioprine, mostly in combination with a glucocorticosteroid (e.g. prednisone). An increased incidence of certain malignant tumours, mainly malignant lymphoma and skin cancer, has been found in patients who have had kidney transplants. However, it is not clear whether this can be ascribed to the immunodepression, or whether it is due to a direct carcinogenic action exerted by the alkylating drug. Since no carcinogenic effect from long-term treatment with glucocorticosteroids alone has been found, the IARC has judged azathioprine to be a human carcinogen. However, the serious nature of the medical conditions involved here means that the risk of cancer may be ignored when there is no equally effective therapeutic alternative.

Cytostatics are also sometimes used in the treatment of non-neoplastic diseases with a good prognosis for survival (e.g. treatment of psoriasis with methotrexate). This usually involves much lower doses than in the treatment of a tumour disease. However, in comparison, although the cancer risk might be low, great restraint is usually exercised in the treatment of such benign disorders with cytostatics, and even for compounds for which no carcinogenic risk has been demonstrated.

HORMONAL THERAPY

Several extensive studies have shown that the treatment of women (usually for disorders connected with the menopause and ovarian insufficiency) with oestrogenic hormones, in particular 'conjugated oestrogens', for a relatively long time (more than 3 years) is associated with an increased risk (4 –10 times excess risk) of endometrial carcinoma. The latency period for induction of neoplasia appears to be remarkably short. In the USA the introduction of this therapy during the 1960s resulted in a significant increase in this type of cancer during the following decade, followed by a drastic reduction to previous levels, linked to the decreased use of this treatment and a reduction in the time over which it was administered. A cohort study recently conducted in Sweden did not produce indications of a similar increase in the incidence of endometrial cancer (Persson et al., 1983). It should also be pointed out that a possible confounding factor in epidemiological studies of this kind is that it is often difficult—sometimes even impossible — to distinguish microscopically between a benign oestrogen-induced hyperplasia and a highly differentiated neoplasia of the endometrium.

The different experiences with oestrogen therapy in the USA and Sweden may have several causes. One is the differences as to preferred types of preparation between the two countries; another that therapy in Sweden has been characterized by lower oestrogen dosages used, a shorter period of administration and—possibly crucial to the outcome— the practice of interrupting oestrogen treatment regularly to induce a periodic shedding of the endometrium (e.g. by administration of gestagen). On the other hand, the follow-up period of the Swedish cohort has, on average, been only 3–4 years, which could be insufficient time for the carcinogenic activity of these hormonal agents to manifest itself. Thus, in Sweden too a certain increase in the incidence of endometrial cancer may have occurred. However, it should be emphasized that—provided an early diagnosis is made—this is a type of cancer characterized by a favourable prognosis.

The issue of a possible increased risk of mammary neoplasia as a result of oestrogen therapy has been intensely debated. Extensive epidemiological investigations have failed to provide clear-cut evidence to support such a fear, and even if there is such a risk, it must certainly be low. The risk of breast cancer is also being studied in the Swedish investigation mentioned above (Persson et al., 1983).

According to the IARC sufficient evidence exists to prove a causal relationship between the administration of conjugated oestrogens and endometrial cancer.

For some progestogens and oestrogens, including norethisterone, mestranol and ethynyloestradiol, it is felt that there is sufficient evidence of carcinogen activity in experimental animals, while for a number of other substances belonging to this class of compounds the evidence is limited. According to the IARC no adequate proof of genotoxicity exists for these substances.

Regarding combined oral contraceptives, the IARC has expressed the opinion that sufficient evidence is available to prove a cause–effect relationship between the use of oral contraceptives and a certain type of rare, histologically benign tumour of the liver (vascular adenomas associated with a risk of internal haemorrhages). A decreased incidence of neoplasia of the ovary and the endometrium has been found in users of oral contraceptives, while increased *and* decreased incidences have been reported for breast cancer. However, recently published epidemiological investigations have lent support to suspicions of an increased risk of breast cancer in women who—from a young age and before the birth of the first child—have used these preparations for long periods of time (Pike et al., 1983; McPherson et al., 1983). From the methodological point of view these studies are somewhat ambiguous, and in an attempt to further illuminate this issue an extensive study is currently being planned in Sweden.

In contrast to the decrease in endometrial cancer found after use of combined contraceptives, there is a certain amount of evidence that sequential contraceptives—in particular preparations containing relatively large quantities of a potent oestrogen (e.g. 100 µg of ethinyloestradiol)—cause an increase in endometrial cancer. Contraceptives of this type are no longer registered for use in Sweden.

The synthetic oestrogen diethylstilboestrol has been proved to be a transplacental human carcinogen. Clear-cell carcinoma of the vagina, a very rare cancer with high mortality, has appeared in young girls whose mothers were treated with diethylstilboestrol during pregnancy. The hormone has been found to be carcinogenic in several animal species, and the IARC regards the evidence of carcinogenicity of diethylstilboestrol in animals and in humans as sufficient. In Sweden one pharmaceutical preparation contains a phosphate ester of diethylstilboestrol (phosphestrol) which is used solely for the therapeutic treatment of cancer of the prostate.

Oxymetholone is a hepatotoxic testosterone derivative with an anabolic effect, which in several studies has been implicated in the induction of liver cancer (hepatocellular carcinoma) in man. Doll and Peto (1981), as well as a group of experts in problems related to cancer, associated with the Office of Technology Assessment of the US Congress (OTA, 1981), have judged these types of anabolic steroids to be human carcinogens, whilst the IARC feels that there is limited evidence of a carcinogenic effect of oxymetholone in humans. As the substance occurs in Sweden only as a constituent of a preparation registered for use in cases of aplastic anaemia, the quantities in use cannot be great.

Even though oestrogens, in particular, are currently responsible for considerable collective doses in Sweden, risk quantification of the kind carried out for genotoxic agents does not seem warranted for steroid hormones with a likely promotive/co-carcinogenic effect.

METRONIDAZOLE

This compound is present in certain drugs used in Sweden for the therapeutic treatment of infections caused by *Trichomonas vaginalis* (colpitis of the vagina) as well as for certain infections such as amoebic dysentery, which are rarer in this country. The treatment periods are relatively short.

In low doses metronidazole induces lung tumours and lymphoma in mice as well as tumours of the liver, pituitary and mammary glands in rats. The IARC considers this sufficient evidence of carcinogenicity in animals. In two epidemiological studies an increased incidence of cervical cancer was found in women treated with metronidazole, mostly for colpitis caused by *T. vaginalis*. On the other hand, it is well known that this infection as such is associated with an increased incidence of this cancer. Therefore the IARC considers that the evidence implicating metronidazole in human neoplasia is insufficient.

In Sweden the medical profession has been alerted by information from the National Board of Health and Welfare (NBHW, 1983) on the carcinogenic and mutagenic effects as well as on the adverse effects on reproduction caused by metronidazole and some closely related drugs. The importance of not prolonging the period of treatment more than that necessary to obtain therapeutic effect is emphasized and a reminder is given that these drugs should be prescribed only when absolutely necessary for medical reasons.

PHENACETIN

Long-term usage of analgesics containing phenacetin has been demonstrated to increase the risk of neoplasia of the urinary tract, especially of the pelvis and the ureter. The effect can probably be ascribed to phenacetin, which is an animal carcinogen. A well-known example of such usage from Sweden is the Huskvarna armaments factory where the workers habitually used 'headache powder' containing phenacetin for long periods of time. Among these subjects, a high incidence of cancers of the urinary tract was later observed. The IARC has included analgesic mixtures containing phenacetin in the group of human carcinogens (phenacetin itself has been classified in group 2A). As noted earlier (Table 4.12), all preparations containing phenacetin were banned in Sweden in 1982.

PHENOBARBITAL AND PHENYTOIN

These compounds are present as active ingredients in drugs used in Sweden for the treatment of psychiatric disturbances and organic neurological diseases, particularly epilepsy. Limited epidemiological evidence is available for the carcinogenicity of these compounds in humans. The statistical association seems most clear-cut for tumours of the central nervous system. However, certain facts point to a link between the actual epileptic condition and an increased incidence of tumours at this site. There are also some indications that phenytoin may act as a transplacental carcinogen. The association is less clear for other types of neoplasia (lymphoma and phenytoin; liver carcinoma and phenobarbital). Phenytoin has induced lymphoma and leukaemia in mice, and phenobarbital has produced liver tumours in rats and mice, which is considered as limited evidence of carcinogenicity in animals by the IARC.

OTHER PHARMACEUTICALS

Considerable exposure to *oxazepam* occurs, but no adequate evidence is available to implicate this substance in the induction of cancer. The compound has not been classified as carcinogenic by the IARC.

Certain data do exist indicating a carcinogenic action with *griseofulvin* (used in the treatment of fungal infections) and *reserpine* (against hypertension). Griseofulvin, in particular, is widely used and usually for relatively extended treatment periods (up to 12 months). However, no evidence of human carcinogenicity exists at present. Among other substances for which there is no proof of human carcinogenicity, and where the relevance of the carcinogenic effects seen in animal experiments appears to be questionable, are *captan* and *selenium sulphide*, which are used against seborrhoea and dandruff. There is also a limited dermal exposure in Sweden to *DDT* (a group 2B substance according to the IARC), present in preparations against skin parasites such as scabies and lice.

4.4.6 Concluding evaluations

As was stated earlier, the aim of the exposure review was not to create a comprehensive survey of all the substances on the lists drawn up by the IARC, the NCI and the secretariat of the Cancer Committee. The actual objectives were:

(a) to investigate the availability of Swedish exposure data for the substances included on these lists;
(b) to study the methods and routines used by the authorities to procure exposure data, and to attempt to evaluate their relevance to Swedish conditions;
(c) to try to demonstrate the levels of exposure of the Swedish population to carcinogens and suspected carcinogens by means of some illustrative examples.

General conclusions concerning exposure data and potential for exposure

In spite of the deficiencies in the documentation available, it seems clear that exposure in Sweden to many of the carcinogens and suspected carcinogens on the IARC and NCI lists is very low. This is particularly true of most substances known to be carcinogenic in humans. For several of the compounds there is no known commercial use.

Fifteen of the substances on the IARC list are reported to be used only in laboratories, and for an additional 14 compounds there is no commercial production in Sweden. Another 41 substances from the survey lists have likewise no known practical use in Sweden outside a couple of research laboratories. However, some of these compounds can be formed during combustion and/or are present as impurities in certain products. In addition, some 20 of the pesticide chemicals on the lists are banned in Sweden, but may be present as residues in imported foods.

Data accurate enough to permit a reliable estimate of individual and collective doses in Sweden are available for only a few compounds. Current information indicates that very little is known about most substances. As illustrated by their responses, the government agencies questioned use collective doses as a basis for risk estimation to only a very limited extent.

The role of the regulatory system in providing a basis for reviewing exposure conditions

Certain chemicals with specialized applications or known to be highly toxic, have long been subject to special regulatory control. Included in this category are chemicals where, *a priori*, a high human exposure can be assumed—such as food additives and pharmaceuticals. Pesticides are another such group subject to regulations over and above the basic rules on chemicals, partly because their mode of use involves a high likelihood of exposure and partly because their (intended) biological effects often imply toxic properties. With a few exceptions (discussed below) these products require approval from a central authority before they are released commercially. Such procedures provide a good basis for obtaining information on function, manner of handling, and other data which can be used in estimating human exposure. For substances present in these products the exposure data are naturally more detailed than for most other substances. For such products, data are also recorded by licensing authorities on actual sales volumes, in computerized registers.

Other substances are subject to special regulations because of their extreme toxicity to man or other living organisms. Regulation of such compounds, by banning certain usages and so on, has been introduced as a preventive measure, sometimes irrespective of whether their exposure may have caused problems or not. In cases of unavoidable exposure, restrictions such as maximum permitted levels in foods and hygienic limit values in the work environment and the like have been introduced in order to keep exposure to a minimum. The more or less extensive surveillance to ensure compliance with these regulations provides good opportunities in principle for obtaining a general view of actual exposure conditions. The same should apply to emissions into air and water of hazardous substances from industrial and similar activities – to the extent that individual pollutants have been specified for a certain emission source.

Information on some groups of products

Through the registration procedure and sales data, the Swedish National Board of Health and Welfare possesses almost completely comprehensive information on exposure to known and suspected carcinogens in pharmaceuticals, although individually related exposure data cannot be obtained from the sales volumes.

In recent years several of the substances of interest here have been eliminated from pharmaceutical preparations which are not used in the treatment of terminal diseases. However, certain questionable uses remain which result in a relatively high exposure to a few compounds which induce cancer in experimental animals.

The present cancer rates reflect the exposure levels of several decades ago. The registration for one preparation containing the well-known human carcinogen arsenic trioxide was cancelled as late as 1971. Since arsenic trioxide was present in a number of vitamin preparations and tonics, previous exposure to inorganic arsenic—expressed as the collective dose—may have been considerable. Similarly, 2.5 million defined daily doses of phenacetin were consumed in 1980, but registrations for preparations containing this substance were withdrawn in 1982. Thiourea was removed as an inactive constituent from a mild sedative for children in the same year.

The available information indicates that the incidence of drug-induced cancer in Sweden is low at present. For the USA, Doll and Peto (1981) estimated that at most a few per cent of the total cancer mortality can be ascribed to 'medicines and medical procedures'. Cancer is, nevertheless, a serious side-effect which as far as possible must be avoided. The correspondence between experimental results and carcinogenic properties is sufficiently well established to enable the identification of potential human carcinogens with initiating and mutagenic properties during the testing of new drugs. This correspondence is probably much less satisfactory for compounds which act as promoters, for example hormones. In so far as a compound, after having been tested, is put to use as a drug, the outcome of a continuous monitoring of its effects through clinical and epidemiological studies will, naturally, be of paramount importance in evaluating the carcinogenic potential of a drug, irrespective of the way it causes tumours. Cancer testing of pharmaceuticals also involves a problem of a diametrically opposite kind: the possible rejection of a valuable drug— the use of which for the therapy of a serious disease would involve only a negligible risk of cancer— on the basis of a rigorous interpretation of the results obtained in experimental animals. The risk–benefit analysis which has to be carried out for all suspected carcinogens for which experimental data are available is often very complicated in the case of pharmaceuticals.

Present regulations require that documentary material for drug registration shall include a report and evaluation of the possible mutagenic and carcinogenic potential of the substance. This requirement is applicable to active as well as to inactive ingredients. The possibility of co-carcinogenic and promoting effects should also be taken into account. Therefore, from experimental data, the National Board of Health and Welfare can evaluate the carcinogenic potential of the ingredients of any new pharmaceutical registered today. However, considerable problems remain for older pharmaceuticals. This has implications also for exposure analysis with regard to potentially carcinogenic agents, since the identification of such agents is the first step.

Of the roughly 2500 pharmaceutical preparations registered in February 1983, some 1300 were granted registration before 1970, at a time when there were no general requirements governing testing of drugs for carcinogenicity in Sweden. Information on the carcinogenic or mutagenic properties of these products is rarely available, and it would be desirable for the relevant authorities to have the power to examine and monitor both active and inactive constituents of these older medicinal products. There is a conflict between the need to deal with applications for registration of new drugs without undue delay on the one hand, and the need to systematically follow and evaluate the effects of products already accepted for use, on the other hand. Besides complaining of lack of resources for the latter purpose, the Pharmaceuticals Department of the Board of Health and Welfare also points out that the agency rarely receives—without a special request—information from registration holders on new findings concerning mutagenic or carcinogenic properties of registered pharmaceuticals.

Similar problems also seem to exist for certain food additives and pesticides. For two of the main pesticides used in Swedish agriculture, with an annual consumption of altogether about 2000 tonnes (dichloroprop and MCPA, which are chlorinated phenoxy propionic and -acetic acids, respectively), the Products Control Board did not in 1982 possess any adequate information on animal studies of the effects of long-term administration (including carcinogenicity). For another pesticide, used as a fungicide in the cultivation of potatoes, lettuce and other produce (consumption 200 tonnes), the data were incomplete in this respect. However, an updating procedure now exists for improving the state of knowledge concerning previously registered products.

A considerable proportion of the cancers seen in the general population appear to be attributable to *dietary factors in general*. Several facts indicate the dominant role played by intake of certain normal major consitutents of foods, such as the proportion of fat in the diet and the amounts present of probable anticarcinogen factors like certain vitamins and selenium. On the other hand, the significance of foreign substances which have been intentionally or unintentionally added—or of compounds generated within the foodstuff—cannot be overlooked. Due to the high potential for exposure which may arise from the presence of carcinogenic substances in foods, analytical data for this type of product, which may be used as a basis for estimating total intakes, are of utmost importance.

In many cases extensive toxicological documentation is available for *food additives*. However, adequate investigations fulfilling modern requirements for the testing of carcinogens are not available for all types of additive. According to the US Food and Drug Administration (FDA) about 2300 'flavouring agents' are used in modern food technology, of which about 1300–1400 are synthetic. For a large number of such substances, toxicological testing has been inadequate (Morgenroth and Rulis, 1984). Within the framework of a programme aimed at improving the supporting documentation for all food additives in accordance with a system of prioritization based on degree of concern, the FDA has systematically evaluated this group of additives (US FDA, Bureau of Foods, 1982). The toxicological evaluation of essences and other flavouring agents appears to be an international problem. In Sweden this group of products is exempted from the requirement of an approval by the National Food Administration, and no comprehensive survey has been made of the occurrence of such substances in food products marketed in the country.

Relatively satisfactory data are available covering current exposures in Sweden to certain *impurities in foods*, like PAHs volatile nitrosamines and heavy metals. For other substances knowledge is more fragmentary, particularly in the area of data serving as a basis for the estimation of total intakes.

Mycotoxins provide an example of an exposure which needs to be more clearly defined (see also Section 4.3). Both past and present mycotoxin exposure may be important from the point of view of cancer induction. Practically no effort had been made to look at this type of exposure in Sweden until about 10 years ago. At that time high levels of mycotoxins could sometimes be found, particularly in certain imported products (aflatoxins in nuts). Today's low levels, for example in peanuts, cannot, however, be taken to reflect the size of current aflatoxin exposure of the Swedish population. Aflatoxins have also been identified in mouldy bread, which together with similar observations in other countries (Hanssen and Hagedorn, 1969) seem to render the issue more serious. Aflatoxins probably occur in other types of foodstuff in Sweden as well.

Exposure to other mycotoxins in foods may also constitute a health problem. Experimental data in animals indicate carcinogenic properties for sterigmatocystin, zearalenone and T-toxin (US National Research Council, 1982). For other mycotoxins (e.g. for a number of toxins derived from *Fusarium* and *Alternaria species*), adequate data on their effects after long-term administration are lacking, and the chemical analysis of several of these toxins is very difficult.

Residues in foods constitute the most important way in which the general population is exposed to pesticides. Here (as in the case of food contaminants from other sources), the possibility of new compounds forming by chemical reactions in the treated products must also be considered.

Certain types of product may give rise to an exposure situation which is analogous to the exposure caused by the registered chemical products discussed above. Here *packaging materials* and similar products are obvious candidates. The levels of vinyl chloride and acrylonitrile—which migrate from food-packaging materials—are regularly monitored, but other possibly carcinogenic substances can also migrate from packaging materials to foods. Sweden, unlike the USA, Holland and West Germany, does not compulsorily control or register food packaging materials.

Maximum acceptable levels in foods

In a Swedish programme for control of pesticide residues in fruits and vegetables, very low levels are found as a rule, which in 1983 were reported to only amount to fractions of the maximum acceptable level for the substance in question. Only in about 3 per cent of the analysed samples are these levels exceeded. On the basis of this, two matters of principle will be raised with regard to exposure analysis.

Firstly, although there exists an extensive and sophisticated programme for analysing chemical impurities in foods, it has not been possible to estimate total intakes for the different substances due to the manner in which the sampling has been conducted. The programme is primarily directed towards enforcing the maximum residue levels. The sampling programme has, therefore, in part focused on product categories where, on the basis of past experience, conspicuous levels can be expected to occur. This policy is sensible for controlling impurities thought to have a dose threshold for toxic effects, but does not lend itself to the estimation of total exposure to carcinogens without a known dose threshold. For the latter purpose, 'directed' surveys must be supplemented by a sampling which is statistically representative of the consumption pattern. Sampling along these lines has recently begun.

Secondly, it is important that the significance of the term 'maximum acceptable level' should be completely clear. In many cases such a concentration level may imply good or very good margins of safety, particularly where actual practical cirumstances permit this level to be set lower than what might be considered acceptable from the toxicological point of view. In other cases tolerance limits have been established in the absence of adequate investigations of the effects of long-term exposure, including possible carcinogenic effects (e.g. for the herbicides dichloroprop and MCPA mentioned earlier; see Swedish Special Panel, 1982). The need, from an administrative point of view, for some kind of standard has here been based on more limited toxicological data as well as on a knowledge of the concentration levels actually present. Such administrative tolerance levels have also been set for pesticides and other foreign compounds which, on the basis of results from long-term tests on experimental animals, should be considered as carcinogens or suspected carcinogens (aflatoxin, ethylthiourea, captan) and where in principle no 'acceptable daily intake' (ADI) can be established from a scientific point of view. Even though no ADI has been fixed for certain foreign substances (ADIs are usually determined as a result of international co-operation), there may still be a need for the control of such compounds in several countries, for example through some kind of tolerance levels. If the linear dose–response model is to be applied here, information concerning the (small) number of samples which have exceeded maximum acceptable levels in Sweden will not suffice to define individual or collective exposure and is, consequently, not an adequate basis for a risk assessment.

Although there are no grounds for alarm over the contamination of foodstuffs by carcinogens, the manner in which the tolerable levels have been arrived at and the scientific background to them should be taken into consideration. If data which could support a decision on a carcinogenic effect are lacking, or if the total exposure via food cannot be estimated even roughly, then no kind of sampling statistics based on maximum acceptable levels will be of any help in risk evaluation.

Other substances

For certain *heavy metals* like lead and cadmium, which have been under special regulation for other reasons than possible carcinogenicity, the government agencies jointly seem to possess quite extensive information on exposure conditions.

As for the use of *carcinogens in the work environment*, 18 of the 19 substances defined by the IARC as carcinogens or probable carcinogens in man are regulated by the Board of Occupational Safety and Health. These compounds only occur rarely in the workplace, partly because many of them are also regulated in other countries and/or are no longer produced commercially. In addition, about 60 experimental carcinogens are subject to special regulation by the Board of Occupational Safety and Health, which likewise ought to facilitate obtaining exposure data for these compounds when needed—at least relative to their use in the home industry. Since an all-inclusive register containing the compositions of various chemical products is not available, information on imported products is primarily dependent on the efforts of control and enforcement bodies (mainly the Labour Inspectorate). In the case of carcinogens with hygienic limit value in the workplace (category C), which may be utilized in a more general fashion, only for a few substances like asbestos, benzene and vinyl chloride have more extensive measurements of exposure been carried out, which may provide a basis for the estimation of collective doses.

As discussed previously, a considerable amount of data from Sweden and other countries is available relating to occupational exposure to pesticides as well as to pesticide residues in foods. In Swedish agriculture and forestry, handling of pesticides is limited to a defined number of application methods and other situations involving exposure to the chemicals in question. Furthermore, the physico chemical properties of the active ingredients are, as a rule, well known. Based on existing data and on experience derived from analogous situations, it should therefore be possible to predict the occupational exposure with sufficient accuracy, even for substances where actual measurements of exposure are inadequate.

Substances for which pre-marketing approval is required, or substances regulated in some other special way, constitute a very minor part of the *total chemical assortment*. This also applies to most carcinogens or suspected carcinogens. For the majority of the chemical substances categorized as carcinogens or suspected carcinogens, available information from authorities has been exceedingly poor. For most of the substances no exposure-related data are available at all, and when such information does exist, it is often very unreliable. Nor are international data on product function and use always applicable to conditions prevailing in Sweden.

From the viewpoint of risk, exposure to carcinogens *via the general environment*, such as urban air or ambient air outside a factory, is usually of less importance. Many of the substances listed by the IARC and NCI are used in Sweden in such a manner and/or in such low volumes as to preclude significant emissions into the environment.

However, among the compounds listed by the National Environmental Protection Board several appear which are handled or formed (e.g. by combustion) in large quantities, implying a considerable potential for exposure. A better picture needs to be obtained of existing exposure levels for these substances, not only from the viewpoint of cancer induction. Data from other countries are not always applicable to the particular situation of interest. Considerable efforts have been devoted to the analysis of combustion products from fossil fuels in Sweden. However, for a number of compounds of importance to health and the environment, current levels have not been adequately determined in terms of representative data for the general environment.

Some additional conclusions concerning information sources

Since fundamental information is lacking to a large degree on the use of products and occurrence of individual substances, directed surveys of particular branches of industry can be a useful tool for some purposes. As reported by the Board of Occupational Health and Safety, a relatively large number of products containing carcinogens or suspected carcinogens were identified in this way. Since it has not been possible to assess whether or not these are linked with significant exposures, a misleading impression may be given as to the real risks involved. In some cases the method of use indicates that a certain exposure may have occurred, as in the use of 1,2-dichloroethane for the cleansing and preparation of offset plates within the printing industry. In many other instances the exposures appear to have been insignificant, for example to certain aromatic amines present as impurities in quantities below 1 per cent in dyes used in the textile industry.

The availability of a *complete products register* would undoubtedly make it easier for the authorities to concentrate their efforts on substances which on the basis of their properties and the degree of exposure are assumed to entail a non-negligible risk. For such a register to be useful the information on composition would need to be supplemented by fairly detailed data on sales volumes, function, and methods of use.

Problems associated with sampling and chemical analysis

There are various problems associated with sampling and chemical analysis for exposure determination. For example, the few existing Swedish exposure data for the general environment which have been obtained under conditions sufficiently standardized to permit meaningful comparisons, still often provide inadequate information on background levels and on parameters necessary for judging whether the data are representative of the polluted environments investigated. As a result it is often difficult, or even impossible, to estimate collective doses for different population groups or for the entire population. With the creation of the National Swedish Environmental Monitoring Programme the situation can be expected to improve in the long term, at least for baseline data. For more polluted environments (e.g. certain bodies of water, and in particular urban areas) additional efforts seem to be needed to improve the quantity of data and the availability of information.

The scarcity of representative analytical data is not only a problem with the general environment. For the few dose estimates which have been provided for the work environment, the impression remains that data for some substances such as ethylene oxide may have been based on non-representative measurements. The difficulties associated with the estimation of collective doses based on analytical data derived from the control of foods have been discussed above. Furthermore, the extremely uneven distribution of damage caused by fungi in infested shipments of foods or raw materials for foods presents a serious problem when taking samples for the analysis of mycotoxins.

The lack of widely adopted standard analytical methods for a number of the substances listed by the IARC and NCI has been said to present a problem. This may be true as regards simple routine methods suitable for most analytical laboratories, to be applied at the request of regional and local authorities. Otherwise, current analytical methodology appears, in general, to be adequate for most of the substances discussed here. The analytical problems involved can most certainly be handled with the required precision by several central laboratories of internationally acceptable standards. The fact that analytical chemistry in Sweden is well developed scientifically, and often has good technical resources, does not contradict the fact that the generation of exposure-related data is generally speaking a neglected area. For this reason, improved central planning is called for, and increased co-ordination of sampling for the purpose of producing such data (related questions will also be discussed in Chapter 11).

4.5 Physical factors

4.5.1 Physical carcinogens—background

In this section the carcinogenic action of different kinds of radiation is discussed. The National Institute of Radiation Protection (NIRP) has reviewed and described the available sources of information on exposure to ionizing radiation in Sweden (NIRP, 1984), that is, supporting material of the same kind as has been requested from the other government agencies in the field of carcinogenic chemicals.

Ionizing radiation and ultraviolet (UV) light are proven carcinogenic agents which are natural components of the human environment, but ones to which certain human activities result in increased exposure. In other cases the radiation is generated by artificial means. These agents will be discussed in Sections 4.5.2 (ionizing radiation) and 4.5.3 (UV light) respectively.

The possibility of an unacceptable cancer risk being caused by low energy radiation like microwaves and radio waves is considered unlikely at current collective doses in Sweden (Anderstam et al., 1983), if indeed these forms of radiation can cause any detectable carcinogenic effect (at intensities that will not cause burns).

A statistical correlation between an increased incidence of cancer in children and of certain cancers in adults and exposure to alternating current fields has been reported from other countries (see the report prepared by IVA/BEEF 1983). An epidemiological study of this question is currently being conducted in Sweden. Further scientific efforts are necessary to clarify whether or not we are dealing with a true causal association in this context.

Non-specific physical agents causing burns and other kinds of wounds, or which may induce a chronic local tissue irritation, may facilitate the induction of neoplasia by means of a mechanism which may be defined, at least in operational terms, as a non-specific promotion.

The types of radiation which are important in the aetiology of cancer are traditionally classified in the two following categories: *electromagnetic waves* (gamma radiation, X-rays, UV light) and *particulate radiation* (alpha, beta, proton, neutron beams, etc.). When such radiation passes through matter, its intensity is diminished by interaction between the radiation beam and the atoms and molecules of the medium. How this interaction occurs depends on the character (charged or neutral particles, electromagnetic waves) and energy (wavelength) of the radiation as well as on the nature of the irradiated material.

UV light loses most of its energy to the molecules of the medium by inducing energetic excited electronic states. X-rays and gamma rays are electromagnetic waves of much higher energy (shorter wavelength), and are therefore much more penetrating. These types of radiation also induce excitations, but the energy is sufficiently high to cause the ejection of electrons from atoms and molecules, which are thus transformed (ionized) into electrically charged ions.

The electrons ejected in the primary ionization events have, in turn, sufficient surplus energy to cause additional secondary ionizations. Particulate radiation, such as alpha radiation from radioactive elements, likewise loses most of its energy by inducing ionization in the irradiated medium.

For this reason, such high-energy radiation is known as *ionizing radiation*. The intensity of electromagnetic waves, such as gamma rays, is gradually attenuated as the radiation passes through matter, and gradually approaches zero. Particulate radiation differs from electromagnetic waves in that it has limited ranges of penetration in different materials.

4.5.2 Ionizing radiation

General aspects of dose–risk relationships

The carcinogenic effects of ionizing radiation have been demonstrated in experimental animals and in populations of exposed humans, primarily the survivors of the nuclear explosions over Hiroshima and Nagasaki and groups of patients exposed to ionizing radiation for medical purposes. Radiation—as a carcinogenic agent—has been the most thoroughly studied of all environmental factors from the dose–response viewpoint, and has been the subject of great public attention all over the world. For this reason, radiation carcinogenesis has played a central role in the evolution of theories and hypotheses about mechanisms of tumour induction (see Chapter 3), and has also provided the basis for a risk philosophy that is of interest in the management of other environmental risks (see Lindell, 1978, 1984; Ehrenberg, 1974, 1984b).

Despite this great publicity, the effects of radiation appear to be rather small compared with the cancer incidence and mortality from other causes (see Chapters 2 and 6). The total number of cancer cases which can be ascribed to exposure to radiation among the 250 000 survivors from Hiroshima and Nagasaki has been estimated at around 500 to date, corresponding to an increase of about 5 per cent over the number of cases that would have been expected to arise from other causes (WHO, 1984). It should be added that an increased cancer incidence would certainly not be the most significant consequence of a nuclear war. Acute casualties and devastating environmental effects would be far more serious (*Ambio*, 1982).

With the aim of preventing unnecessary risks to individuals and groups, strict rules have been introduced in most countries during the last few decades to prevent occupational exposure as well as exposure of the general population to radiation. In Sweden this task falls under the jurisdiction of the National Institute of Radiation Protection.

Types of ionizing radiation

Gamma radiation and X-rays are in principle identical and differ only in their source: X-rays are generated by the impact of fast electrons on the heavy anode material of the X-ray tube, while gamma radiation originates from the decay of radioactive elements.

Particulate radiation is mainly produced from various types of radioactive decay, but it is also formed from the absorption of electromagnetic waves by matter as follows:

Type of particles	Formed by	Origin/occurrence, examples
Heavy particles (alpha particles, etc.)	Alpha decay of certain radioactive elements in the body	Radium, radon, radon daughters in the environment
	Interaction of neutrons with matter	Formed by certain nuclear reactions, e.g. fission of uranium; component of cosmic radiation
Light particles (electrons, including beta particles)	Beta decay of radioactive elements in the body	Many elements, including potassium-40 (naturally occurring in tissues), carbon-14, phosphorus-32
	Interaction of electromagnetic radiations with matter	X-rays generated by X-ray tubes; gamma radiation, formed from the decay of certain radioactive elements, e.g. potassium-40

The most important types of radioactive decay are the following:
Alphadecay – a positively charged helium nucleus (alpha particle) is emitted from an unstable atomic nucleus.
Beta decay – an electron (betaparticle) is emitted.
Gamma radiation – excess energy, the release of which often accompanies radioactive transformations.
Neutrons – generated in certain nuclear reactions, in particular the fission of the uranium isotope ^{235}U and the plutonium isotope ^{239}Pu.

Particulate radiation emitted from radioactive decay has a short penetration range (for alpha radiation just a few hundredths of a millimetre) and unless the radioactive elements have been taken up by the body this type of radiation consequently has a low efficiency of tumour induction. Neutrons and electromagnetic waves, which in general produce the same types of particle (electrons and heavier particles) by secondary processes as are emitted upon radioactive decay (see above), are considerably more penetrating.

The concept of dose

As mentioned earlier, gamma radiation, X-rays and particulate radiation generate electrically charged molecules (ions) and excited states when they pass through tissue. These ions are unstable and take part in fast chemical transformations, often in the form of what are known as 'free radicals'. If such reactions take place in the cell's DNA, they may result in inheritable damage (germ cells), initiation of cancer (somatic cells), or in cellular damage or death (all cell types). The replacement of dead cells by tissue regeneration appears to facilitate the formation of tumours by unspecific promotion (see Holmberg and

Box 2

Dose–risk

DOSE
Radiation dose is expressed as the amount of energy absorbed in joules per kilogram (J kg^{-1}) of tissue, the unit being called the gray (Gy). Previously, dose was expressed in rads (=100 erg g^{-1}); 100 rad=1 Gy.

DOSE EQUIVALENT
At identical dosage levels, different kinds of radiation are capable of inducing varying frequencies of mutations and tumours. Thus, neutrons have a 5–10-fold, and alpha radiation a 20-fold higher biological activity than gamma radiation for many radiation effects. In order to define the absorbed dose in a unit (dose equivalent) proportional to risk, the dose is multiplied by a quality factor for the relative biological effectiveness (RBE) in relation to gamma radiation, the relative effectiveness of which is given the value 1.0. The unit for dose equivalent is known as the sievert (Sv):

dose equivalent in sieverts (Sv) = RBE × dose in grays (Gy).

In a similar way, the unit rad was formerly converted into the dose equivalent rem. For alpha radiation (RBE = 20), the dose equivalent upon irradiation with a dose of 1 Gy is

$$20 \times 1 = 20 \text{ Sv.}$$

Similarly, 1 rad of alpha radiation will give a dose equivalent of 20 rem.

EFFECTIVE DOSE EQUIVALENT
As a rule, the dose is not uniformly distributed in the tissues of the body. In order to facilitate risk estimation, the dose in each organ is weighted in relation to the proportion of the total risk which that organ would contribute in the case of an evenly distributed dose throughout the body. With whole-body irradiation, the risk of lung cancer is estimated to be 12 per cent of the total risk. Thus, for alpha radiation in the lung (see previous example) the effective (or weighted) dose equivalent, expressed in Sv, will be

$$1 \text{ Gy in lung} = 20 \times 0.12 \text{ Sv} = 2.4 \text{ Sv.}$$

COLLECTIVE DOSE

Multiplication by the number of individuals exposed to a certain average dose, dose equivalent or effective dose equivalent yields the corresponding:

Collective
- dose, expressed in man Gy
- dose equivalent, expressed in man-Sv
- effective dose equivalent, expressed in man-Sv

RISK ESTIMATION

The risk coefficient constitutes a measure of risk:

$$\text{risk coefficient} = \frac{\text{number of expected injuries}}{\text{effective man-Sv}}$$

The following relationship between dose and cancer mortality has been postulated on the basis of epidemiological data (see text):

Dose equivalent　　　　　　　*Risk*
1 Sv (whole-body irradiation)　0.02
or effective dose equivalent

Thus, the *risk coefficient* for death from cancer is equal to 0.02 man-Sv^{-1}. (This represents a mean value in a population characterized by a normal sensitivity and age distribution.)

When the collective (effective) dose equivalent is multiplied in the same way by the number of persons in the exposed population, an estimate of the *expected number of injuries* (mainly deaths from cancer) is obtained. Thus if a population of 1000 individuals is exposed to an average radiation dose of 1 Sv, this will be expected to result in 1000×1 man–Sv $\times\ 0.02$ man-Sv^{-1} = 20 cases.

Ehrenberg 1984; for further information on excited molecules see Section 4.5.3).

The instantaneous formation (within 10^{-16} seconds) of ionized and excited molecules when a tissue is irradiated is the primary process in a complex sequence of events, which under certain conditions may result in a cancer tumour after a decade or more.

From what has been said above, it is obvious that a relation exists between the *amount of energy* dissipated upon passage of a certain kind of radiation through tissue, and the number of ionizations and excitations produced. The number of ionizations will, in turn, decide the degree of biological damage induced: the biological effect is a function of the absorbed dose expressed as energy absorbed per unit mass.

However, the biological effectiveness is not determined solely by the absorbed dose. Biological action is also dependent on ionization density, that is the amount of energy dissipated per unit length along the particle's trajectory. As a rule, densely ionizing radiation is more effective per unit dose than sparsely ionizing radiation: beta and gamma radiation, and X-rays. Heavy particles, as in alpha radiation, are for this reason more effective than light particles (like beta particles). At identical dose levels and in the presence of oxygen (which increases the effectiveness of light particles by approximately a factor of three), fast neutrons are 3–10 times and alpha radiation 5–20 times more effective than electrons. In order to compensate for such differences in radiation quality, a generalized *dose equivalent* (the sievert, (Sv); a formerly used unit is the rem)—obtained by multiplying the dose in Gy by a quality factor for the 'relative biological effectiveness' (RBE)—is used for risk estimations in radiation protection. RBE is thus a measure of the biological effectiveness compared with that of X-rays (gamma radiation) with defined characteristics (RBE = 1). If the dose is not evenly distributed throughout the body, the dose equivalent is often weighted by multiplication by a proportionality factor for cancer risk per unit dose with homogeneous whole-body irradiation. The unit derived thus is called the *effective dose equivalent* and is expressed in sieverts (see Box 2). By multiplying the effective dose (dose equivalent) by the number of individuals irradiated, the corresponding *collective dose* is obtained (man-sieverts (man-Sv)).

Dose–risk estimates

The number of expected injuries per collective dose equivalent constitutes the *risk coefficient*.

When individual doses (expressed in terms of effective sieverts) and collective doses (expressed in terms of effective man-sieverts) are multiplied by the risk coefficient, an estimate of the individual risk and the expected number of injuries in the exposed population, respectively, will be obtained (see Box 2). Although the risks in most cases are so low that they cannot be directly demonstrated epidemiologically, this formal approach to risk estimation is universally accepted as the basis for introducing various kinds of protective measures in the area of radiation protection.

The risk coefficient used by the Swedish authorities of 0.02 late injuries (deaths from cancer as well as inheritable defects manifested in the next two generations) per man-sieverts (implying two induced injuries per 100 man-Sv) has been based on detailed analyses of dose–response relationships in all available documentation, in particular that of UNSCEAR (the United Nations Scientific Committee on the

Effects of Atomic Radiation) and BEIR (Committee on the Biological Effects of Ionizing Radiations of the US National Research Council). This coefficient probably suffers from an uncertainty factor of two at doses exceeding 1 Sv, and even greater uncertainty for the very low doses characterizing most radiation exposure. In the latter case this may be ascribed to the fact that it has not been possible in practice to detect effects at these low radiation levels by epidemiological methods. In the opinion of many experts, the application of this risk coefficient to low doses may result in a certain overestimation of risk. UNSCEAR (1977) and the International Commission for Radiation Protection (ICRP, 1977) therefore give a risk coefficient of 0.01 man-Sv^{-1} in round numbers as the most probable estimate. This also represents an adequate expression of risk at low doses according to the linear – quadratic model proposed by the majority of the delegates of BEIR III (1980). On the other hand, there are also indications that this figure may involve an underestimation of risk at low doses (Ehrenberg, 1978; Radford, 1980). The higher value of 0.02 man-Sv^{-1} was based on results from work carried out by the Swedish Energy Commission (SEC, 1978). Bearing in mind the great uncertainty involved, the Cancer Committee has chosen to use this coefficient of 0.02 man-Sv^{-1} as the cancer mortality risk. The average cancer *incidence* is about twice as high as the *mortality* from the disease (lung cancer being an important exception, where mortality and incidence are practically identical). From this basis it follows that the coefficient for cancer morbidity due to radiation exposure should be set at 0.04 man-Sv^{-1}.

On passing through a cell nucleus, one alpha-particle—for example, from a radon daughter nuclide—will deliver such a high dose to this structure (about 1 Gy), that the dose– response relationship can be claimed to be linear down to the lowest doses, with a higher degree of certainty than for gamma radiation.

Swedish exposure data

In Table 4.19 collective doses estimated by the National Institute of Radiation Protection, the size of the populations exposed, and the number of expected injuries (mainly deaths from cancer, see above) per year in Sweden are presented (NIRP, 1984). The approximately 1100 injuries predicted by NIRP to be caused by exposure to radon (category 7), refer to cases of lung cancer. It should be emphasized that this table refers to the 'environment of today' and the 'injuries of tomorrow'. The *current* cancer incidence and mortality caused by previous exposures provide the basis for analysis elsewhere (including Chapters 5 and 6, where 'explainable' proportions of induced injuries are discussed). In general, the figures agree closely with those computed in 1981 by G. Bengtsson of NIRP. The marked upward adjust-

Table 4.19 Expected yearly collective dose for different populations at the beginning of the 1980s. The computed number of injuries is based on a risk coefficient of 0.02 future deaths from cancer or serious hereditary defects per man-sievert. The listed estimates may have an uncertainty amounting to a factor up to 2.

	No. of individuals concerned per year	Yearly collective effective dose equivalent[1] per man		Total no. of estimated cancer deaths or serious hereditary defects from doses during one year	
		According to Bengtsson (1981)	After revision	According to Bengtsson (1981)	After revision[a]
1. Cosmic radiation	8 million	2000	(2400)	40	(48)
2. Natural radioactive elements in the body	8 million	3000	(3500)	60	(70)
3. Natural from ground	8 million	2000	(800)[6]	40	(16)
4. Nuclear power, external natural environment	8 million[2]	200[7]	(0.3)[8]	4	(0.006)
5. Nuclear power, internal occupational environment, staff	3000	10	(15)	0.2	(0.3)
6. Fallout from from nuclear tests	8 million	100	(100)	2	(2)
7. Homes, radon	8 million	20 000	(57 000)	400	(1 140)
8. Homes, gamma radiation	8 million	2000	(4000)[6]	40	(80)
9. Workers in mines and rock chambers	5000	100	(75)	42	(1.5)
10. Consumer articles	8 million	10	(1)	0.2	(0.02)
11. Other industries, staff	30 000	10	(2.5)[9]	0.2	(0.05)
12. Research, education	60 000	10	(10)	0.2	(0.2)
13. X-rays, dental staff	20 000	5	(0.3)	0.1	(0.006)
14. X-rays, dental patients	8 million	500	(600)	10	(12)
15. Radiation therapy staff	1000	1	(1)	0.02	(0.02)
16. Radiation therapy patients[3]	20 000	–	–	–	–
17. X-rays, diagnostic, staff	10 000	5	(2.3)	0.1	(0.05)
18. X-rays, diagnostic, patients	8 million	5 000	(5 000)	100	(100)
19. Medical use of isotopes, diagnostic, staff	10 000	1	(2.2)	0.02[5]	(0.04)
20. Medical use of isotopes, diagnostic patients	100 000	500[4]	(580)	10	(12)
21. Veterinarians: X-rays, staff	500	–	(0.4)	–	0.008

22. Veterinarians: X-rays, animal owners	20 000	–	(0.4)	–	(0.008)
Total		~35 000	~74 000	~700	~1500

a Figures calculated by the Cancer Committee from the revised dose estimates and using the same risk coefficient as the NIRP, namely 0.02 cases man-Sv^{-1}. In the further analyses those figures have been regarded as estimated numbers of cancer deaths. Notes 1–9 are according to the NIRP:

[1] Doses refer to effective dose equivalents generally calculated from the weighting factors supplied by ICRP. A total collective dose of about 35 000 man-Sv^{-1} year^{-1} corresponds to 2.5 MJ year^{-1} of absorbed gamma radiation energy.

[2] Because emissions are dispersed globally, large populations outside Sweden are also affected. In the emission regulations this fact is taken into consideration.

[3] Patients' radiation therapy accounts for high collective doses, but these are not relevant from the point of view of risk. The collective dose corresponds to approximately 1 MJ year^{-1} of absorbed gamma radiation energy.

[4] Of the total dose equivalent, approximately 400 man-Sv may be ascribed to iodine-31. In a study of patients in Stockholm having received this isotope, no increase in cancer incidence could be detected.

[5] Listed as 100 by Bengtsson (printing error).

[6] The large discrepancy in relation to Bengtsson's figure is due to the fact that indoor collective doses relating to radioactive elements in the ground now appear within the category 'homes, gamma radiation'.

[7] Refers to the global collective dose to be distributed over the next 500 years from the present operation of Swedish nuclear power reactors during 1 year. About 1 man-Sv of this will affect Sweden, plus an approximately equal contribution from nuclear power plants outside the country.

[8] Refers to the present yearly collective dose in Sweden before emission of very long-lived nuclides has reached equilibrium. May be compared to the value 1 man-Sv year^{-1} in footnote 7, plus an approximately equal contribution from nuclear power plants outside the country.

[9] In addition, staff exposed to radiation from smoke detectors should be included. This extra collective dose has been included in the value given within parentheses.

From NIRP, 1984.

ment of doses and expected number of injuries due to exposure to radon daughters in homes is discussed in more detail below.

Specific exposures (other than radon daughters in homes)

In certain cases there remains considerable uncertainty in the dose estimates. However, this problem mainly concerns sources like consumer goods (Table 4.19, category 10) such as watches with luminescent dials, television sets and smoke detectors, where available data—in spite of the uncertainties involved—are sufficient to demonstrate a negligible level of risk. A considerable degree of uncertainty regarding the size of risk computed here may, therefore, be considered acceptable.

The background radiation (Table 4.19, categories 1, 2, 3; part of the gamma radiation in homes, category 8; unavoidable but low exposure to radon and radon daughters outdoors and indoors) will, in theory, produce about 150 deaths from cancer per year in Sweden, and these exposures cannot, in general, be prevented.

The number of expected injuries due to occupational exposure (Table 4.19, categories 5, 11, 13, 15, 17, 19, 21) is very low. Today this also holds true for miners (category 9), where great improvements in the work environment were introduced during the 1970s (see for example Snihs et al., 1981).

A few cases of cancer per year can be expected due to previous nuclear weapon tests conducted in various parts of the world (category 6). Under present operating conditions, the production of nuclear energy in Sweden and abroad will induce a negligible number of cases per year (category 4).[9] However, due to the long half-lives of certain radioactive elements which are dispersed throughout the biosphere, additional dose contributions will be present for a long time (see also Box 3).

Box 3

Dose commitment

In radiation protection work, efforts are made to keep the total dose as low as possible, or below a certain yearly maximum. It must be remembered that certain human activities, such as nuclear weapon tests and the production of nuclear energy, will result in long-lived radioactive material being introduced into the biosphere and generating dose contributions for a long time into the future. Part of the yearly maximum dose—which we are endeavouring not to exceed in the future—will, thus, already be 'committed' by our current activities leaving us less latitude for action. For this reason, the concept of *dose commitment* has been defined as the total dose per individual for all future time due to a certain activity (or activity per year). Because of the uncertainty of predicting conditions in the distant future, what is known as an incomplete dose commitment covering the next 500 years is often used.

As an example, under normal operating conditions, the production of 1 GW of nuclear power has been estimated to result locally and regionally in a *collective effective dose equivalent commitment* of 6 man-Sv. In addition, 18 and 70 man-Sv respectively will affect the world population during the next 500 (incomplete commitment) and 10 000 years. UNSCEAR (1982) has, however, estimated that during normal operating conditions, the yearly dose contributions will be very small in comparison with the background radiation even from a fully developed worldwide nuclear energy programme running for hundreds of years.

The use of X-rays and isotopes for diagnostic purposes in patients has been estimated to result in slightly more than a hundred cases per year. This could be used as an incentive for reducing doses (see the report from the National Board of Health and Welfare (NBHW, 1976), and Åsard (1982) by introducing improved techniques (e.g. picture amplification) and, in particular, by education. At the same time it must be emphasized that we are in this instance dealing with measures aimed at improved diagnosis in sick individuals where, as a rule, a very small personal risk is offset against greatly improved chances of recovery. (For the diagnosis of breast cancer and mammography, see Section 13.2.3.) Evidently, the *individual risk* is of greater significance here than the collective risk. It should also be stressed that part of the diagnostic medical exposure affects elderly patients or those suffering from terminal disease, so that carcinogenic effects need not be taken into consideration. Therefore, the estimate of about 100 fatal cases per year probably exaggerates the risk. Radiation therapy mainly involves patients suffering from a malignant disease (cancer). Although this collective dose is substantial, it should clearly not be considered in this context.

Radon and radon daughters

The earth's crust contains the heavy elements uranium and thorium in small but varying quantities. The decay of these unstable elements is so slow (half-lives of 4500 and 14000 million years, respectively) that they have been present since the formation of the earth's crust about 5000 million years ago. Primary rock formations, such as certain granites occurring in Sweden, may contain relatively high levels of uranium. Uranium-238 and thorium-232 decay (see Box 4) through the emission of alpha, beta and gamma radiation in a series of steps via isotopes of radium with the masses 226 (half-life of 1600 years) and 224 (half-life of 2 days) to the stable lead iostopes, lead-206 and lead-208. Alpha decay of the radium isotopes leads to radon with masses 222 and 220; the latter is often called thoron due to its appearance in the disintegration series of thorium.

Radon is one of the noble gases, which means that the element is almost chemically inert. Part of the radon formed is therefore released from the earth's crust (and any minerals derived from it) to air and water. Radon-222, which has a relatively long half-life (3.8 days) is more important from the viewpoint of risk than thoron (radon-220) with a half-life of barely a minute. Further disintegration of radon and thoron takes place via alpha-and beta-emitting radioisotopes of heavy elements, in particular, of the metals polonium, bismuth and lead. The products of these decays are called radon daughters and thoron daughters, respectively. They occur in air partly as free ions, and partly bound to dust particles. Due to their chemical properties they are easily retained at the site of uptake, e.g. in bronchi and lungs upon inhalation. Because the radon daughters have short half-lives and also emit alpha radiation (which has a short range of penetration and a high biological effectiveness) damage is induced locally at the site of uptake. This is why radon daughters are a health problem.

Radon itself is not bound locally but can be distributed through the body. Being a heavy noble gas, it is soluble to some extent in fat and blood and may therefore be retained in the tissues. However, the dose delivered from this small amount of radon is negligible.

Radon and radon daughters are generally present in the air and are therefore one of the unavoidable sources of background radiation. The concentrations are highest in the vicinity of the sources (uranium and radium deposits), but nuclides can travel far from the point of emission. The level above the oceans is, on average, 100 times lower than over land. Particularly high levels are found in the air in uranium mines, and also in other types of mine when the rock contains uranium or thorium, as well as in the vicinity of waste deposits from uranium mining. Radon is also liberated during the burning of coal, in the production of geothermal energy and, locally, from water with high concentrations of radium or radon. However, outdoor levels of radon are generally very low in comparison with those found in many homes.

The measurements of Hultqvist (1956) during the 1950s revealed that certain building materials could release radon, resulting in increased radiation doses indoors. In addition, it was discovered as late as 1981 that diffusion from the ground and uptake through the foundations of buildings could result in high radon levels. Changed construction techniques, including energy-saving measures, have over recent years produced houses with better insulation and reduced ventilation, but also higher indoor levels of radon daughters.

Since radon and its disintegration products are also present naturally in water, the general water supply may under certain conditions contribute to an increased exposure to radon, mainly by inhalation.

Measures in 500 randomly selected homes, conducted during the summer of 1982, indicated higher levels than had been assumed previously (see Table 4.19), which implied a risk of about 1100 cases of lung cancer per year from this cause in Sweden. Such a risk would constitute the most serious problem in the area of radiation protection in Sweden.

Due to the difficulties in determining the radiation doses in the affected target cells—primarily the so-called basal cells which normally are coated with a mucous layer and a layer of columnar cells—exposure to radon is much harder to analyse than other radiation hazards. Since the penetration range of alpha radiation in tissue is no more than a few cell diameters, the dose distribution in the lungs becomes very uneven. Estimating the true radiation dose at a certain exposure to radon for the cells that are relevant in carcinogenesis is consequently very difficult and depends on several things, including the state of the epithelium, the physiological conditions of respiration and the amount of dust in the air (dust particles can serve as transporting vehicles for radon daughters). This makes any extrapolation of animal experimental data and epidemiological findings—where a more homogeneous irradiation to the lung with X-rays and gamma radiation has been used—extremely uncertain. Since the dose in the relevant target cells cannot be determined, no generally accepted risk coefficient can be applied. For this reason, risk estimates have been based on dose–response relationships found in epidemiological studies of radon-exposed populations. The relation between radon exposure levels and the incidence of lung cancer has been determined with adequate accuracy only for certain groups of miners.

In Sweden a few investigations of the correlation between the type of dwelling (in relation to exposure to radon in the home) and cancer incidence have been carried out (see Edling, 1983). Because the samples were small and the exposures not determined with sufficient accuracy, these studies do not permit any determination of the size of the risk involved, and should be regarded merely as methodological trials. In comparisons between the different counties of Sweden, a certain correlation between average gamma radiation levels in homes and the incidence of lung cancer was found. This observation needs to be followed up by additional studies.

UNSCEAR in 1977 estimated that the risk of lung cancer was 200–450 cases per million man-working level months (see Box 4). By converting this value to SI units—while taking the respiration rates in homes (about 0.8 m^3 h^{-1}) and during work in mines (about 1.2m^3 h^{-1}) into consideration—a risk coefficient in the range 1.9–4.2 per 10^6 man-Bq-year m^{-3} is obtained. The 'reference value' of 2.5 cases of lung cancer per million persons exposed to 1 Bq year^{-1} and 1 Bq m^{-3} which has been used by the Swedish National Institute of Radiation Protection thus lies at the lower end of this range. The average exposure level for radon daughters in modern Swedish homes is estimated to amount to 53 Bq m^{-3}. These values yield the following estimate of future annual lung cancer incidence from today's exposure:

$$53 \text{ Bq-year m}^{-3} \times 8.3 \text{ million persons} \times \frac{2.5 \text{ cases}}{1 \text{ million man-Bq-year m}^{-3}} \approx 1100 \text{ cases.}$$

    collective exposure dose   risk coefficient

The annual dose which corresponds to the present hygienic limit, or 'action level' of 400 Bq m^{-3} in Sweden is exceeded in an estimated 40 000 homes.

This problem is causing great concern, but there is, at the same time, great uncertainty over this risk estimate. According to the NIRP, this uncertainty may amount to a factor of three either way, which corresponds to a range of 300–3000 cases per year. However, for several reasons the estimate of 1100 cases per year and, in particular, the upper confidence limit (3000 cases per year) appear to be overestimates.

In the latter part of the 1970s, about 2200 cases of lung cancer were being reported each year in Sweden. The risk estimate mentioned above does not relate to present lung cancer rates but rather to current levels of radon daughters, and these were about four times lower around 1950. Due to changes in building techniques and energy conservation measures, indoor radon daughter levels increased by a factor of two up to 1970, and by an additional factor of two during the 1970s. Even if the number of cases induced 20–30 years ago were three to four times lower than at present (corresponding to 300–400 cases per year or about 1000 cases per year at the upper limit in the NIRP's estimate), it would be surprising if such an increase could remain undetected by the epidemiological comparisons which have been carried out between different regions in Sweden and in neighbouring Nordic countries. The increases in lung cancer in Sweden and Norway have been virtually identical, and in comparison with Denmark, where exposure to radon is quite low, the differences appear to be fully accounted for by existing differences in smoking habits (see Saxén et al., 1977; Kvåle, 1982).

The BEIR committee of the US National Research Council (BEIR III 1980) proposed a risk coefficient corresponding to 6×10^{-6} per man-Bq-year m^{-3} in homes, an estimate 2.4 times higher than that applied by NIRP. Cohen (1982) has advanced a number of objections to the effect that this value represents a considerable overestimate, perhaps by a factor of 20. Some of these arguments are relevant to Swedish conditions. Much of the carcinogenic effect of radiation from radon daughters seems to be due to an interaction with cigarette smoking (Damber and Larsson, 1982; Larsson and Damber, 1982 and cited publications; see also Section 4.6). In the groups of miners studied with respect to dose–response relationships, the proportion of smokers appears to have been at least twice as high as in the general Swedish population. This would result in an overestimation by a factor of two. Furthermore, it has been demonstrated that certain histological types of lung cancer (in particular, oat cell cancer) are more common among miners exposed to radon than in the population at large. Even if the difference is not as large as suggested by Cohen (see Damber, and Larsson 1982), the implication is that the proportion of lung cancer which can be ascribed to exposure to radon daughters in homes is reduced, possibly by a factor of two to three. The environmental differences between mines and homes represent the largest uncertainty introduced by applying a risk coefficient based on populations of miners. At the time when the cases of lung cancer studied epidemiologically in recent decades were induced, the levels of dust and particles were very high, particularly during the 1940s and 1950s. Such pollutants might have increased the biological efficiency of radiation from radon daughters in combination with smoking, due to the presence of carcinogenic metal compounds or through physical damage. A chemical and physical causal contribution of this kind from particles in the air of mines might in certain cases result in dose–response curves which are concave when seen from below, that is the risk coefficient appears to be greater at low concentrations of radon daughters (see UNSCEAR, 1982).

In view of these considerations, the lower limit of the risk interval suggested by NIRP (about 300 cases of lung cancer at present levels of radon daughters in indoor air) appears more realistic than the estimate of 1100 cases per year, and the value could be as low as 100 cases per year in accordance with the estimations made by Cohen (1982). Some support, though weak, for this estimate may be derived from the most probable value for the effective dose equivalent per Bq-year m^{-3} for the epithelium of bronchi and lungs (see Box 4). Based on today's exposure, such an estimate gives about 200 cases per year in Sweden. In conclusion, these considerations lead to the assumption that the interval of 100–1000 cases per year covers the true risk.

This analysis has above all aimed at illustrating the uncertainty of any risk evaluation for radon carried out at present. It should be emphasized that it is not possible to confirm scientifically whether the true risk is really lower than the 1100 estimated lung cancer cases, so long as the risk assessment has not been based on sufficiently extensive epidemiological studies of the association between cancer incidence and levels of radon daughters in homes.

4.5.3 UV light

Properties and biological effects

UV light is composed of electromagnetic waves of wavelengths between about 10 and 400 nm. From the point of view of energy content it thus occupies an intermediate position between X-rays and visible light. UV light is generated by such equipment as electric arcs, lasers and mercury-vapour lamps. Most of the solar UV light with wavelengths

Box 4

Radioactive disintegration

In a population of unstable atomic nuclei, the proportion which will disintegrate within a certain period of time is characteristic of the radioactive element in question. The time elapsing before one half of the radioactive nuclei have disintegrated is known as the *half-life*. Half-lives of radioactive elements vary from fractions of a second to thousands of millions of years.

The radioactive noble gas *radon* is at an intermediate level in the disintegration series that starts with uranium and ends with stable lead.

Radioactive disintegration

In a population of unstable atomic nuclei, the proportion which will disintegrate within a certain period of time is characteristic of the radioactive element in question. The time elapsing before one half of the radioactie nuclei have disintegrated is known as the half life. Half-lives of radioactive elements vary from fractions of a second to billions of years.

The radioactive noble gas radon is at an intermediate level in the disintegration series that starts with uranium and ends with stable lead.

Nucleide	Half-life
Uranium-238	4.5 billion years
Radium-226	1 600 years
Radon-222	3.3 days
Radon daughters (Isotopes of polonium, bismuth and lead)	Fractions of a second– 27 minutes
Lead-210	21 years
Polonium-210	138 days
Lead-206	Stable

Activity

The number of disintegrations per second of a radioactive material can be measured precisely and is referred to as the *activity* of the material in question. The activity of a medium is therefore a measure of the concentration of the radioactive elements present.

The unit of activity is the *becquerel* (Bq):

1 Bq = one disintegration per second.

The unit *curie* (Ci) was used formerly:

1 Ci = 3.7×10^{10} Bq.

The concentration of radioactive atoms in air is represented as becquerels per cubic metre (Bqm^{-3}).

A given amount of radon exists in equilibrium with defined amounts of each of the radon daughter nuclides. In the air in buildings or mines this equilibrium is not reached because of the relatively rapid elimination of the radon daughters (which are not gaseous) through absorption onto walls, fan blades or other solid materials, or through absorption by living organisms. The radon daughter level is, as a rule, determined by analysis of the level of radon—which is most easily accessible for measurement followed by estimation of the concentration of radon daughters.

For the control of the concentration of radon daughters in mines, the levels were formerly expressed in terms of 'working levels' (WL), defined as the concentration of radon daughters which exist in equilibrium with 3700 Bq per m^{-3} radon. The exposure dose in 'working level months' (WLM) was obtained by multiplying the concentration in WL by a monthly working time of 170 hours.

UNSCEAR (1977) has estimated the cancer risk for miners to be 200–450 cases per 10^6 man-WLM.

UNSCEAR has further estimated the correlation between the concentration in bequerels of a radioactive substance in inhaled air and the effective dose equivalent (see Box 2) in the epithelium of the bronchia and lungs to be in the range of 1.5–3 (below expressed as 2($\pm$1) per 10^{-5} Sv for 1 Bq-year/ m^3).

At an average of 53 Bq m^{-3} for 8.3 million individuals (the population of Sweden) this corresponds to an effective collective dose equivalent of

$8.3 \times 10^6 \times 53 \times 2 (\pm 1) \times 10^{-5}$ man-Sv year^{-1}

$= 9000 (\pm 4500)$ man Sv year^{-1}.

Using a risk coefficient of 0.02 man-Sv^{-1}, a calculation of the risk of cancer death from the dose in the epithelium of the bronchia and lungs would then yield

$9000 \times 0.02 = 180$ cases per year.

below 280 nm ('UV-C') is absorbed by the ozone layer of the stratosphere. However, light of these wavelengths is generated by certain artificial light sources such as older types of 'sun-lamps'. In Sweden, detailed regulations for sun-lamps cover the radiation quality, maximum effect at different wavelengths, technical protective devices, and other matters. Solar UV light is also UV-B (280–315 nm) and UV-A (315–400 nm), both of which induce pigmentation of the skin (sun tanning).

UV-B can cause skin damage and is the factor responsible for skin cancer insofar as this can be related to UV light. High doses of UV-A may severely damage the tissues of the eye, including the retina and the lens (cataracts) (Ham et al,. 1976; Lerman, 1980). UV-A can also induce severe dermal reactions (phototoxicity, photoallergies), as well as cancer, when irradiation is accompanied by intake of certain drugs and other chemical compounds (Magnus and Young, 1981).

As mentioned before, because of its low energy UV light does not produce ionization, and absorption of the energy causes excitation of the molecules. An excited molecule may return to its original state by fast physical deactivation processes (emission of fluorescence, conversion of radiation energy into thermal energy, etc.). However, under certain conditions the excited molecule may induce chemical changes in the hereditary material (DNA) of cells, often via free radicals.

Thus, UV light of wavelengths between 250 and 300 nm has been used as a standard agent in the study of induced mutations as well as of repair of DNA damage. In the elucidation of the role of DNA as the target molecule in the initiation of cancer, important clues have been obtained from the study of the effects caused by UV light (see Holmberg and Ehrenberg, 1984). For example, it has been demonstrated that individuals suffering from a rare hereditable defect in the ability to repair lesions in the DNA (patients with xeroderma pigmentosum) are extremely sensitive to the carcinogenic action of sunlight, and these patients usually die at a young age from skin cancer. For one kind of alteration in DNA caused by UV light, pyrimidine dimer formation (particularly thymine dimers), it has for the first time been possible to prove the existence of a causal association between a chemical change in the hereditary material and the induction of cancer.

UV light has a short penetration range in biological material, and its carcinogenic effects are therefore restricted to the illuminated parts of the skin. There is strong evidence that UV-B is an aetiological factor—partly through interaction with other agents—in the induction of various types of cancer of the skin and lips.

The ozone layer in the stratosphere is our most effective protection against dangerously intense UV radiation reaching the surface of the earth. Human activities which damage the ozone layer may indirectly result in an elevated risk of cancer due to an increased intensity of UV radiation (Crutzen, 1974; US National Research Council, 1982). Organic chemicals known as 'freons' used as propellants in spray cans and as refrigerating fluids, and also dinitrogen oxide (N_2O, 'laughing gas'), produced microbially from nitrogen-based fertilizers and from other nitrogen oxides produced by combustion, are sufficiently stable to diffuse into the stratosphere and react with ozone. Nitrogen monoxide (NO) and nitrogen dioxide (NO_2)—together known as NO_x—are found in exhausts of supersonic jets (Crutzen, 1971) and formed in nuclear explosions (Crutzen and Birks, 1982) and rapidly react with ozone when introduced into the stratosphere.

Cancer induced by UV light

Malignant melanoma and *squamous cell carcinoma* are two forms of skin cancer to be considered in connection with UV light. Squamous cell carcinoma is somewhat more common than malignant melanoma in Sweden (in 1979 about 1000 cases of squamous cell carcinoma and about 800 cases of malignant melanoma were reported), but it is far more curable. During the period 1961–73 the mortality from squamous cell carcinoma was some 10–20 times lower than from malignant melanoma; (Swanbeck and Larkö, 1982). Of all skin cancers, squamous cell carcinoma is most readily induced by UV light in experimental animals. In addition to these types, *basal cell carcinoma* of the skin, which also is associated with exposure to UV light, is probably the most common of all cancers (approximately 5000 cases per year in Sweden), but is a relatively innocuous disease and is therefore not reported to the Swedish Cancer Registry. In addition to pipe smoking, UV light appears to constitute an aetiological factor in *cancer of the lips*, which is relatively frequent among outdoor workers (about 200 cases in Sweden in 1979). The decline in pipe-smoking may be a contributing factor in the fact that the incidence of this type of cancer is not increasing at present.

The correlation between squamous cell carcinoma and exposure to sunlight is evident from the correlation between cancer incidence and outdoor work, as well as from the striking localization on the head (on the ears among men, in particular) neck and face (more than two-thirds of the tumours are at these sites). The face is also the most common site for basal cell carcinoma. Among white-skinned races all the types of skin neoplasia mentioned occur more frequently close to the equator, increasing progressively with the intensity of the sunlight.

The incidence of malignant melanoma shows certain discrepancies in comparison with the other skin cancers that are clearly sunlight related, and the role of UV radiation has therefore been questioned by some scientists. Although more complex than with squamous cell carcinoma, an association with exposure to sunlight most probably does exist. Of all forms of cancer, the malignant melanomas appear to be showing the most rapid increase in Sweden (see Eklund 1984). A similar trend has been observed in the other Nordic countries, in the USA and in other European countries. In women (but not in men) the mortality from this disease is increasing rather more slowly than the morbidity (Magnus, 1977a). Earlier diagnosis seems to be the most important reason for this.

Due to the rapid increase in malignant melanoma (in Sweden it tripled between 1960 and 1978, when it reached about 10 cases per 100 000), it will probably become a serious problem among people who are now young or middle aged. This rapid increase clearly does not seem to be caused only by better diagnosis and reporting (Magnus, 1982).

More detailed analysis of this trend has been carried out by Magnus for Norway (Magnus, 1981) and for the five Nordic countries (Magnus, 1977b). The incidence of malign melanoma on the head–face–neck exhibits the same moderate increase per year (about 3 per cent) as other reported forms of skin cancer, and also shows the same typical age dependence as for many other forms of neoplasia, characterized by a marked increase of the incidence in higher age groups. This is demonstrated in Figure 4.11, which shows the Swedish melanoma incidence for 1979 for different age groups. A large proportion of the melanomas, however, appear on the trunk and legs. At these sites melanoma has exhibited a marked increase amounting to about 10 per cent per year, which is greatest in the age group born between the turn of the century and the beginning of World War II. Due to this development, the relatively large—and increasing—contribution to the total incidence of melanoma from tumours on trunk and legs is affecting younger age-groups than is the case for tumours of the head, face and neck.

Magnus has discussed a possible association between the increase in malignant melanoma on the legs (particularly in women) and trunk (initially men, later also in women) and changes in sun bathing habits and fashion, particularly in sports-wear. Several factors appear to favour the existence of such a relationship. The increase in the incidence of tumours on the legs of women appears to be related to a change to shorter skirts and to stockings permeable to UV-B. The fact that this increase is lower in cohorts born around 1900 and earlier seems to be a result of these age groups not having acquired the same habits. Similarly Eklund (1984) has observed a lower increase in the total incidence of malignant melanoma in the highest age groups than in younger individuals.

Different types of exposure 241

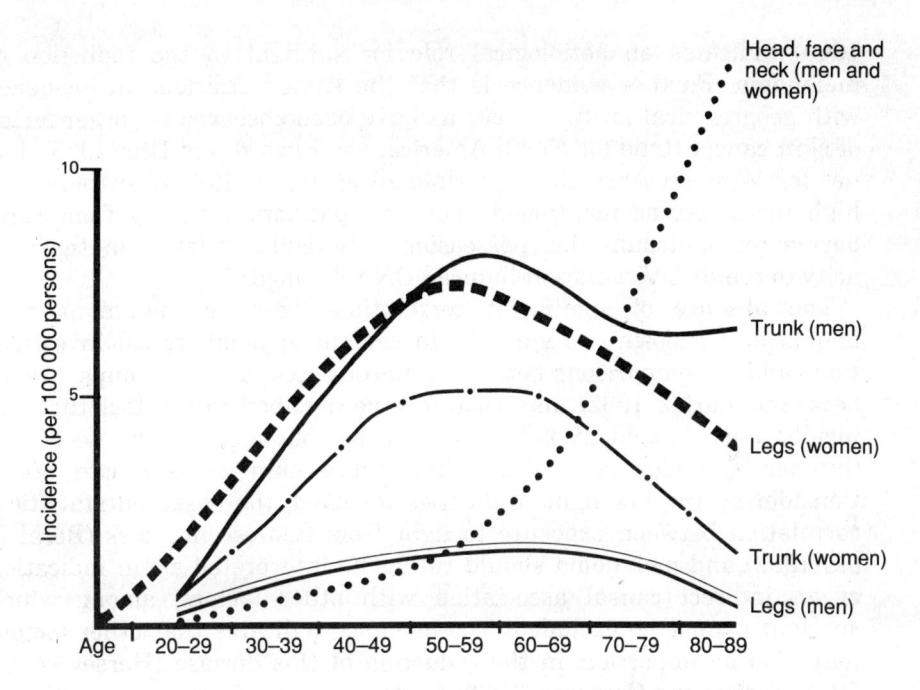

Figure 4.11 Incidence of malignant melanomas in different parts of the body and in different age groups. Smoothed curves based on Cancer Incidence in Sweden, 1979
Note: Head, face and neck comprise sites ICD no. 190. 1–4; trunk, ICD no. 190.5: legs; ICD no. 190.7.

In his study of the Norwegian data, Magnus (1981, and earlier works; see also Elwood and Lee, 1975) observed that in cohorts born after 1930, the incidence per unit area of the skin is higher for the legs and trunk than for the face, neck and head, in spite of the fact that the accumulated UV radiation dose to legs and trunk certainly never exceeded that to the face, neck and head. As suggested also by some Australian scientists (Holman *et al.*, 1980), malignant melanoma seems to be aetiologically distinguishable from squamous cell carcinoma in that not only is the cumulative UV-B dose of importance, but also the skin damage ('sun-eczema' with erythema, urticaria and scaling) caused by the sudden exposure of unpigmented and not yet thickened areas of the skin to high doses of sunlight. A statistical correlation between malignant melanoma and such skin damage incurred at an early age has been demonstrated in a case-control study of patients (Sober *et al.*, 1979). This type of skin damage—leading to tissue regeneration—may in these instances have a promotive effect, or amplify the initiating action of the radiation by stimulating cell division (Farber and Cameron, 1980).

The fact that the risk is highest in individuals with fair skin, pale eyes and red or blond hair (Lancaster and Nelson, 1957; Gellin *et al.*,

1969) indicates an aetiological role for sunlight in the induction of melanoma. Further evidence is that the same variations in incidence with geographical latitude occur as have been observed for other forms of skin cancer (true for North America, see Elwood and Lee (1975), but not for Western Australia, see Holman et al., (1980)). Also there is a high incidence, as mentioned above, in patients suffering from xeroderma pigmentosum—i.e. possessing a hereditary defect in the capacity to repair UV-radiation-induced DNA damage.

The absence of significant correlations between malignant melanoma and exposure to sunlight in certain epidemiological investigations and in comparisons between different occupational groups (Swanbeck and Larkö, 1982) may therefore be ascribed to the fact that the incidence is dependent not only on dose, but also on the dose rate (intensity), under conditions when acute skin damage can occur. Considering the low light intensities involved, the observed statistical correlation between exposure to light from fluorescent tubes (Beràl et al., 1982) and melanoma should rather be interpreted as an indication of an indirect causal association with other factors, among which sunlight cannot be excluded. The evidence indicates that other factors may also be important in the induction of this disease (Hersey et al., 1983; Farber and Cameron, 1980; Astrup Jensen, 1982).

The role of sunlight—in particular when associated with sudden and intensive sunbathing—cannot be discounted as an important causal factor in malignant melanoma, despite the fact that, compared with other forms of skin cancer, the aetiology of melanoma is partly unknown and appears to be very complex. Partly for social reasons (particularly a wish to obtain a sun-tan in the shortest possible time), a changed exposure pattern has in recent years affected certain age cohorts. The incidence trends therefore bear a resemblance to the changes in incidence of lung cancer. (In the latter case, however, the incidences mirror the changes in smoking habits which have occurred; see Section 4.2.) The increase in the incidence of malignant melanoma can, therefore, be expected to continue as these cohorts reach higher ages (Magnus, 1981).

From a preventive point of view, it would appear that sudden and intensive sunbathing resulting in skin damage should be avoided. In addition, caution during the initial phase of sun bathing seems to be the safest way to acquire a nice sun-tan.

The proportion of the total number of cases of lip cancer, squamous cell carcinoma, and malignant melanoma which can be ascribed to the action of sunlight cannot be ascertained with a high degree of accuracy. In view of what has just been said, an assumption that about three quarters of the roughly 2000 cases in Sweden—about 1500 cases per year — share this aetiology appears to be reasonable. This figure is rather uncertain but should, nevertheless, be of the right order of magnitude.

4.6 Interaction effects

General points of view

As was described in more detail in Chapter 3, the induction of tumours involves a multi-stage process where at least two necessary steps have been identified: initiation and promotion. Tumour induction in itself could thus be characterized as an interaction effect.

Whereas initiation is considered to be mainly an irreversible process, promotion is reversible. The effects of initiators and promoters or promoting conditions may in turn be modified by other factors which may increase or decrease the risk of a tumour disease in a given initiator–promoter situation.

In disease processes less complex than cancer induction only purely modifying factors usually have to be considered as concerns interactive effects. From the scientific point of view, the identification of modifying agents often presents great difficulties. For this reason it is particularly important to try to form an opinion as to whether in a given situation a large increase or decrease of risk is involved. The latter situation may be of importance when dealing with agents that have a protective action against some risk factor which may be difficult or impossible to avoid.

Several illustrative examples of the type of interaction referred to above, which constitutes a *prerequisite* for the induction of cancer, have been provided in other sections of this chapter. Such interactions include initiators, promoters or promoting conditions. Man is and always has been, exposed to a broad spectrum of initiators of different origin, including initiators produced within the body. The concentrations in the human environment are mostly very low in comparison with the levels used in animal studies, where chemical carcinogens are investigated for initiating effects. The effect of individual initiators can, therefore, often be of less importance (except for special risk situations) than that of certain promoters which affect already initiated cells independently of the initiating agent. Furthermore, certain types of promoter are probably common and may be implicated in considerable numbers of cases. Thus, part of the effect ascribed to a high intake of fat (see Section 4.3) can probably be attributed to an indirect promotive action mediated by hormonal factors. The observation that the risk of lung cancer in smokers who have stopped smoking decreases quite rapidly (Figure 4.9) indicates that continuous exposure to promoters in tobacco smoke (together with known initiators in the smoke) plays a decisive role in the induction of lung cancer.

A special issue with regard to the action of initiators is to what extent agents from different sources act additively. In this context we are not dealing with a truly interactive effect, but with an increased risk of initiation resulting from exposure over time to any one of a number of initiators. When relying, as here, on the linear dose–response model, it is justified to add risk contributions from different sources when considering exposure to initiators. However, this generalized assumption cannot be extended to promoters and other modifying factors without further qualification. We are in these cases often dealing with specific effects in particular organs of the body where threshold doses for promotion have sometimes been determined. On the other hand, it must be emphasized that our knowledge is incomplete in this area (see Chapter 3). When interaction between different factors results in an overall effect which is greater than the sum of the individual risk contributions for each factor, this is usually described as 'synergism'

In practice, it may be difficult to distinguish between a promotive action and other actions which modify the level of cancer risk. This consideration provides an additional basis for dealing with the issues related to interaction in a broad fashion.

With a few examples from animal experiments and epidemiological investigations, different mechanisms for interaction are illustrated below.

Examples

In Chapter 3 the multi-stage nature of cancer induction is illustrated (Figure 3.1). Although this only provides a schematic and by no means complete picture of the more important stages involved in chemical carcinogenesis, it may serve as a basis for a discussion of the interaction of different factors in tumour induction. In principle, two types of interaction exist:

(1) An interaction which constitutes a prerequisite for the formation of a tumour: interaction between causative factors associated with specific stages in the chain of events which links a normal cell (A) to a tumour (D) as described in the diagram below.

Different types of exposure

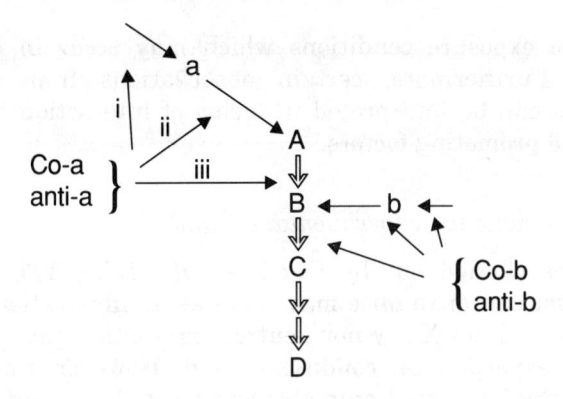

```
            a
         ↗
     i  ↑
        ii ↗
              A
  Co-a  ⎫  iii    ⇓
  anti-a ⎭ ────→  B  ←── b ←
              ⇓      ↖  ↑
              C  ←────  ⎧ Co-b
              ⇓         ⎩ anti-b
              D
```

The initiator a induces a transformation of a normal cell (A) into a cell possessing a latent defect (B)—an initiated cell. Factor b, a promoter, transforms the 'dormant' cancer cell (B) to an intermediate (pre-cancerous) stage (C) which eventually results in a tumour (D). In this process, a and b are interactive factors essential to the formation of the tumour. The initiator may have been formed metabolically from a pro-carcinogen, or in certain cases by means of an interaction which requires the simultaneous administration of two separate compounds. The formation of carcinogenic nitrosamines from nitrite (from certain foods or from nitrate) and from secondary amines (in the diet) in the gastro-intestinal tract is an example.

It should be emphasized that b in the diagram may be either an internally or an externally supplied factor. In animal experiments it has been demonstrated that the same agent (at high doses) may act both as a- and b- type Factors.

(2) Interaction between agents where certain factors increase ('co-a in the diagram) or decrease ('anti-a) the effect of the initiator A. The arrows i–iii on the diagram indicate that co-a and anti-a may modify the transformation of (A) into (B) in different ways: (i) by increasing or decreasing the dose of the initiator (e.g. by an alteration in its bio-activation or detoxification); (ii) by a change in the number of initiating reactions which occur between a and the hereditary material of (A) (by altering the frequency of cell division, etc.); or (iii) by changing the capacity of cell (A) to repair DNA damage. Though not of crucial importance for the transformation of (A) into (C), this kind of interaction results in a modification of the effects of a. In a similar way the effect of the promoter b can be modified by potentiating ('co-b') or inhibiting factors ('anti-b').

Mechanisms of interaction have been investigated in animal experiments under circumstances which are more or less comparable to exposure conditions which may occur in human populations. Furthermore, certain observations from epidemiological studies can be interpreted in terms of interaction between initiating and promoting factors.

Type (1) interactions—experimental animals

The studies carried out by Curtis *et al.* (1968, 1972) on radiation-induced liver cancer in mice may serve as an illustration of this kind of interaction. Neither X-ray nor neutron irradiation gave rise to tumours under the experimental conditions used. However, tumours could be induced if the irradiated animals were treated at some later time with a one-shot dose of carbon tetrachloride, which itself was insufficient to cause such an effect. The radiation may in this case be designated as an initiator (*a*) and the carbon tetrachloride as a promoter (*b*), and their interaction as obligatory. The development of liver cancer (in the absence of other initiators or promoters) may be prevented to the same extent by eliminating exposure to *either* of the two agents.

After oral administration of the substance urethane, skin tumours will be induced only after direct application of a promoter—in these experiments usually croton oil or phorbolic esters (the active constituents isolated from this oil)—to the skin of the experimental animals. If, on the other hand, a section of the liver is removed, inducing rapid cell division in this organ, liver tumours will appear. Similarly the administration of 2-acetylaminofluorene (2-AAF) via food to experimental animals will not induce skin tumours unless the skin is treated with croton oil. These are classical examples of the initiator (urethane, 2-AAF)–promoter (croton oil) situation (see review by Saffiotti (1980)).

Although observed dose–response relationships cannot be directly extrapolated to man, certain animal models are more relevant than others with respect to the pattern and conditions of exposure when taking into consideration how man actually is being exposed.

The ability of BaP to induce skin tumours in mice at low concentrations increases by a factor of 1000 in the presence of a non-carcinogenic hydrocarbon like n-dodecane. The poor correlation between the concentration of initiators like PAHs, present in mineral oil-based lubricants, and their carcinogenic potency when directly applied to mouseskin has been ascribed to differences in promoting activity (Bingham and Falk, 1969). These findings could also be important when assessing the relative risk associated with the use of products based on mineral oils. The observations that high levels of fat in the diet increase the colon tumour incidence induced by carcinogens like dimethylhydrazine and methylnitrosourea in rats (Reddy *et al.*, 1976, 1977) and that a high-fat diet stimulates the induction of mammary cancer in rats initiated by 7,12-dimethylbenzanthracene (Hopkins and Carroll 1979) may also be findings of fundamental significance to man.

Type (2) interactions—experimental animals

A number of factors modify the effects of various carcinogenic agents. The influence of externally administered hormones, or of the hormonal status of the organism, has been well documented and may be associated with interactions of type (1) as well as type (2). In rodents the administration of testosterone or the removal of the ovaries will cause an increase in the incidence of hepatic tumours induced by certain carcinogens in females, while administration of oestrogens or removal of the testicles combined with the administration of oestrogen suppresses the hepatocarcinogenic effect of ethylnitrosourea, while adrenalectomy protects (Warwick, 1971) against tumour induction at this site by 2-AAF. The increase in the frequency of liver tumour caused by 2-AAF in combination with hormones from the adrenal cortex (corticosteroids) completely supports this last observation. These hormones probably stimulate the metabolic activation of 2-AAF (Weisburger and Weisburger, 1963); an effect corresponding, in the diagram above, to a modification of the dose of a symbolized by the arrow 'i'.

Returning to the interaction between radiation and carbon tetrachloride mentioned above as a type (1) interaction, the initiating effect of radiation (at a given exposure level of carbon tetrachloride) can be modified by agents with radiation-protecting or -sensitizing properties, including factors which influence DNA repair, the diet administered to the experimental animals, etc. (factors co-a and anti-a in the diagram). The promoting action of carbon tetrachloride and the further progression of the tumour may likewise be modified by factors which affect the capacity of the animal to metabolize the chemical, influence the immunological defence, etc.

Factors which inhibit the formation of neoplasia, called anticarcinogens, have been illustrated by certain dietary factors for example in Chapter 3. Selenium and vitamins A and E belong to this category. However, the effects of such anti-carcinogens are ambiguous. Thus, butylated hydroxytoluene (BHT) possesses anti-carcinogenic properties in several systems (Wattenberg, 1977), but on the other hand increases the rate of growth of pulmonary tumours induced by urethane (Witschi *et al.*, 1977, 1981).

Interactions—human data

In considering the induction of cancer in man, this report has particularly focused on the interaction between smoking and other environmental factors. The importance of interaction has also been underlined in relation to the role played by dietary factors, and various possible mechanisms have been discussed. However, the complex relationships between initiators, promoters and co-carcinogens have not yet been clarified.

As previously mentioned, tobacco smoke contains both initiators and promoters. Besides acting as a complete carcinogen, tobacco smoke may thus also promote the development of cancer initiated in a different fashion, or function as an initiator in a situation where another factor acts as a promoter. Evidence of such interactions has been obtained in several epidemiological studies:

(a) smoking and exposure to radon daughter nuclides in mining (lung cancer);
(b) smoking and arsenic, probably a causative factor associated with work in smelters (lung cancer);
(c) smoking and alcohol consumption (oral cancer, cancer of the pharynx and oesophagus);
(d) smoking and asbestos (lung cancer, but not mesothelioma).

Smokers exposed to other air pollutants (e.g. in the workplace) often run higher risks of lung cancer than other smokers. The same may also apply for passive smoking. However, because smoking is so prevalent, and in addition varies among populations (defined by profession, geographic location, etc.), the identification of other interacting factors is difficult unless detailed data are available on smoking habits at the individual level. Possible interaction effects from the combination of tobacco smoke and urban air pollution have been discussed, but studies have encountered considerable methodological difficulties.

Rather than being exceptional, interactions of this kind are common in the aetiology of cancer in man (see Figure 3.1). Although some evidence of interaction may be available, the causal association is insufficiently known in many cases. This can be ascribed to the following facts. In contrast to experimental organisms, human populations are exposed to an extremely broad and variable pattern of initiators, promoters, and other co-carcinogens, including modifying factors of genetic origin. A co-carcinogen, for example an inhibitor of DNA-repair to which a population is exposed, will epidemiologically also be perceived as a causal factor. Further, epidemiological methods used in the past have only seldom (e.g. for study of the tobacco-related associations mentioned above) been based on statistical models which permit the identification of interaction. However, the lack of knowledge about interactions is primarily due to an absence of adequate measurements of the agents whose interaction is crucial in the aetiology of important neoplasias—agents, which have been identified only in a few cases.

Only scarce epidemiological data are available illustrating interactions associated with exposure to *defined* chemical and physical agents in man. In Figures 4.12 and 4.13 four examples are depicted where smoking has been implicated as one of the factors.

SMOKING AND EXPOSURE TO RADON DAUGHTERS IN MINERS

The mortality from lung cancer as a consequence of the combined action of exposure to radon daughters and smoking has been subjected to detailed investigations in North American uranium miners. The progressive shortening of the latency time for induction of tumours of the lung with increasing number of cigarettes consumed at a given level of radon daughters is one effect which has been reported (Archer et al., 1976). This observation corresponds with the kind of promotion by smoking which has been demonstrated in animal experiments. In studies where the follow-up time for exposed and non-exposed groups has been sufficiently long, and where, in addition, detailed individually related data concerning smoking habits have been available, a synergistic interaction between the two causative factors is also evident. This fact is in agreement with the adaptability of a multiplicative model to the data (see Larsson and Damber, 1982).

SMOKING AND ARSENIC

In a study of workers employed at the smelters of Rönnskärmärsverken, a pronounced interaction between exposure to arsenic and smoking in the induction of lung cancer has been demonstrated (Pershagen et al., 1981). The results tend to support a multiplicative effect. The mechanism underlying this interaction has not yet been fully clarified. Modifying influences of other chemicals associated with arsenic exposure cannot be excluded. In experimental systems it has been demonstrated that arsenic (as well as some other metals) may act by inhibiting the 'error-free' repair of damage in DNA. The operation of such a mechanism implies that arsenic could modify the effect of initiators of other origins, including components of tobacco smoke.

SMOKING AND ASBESTOS

The carcinogenic action of asbestos was mentioned in Section 4.4.5. As seen in Figure 4.12, smoking can cause a 10-fold increase in the risk of lung cancer compared to exposure to asbestos alone. If asbestos acts as a promoter (which is possible) in relation to the effect caused by initiators in tobacco smoke, it may seem surprising that interaction (synergism) does not occur with the mesothelioma induced by asbestos. A localization of the interaction at the pulmonary epithelium directly in contact with the tobacco smoke may provide an explanation.

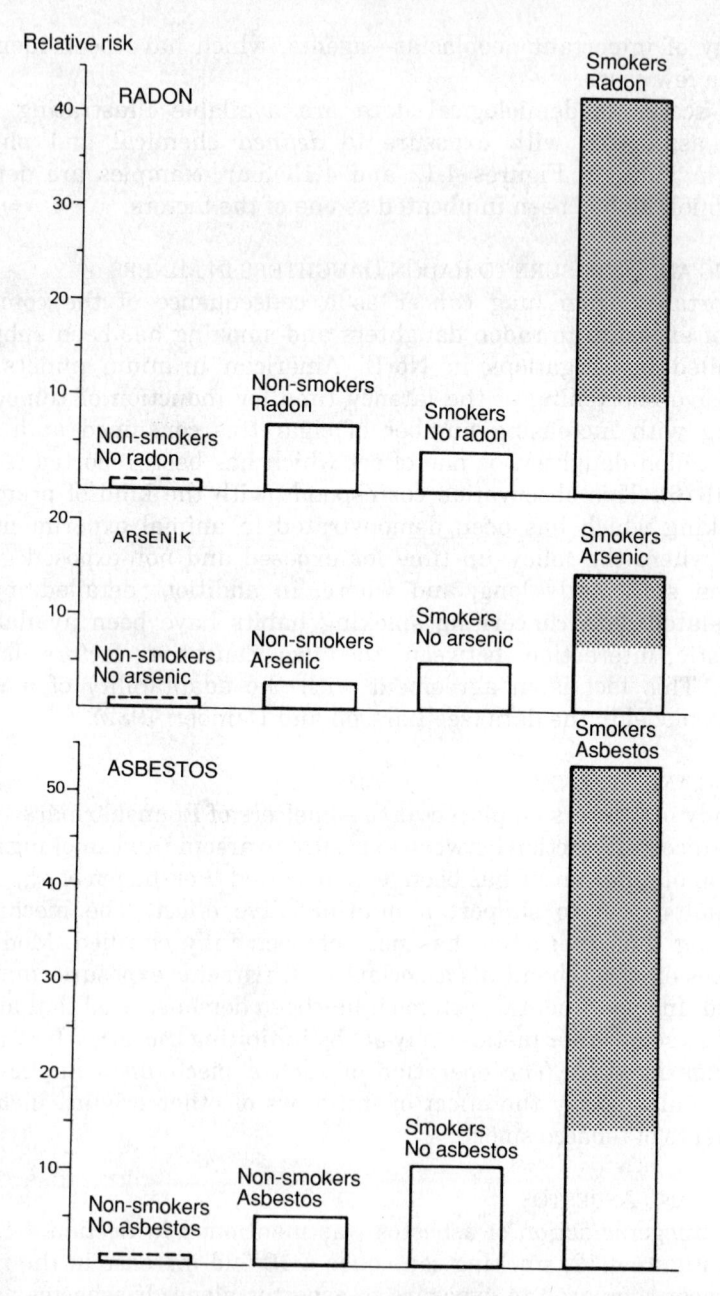

Figure 4.12 The risk of lung cancer from smoking and simultaneous exposure to radon, arsenic and asbestos (Archer et al. 1973; Pershagen et al. 1981; Hammond et al. 1979). The risk for non-smokers who have not been exposed to these agents has been given the value of 1, and the relative risk for the other exposure combinations adapted accordingly. It should be noted that the populations studied are not comparable with respect to factors such as smoking habits. The shaded areas represent the excess risk due to interaction.

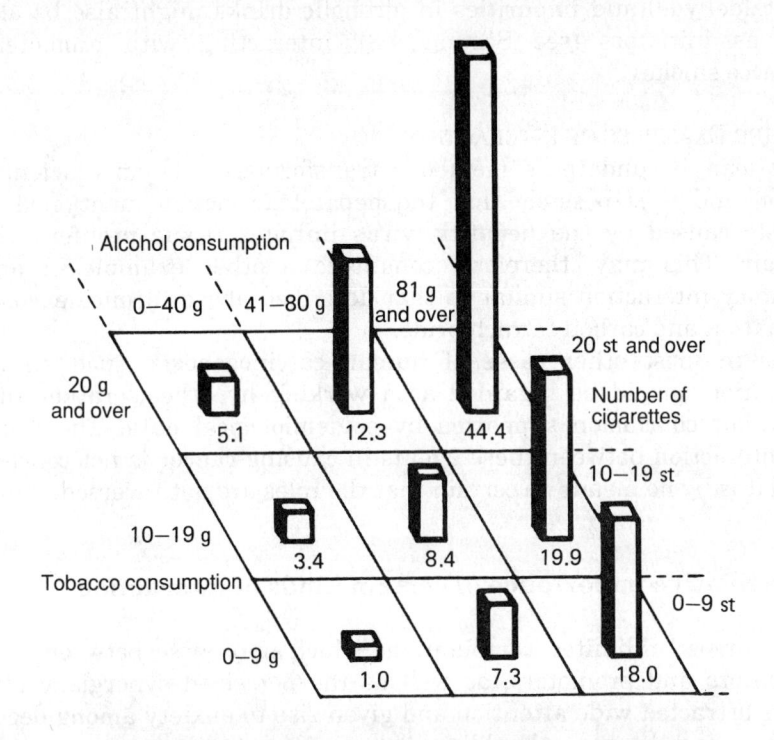

[Figure: 3D bar chart showing relative risk by alcohol consumption (0–40 g, 41–80 g, 81 g and over) and tobacco consumption (0–9 g, 10–19 g, 20 g and over), with values: 1.0, 7.3, 18.0; 3.4, 8.4, 19.9; 5.1, 12.3, 44.4. Axis also labeled "Number of cigarettes" with 0–9 st, 10–19 st, 20 st and over.]

Note: The height of the columns indicates the relative risk compared with persons with low or no consumption of alcohol and tobacco (relative risk (RR) = 1.0)

Figure 4.13 Relative risk for oesophageal cancer in relation to the daily consumption of alcohol and tobacco. From the Office of Technology Assessment (1981).

SMOKING AND ALCOHOL

In a number of investigations the pronounced synergistic effect of a combination of high alcohol consumption and smoking has been demonstrated for the induction of oral cancer and for cancer of the pharynx and oesophagus. In Figure 4.13 the incidence of oesophageal cancer is illustrated as a function of the amount of alcohol and the number of cigarettes consumed per day. In heavy smokers the majority of such cancers could, obviously, be avoided by abstaining from alcohol. Conversely, the risk of oesophageal cancer in heavy drinkers is much greater when drinking is combined with smoking.

The interaction between smoking and alcohol has been interpreted in terms of interactive effects between initiators in the tobacco smoke and a promotive effect of alcohol when consumed in the form of strong liquor. Alternatively the alcohol may facilitate the uptake of carcinogens present in the smoke. However, alcohol (after conversion to acetaldehyde) and impurities in alcoholic drinks might also be able to act as initiators (see Section 4.3), interacting with promoters in tobacco smoke.

OTHER EXAMPLES OF INTERACTION

Aflatoxin B_1 undergoes metabolic transformation to an efficient initiator, and it is possible that the hepatotoxic action mentioned previously caused by the hepatitis virus initiates tissue proliferation for repair. This may, therefore, constitute another example of an obligatory interaction similar to that described above in mice exposed to radiation and carbon tetrachloride.

As in most other cases of human carcinogenesis, such an interpretation should be regarded as a working hypothesis rather than a clear-cut conclusion supported by epidemiological data. The evidence of interaction between these agents in causing cancer is not conclusive, and it is by no means be certain that the roles are not reversed.

The relative importance of certain kinds of interaction

The almost unlimited combinations which may arise between various initiators and promoters, as well as the perceived synergistic effects, have attracted wide attention and given rise to anxiety among decision-makers and the general public.

Data are scarce in this huge field and scientific difficulties abound, including 'traditional' ones of applying various research findings to current conditions and exposures of a human population.

In connection with the interactions between smoking and exposure to radon daughter nuclides, between smoking and arsenic, and between smoking and asbestos, the observed effects are multiplicative. This means that if one agent increases the risk by a factor of four and the other by a factor of 10, exposure to both factors will result in a 40-fold elevation of risk (see Saracci, 1981). However, a statistical correlation of data fitting a multiplicative model by no means constitutes a sufficient criterion for interaction. If certain individuals exhibit an increased sensitivity towards both factors, statistical correlations of this kind may, in fact, arise without any interaction being involved (Miettinen, 1982).

When two causal factors are interacting the number of cases which can be ascribed to each factor will be greater than the number of aetiological cases which can be associated with the two factors together. This situation can be illustrated (Table 4.20) by an example from the work of Wall and Taube (1983) who analysed the effects of smoking and work at roasting kilns. Out of 76 cases of lung cancer, a total of 61 may be associated with the two causal factors. Among the kiln workers who smoked, 29 cases occurred, of which 27 may be ascribed to the pair of exposures in question.

Table 4.20 The number of cases of lung cancer in the so-called Rönnskär study due to exposure to arsenic (work at roasting kilns), tobacco smoking and the interaction between these two factors (see text).

Smoking	Roasting kilns	Number of cases			
		Total	Smoking as a cause	Roasting kilns as a cause	Both factors together
No	No	3	0	0	0
No	Yes	5	0	3	0
Yes	No	39	31	0	0
Yes	Yes	29	23	17	27
Sum		76	54	20	
Sum of aetiological cases		61	(31)	(3)	(27)

From Wall and Taube (1983).

The sum of cases which can be ascribed to smoking (23) and to work at the kilns (17) is greater than the number of aetiological cases (27) because 13 cases (23+17−27) are associated with interaction between the two factors. In the group of roasting kiln workers who smoked, 10 cases (23−13) can be ascribed to smoking alone, and four cases (17−13) solely to working at the kilns. Among the 76 cases of lung cancer, 61 cases can be explained, taking the prevailing smoking habits into account: 41 cases (54−13) can be ascribed purely to smoking, seven cases (20−13) solely to work at the kilns, and 13 cases to interaction between the two factors.

How much importance should be attached to such interaction? Available data indicate that the effects of promoters and co-carcinogens are characterized by a minimum level of exposure below which the effects on the induction of tumours may be taken as negligible (Bohrman, 1983). In reality this seems to imply that for effects to have sufficient impact to influence the overall picture, the causative agents should be primarily commonly occurring promoters or co-carcinogens. In the case of chemical substances this would include agents which are often present at appreciable concentrations, and where exposure is frequent or continuous. Judging from epidemiological data, tobacco smoke, alcoholic beverages, and components in the diet constitute such agents, although the active compounds have not yet been clearly identified; other agents with similar effects will no doubt be identified in the future.

Fears have been expressed that the multitude of combinations including exposure to all the possible chemicals on the market will cause interactions, primarily synergism (multiplicative interaction), which could be responsible for a considerable proportion of the current cancer incidence. Although interaction in the form of promotion undoubtedly plays an important role under certain conditions, for example in association with smoking, consumption of alcohol, dietary factors, etc., it seems very unlikely that such a notion has any real substance with respect to industrial chemicals in general. Estimates of the size of risk contributions from various environments further support this conclusion. On the other hand this does not exclude significant effects from interaction in individuals or in limited populations caused by exposure to a combination of agents in the workplace or with certain types of drug therapy.

Notes

1. A new evaluation of tobacco smoking, by the International Agency for Research on Cancer, is now available as Vol. 38 of the *IARC Monograph Series*. Its main conclusions are that:

    (a) There is *sufficient evidence* that inhalation of tobacco smoke as well as topical application of tobacco smoke condensate cause cancer in experimental animals.

    (b) There is *sufficient evidence* that tobacco smoke is carcinogenic to humans.

    The occurrence of malignant tumours of the respiratory tract and of the upper digestive tract is causally related to the smoking of different forms of tobacco (cigarettes, cigars, pipes, *ibid*). The occurrence of malignant tumours of the bladder, renal pelvis and pancreas is causally related to the smoking of cigarettes. [*Ed. note.*]

2. Now available as *IARC Monograph* Vol., 37 (September 1985), 'Tobacco habits other than smoking; betel-quid and areca-nut chewing; and some related nitroamines'. [*Ed. note.*]

3. In this book, the terms 'mutation' and 'mutation-like' change are often used to cover all the effects referred to here.

4. In principle, a pharmaceutical speciality must not be marketed in Sweden unless it has been approved ('registered') by the National Board of Health and Welfare, which should take efficacity of the product as well as safety aspects into account. [*Ed. note.*]

5. The National Environmental Protection Board points out that the choice of BaP as an indicator substance is subject to many uncertainties, of which one is the fact that the pattern of polycyclic organic compounds varies with the emission source. The concentration of BaP can therefore only serve as a crude estimate of

Different types of exposure

the degree of air pollution for this class of substances. Furthermore, BaP is easily transformed in the atmosphere by photochemical reactions (see also Section 4.4.5)].

6   The hygienic limit in the workplace in Sweden; later lowered to 0.5 fibre ml^{-1} [Ed. note.]

7   The number of cases originally stated was erroneous and has been corrected here. [*Ed. note.*]

8   Reduced to 2.5 mg m^{-3} in 1984. [*Ed. note.*]

9   The Chernobyl accident in the USSR in Spring 1986, although increasing radioactive pollution considerably in some parts of Sweden, is thought to have a limited impact on the total number of expected deaths or serious injuries. One official report (No. 87–13 by the Swedish National Institute of Radiation Protection) arrives at an estimate of 2–4 cancer deaths per year during the next 50 years. [*Ed. note.*].

5
Studies of variations in cancer mortality and incidence in Sweden

5.1 Introduction

This chapter is based partially on studies carried out for the Cancer Committee by Lars Ehrenberg and colleagues at The University of Stockholm. The details of the methods and results of these studies are described in Ehrenberg and Ekman (1984), von Bahr et al. (1984a), Ekman et al. (1984), Berglund et al. (1984) and Eklund (1984).

5.1.1 Background

The incidence of various tumour diseases, and the mortality from them, varies between subpopulations in Sweden characterized by place of domicile, social conditions, occupational status and and other factors. Furthermore, variations occur over time, as illustrated in Figures 2.4a and 2.4b, 2.6, 2.11 and 2.12, and Tables 2.1, 2.2 and 2.6 in Chapter 2. Comparative studies of this kind betweeen regions and population groups in various countries with respect to the occurrence of specific types of tumour, have indicated that the majority of all cancers are caused by environmental factors. This conclusion has sometimes been misinterpreted to mean that environmental factors include only man-made pollution at places of work, in the air, water and food, etc. Environmental factors must however, be interpreted in a broader sense to include 'life-style', a concept which plays an important role[1] (see Chapter 2, Tables 2.7 and 2.8). Variations between subpopulations can help in identifying causes of tumour diseases, and provide a better point of departure for preventive measures.

5.1.2 Information sources

In Sweden and the other Nordic countries all inhabitants are registered by means of a census identifier, the so-called personal number. This number provides a unique possibility of linking information concerning diseases and deaths with environmental descriptors such as place of domicile, occupational status, etc., in order to provide a basis for investigations into the causes of cancer and other diseases. The use and construction of data-bases for epidemiological purposes are treated in Chapter 8.

In Sweden two data-bases of national scope are available which can be used in mapping the occurrence of cancer in various environments and its role in the disease pattern and as a cause of death. These are the Cancer Registry of the National Board of Health and Welfare and the Cause-of-Death Registry of Statistics Sweden (Statistika Centralbyråns, SCB; earlier named the Central Bureau of Statistics) (see also Swenson (1984) and Chapter 8). These data-bases constitute the most important sources of information for describing and investigating the variations with time of tumour diseases as well as variations between subpopulations. The potential for studying variations over time is limited, however, since death certificates have been centrally filed only since 1951, and the Cancer Registry was set up as late as 1958.

Certain environmental descriptors related to individuals such as place of domicile (municipality and parish) and occupational status (according to standard codes) from the national census of 1960 have been merged with data from the Cancer Registry to form the Cancer–Environment Registry (Einhorn et al., 1978) and with data from the Cause-of-Death Registry to form the Mortality–Environment Registry (SCB 1981a).

5.1.3 Objectives, related investigations, etc.

The Cancer–Environment Registry and the Mortality–Environment Registry have been used to examine variations in cancer incidence and mortality in Sweden, as described by von Bahr et al. (1984a), Ekman et al. (1984), Berglund et al. (1984) and Eklund (1984), and summarized by Ehrenberg and Ekman (1984). This chapter reviews these investigations, which are certainly not exhaustive, but should be considered as examples of registry studies aiming to show to what extent it is possible to describe variations and pinpoint their causes by carrying out analyses of data existing in various data bases. The methods and results of these studies have been described in more detail by Ehrenberg and Ekman (1984).

One specific aim of the analyses has been to investigate and as far as possible describe the structure of the 'urban factor', i.e. the complex of factors underlying the well-known phenomenon of higher incidence and mortality in many tumour diseases in urban districts, expecially in large cities, than in rural districts. From the point of view of preventive measures it has been considered important to establish the existence, and order of magnitude, of the effects of general air pollution in urban areas. A further general aim has been to estimate the proportion of the incidence of various tumour diseases attibutable to, or in a statistical sense 'explainable by', environmental descriptors in a broad sense.

> Investigations of the type indicated here do not generally permit conclusions concerning risks run by *individuals*. It is rather a matter of statistical correlations at the *group* level. However, if groups of individuals differ with respect to aspects of life-style which are known to influence cancer incidence, such as smoking, certain sexual habits or fertility pattern, such individual habits may imply differences in the individual risk.

The possibilities of determining causes of disease by these methods are extremely limited, mainly because the *available* environmental descriptors are mostly of an 'indirect' nature. Thus the marital status descriptor and the variables describing socio-economic conditions of domicile—variables used in the investigations—do not directly reflect cause of disease. If statistically significant interdependence is found between incidence or mortality as concerns a particular disease and such an indirect environmental descriptor, this only points to the fact that the direct cause of the disease could be some factor which is in turn related to the descriptor (Ehrenberg and Ekman 1984). For example, differences in marital status could reflect different life-styles, and differences in socio-economic conditions between residential areas could reflect different degrees of industrialization with resulting differences in pollution. Furthermore, in studies of interrelationships between a large number of variables, a certain number of relationships are found which though statistically 'significant' are spurious (the so-called mass significance problem).

Because of the indirect nature of the data-base descriptors, analytical data-base studies should mainly be considered as *identifiers of problems*, not as *solutions* to them: the discovery of statistical relationships provides reasons for further investigations into the true causes; such studies should preferably be carried out at the level of individual cases. Clarification of the causal patterns will involve testing hypotheses generated by the data-base studies or by other research, but an unprejudiced approach should always be adopted as well.

An investigation by Wall and Taube (1983) into the association between cancer risk and occupational exposure at the Rönnskär copper smelter provides a good illustration of the type of problems and the methodology involved in such studies of causality. This study shows how a question of this kind may be approached by different methods, also using data concerning the individuals' exposure situations.

The investigations treated here include:[2]

(a) Mortality from tumour diseases, classified according to the so-called A-list[3], by sex, age, marital status and region of domicile (the three metropolitan areas of Stockholm, Gothenburg and Malmö, and the rest of Sweden), for the periods 1969–1973 and 1974–8. The data have been extracted from the Cause-of-Death Registry. This basic information has been published by SCB (1981b) by marital status and region separately. The data have been statistically processed, using a classical statistical model (see Johansson and Ekman, 1983) as well as a method developed by B. von Bahr (Stockholm University) using a weighted multiplicative Poisson model (von Bahr et al., 1984).

(b) An investigation of the possible *influence of the diagnostic routines in hospitals* (and variations in related reporting frequency) upon *incidence* was included in the studies of cancer incidence using the Cancer–Environment Registry. Both a classical analysis of variance and a Poisson model were employed in this study (Ekman et al., 1984).

As discussed in Chapter 2, the improvement in methods and routines for diagnosing cancer has often been suspected of contributing to the observed increase in incidence of certain tumour diseases over time. If such improvements are not uniform, or there are differences in diagnostic efforts for other reasons in different hospitals, then epidemiological comparisons between various geographical or occupational groups of persons may lead to erroneous conclusions about the true variations in cancer incidence.

In this investigation the parishes in Sweden have been characterized according to the proportion of cancer cases diagnosed by advanced methods (pathological anatomical diagnosis—'PAD'—of biopsy or autopsy material, as well as cytological methods) according to the coding in the Cancer–Environment Registry. Using this information, a variable called *diagnostic intensity* has been constructed. In computing the variations in incidence attempts have been made in various ways to estimate the magnitude of this confounding influence and to eliminate this 'noise'.

(c) Particularly to study the 'urban factors' behind various tumour diseases, the incidences in the Swedish municipalities (a total of 279 according to the 1979 sub-division) have been examined with respect to various socio-economic variables (Berglund et al., 1984). Besides the degree of urbanization itself, calculated according to generally used classification systems in Sweden, these variables include the proportion of the population employed in certain occupations, and car density (owners per 1000 inhabitants). Futher 'explanatory' variables used are the above-mentioned diagnostic intensity (in which connection municipalities are characterized using a weighted mean value of hospitals visited by the inhabitants) and the proportion of 'habitual smokers' (based on a large-scale postal survey in 1963 of smoking habits of persons aged 18–69 years, using a random sample of 55 000 inhabitants (men and women) (SCB, 1965)).

The variables employed in the present study have been selected, using factor analysis of some 30 variables, as relevantly expressing the socio-economic conditions in the municipalities. It should be pointed out that the use of the proportion of the population employed in certain occupational categories to characterize the municipalities by no means implies that those occupations as such entail an increased cancer risk. The variables to a large extent indirectly reflect aetiological factors, which are summarized in Table 5.1. Obviously these variables are not independent of each other but are partially redundant, and the main features of this interdependence are also included in Table 5.1.

Teppo et al. (1980) have studied cancer incidence in Finnish municipalities as a function of various socio-economic variables in a similar investigation, but the dependence of incidence was examined one variable at a time. Study (c) therefore goes one step further, since the multiple regression analyses employed compute the total dependence on several variables while also recognizing their interdependence.

(d) *Occupationally induced cancer*, especially the total number of cancer cases which may be attributable to occupational exposures, has been discussed by Ehrenberg and Ekman (1984) after a preliminary analysis of the Cancer–Environment Registry, and using some other sources as well.

(e) In order to extract *trends from the development of cancer incidence* over time, and to examine fluctuations and possible errors in their assessment, Eklund (1984) has analysed the Cancer–Environment Registry for the years 1960–78 (see also Ehrenberg and Ekman, 1984).

Table 5.1 Variables used in the study of cancer incidences in Swedish municipalities (for details see Berglund et al. (1984).

Variable	The variable expresses:	Positive or negative linear correlations with other variables[a]
1. Diagnostic intensity	Mainly the influence of diagnostic routines upon reported incidence; maybe also 'big-city' character	Var. 6 (+) Var. 3 (−)
2. Degree of urbanization (population density)	Air pollution? Also life-style factors, including smoking and alcohol habits	Var. 4 (− −); Var. 5–8 (+)
3. Cars density	Probably not exhaust emissions. Socio-economic conditions	Var. 5 (+ +); Var. 4, 7 (+); Var. 1 (−); No correlation with Var. 2
4–7. Proportion of population employed in		
4. Agriculture, forestry (men)	Rural character (also absence of urban character)	Var. 2 (− −); Var. 5–8 (−)
5. Manufacturing industry and mining (men)	Factory districts	Var. 2, 3 (+); Var. 4, 6, 7 (− / − −)
6. Banking and insurance (men)	Certain characteristics of 'big cities'	Var. 1, 2 (+); Var. 4, 5 (−)
7. Public service (women)	County centres, hospital towns	Var. 2, 3 (+); Var. 5 (− −); Var. 4 (−)
8. Proportion of 'habitual smokers' (men and women)[b]	Smoking habits and other related habits (highest values in 'big cities')	Var. 2 (+)

[a] Only correlations remaining after elimination of the effect of the other variables, i.e. partial correlations, are given: − −, strongly negative; −, negative; +, positive; + +, strongly positive.
[b] This variable is uncertain for small municipalities.

With regard to the influence of environmental descriptors, the results of these studies are summarized in Section 5.2 (demonstrated correlations) and in Section 5.3 (estimates of the magnitude of demonstrated correlations, 'explainable' fractions, etc.). The relationships between occupational data and cancer incidence or mortality are treated quite briefly in Section 5.4. As concerns specific occupational factors, there have been many Swedish and non-Swedish studies (see Section 4.4).

The relation of cancer to other diseases and causes of death is treated in Section 5.5. No more penetrating analyses have been carried out, partly because cancer as such is not one unique disease. The question is posed whether various socio-economic groups are associated with different risks for cancer as a cause of death as compared with other causes of death.

The special study of cancer development over time is summarized in Section 5.6.

In Section 5.7, lung cancer, and its relation to smoking as an aetiological factor, is examined as a case study of the consequences of changes in an environmental factor.

5.2 Demonstrated relationships between incidence of mortality and certain environmental variables

5.2.1 Diagnostic routines

The influence of the diagnostic intensity on the reported incidence of certain types of cancer has been examined, together with the parallel influence of age and degree of urbanization. Two complementary statistical methods were employed. This section summarizes some of the conclusions drawn by Ehrenberg and Ekman (1984) from these studies. The results, highly compressed and simplified in Table 5.2, shows that, besides a more or less marked influence of the degree of urbanization (except as concerns stomach cancer and leukaemia), correlations of reported cancer incidence with the diagnostic intensity appear which are partly dependent and partly independent of age and degree of urbanization. The dependence of this correlation on age is illustrated in Figure 5.1, in which the age dependence for all male cancer incidence is given at different degrees of diagnostic intensity as interpreted by a scale from 1–9 with increasing degree of diagnostic sophistication. From these results it may be concluded that the influence of this diagnosis factor is, above all, that at a lower diagnostic intensity there is a deficit of reported cancer cases at higher ages. This differing influence of the diagnosis factor between age groups gives rise to the significant interaction effects in Table 5.2 (penultimate column). The same relationships may be illustrated by a parameter

Table 5.2 Dependence of incidence of certain types of tumour on the degree of urbanization and 'diagnostic intensity' (for details see Ekman et al. (1984).

		Correlation [a] demonstrated with			
		Urbanization	Diagnosis	Age × diagnosis[b]	Urbanization × diagnosis[b]
Stomach	M	–	(+)	+	–
Colon and rectum	M	(+)	+	++	+
Pancreas	M	+	+	+[c]	–
Pancreas	F	(+)	–	+[c]	–
Lung	M	++	++	++	+
Lung	F	(+)	++	–	(+)
Breast	F	+	+	–	–
Cervix	F	++	++	–	+
Prostate	M	+	+	++	+
Kidney	M	+	+	++	+
Urinary bladder	M	+	+	–	+
Leukemia	M	–	+	–	–
Leukemia	F	–	–	–	–
All tumours	M	+	+	+	+
All tumours	F	+	+	+	–

[a] Correlations: –, small or not significant; (+), almost significant; +, significant; ++, strongly significant.
[b] Significant interactions age × diagnosis and urbanization × diagnosis imply that the dependence of incidence on diagnostic intensity varies with age and degree of urbanization respectively.
[c] As regards cancer of the pancreas, this interaction varies with the degree of urbanization (i.e. the symbol '+' signifies a so-called second-order interaction.

matrix with numerical values for deviations from the average, which may be used when correcting for underreporting of cancer cases.

A significant influence of the diagnosis factor was also discerned for most types of tumour in the analysis of the statistical relationships between socio-economic variables and cancer incidence (Berglund et al., 1984). As in the former investigation, stomach cancer and leukaemia were exceptions and, furthermore, no influence of the diagnosis factor could be detected for cancer of the pancreas, breast and corpus uteri in the latter study.

Differences in diagnostic intensity result in varying proportions of actual cancer cases being diagnosed and/or in a reduced tendency to report to the Cancer Registry when diagnosis is uncertain. This effect is quite small at ages below 65 years, but can be of great importance at higher ages. Since a large proportion of cancer cases occur in elderly people, errors may result from comparisons between populations based on traditionally age-standardized incidences, or between periods of time which may have different reporting probabilities. In certain areas there has been a tendency for under-diagnosis or under-

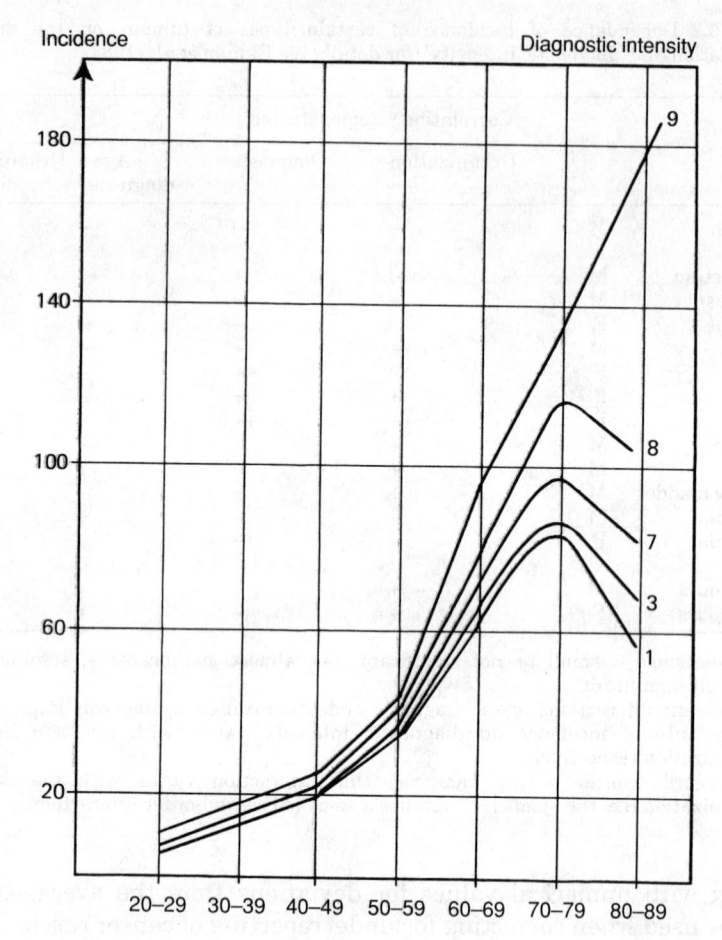

Figure 5.1 Dependence of cancer incidence (all tumour types between 1961 and 67) in men at varying diagnostic intensities, represented by a scale 1–9. (Age by intervals, year 1960).
From Ekman et al. (1984).

reporting to decrease during recent years, which can cause trends to be over-estimated and even the incidence of a certain tumour to be judged to be increasing when in fact it is decreasing.

Doll and Peto (1981), in their overview of the causes of cancer in the USA, have attempted to solve this problem by examining trends only on the basis of data for ages below 65 years. In his report to the Cancer Committee Eklund (1984) arrived at a similar conclusion under Swedish conditions and proposed exclusion of data for persons over 75 years of age. (Doll and Peto furthermore make use of mortality data, where noise dependent on variations of diagnostic routines with time and place is not so great, for their estimates of changes of incidences.)

Valuable information is lost by such procedures, however, since so many of the cases occur at higher ages. The so-called Poisson model may provide an acceptable solution to these problems (von Bahr et al., 1984a; Ekman et al., 1984).

Part but not all of the influence of the diagnostic factor derives from variations in time and place of frequency and methods of autopsy. In particular in the southern Swedish city of Malmö, which shows the highest diagnostic intensity in Sweden, it is notable that a greater proportion of the cancer incidence is represented by latent tumours discovered unexpectedly at autopsy than in the rest of the country. This, for example, affects the reported *incidence* of prostate cancer (see Saxén, 1982), which was nearly twice as high in Malmö as in Stockholm, whereas the *mortality* with prostate cancer as the primary cause of death was somewhat lower in Malmö than in Stockholm. An improvement, if not a solution, to the problem of the confounding influence of the diagnostic factor would result if cases detected unexpectedly after death (and where the tumour was judged neither to have constituted a disease nor to have been a contributory cause of death) were removed from the incidence data used for the estimation of trends and in statistical comparisons between populations. However, such autopsy findings are of considerable scientific value in the overall description of cancer diseases and their causes.

5.2.2 Socio-economic factors and life-style

Examination of the dependence of cancer incidence and mortality on certain socio-economic variables reveals certain characteristic patterns. The variations in mortality are summarized in Table 5.3.

The remainder of this section is taken directly from the report by Ehrenberg and Ekman (1984).

The types of tumour for which a causal relationship with tobacco smoking has been demonstrated or proposed occur in relationship patterns which differ radically from the patterns of tumours at other sites. The fact that, in the investigation of incidences using the Cancer–Environment Registry, a positive correlation appears for exactly those types of tumour, in spite of the uncertainty of the variable reflecting the proportion of smokers in the municipalities as derived from a survey sample, indicates that the results are reliable and permits a cautious conclusion that a real causal relationship with smoking exists. The incidences of cancer of the oesophagus and of the lung in men furthermore show a correlation with degree of urbanization and with the variable reflecting 'big city environment', undoubtedly in part a consequence of differences in smoking habits between urban areas, especially large cities, and the rest of the country (Table 5.4). The mortality study (Table 5.3) shows the highest mortality rate, together

Table 5.3 Cancer as cause of death. Significant variations between regions and civil status expressed as the ratio between the highest and lowest death rate; in parentheses is the group with the highest value. (For details see Ehrenberg and Ekman (1984) and von Bahr et al. (1984a).)

	Comparison between regions		Comparisons between civil status	
	Male	Female	Male	Female
Tumours related to smoking				
Oral cavity, pharynx	2.4(SM)		3.0(d)	
Oesophagus	2.4(SM)		2.7(d)	
Larynx	2.9(SM)		2.8(d)	
Lung, etc.	2.0(SM)	1.8(SM)	2.1(d)	1.6(d)
Cervix uteri[a]	–	1.4(SM)	–	2.8(d)
Tumours of the alimentary tract				
Stomach			1.2(d)	
Small intestine and colon	1.3(MÖ)	1.3(MÖ)	(w)	1.2(u)
Rectum	1.4(MÖ)	1.3(MÖ)	1.2(w)	1.3(u)
Tumour of the sex-related organs				
Corpus uteri	–		–	1.4(u)
Breast	–	1.1(SM,GG)	–	1.4(u)
Prostate	1.2(SM)	–	1.3(d)	–
Other tumours[b]				
Skin	1.4(MÖ)		1.1(m)	
Leukaemia			1.1(m)	
Other lymphatic		1.3(MÖ)		
Benign	1.8(SM)			1.4(u)
All cancer forms	1.4(SM)	1.1(SM)	1.4(d)	1.2(d)

SM, Stockholm metropolitan area
GG, Gothenburg metropolitan area
MÖ, Malmö metropolitan area

Number noted, significant variation
No notation, variation not significant
–, comparison not relevant

u, unmarried
m, married
d, divorced
w, widow/widower

[a] Tobacco smoking can be an aetioligical factor (see Table 4.6b), but statistical correlation with smoking may be mainly attributed to the connection between smoking and such sexual habits as deficient hygiene, furthering the induction of a tumour.
[b] The 'cause-of-death' group A58 (tumours in 'other unspecified organs') is not included.

with cancer in the oral cavity and pharynx and larynx, in the Stockholm area—two to three times higher than in the area outside the three largest cities (denoted 'the rest of the country'). This is compatible with the fact that the proportion of smokers is highest in the Stockholm area (Table 5.5). The comparison with marital status shows a considerably increased risk for divorced people, probably

Cancer mortality and incidence in Sweden

Table 5.4 The proportion of habitual smokers by degree of urbanization.

		Men, age in 1963 (years)		Women, age in 1963 (years)	
		18–49 (%)	50–69 (%)	18–49 (%)	50–69 (%)
Habitual smokers	Big cities	57.4	55.9	38.6	19.1
	Other urban areas	55.5	50.8	30.8	10.9
	Rural areas	47.3	37.0	21.7	4.9
Heavy smokers (more than 16 cigarettes/day)	Big cities	17.0	11.3	5.5	2.1
	Other urban areas	10.6	5.3	2.5	0.5
	Rural areas	5.7	1.0	0.9	0.1

From the postal survey (1963), SCB (1965) and Cederlöf et al. (1975).

Table 5.5 Proportion of habitual smokers in the three metropolitan areas and the rest of Sweden in 1963. Weighted means for municipalities of the smoking variable in the study of the dependence of cancer incidence on socio-economic variables. (For details see Ehrenberg and Ekman (1984).

Area	Number of persons[a] (thousands)	Proportion of habitual smokers [a](%)
Stockholm area	833	44
Gothenburg area	394	40
Malmö area	264	43
Rest of Sweden	3830	37
Sweden in total	5320	39

[a] Both sexes, ages 18–69 years

Table 5.6 Smoking habits by marital status.

	Proportion of smokers (%) among			
	Unmarried	Married	Divorced	Widowers/Widows
Men	30	41	65	47
Women	9	12	23	13

From Mellström's (1981) study of persons aged over 70 years.

because they are on average the heaviest smokers (Table 5.6). In contrast to the other types of tumour associated with smoking, lung cancer exhibits the lowest frequency amongst the unmarried, a phenomenon which could be related to the lower smoking prevalence in this group (Table 5.6), but which is less distinct in the larger cities than the rest of Sweden. It should be recalled, however, that this correlation with smoking habits does not exclude other causes, alternative or complementary. For example it is probable that alcohol habits contributed to the considerable variation in incidence of and mortality from oesophageal cancer and cancer of the upper respiratory tract, in accordance with the aetiological role generally ascribed to alcohol for these types of tumour; further available statistical data show that abuse of alcohol in Sweden is strongly correlated with tobacco smoking (Table 5.7).

Table 5.7 The proportion of men aged 18–69 years, recorded in the Alcohol Registry for law violations related to the use of alcohol, in various categories of smokers in 1963.

Smoking category	Proportion in the Alcohol Registry[a] (%)
Never smoked	9.4
All who smoked in 1963	19.9
Smoke 16 cigarettes or more per day	27.6
Former smokers	11.8
All men, irrespective of smoking habits	16.6

[a] Law violations recorded include being drunk in public, drunken driving, committing crimes while under the influence of alcohol and its illegal sale or manufacture.
Data from Cederlöf et al. (1975).

Significant statistical correlations are also found between smoking habits and incidences of other tumour forms for which evidence has been put forward for an aetiological role for tobacco smoking. This concerns the pancreas, kidney, possibly the urinary bladder, and also stomach cancer. Indicated correlations with the incidence of leukaemia call for further investigations. A particularly strong correlation with the smoking variable is seen for cervical cancer, where the pattern of incidence also includes a positive correlation with the degree of urbanization.[4] As for cancer of the lung, the mortality in cervical cancer is highest in the Stockholm area and among divorced people. The fluctuations in the occurrence of cervical cancer could be considered to support the hypothesis concerning a direct role played by tobacco smoking, but should be attributed above all to the connection between smoking habits and sexual habits that further the development of this tumour.

The types of tumour for which an aetiological influence of dietary habits and fertility pattern has been surmised exhibit a completely different spectrum of statistical dependences on the variables studied when compared with cancer of the respiratory tract and the oesophagus. Thus the incidences of colorectal cancer and breast cancer are positively correlated both with urbanization and with variables associated with rural and semi-rural characteristics such as the proportion of employees in farming and forestry, in the manufacturing industries and (for colorectal cancer) the density of car ownership (see Table 5.1).

Mortality for such tumours is highest in the Malmö area and among unmarried women and widowers. Similar correlation patterns are found for incidence and mortality in cancer of the corpus uteri, but with a slight positive correlation with an increased degree of urbanization. In addition the incidences of pancreatic and prostate cancer seem to have a 'rural component' in their correlation spectra, besides associations typical of cancers of the respiratory tract, with mortality peaks in highly urbanized areas (prostate cancer shows its highest mortality in the Stockholm area), and among the divorced group.

The 'bi-polar' correlation patterns found in the epidemiological analyses for these types of cancer correspond, for colorectal and breast cancer, to relatively high incidences in the big cities as well as in certain rural areas of southern and middle Sweden. The results of the analysis allow some reflection over the role played by factors such as different dietary habits on the one hand associated with relative affluence, and on the other associated with the opposite among single persons (divorced, widowers). The incidences of these types of tumour show no correlation with the smoking variable used, except for the correlations indicated above for pancreatic and possibly prostate cancer. For a couple of tumour types (colorectal, corpus uteri) the correlation with smoking is negative. In a multiple regression analysis there is always the possibility that a true positive correlation appears instead as a negative correlation with another variable which is negatively correlated with the first one (e.g. with respect to the two variables 'rural character' and 'proportion of smokers'), but apart from this it cannot be excluded that these statistical correlations are genuine. In for example Hammond's (1966) large-scale investigation covering 1 million US citizens, a lower mortality in colorectal and breast cancer for smokers than for non-smokers was found, while former smokers showed a higher risk. These correlations may indicate that dietary habits of a kind that favour the induction of such tumours are more frequent among non-smokers than among smokers.

As concerns both incidence and mortality for leukaemias, no relationship with the variables examined was evident. This is also the case for stomach cancer except possibly for a certain variation with marital status (highest figures among divorced men) and for a suggested correlation with the proportion of smokers.

The mortality and incidence for cancer as a whole is an aggregate of the patterns for the individual sites, and this is reflected in the correlations obtained, although the aggregate correlations obviously are weakened to the extent that the correlations between incidences of individual tumour types and the variables examined go in opposite directions. The total cancer mortality is higher in the three metropolitan areas than in the rest of Sweden (Table 5.3), especially in the Stockholm area, by 40 per cent for men and 10 per cent for women, and a comparison of marital status shows the highest excess risk to be among divorced people (40 per cent and 20 per cent greater than among married men and women respectively). For the period 1968–73, the total cancer incidence is positively correlated in both sexes with most of the descriptor variables, including variables expressing rural and 'big city' character as well as the proportion of smokers.

5.3 Estimates of the magnitude of demonstrated correlations

In planning preventive measures to be taken and studies of causal relationships, it is usually important to have some idea of the proportion of mortality or incidence which may be attributed to specific environmental variables or to groups of such variables. The fact that a certain proportion of a death rate from a given disease is 'attributable' to specific environmental descriptors implies that this rate is 'explainable' in a statistical sense by these descriptors. This holds regardless of whether the variable directly indicates a causal factor or whether, as is usually the case, it is an indirect expression of causal factors. The strength (the statistical significance) of a relationship, as discussed in the preceding section, has little to do with the magnitude of the relationship in the sense of the 'explainable' proportion of incidence or mortality (or the corresponding number of cases per year). On the other hand the fact that significance has been obtained justifies an attempt to calculate the proportion that is 'explainable' by the variables under consideration. Using data from the data-base analyses described in Section 5.2, Ehrenberg and Ekman (1984) calculated the proportion of observed cancer cases 'explainable' in this sense, firstly for specific 'explanatory' variables, primarily degree of urbanization, proportion of habitual smokers and diagnostic intensity, and secondly (tentatively) the total proportion of

Cancer mortality and incidence in Sweden 271

the incidence which may be 'explained' by the whole set of variables examined. The methodology employed is depicted in Figure 5.2.

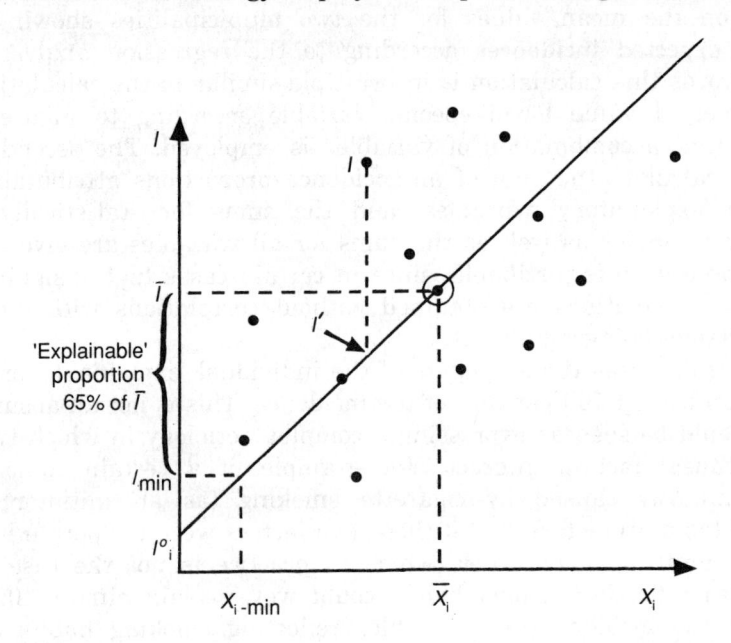

Figure 5.2. Illustration, using a hypothetical example, of the method for estimation of proportions of the average incidence, $\bar{I}$, 'explainable' by variables x_i in the multiple regression analysis. ● observed incidences I; ⊙ average incidence (= incidence in Sweden). The most likely parameter values, e.g. the slope B, for a regression line ($I' = I^0 + B\,x$), are computed from the dual values of the incidence (I) and the explanatory variable (x, i.e. the percentage of habitual smokers). I' is the value on the line (expected value) corresponding to the values of x for the incidences I. I^0 is the expected value of the incidence for $x = 0$. (When analysing the dependence on several variables x_i simultaneously, the calculations are performed in a similar fashion using partial regression coefficients B'_i.) The explainable proportion of the incidence is the proportion of the national incidence (which could be equal to the mean incidence $\bar{I}$ that may be attributed to the dependence on x in a statistical sense. If x_{min} is the lowest possible value of x (for the proportion of habitual smokers this value could theoretically be zero), and I'_{min} is the expected value associated with x_{min}, the explainable part of the incidence will be $\bar{I} - I'_{min}$ and the explainable proportion ($\bar{I} - I'_{min})/\bar{I}$ (expressed for example as a percentage of I). In the example in the figure, this proportion had been set to 65%.
Based on Ehrenberg and Ekman (1984).

When positive correlation occurs, the 'explainable' proportion is calculated, as shown in this diagram, as the difference (as a percentage) between the mean incidence in Sweden and the incidence value on the regression line corresponding to the lowest value (determined as the average for two municipalities) of the 'explanatory' variable. (By choosing the incidences expected from the regression line and not the lowest municipality incidence in Sweden, the considerable statistical error associated with the latter is reduced.) The calculation of the total 'explainable' proportion has been carried out in two ways. One was based on the mean values for the two municipalities showing the lowest expected incidences according to the regression analyses; in other words this calculation is in principle similar to the calculation of the expected value for a specific variable according to Figure 5.2, except that a combination of variables is employed. The second way was to calculate the sum of all incidence proportions attributable to specific 'explanatory' variables, and the sums for statistically significant variables as well as the sums for all variables are given. The latter procedure is justifiable, since in certain cases highly significant multiple correlations are obtained without correlations with individual variables being significant.

In certain cases the aggregate of the individual 'explainable' proportions can exceed 100 per cent of the incidence. This is not an absurdity, and should be seen as expressing a complex aetiology in which two or more causal factors interact. For example, if a certain tumour is predominantly caused by cigarette smoking (as an initiator) and alcohol (as a promoter), and if these two factors were to operate highly independently of each other (which in practice is not the case), the variables reflecting alcohol habits could well explain almost 100 per cent of the incidence and variables reflecting smoking habits could also explain almost a further 100 per cent, giving a sum of nearly 200 per cent. From a preventive point of view this would mean that the disease in question could be prevented by an abstinence from either smoking or alcohol.

5.3.1 Diagnostic intensity

A majority of the types of tumour examined in the study of socio-economic variables show a significant dependence on the diagnosis factor. Exceptions here are cancers of the stomach, pancreas, breast and corpus uteri as well as leukaemias. The magnitude of the dependence, computed as a percentage of the incidence, is presented for some tumours in Table 5.8.[5] In this table parallel estimates from the special study dealing with diagnostic intensity are also given; the calculations here are based on a Poisson model and are thus independent of the regression analysis. The agreement between the two is comparatively good. On average some 10 per cent of the total cancer incidence appears to be attributable to the diagnosis factor (as a proportion of cases not detected or reported).

Table 5.8 Percentages of cancer incidences during 1961–67 attributable to the variable diagnostic intensity. Estimates are given for certain sites for which significant correlations occur. As a comparison, values estimated using an independent method based on a Poisson model are given. These proportions have been calculated as the percentage of cases not detected for reasons of under-diagnosis or under-reporting at the prevalent diagnostic intensity as compared to the highest diagnostic intensity in Sweden.

Tumour site	Proportion attributable to diagnostic intensity (%)	
	From regression model	From Poisson model
Colon and rectum, men	8	
Colon and rectum, women	7	
Lung, men	12	29
Lung, women	(7, not significant)	16
Cervix uteri	11	
Prostate	6	9
Kidney, men	15	
Kidney, women	9	
Urinary bladder, men	14	
Urinary bladder, women	20	23
All cancer, men	5.3	11
All cancer, women	5.0	11

From Ehrenberg and Ekman (1984).

5.3.2 Total 'explainable' proportions of incidences

The total 'explainable' proportions of the incidences for the tumour types studied by Berglund et al. (1984) have been summarized by Ehrenberg and Ekman (1984) (Table 5.9). When the estimates are based on comparisons with the municipalities with the lowest incidences, some 25 per cent–50 per cent, in general, of the total number of cases in the country are 'explained', and this figure is 90 per cent for lung cancer in men. When all explanatory proportions are added together, 'degrees of explanation' of well over 50 per cent are obtained for most of the important sites. According to Ehrenberg and Ekman these results suggest that the majority of all present incidences may be attributable to specific causal factors, and that efforts to identify them are meaningful and would probably provide a basis for more effective prevention.

In some cases the total 'degree of explanation' exceeds 100 per cent, which should be interpreted as being due to interacting factors in the aetiology of the respective tumours. The 'explainable' proportion estimated from the regression analyses of all cancer (as a mean of the figures for the two methods of calculation at the bottom of Table 5.9, namely 50 per cent for men and 30 per cent for women) are undoubtedly underestimates, since the different types of tumour depend in different patterns on the variables considered. Weighted means of the

Table 5.9 'Explainable' proportions (per cent) of selected cancer incidences. Mean of values for 1961–7 and 1968–73.

Tumour site	Sex	Sum of specific proportions from the regression analysis		Comparison with current minimum incidences
		Significant	All	
Oesophagus	M	225	265	50
	F	115	300[a]	20
Stomach	M	70	85	22
	F	30(0–55)	60	12
Colon and rectum	M	45(60)[b]	65(90)[b]	39
	F	40(90)[b]	65(115)[b]	24
Pancreas	M	35	85	35
	F	30(0–60)	80	17
Lung, etc.	M	160	160	90
	F	35	90	48
Breast	F	40(60)[b]	50(70)[b]	23
Cervix uteri	F	95	110	50
Corpus uteri	F	40	65	20
Prostate	M	75	80	30
Kidney	M	40	75	39
	F	50	80	30
Urinary bladder	M	45	90	54
	F	60	110	41
Leukemia	M	25(0–50[c])	80	20
	F	10(0–20)	65	18
Weighted mean[d]	M	75(80)[b]	93(97)[b]	43
	F	60	86(97)[b]	30
All cancer	M	63	65	30
	F	38	40	20

[a] Value uncertain due to low incidence.
[b] Sum of explainable proportions in investigations including variable 4 according to Table 5.1.
[c] This value, from 1968–73, holds provided that smoking is an aetiological factor.
[d] The sum of the incidences of the tumours examined represents somewhat more than 70 per cent of the total cancer incidence.

From Ehrenberg & Ekman (1984).

aggregated 'explainable' proportions of the incidences for the specific tumours reach 60 per cent or more.

The proportions of cancer incidences attributable to the variable 'diagnostic intensity' contain a source of error, inasmuch as the proportions in question may be interpreted as the proportion of non-detected or non-reported cancer cases. It would therefore have been appropriate not to include these proportions in the aggregate explainable proportions. They have, however, been included since this variable doubtless expresses other socio-economic conditions. The estimated values are furthermore little affected by the method of calculation.

5.3.3 Proportions of incidences attributable to urbanization factors and tobacco smoking

The calculation of the proportion of cancer cases attributable to the smoking variable provides a test of the reasonableness of the model. A corroboration of a qualitative kind is immediately obtained, since the dependence on the smoking variable appears for just those types of tumour for which smoking has previously been regarded as an important causal factor. The calculations of Ehrenberg and Ekman (1984) of the magnitude of the influence of smoking show that approximately one-third of the lung cancer incidence for men and approximately 10 per cent of all cancer (15 per cent for men in both periods studied and 0 per cent and 9 per cent respectively for women) appears to be attributable to smoking. The incidence of lung cancer among non-smokers is estimated to be about six per 100 000 person years for both men and women (Section 4.2). The proportion of lung cancer incidence where tobacco smoking is the causal factor may then be estimated as 80–85 per cent among men and 20–40 per cent among women for the period 1961–1973. It is estimated that at the end of the 1970s some 25% of all cancer for men and some 7 per cent of all cancer for women had tobacco smoking as an aetiological factor. Compared with these figures, the calculations based on the regression model result in lower 'explainable' proportions. This is probably because the smoking variable used in these studies expresses only the proportion of habitual smokers in the municipality and does not reflect characteristics which can be important for cancer incidence such as the number of cigarettes per day, the depth of inhalation and the age of starting to smoke. All these factors are responsible for higher risk contributions in urban areas, especially the big cities (see for example the proportion of heavy smokers in Table 5.4), and in the statistical analysis their impact will therefore be transferred to the urban and big-city descriptors (especially Nos. 2, 6 and 7 in Table 5.1). Furthermore the influence of the smoking variable is weakened by the fact that it is based on a postal survey of a small sample of the population, implying a statistical error which may be considerable for small municipalities.

For these reasons Ehrenberg and Ekman (1984) have especially pointed out that the influences of the smoking habit variable and the urban descriptors should be viewed together. The proportions of the incidences of lung cancer and of all cancer which are 'explainable' by these variables are summarized in Table 5.10. The proportions of each respective incidence attributable to the urban and smoking descriptors together are much higher than the aetiological fraction for tobacco smoking calculated as above (and in Section 4.2). If it is thus assumed that 85 per cent of the lung cancer incidence among men has tobacco smoking as a causal factor, room for some 40 per cent of the incidence is left for the other variables associated with urbanization or big cities. For women the comparable figure is much more uncertain, but probably about 20 per cent of the incidence could fall on urban and big-city descriptors other than smoking. An analysis of this type obviously cannot pinpoint air pollution that is characteristic of urban areas (including 'passive smoking') as a contributing causal factor. It does, however, permit the conclusion that the results are compatible with the existence of an influence of general air pollution upon the risk of lung cancer.

Table 5.10 Proportions (per cent) of incidences of lung cancer and all cancer attributed to urbanization and smoking habit descriptors.

Variable (Nos. as in Table 5.1)	Lung cancer Men	Lung cancer Women	All cancer Men	All cancer Women
High degree of urbanization (2)	44	(15)[a]	6	9
'Big-city' character (6)	32	22	15	10
County centres, hospital towns (7)	20	(10)[a]	12	6
Tobacco smoking (8)	31	(5)[a]	15	5
Sum	127	50	≈ 50	≈ 30
Minus: Tobacco smoking, assuming an age-standardized risk of 6×10^{-5} in non-smokers	85	20–40	≈ 25	≈ 7
Other factors related to urbanization	≈ 40	≈ 20	≈ 25	≈ 25

[a] Parentheses denote that the dependence is not significant.
Mean values for the periods 1961–67 and 1968–73; extracted from Ehrenberg & Ekman (1984).

The proportion of the incidence that seems to be due to factors other than smoking is considerably greater than that which has been, in other studies, considered to have air pollution as an aetiological factor (about 5 per cent of the total lung cancer incidence, as may be deduced from Section 6.6). It is thus indicated that other factors (e.g. occupational exposure characteristics of urban and big-city areas, and dietary habits) play a role, in part, in interaction with tobacco smoking.

Similar reasoning may be applied to the proportions of the total cancer incidence attributable to tobacco smoking and to other factors associated with a high degree of urbanization. Since significant correlations with the smoking variable occur in addition to correlations with urban and big-city descriptors in analyses with seven or eight explanatory variables, it is probable that they do reflect causal relationships with tobacco smoking. It is also probable that the above mentioned weakness of the smoking variable leads to underestimation of the contribution of smoking to cancer incidence. The results of this analysis are thus compatible with the estimate in section 4.2 of the proportion of cancer cases in Sweden which have smoking as a causal factor (see Table 5.10). The relatively high proportion of the total cancer incidence—itself probably underestimated—attributable to other factors associated with urban areas includes the strong big-city component in such quantitatively important sites as colorectal and breast cancer.

The underlying data upon which the reasoning presented here is based have considerable uncertainty, both statistical and theoretical, and the evaluation of these margins of error has only just started.

5.4 Working conditions and occupational exposure

Einhorn et al. (1980) have carried out a comprehensive analysis of the influence of variables in the Cancer–Environment Registry describing occupation, employment and branch of industry. This work helps in generating hypotheses and pinpointing important problem areas to which more penetrating analysis should be applied. The degree of urbanization and some other factors have so great an influence on the occurrence of the majority of forms of tumours, as just described, that one must take these relationships into consideration when analysing effects specific to occupations. One step in this direction has been taken by the construction of a computer program at the National Board of Occupational Safety and Health, in which routine age and sex standardization is carried out at county level (Malker and Weiner, 1984).

From the previously mentioned Mortality–Environment Registry of Statistics Sweden, created by the merging of information from the Cause-of-Death Registry with, among other things, occupational data from the 1960 population census, distributions by occupation of causes of death have been published (SCB, 1981a). The data, presented without statistical analysis, cover the years 1961–70 and persons in their active years, i.e. born after 1896. The occupations are classified according to a two-digit code. The causes of death are specified as 'all diseases', and within this group are cancers and cardiovascular diseases, and, furthermore, injuries due to violence and poisoning. A conspicuous excess risk for tumour diseases as the primary cause of death is seen among those 'not economically active'. This will be discussed in Section 5.5. Furthermore, noteworthy differences between various occupational groups appear, with low death rates for all causes of death for occupations within the farming, forestry and fishing sectors. The highest excess risks occur in certain occupations entailing much entertaining, and in service occupations for which it is probable that life-style factors, partly associated with smoking habits, could have an influence.

In some analyses of the Cancer–Environment Registry, an occupational variable reflecting possible exposure to chemicals has been studied alongside the degree of urbanization and the diagnostic intensity (Ehrenberg and Ekman, 1984). An excess risk for lung cancer and leukaemia in the group 'exposed' was observed in this study, but with a considerable margin of error. The incidence of all cancer is, however, higher among the 'non-exposed' (which includes persons in administrative work) than among the 'exposed' (which include the majority of groups in manufacturing industry).

5.5 Cancer in relation to other diseases and causes of death—population group correlations

The increased risk among persons living alone, especially the divorced (Section 5.2.2), for lung cancer and other types of cancer more or less associated with smoking, should be interpreted as due to the existence within these family status categories of a relatively large risk population characterized by certain living habits. However, such variations between family status groups apply to the majority of causes of death as well as for the total death rate (Figure 5.3). Lung cancer accounts for only about 5 per cent of the total death rate. A category with a similar risk pattern consists of persons denoted as 'not economically active', although normally of active age at the time of a census. This category as a whole shows a highly increased mortality from several causes (Table 5.11). Although men not economically active and below the age of 65 years constitute only 9 per cent of the male population in Sweden, they accounted for more than 22 per cent of the male death rate. For this reason the mean mortality in specific age intervals in this group is greater than the mortality among the economically active. This illustrates the so-called healthy-worker effect, an important factor to consider when choosing control groups in investigations dealing with occupational diseases. Economically active persons with

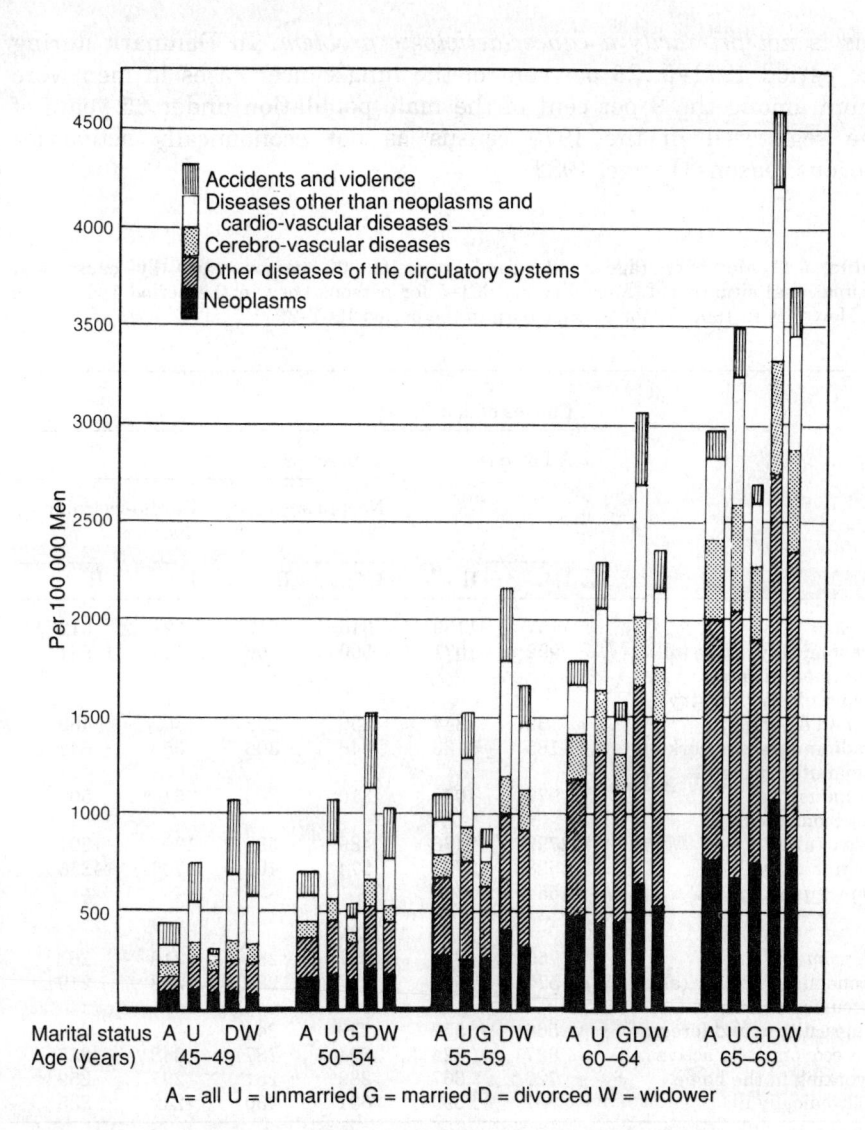

Figure 5.3 Death rates by cause per 100 000 men in age intervals, by marital status, during the period 1974 to 78.
(From Bolander and Lindgren, 1981.

good health in an occupational branch under investigation should thus only be compared with persons with a similar health status.

The relative excess risk for tumour diseases in the group of men not economically active is less (14 per cent of the total cancer mortality) than for the total mortality from all causes, which demonstrates that this is *not primarily a cancer-aetiologic problem*. In Denmark during the period 1971–5, 28 per cent of the lung cancer cases in men were found among the 9 per cent of the male population under 65 years of age registered in the 1970 census as not economically active for various reasons (Lynge, 1982).

Table 5.11 Mortality (age-standardized, per 100 000 person-years) by cause and occupational situation: I, Mortality in 1961–5 for persons born in the period 1896–1915; II, Mortality in 1966–70 for persons born in the period 1901–20.

	All diseases		Neoplasms		Cardio-vascular diseases	
	I	II	I	II	I	II
All men	1157	1139	316	310	621	612
Economically active (all)	992	1071	300	306	534	581
occupied within agriculture, forestry and fishing	762	844	230	238	402	460
administrative work	1185	1133	346	306	658	647
manufacturing industry	976[a]	1050	310[a]	303	516[a]	569
Not economically active (all)	2799	2476	489	392	1391	1201
chronically ill	3528	2751	574	401	1709	1336
unemployed	1554	1864	–	–	–	–
All women	756	679	297	285	310	261
Economically active (all)	570	592	277	281	208	219
occupied within agriculture and forestry	566	557	249	241	–	207
Not economically active (all)	827	724	304	287	348	285
working in the home	720	667	289	281	297	259
chronically ill	2887	2099	631	430	1242	835

Causes of death: All diseases; Subgroups: Neoplasms, Cardio-vascular diseases.

[a] Mean value for Scandinavian occupational codes 7 and 8, which are close to the International Standard Classification of Occupation, ISCO (see SCB, 1981a).
From SCB (1981a).

The group 'not economically active' according to the registry definition is a heterogeneous group. The highest risks among men for various causes of death are found among the chronically ill and persons on disability pension (about 40 per cent of the group), but an increased risk is apparent also within the remainder of the group, which consists of the unemployed and persons receiving social security payments. It is probable that within this group, complex causal relationships exist between life-style and diseases (possibly also including tumours already growing, which result in increased cancer mortality (Ehrenberg and Ekman (1984)). The risk pattern makes it probable that the group described as 'drop-outs from society' is included as an extreme risk group. The extent to which the high risk figures for divorced people could also be due to a predominance of such 'drop-outs from society' in this category needs to be investigated.

The total mortality is also lower for women among the economically active than among those not economically active but of active age. The discrepancy is, however, much smaller than for men. With regard to tumour diseases, there is hardly any difference at all. It may be relevant that most of the women classified as not economically active are engaged in household work.

These circumstances indicate the need, in epidemiological studies, to take other diseases and causes of death into consideration, with respect both to common causal effects and to competing effects on incidences and death rates.

In the economicially active groups, the occupational characterization constitutes a basis for a socio-economic classification. Information concerning some different groups is presented in Table 5.11. The group of economically active men employed in farming and forestry shows—in parallel with its low cancer incidence—a low mortality for cancer but also for other diseases, in comparison to the other groups. Whereas men in manufacturing industry show about the same mortality as the average for the economically active, the death rates for men in administrative work are visibly higher, for death due to cancer as well as other diseases. These results also point to the importance of distinguishing between disease risks—including cancer risks—due to the occupational environment itself, e.g. occupational exposure, on the one hand, and risks run by occupational groups on the other hand. The latter risks are to be ascribed to the entire complex of circumstances of life for the group, including personal life-style.

The investigation by Teppo et al.(1980) of cancer incidence in Finland also made use of a classification according to 'standard of living' with respect to income, social class, education, housing conditions, etc. Several common types of cancer examined showed a higher incidence for values of the individual components reflecting a high standard of living according to the definition in this study.

5.6 Trends in cancer incidence and mortality

The developments over time of incidences of cancer, derived from the Cancer Registry, have been published at intervals (*Cancer Incidence in Sweden*), and corresponding death rates are available in the Cause-of-Death Registry. Changes with time in cancer incidence or mortality provide important information which can be used for determining both the causes of disease and the effectiveness of any preventive measures taken. The monitoring of trends is an important component in epidemiological monitoring systems.

The *number* of registered cancer *cases* in Sweden during the period 1960–78 increased from about 10 000 to about 16 000 per year for both men and women, that is by 3 per cent per year (see Chapter 2). Since the probability for the occurrence of a tumour clearly increases with age, a large part of the increased number of cases is due to the change in the age structure of the Swedish population. However, after adjustment by age standardization, an increase of 1 per cent per year in women and 2 per cent per year for men remains as an average for the period considered. Hidden within these increases are increasing as well as decreasing trends for individual types of tumour.

Corresponding trends for cancer *mortality* can be studied for another decade backwards in time in the Statistics Sweden Registry. Over the period 1951–78 a gently falling trend is seen with regard to women, except possibly in the highest age bracket (80–84 years) (Chapter 2, Figure 2.6 and Table 2.1b). The trend is also falling slightly for younger men, but is rising for those aged above 60 years. Significant differences in mortality are evident for certain tumour diseases between the periods 1969–73 and 1974–78 (von Bahr et al., 1984a). Since these figures take the distribution over marital status and regions into account, they would seem to be adequate estimates of trends in cancer mortality during the 1970s.

Forecasting of changes in cancer incidence during the next few decades depends on several circumstances. It is rendered more difficult if different age groups may not be uniformly affected by the reasons for the trend, which is the case if factors influencing the incidence vary with time. For example, prediction of incidences is made harder if changes in smoking habits occur only in certain age groups. Furthermore it must be possible to make adjustments with respect to changes in the effect of diagnosis and reporting routines.

Eklund (1984) has compared incidences of tumour diseases in 10-year age intervals (35–44 up to 75–84 years of age) for the 4-year periods 1960–3, 1968–71 and 1975–8. In the 1960s in particular an extremely large increase for several types of tumour in the highest ages is observed, whereas during the latter part of the period this effect is much smaller. This phenomenon seems to be due to a rapid improvement in diagnosing and/or reporting, especially during the earlier part of the 1960s. In order to evaluate the true development of a disease over time, the effects of such changes in the diagnosis factor must be eliminated (see Section 5.2.1).

The development over time of incidences of most types of tumour has been rather uniform for all age categories during the period 1968–78 (Eklund 1984). An exception here is lung cancer in men, where the increase was lowest for ages around 60–64 years, an effect also observed by Kvåle (1982), which seems to be due to changes in smoking pattern. Another noticeable exception is cervical cancer, where the decrease mainly occurs in the lower age groups, but where a certain increase is still noted for the higher age groups. This effect is probably partly the result of health screening, which has in particular been directed towards younger women (Pettersson et al. 1982; see also Chapter 13). This analysis also confirmed the previous observations that malignant melanoma is the tumour disease which undergoes the most rapid increase. This increase has also been discussed in connection with ultraviolet radiation in Section 4.5.3.

The increase recorded since the beginning of the 1950s of the total mortality for men in tumour diseases is due mainly to an increase for two sites, lung and prostate cancer, in both of which cases much of the increase could be attributed to better diagnosis. In the case of prostate cancer it would often seem to be a matter of reclassification of prostate hyperplasia to prostate cancer. These two causes of death show opposing time dependence, while the trend for both taken together has been practically constant (Figure 5.4). This is probably also the case for the incidence of prostate cancer, which showed a 70 per cent increase from 1960 to 1979, mainly before 1975. The average annual increase of 2.6 per cent during the whole period 1959–79 (NBHW, 1982) is probably a gross over estimate. In all probability the mortality as well as the incidence of prostate cancer has been practically constant during this period. The considerable increase in lung cancer incidence among older men must be attributed to two causes, one being that smokers now attain a higher age, and the other being better diagnosis. Taking these factors into account the true increase in the incidence during the 1960s and 1970s among men would be only around 2 per cent per year (Ehrenberg and Ekman, 1984). Among women the increasing use of tobacco seems to have led to an increase in lung cancer incidence of about 4 per cent per year.

The decrease in incidence and mortality for lung cancer among men observed during the latter 1970s seems to have begun earlier in Stockholm and probably in Malmö. In these metropolitan areas a decrease is seen for 1971–76, while the figures were still on the increase in the rest of the country and in the Gothenburg area (Table 5.12).

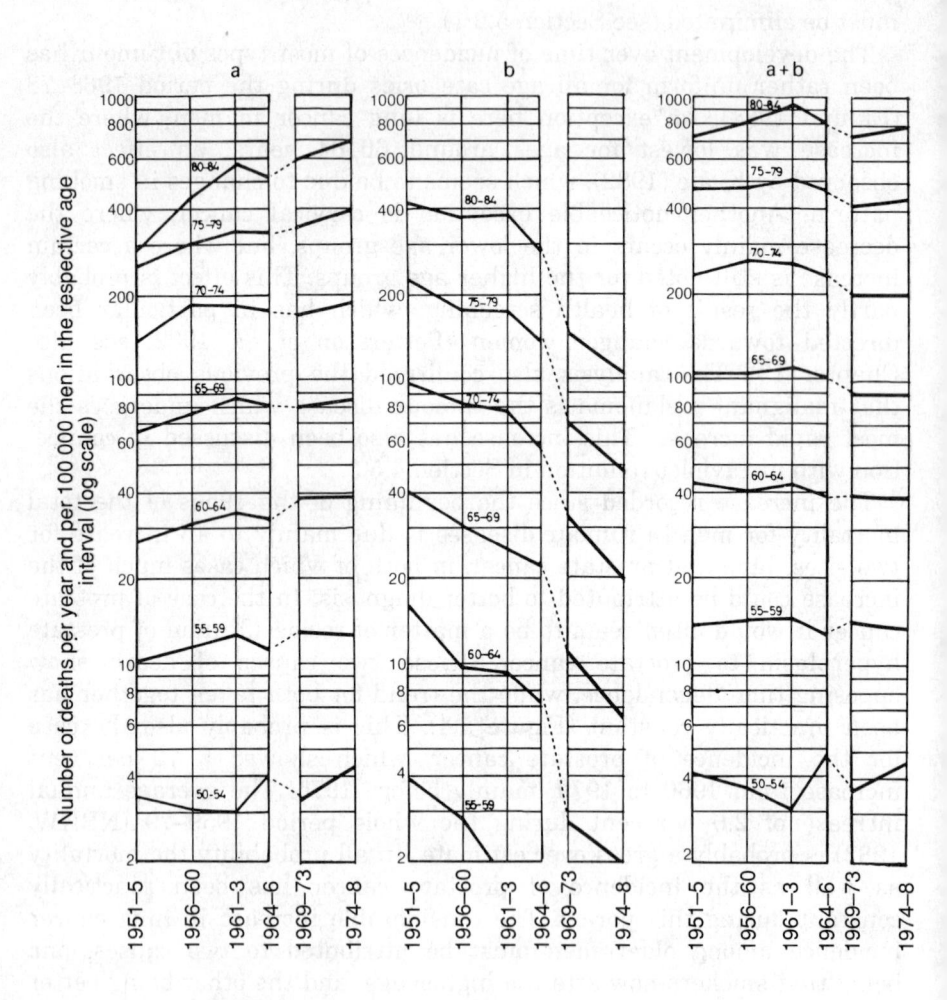

Figure 5.4 Trend during the period 1951–78 of the mortality from malignant tumour of the prostate (a), of prostate hyperplasia (b) and of these diseases taken together (a + b), among men at 5-year age intervals.
From Bolander and Lindgren 1981.

Table 5.12 Mortality rates from lung cancer in men by region (the Stockholm, Gothenburg and Malmö metropolitan areas and the rest of Sweden), and by period (5-year periods 1969–73 and 1974–8). Data from von Bahr et al. (1984a). Relative risks, per thousand, calculated from the matrix for interaction period/region. This interaction is significant.

Period	Region: Stockholm area	Gothenburg area	Malmö area	Rest of Sweden
1969–73	1016	964	1042	907
1974–8	961	1008	1021	993
Trend (% per year)	−1.1	+1.0	−0.4	+1.9

From Ehrenberg & Ekman (1984).

This difference in temporal development between different regions (Wiman and Jansson, 1980) is possibly an expression of the fact that changes in life-style occur most rapidly in the capital city and other urban centres. In this case it is a question of a decrease in cigarette smoking—in the same way as when this habit was earlier being taken up. Any similar beneficial decrease in the lung cancer incidence for women cannot yet be detected.

5.7 Attempts to forecast future lung cancer incidence

Lung cancer is the tumour disease for which the causal relationships are clearest and for which a forecast is most immediately called for from a preventive point of view. A forecast of future lung cancer incidence must take several factors into consideration. The lung cancer risk, above a relatively low background level, is dependent above all on smoking habits, especially with respect to the age of starting to smoke (since the number of years of smoking plays a considerable role), how much tobacco is smoked per day as well as what sort and how it is smoked (see Section 4.2). Furthermore, the age distribution of the population is of great importance, since the risk increases considerably with age. Different changes in smoking habits between the sexes make it necessary for men and women to be treated separately.

5.7.1 Men

Hakulinen and Pukkala (1981, 1982) have forecast the incidence of lung cancer among men in Finland under various assumptions of possible changes in smoking habits. Whereas cessation of smoking leads to immediate effects, the effects of a change of the proportion of smokers starting to smoke at the age of about 20 years become apparent only about 25 years later, when the smokers approach the 'critical' age when lung cancer incidence becomes high. Specially noteworthy is the great effect of a postponement of starting to smoke, even by as little as 5 years, on the incidence 25–50 years later.

Finland differs from Sweden in that the lung cancer incidence in men was higher in the 1960s—undoubtedly because of the higher consumption of cigarettes in Finland (Kvåle, 1982)—but a significant decrease in the incidence was observed already about 1970. The methods of computation employed by Hakulinen and Pukkala should nevertheless in principle be applicable to Swedish circumstances.

In Section 4.2 the temporal developments of Swedish smoking habits and their relationship to lung cancer incidence have been discussed (see also Ehrenberg and Ekman 1984). The proportion of habitual smokers among men was 49 per cent in 1963 (cigarette and pipe smokers), reached a peak in 1969 and then declined. Lung cancer incidence peaked in 1976 (46 per 100 000 man years) and then declined (by 1980 the figure was about 40 per 100 000). This latter figure and other data are consistent with the expected increase, assuming about 60 per cent smokers in total (of cigarettes and pipes) during the preceding decade and assuming a lung cancer risk about 10 times higher among smokers than among non-smokers, whose risk seem to be about 6 per 100 000 person years (table 4.5). In the non-smokers' figure, the effects of passive smoking may account for about one case per 100 000 person years (see section 4.2.5). This implies that smoking directly or indirectly is the cause of approximately 35 out of 40 lung cancer cases per 100 000 person years, i.e. about 85 per cent of the present incidence, and that a total cessation of smoking would bring the incidence down to about 5 cases per 100 000 person years. This assumes that the risk contributions due to changes in exposure to radon daughters and to general air pollution in urban areas is negligible. How rapidly this lower incidence could be attained would depend of course on the rate at which smoking is given up (Hakulinen and Pukkala, 1981). Even if such a highly improbable situation as a total end to smoking could be achieved instantaneously, the smoking-independent level of incidence would not be reached for some 50 years, as long as former smokers were still alive. A considerable reduction in incidence, to about 50 per cent of the present number of cases, could nevertheless be attained after only about 10 years (Hakulinen and Pukkala, 1982).

The decrease of about 10 per cent in lung cancer incidence observed in Sweden during the latter part of the 1970s for all age groups (see Table 5.13), cannot be attributed exclusively to a decrease in the total consumption of cigarettes, but is also partly related to changes in the age distribution of smokers—an effect operating in the opposite direction—as well as to the transition to other types of cigarettes, such as filter cigarettes. It should be added here that a certain increase in the lung cancer incidence among men has again been observed lately.

Table 5.13 The incidence of lung cancer, etc. (ICD code 162), in Sweden during various periods of time. Age-standardized incidences calculated at the 1970 age distribution according to a procedure employed in the Cancer Registry (see *Cancer Incidence in Sweden*, e.g. 1980).

		Age-standardized incidence (per 100 000)	Incidence in the age groups (per 100 000)			
		(0 years)	40–44	45–49	65–69	75–79
1959–69	M	28.7	6.6	12.5	126	110
	F	6.5	2.5	4.5	23	34
1972	M	41.9	6.8	20.6	167	211
	F	9.2	3.9	4.3	28	53
1977	M	44.3	7.6	19.4	165	296
	F	10.2	3.2	9.2	40	46
1978	M	43.8	10.1	17.9	163	249
	F	10.7	6.3	8.5	35	47
1979	M	42.2	9.4	17.7	155	234
	F	11.1	5.7	10.9	40	39
1980	M	45.0	7.0	21.5	168	241
	F	12.7	7.8	15.2	41	47

M, males
F, females.

5.7.2 Women

Around 1960 the lung cancer incidence among Swedish women was probably not much higher than could be expected for non-smokers (Table 5.13; about six per 100 000 over the whole population, corresponding to somewhat more than twice that rate for ages over 35 years). Similarly, the incidence among women shows the same smaller dependence on age as is characteristic of non-smokers (Doll, 1978). Around the middle of the 1970s the rate of increase in mortality and incidence of lung cancer in Sweden was greater for women than for men, and the decrease in incidence which occurred for men towards the end of the 1970s has not been detected for women (Table 5.13).

288   Cancer: causes and prevention

These differences between the sexes have also been illustrated in the cohort analysis by Kvåle (1982). In age cohorts born during the first decade of this century the incidence ratio between the sexes (male/female) is as high as 6, but it decreases to about 2 in the youngest cohorts, and is tending to become even smaller. This is illustrated by the data from the Cancer Registry in Table 5.13. For the age categories 40–44 and 45–49 years the ratio between the sexes is about 2, whereas at higher ages the incidence among men is 4–6 times higher than for women. The incidence increase among women since the beginning of the 1960s is greatest in the youngest groups, and would seem to be due to the fact that they acquired the smoking habits that men had about 20 years earlier. The well-known diagram of Figure 5.5, based on

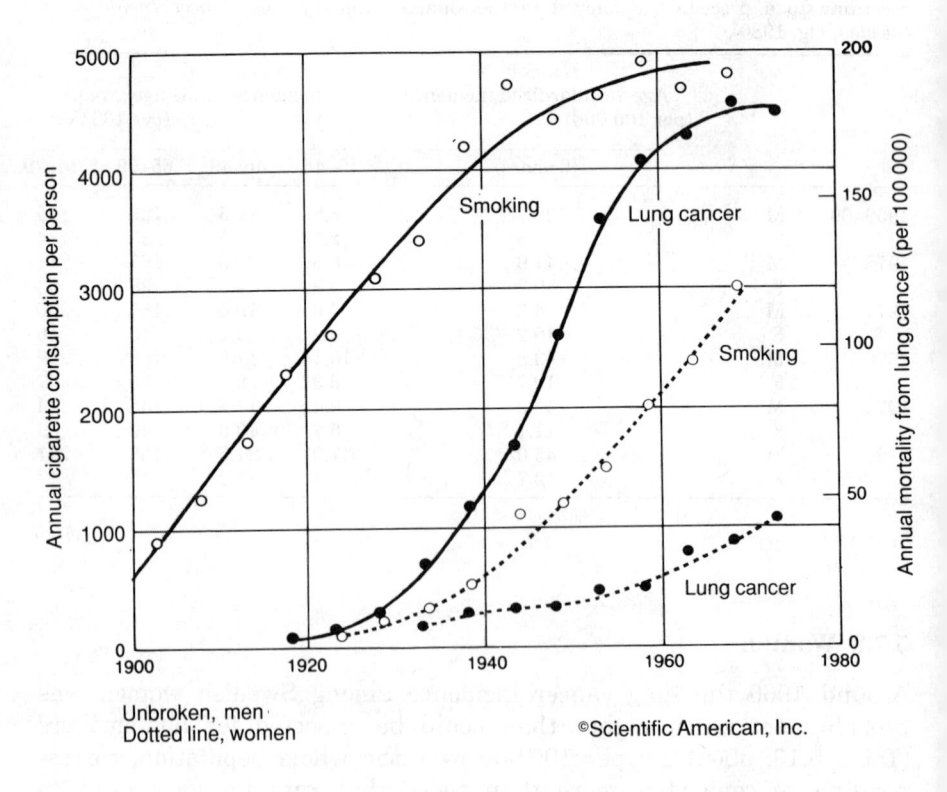

Figure 5.5 The development over time of annual cigarette consumption and of lung cancer mortality among men and women in England and Wales.
From Cairns, 1975.

British data, illustrates the relationship over time between smoking habits and lung cancer incidence.

How seriously this development must be viewed is evident from the fact that lung cancer incidence in Sweden for women aged 40–49 years is now as high as it was for men in this age group 15–20 years earlier (Table 5.13). Unless a substantial reduction of the proportion of smokers occurs among these women, there would be a very great increase in the number of lung cancer cases when the cohorts in question reach the ages, during the next 10–30 years, at which the risk of lung cancer caused by smoking increases rapidly. What may be feared here is a development paralleling that already noted among men. Similar misgivings are supported by analyses of a similar development in Norway (Sandstad 1982). Recent information from the USA seems to confirm such an alarming development among women.

This increased future risk undoubtedly also holds true for the younger age cohorts, which have not yet reached the ages at which the lifelong dosage of tobacco smoke leads to cancer cases appearing in the Cancer Registry. For a long time the proportion of Swedish school-girls starting to smoke has been increasing. Although in the 1970s smoking decreased among the young, in 1981 still over a third of 15–16 year old girls were smokers (compared with 23 per cent of boys). For women this could—unless there is a change in present smoking habits—lead to a serious cancer increase in the next few decades, unaffected by the fact that the trend towards an earlier start of smoking seems to have been reversed during the last few years (see Section 4.2).

5.8 General experience from the data-base analyses described

Results from the investigations described above using data from the Cause-of-Death Registry, the Cancer Registry and the Cancer–Environment Registry are used in Chapter 6 to obtain quantitative estimates of the importance of different causes in terms of numbers of cancer cases. This is also the case for relationships with occupational variables (see Section 5.4). Only some very general observations will be given here, as a summary of conclusions from Ehrenberg and Ekman (1984).

The main conclusions of the epidemiological approaches are the following:

(a) A large proportion of present cancer incidence and mortality may be 'explained' in a statistical sense with the aid of a number of available 'environmental descriptors'. More than half of the total cancer incidence, and for some specific tumour diseases three-quarters or more, may be 'explained' in this fashion. This is remarkable and undoubtedly an underestimate, since for example the geographical units examined—municipalities and certain metropolitan areas—are particularly heterogeneous with respect to the occurrence of known causal factors.

(b) The data-base 'environmental descriptors' which have been used are predominantly of an indirect nature, i.e. they are not actual causes of the diseases. The results are thus primarily useful to help generate hypothesis, but do indicate that efforts to clarify the true causal relationships are worthwhile.

(c) Further work in identifying the causes of disease should mainly be carried out on a personal level. Macroepidemiological analyses of registry data of the type described here provide indications as to the factors which must be taken into consideration in such future work and also as to the magnitude of the effects of these factors.

(d) These circumstances point to the importance of recording both medical data and environmental descriptors in personal-data registries of good quality.

(e) The demonstrated influence of the diagnosis variable, here termed 'diagnostic intensity', points to geographical variations in the proportion of cancer cases detected (or variations in reporting them). This influence was greatest during the 1960s and mainly concerns elderly persons, and it makes great caution essential when making comparisons and carrying out trend analyses with the aid of age-standardized incidences.

Statistical relationships and real causal relationships

Statistical relationships (correlations) between the occurrence of or mortality from tumour diseases and various variables expressing environmental and life style factors have been discussed in Chapter 5; furthermore, attempts have been made to estimate, from these statistical relationships, how great a proportion of the cases of disease are in—a statistical sense—'explainable' by or 'attributable' to such environmental descriptors.

In the next chapter attempts are made to estimate what proportions of cancer cases are attributable to various causal factors.

It is important to distinguish between the concepts of statistical relationships or correlations and causal relationships. The occurrence of a statistical relationship only means that the groups compared differ with respect to some factor. The statistical relationship cannot pinpoint causal factors without extensive further investigations—it can only point to the fact that the causal factor is correlated with the factor studied. Such a factor 'explains' the frequency of a disease in a statistical sense only.

A few examples can illustrate this. Certain statistical relationships between cancer mortality and marital status have been found, and for some types of cancer the highest mortality is found among the divorced (and for certain other tumour types among the unmarried). It is obviously not the circumstance of being divorced that leads to the elevated risk, but some factor(s) such as tobacco, alcohol, sexual and other living habits, by which divorced people *on average* differ from other groups of people. This increase in risk could in some cases be due to the fact that minorities within each respective group live under extreme conditions.

Certain statistical relationships found in international comparisons between the incidences of special forms of cancer and a high fat intake could just as well be described as relationships between these risks and the gross national product, as an expression of material affluence. The fact that it is now beginning to be seen that high fat intake could be an important causal factor in the developed countries is the result of comprehensive experimental studies, including attempts to clarify the mechanisms of the effects of fats in the induction of cancer. But as long as there is an uncertainty, it is prudent to talk not just about 'high fat intake' but to add 'and/or associated dietary factors'.

In order to accentuate the difference between statistical relationships and causal relationships, the terms 'explanatory' variable, 'explainable' proportion are placed in inverted commas throughout, when these concepts only refer to statistical relationships.

Notes

1. The World Health Organization definition of environmental factors is given in Section 3.2, and it is in this broad sense that this term is used consistently here.
2. Investigation (a) was carried out upon the initiative of the Cancer Committee as a cooperative project between Statistics Sweden and the Committee with the assistance of instiutions at Stockholm University; investigation (b) and in part (c) are included in research projects at Stockholm University supported by the Work Environment Fund and the National Environmental Protection Board; investigation (c), also upon the initiative of the Committee, has been carried out in cooperation between the National Institute of Environmental Medicine and Stockholm University; (d) certain analyses are extracts from projects at Stockholm University supported by the Products Control Board; investigation (e) was carried out by G Eklund of the Karolinska Institute upon the initiative of the Committee.
3. The A-list of the eighth version of the International Classification of Diseases (ICD 8) consists of a grouping of the diagnostic codes for 150 causes of death, of which 17 refer to tumour diseases. This classification is primarily intended to facilitate international and other comparisons, and is therefore not particularly well adapted to analyses of causes of death.
4. In these studies the incidence also includes 'carcinoma *in situ*', i.e., a pre-cancerous lesion, not normally included in figures for the total cancer incidence.

6
Attempts to quantify the importance of different causes of the number of cancer cases in Sweden

6.1 Introduction

The magnitude of the contributions to the total cancer incidence from various factors will be discussed in this chapter. The basis for such calculations varies greatly with the different factors with respect to the confidence with which statements about the nature of the factors may be made and the magnitude of their effects. There is a range of factors, from well-established ones, such as tobacco smoking, to factors of which the importance is difficult to assess due to the vagueness of knowledge about them. Our picture of the relative importance of various factors is thus built up of components with widely differing degrees of reliability.

Chapter 5 has shown that a considerable proportion of the present incidence or mortality of tumourous diseases in Sweden is in a statistical sense 'explainable' by environmental descriptors of geographical, socio-economic or other kinds. The term 'explainable' is put between inverted commas to denote that variables available from databases or registries in relation to various groups in the population are usually not the direct causal factors.

Nearly all lung cancer and about three quarters of the incidences of some other quantitatively important tumour sites seem to be 'explainable' in this sense by variables such as smoking habits, degree of urbanization and socio-economic factors, provided that these variables are expressed as averages for areas such as municipalities. In relation to cancer prevention, however, it must be borne in mind that the proportions which may be ascribed to *specific* causal factors—with the exception of tobacco smoking—are only a small part of the incidence 'explainable' in a statistical sense, since the actual causal factors are yet not known with certainty.

Attempts to assign cancer incidence to various causal factors have been made during recent years by, for example, Wynder and Gori

(1977) and Higginson and Muir (1979) (see Chapter 2, Table 2.7); these approaches were discussed and developed by Doll and Peto (1981) in their review of causes of cancer mortality in the USA (see Table 2.8). The Swedish investigations referred to in Chapter 5 confirm, although partly by a different approach, the conclusion of these studies from other countries that environmental variables taken in a broad sense (i.e. including living habits) are of importance for the induction of cancer in a major proportion of cases.

A large part of the variation in cancer incidence between geographical areas and segments of the population has during recent years been attributed to differences in life-style. This concept is viewed broadly and concerns factors discussed in the following pages. Life-style factors that show statistical correlations with incidences of several cancer diseases are dietary, tobacco and alcohol habits. Living habits are determined by hereditary factors, tradition (including religion) and environment, in which context economic conditions are an important component. Living habits in a wide sense include people's choice of profession, their domicile, their hobbies, even their attitude towards sickness and ailments, and their disposition to consult a doctor. Life-style also influences the risk of infections and other illnesses which could have a bearing on the induction and development of cancer. This demonstrates the complexities of the relationships and provides a background to the difficulty, maybe even impossibility, of identifying various causal factors or quantifying their importance by means of crude epidemiological methods only, such as register or data-base analyses and correlation studies. Not even for 'drop-outs' from society, a risk group which is obviously extreme with respect to several causes of death including cancer, and which seems to contribute to the excess risk among 'divorced' and among 'not economically active' persons (Section 5.5), is it possible to characterize clearly the quantitative importance of alcohol, tobacco and sub-optimal or inappropriate food intake, although these factors certainly are important components in a very complex chain of relationships.

Among the possible environmental factors responsible for the occurrence of cancer, a proper understanding of specific agents exists only in exceptional cases (e.g. radiation, certain occupational exposures and certain iatrogenic factors). With regard to the proven carcinogenic influence of tobacco smoking or certain occupational environments and the probable carcinogenic effect of pollution in urban areas, we are dealing with complex, mixed exposures in which the most important active agents have not been identified with certainty, even though the sources can be located. Among the factors grouped under living habits are both endogenous agents (such as natural hormones of the body) and exogenous agents, the identities and effects of which are still a

Different causes of cancer cases in Sweden

matter for discussion and research. Products of the intestinal bacteria are on the border-line between endogenous and exogenous agents.

Certain cancer cases will be assigned to more than one causal category when one attempts to quantify the importance of various factors for cancer incidence. This is because cancer often has multiple causes which interact.

In the following sections discussions on some causal factors such as tobacco smoking are deliberately brief; risk quantifications for these have been carried out in conjunction with the discussion in Chapter 4. Other factors which previously have not been treated from a quantitative point of view are discussed in more detail. This is based on considerations concerning mechanisms and dose–response relationships, exposure data and so on in Chapter 4 and certain international reviews referred to earlier in Chapter 2. In addition to this, the possibilities for verification of assumptions made according to the studies described in Chapter 5 are discussed. The estimates refer to cancer incidences for the last few years, which to a large extent are assumed to be the result of causal factors which existed years or decades ago.

The investigations forming the basis for the risk evaluations are mainly based on aggregated data, that is group means. In some cases a carcinogenic factor (e.g. one with promoter effect) may have a dose–response relationship such that the risk per dose unit increases with increasing dose. This often leads, for a given average dose with variation of the dose within the group, to a higher *average risk* for the group (Ekman, 1983) as well as to extremely high individual risks within the most heavily exposed part of the group. As discussed in Section 5.5, it is probable that the elevated average mortality in cancer and in other diseases among persons not economically active mainly depends on the extreme living circumstances of a small section of the group (e.g. 'drop-outs') In a similar manner the relatively low cancer incidence or mortality of religious groups with strict living habits (Mormons, Seventh Day Adventists) would seem in part to be due to the relatively small variability *within* the groups with respect, for example, to dietary habits.

6.2 Tobacco smoking

The estimates in Section 4.2.4 indicate that in Sweden about one quarter of all cancer cases in men and about 7 per cent of the cases in women (an average of 15 per cent for the two sexes, with a margin of error of 12–20 per cent) is caused by tobacco smoking. Included in these figures for men are about 1500 cases per year of lung cancer, which is clearly associated with smoking, a similar number of cases of other forms of cancer which are probably associated with smoking, and about 1200 cases of other cancer forms. For women the corresponding numbers are approximately 250, 550 and 450 cases per year. Altogether, therefore, there are about 5500 cancer cases per year.

Since tobacco smoking often interacts with other causal factors (see Section 4.6), a certain proportion of these cases will be ascribed to the occupational environment, the diet and other living habits.

The epidemiological studies referred to in Chapter 5 take into consideration the smoking habits of inhabitants of Swedish municipalities, through the inclusion of a variable reflecting the proportion of 'regular smokers'. This does not take into consideration the fact that in areas such as big cities with a high proportion of smokers these persons also smoke more cigarettes per day, inhale more deeply and start to smoke earlier in life. The smoking variable employed will, therefore, underestimate the importance of smoking as a causal factor. The influence of such characteristics will instead be ascribed to urbanization and 'big-city' variables, with which they are correlated. However, the proportion of the lung-cancer incidence, as well as of the total cancer incidence, which in a statistical sense 'is explained' by the proportion of 'regular smokers' and by the urbanization and 'big-city' descriptors, is compatible with the estimate cited above of the importance of tobacco smoking as a causal factor.

There has been much debate on the risks from tobacco smoke to non-smokers, in particular the effects of passive smoking (Section 4.2.5). However, there are no data available on the exposure in Sweden to environmental tobacco smoke. The cancer risk due to passive smoking can without doubt be substantial in extreme individual cases, but on a whole there seems to be no reason to adjust the estimated number of cases due to smoking given above.

The development of the smoking pattern in Sweden described in Chapter 4 implies a reduced future incidence of cancers associated with smoking for men, but an increasing incidence for women.

Other consumption of tobacco (snuff, chewing tobacco) entails a certain cancer risk, the magnitude of which could not be determined. The type of cancer most usually associated with such habits (cancer of the oral cavity) seems to account for only a few cases per year.

6.3 Dietary factors

General aspects

As seen in Section 4.3, considerable importance with respect to the occurrence of cancer is ascribed to dietary factors. This conclusion is based on epidemiological comparisons between countries and subpopulations, such as groups that have moved from one cultural environment to another, and it is also supported by data from animal experiments.

Quantitative estimation of the importance of diet is beset with great difficulties. No Swedish epidemiological studies of the relationship between dietary variables and cancer incidence exist, largely because of a lack of information concerning the intake of different food components on an individual level and over time.

In the estimates of the importance of diet for cancer mortality and incidence in the USA and the UK, referred to in Chapter 2, dietary factors or 'life-style' factors (probably mainly dietary habits) are stated to account for about a third to a half of all cancer. The magnitude of the uncertainty might amount to a factor of 2 (see Sections 2.4.2 and 4.3). If this estimate is correct, it should in all probability also be valid for Sweden, for which the cancer pattern closely resembles that of other western industrialized countries. The Swedish investigations referred to in Chapter 5 do not contradict such an assumption.

Specific dietary factors

A high intake of fat has been attributed a substantial aetiological importance. Although the view that the fat itself is the active component is supported by animal experiments and, by present understanding of its mechanisms of action, one cannot, because of the chemical complexity of foods, dismiss a role, in epidemiological relationships, of other dietary factors that are correlated with the fat intake.

In several investigations (see Section 4.3.2) a high fat intake has been judged to be of importance in the occurrence of several tumour diseases, in particular *colo-rectal* and *breast cancer*. Almost linear relationships between fat intake and mortality in colon and breast cancer have been demonstrated in examinations of statistical data from various countries. The relatively high incidences in Sweden, where close to 40 per cent of the energy intake consists of fat, are compatible with these dose–response curves. Although the linear relationships are only an approximation of reality, they support the notion that a substantial number of these cancers in Sweden could have a high fat intake and/or associated dietary factors as a cause. It would not appear unreasonable to assume that about half of the cases out of some 8 000 each year could be due to this factor. This view is not contradicted by the epidemiological studies cited in Chapter 5 together with statistical data on food consumption patterns.

The excess risk for breast cancer, which has been correlated statistically with a high fat intake, is probably among other things related to an elevated level of certain hormones caused by dietary habits. The incidence of breast cancer is also affected by the fertility pattern, with a reduced risk if the first pregnancy occurs relatively early in life (see Section 6.4). A similar covariation with fertility pattern is shown by *ovarian* and *uterine cancer* (see Chapter 5), which are each responsible for about 6 per cent of the total cancer cases among women in Sweden (about 950 and about 1 100 respectively per year). It is likely that dietary factors play a similar aetiological role for these cancer types (see US National Research Council 1982). This may be possible also for *cancer of the pancreas*, of which there are some 1 200 cases per year in Sweden. In international studies both pancreatic and endometrical cancer (cancer of the pancreas and corpus uteri) show tendencies to geographical and other variations similar to those of intestinal and breast cancer, and the same tendencies are seen for *prostate cancer* (about 3700 cases per year in Sweden).

Even if about half of the cases of breast and colo-rectal cancer may have fat intake and/or associated dietary factors as a cause, this cannot be taken to imply a correspondingly high causal proportion of the other mentioned cancer forms (cancer of the ovary, corpus uteri, pancreas and prostate), because of their complex aetiology. Against the background of the international reports referred to and the Swedish cancer pattern, it is not unreasonable to assume that *in total* some 5 000 cancer cases per year in Sweden are caused by a high fat intake and/or associated dietary factors.

It appears from the large-scale US investigations of the mortality and causes of death due to smoking that the risks for intestinal and breast cancer are relatively low among smokers, in certain cases lower than among non-smokers (Hammond, 1966). Norwegian data (Lund and Zeiner-Henriksen, 1981) suggest that this is also the case for corpus uteri and ovarian cancer. On the other hand former smokers exhibit a certain excess risk compared to smokers (Rogot and Murray, 1980). It is possible that these circumstances are due to differences in dietary habits between smokers and non-smokers. Further research on these matters is called for, especially to avoid negative consequences of a recommendation to stop smoking.

Undoubtedly other factors than fat and/or associated dietary factors play an aetiological role in the occurrence of cancer. Animal experiments suggest that a high total food intake can also advance the induction of tumours, but it is difficult to isolate such effects from the effects of total intake of such specific components as fat. *Lack of certain dietary factors* may also lead to an increase in tumour diseases.

Among natural food-product components, variations in the intake of vegetables may be of importance with respect to the supply of fibre (which is considered to counteract colon cancer), and vitamins A, C and E (which are considered to have a certain anticarcinogenic effect);

the latter is also true for selenium (see Section 4.3.4). A lack of such factors could be the result of an unbalanced diet.

The effects of fat intake may in part be promotive in character, and, as Section 4.3.2 indicates, in part be of a direct initiator nature. Food products also contain *specific initiators*, but a sound basis for assessing their importance in risk estimates is lacking (see in particular Sections 4.3.3, 4.4.4 and 4.4.6). A large part of the total initiator exposure of the Swedish population is through food intake. These initiators will then contribute to the risks in conjunction with promoters and cocarcinogens, whether the latter are due to dietary habits or to other sources. Pesticide residues and food additives (in such cases where the product has been tested for genotoxicity at high concentrations) are apparently of insignificant importance in the total initiator activity of the food intake in Sweden (with the possible exception of nitrite). On the other hand it seems justifiable to take certain kinds of naturally occurring substances into consideration as well as mycotoxins, substances formed during preparation processes including heating (pyrolysis products, nitrosamines), fermentation (urethanes) and smoke-curing (polycyclic aromatic hydrocarbons), certain food additives without licence requirements and contaminants from the atmosphere and water.

Drinking water may also be regarded as a dietary factor. However, its contribution to the total cancer incidence in Sweden is probably very small.

The incidences of the forms of cancer mentioned in this section mostly exhibit only small fluctuations with time, although all of them show an increase. However, *stomach cancer*, long considered to be to a great extent caused by dietary factors (Section 4.3.2), exhibits in Sweden, as in other industrialized countries, a decided downward trend. Since this decrease is still in progress, and considerable differences between geographic areas exist, it is probable that a substantial part of the still rather high incidence of stomach cancer (more than 1800 cases in Sweden in 1980) is caused by dietary factors. Among these a high intake of nitrates and table salt and a sub-optimal intake of foods containing vitamin C have been suggested.

Certain possibilities also exist to estimate the number of cases of cancer associated with *alcohol (ethanol)*, to a great extent in conjunction with tobacco smoking (see Section 4.3.5). According to available data it may be a matter of about 500 (at the most 1000) cases, not a negligible number.

Summary

It appears that about one third of the total incidence of cancer in Sweden could be the result of dietary factors (partly in interaction with other factors). This corresponds to an incidence of roughly 10 000 cases per year, but there are great uncertainties attached to this figure.

About half of the colo-rectal and breast cancer cases could have a high fat intake and/or associated dietary factors as a cause. A certain additional risk with the same aetiology probably also concerns cancer of the corpus uteri, ovary, pancreas and prostate.

A considerable fraction of the cases of stomach cancer probably also have dietary factors as a cause, but the specific causal factors here are with great certainty of a different kind.

The estimates made here of the total role played by diet as well as the significance of a high fat intake (and/or associated dietary factors) are obviously uncertain, but should indicate a reasonable order of magnitude based on the present state of knowledge.

6.4 Other life-style factors, especially sexual habits and fertility pattern

There are strong indications that factors associated with reproduction and fertility influence the incidences of *cancer of the breast, ovary and corpus uteri*. The study referred to in Chapter 5 concerning a statistical connection between marital status and cancer mortality showed a considerable risk among unmarried women in Sweden, compared to those of other status, of cancer of the breast and corpus uteri, in agreement with studies in other countries. Cancer of the ovary was not studied here, but investigations in other countries have reported a similar dependence on marital status. As has been shown in the case of breast cancer, the risk increases with the age at the first full-term pregnancy. This indicates, as do experimental data, that hormonal factors are of importance for the induction of these diseases.

These hormonal factors are probably affected both by the fertility pattern and by dietary factors, in particular the intake of fat and/or associated dietary factors. (From the point of view of cancer prevention dietary habits can much more easily be altered than fertility patterns). To the extent that there is an interaction, some cancer cases will be accounted for as due to both dietary habits and the fertility pattern.

A total of some 6 500 cases of cancer of the breast, ovary and corpus uteri were recorded in Sweden in 1979. Judging from the strong influence of the age at first pregnancy on breast cancer incidence shown by MacMahon *et al.* (1973), it would seem that a not insubstantial proportion of the cases of breast cancer could be related to the fertility pattern. Since the three diseases quantitatively exhibit about the same differences in incidence between women of different marital status, a large proportion of the cases of cancer of the ovary and corpus uteri might also be related to the same causal factors. It should be pointed out that Swedish epidemiological studies have not unequivocally confirmed the same relationship between breast cancer incidence and fertility pattern (Adami, 1977). Considering the above, it would, however, seem reasonable to assume that about half of the cases, with a large uncertainty interval, are related to the fertility pattern.

Cancer of the *cervix* exhibits a different incidence pattern. This form of cancer shows statistical relationships with factors used to characterize 'big cities' (see Chapter 5), and the incidence is highest among divorced women. Several epidemiological studies have demonstrated the relationship between this disease and the number of sexual partners, and a recent study has even shown a relationship with the number of sexual encounters of the male partner (Skegg et al. 1982). The incidence is very low for nuns and very high in certain South American big cities where, although the women are to a great extent monogamous, the custom of using prostitutes is prevalent among men. These observations indicate that cancer of the cervix is to a large extent a hygienic problem; among other things it is suspected that a herpes virus transmitted during intercourse is a causal factor. Certain epidemiological studies indicate, furthermore, that cigarette smoking could be another aetiological factor (Buckley *et al.*, 1981).

In 1979, 543 cases of invasive cervical cancer were reported in Sweden, that is, approximately 3 per cent of the total cancer incidence for Swedish women. This incidence figure has shown a large decrease since the 1960s, as in other industrialized countries (see Chapter 5), doubtless due at least in part to mass health controls (see Chapter 13). At the same time, a very considerable increase in reported premalignant changes (dysplasia and cancer *in situ*) has been observed.

To sum up, sexual habits and the fertility pattern are assumed to be linked with some 3500 cases of cancer per year in Sweden, almost exclusively among women.

Other possible causal factors which may be more or less strongly related to the conditions of life are contained in the following sections of this chapter. There is even good reason for not precluding the existence of still more, unknown, factors linked to life-style, for example related to psycho-social circumstances (see Kasl (1984) and references cited therein), but at present all prerequisites for quantifying their importance are lacking.

Jenkins (1983) has shown in a study from Massachusetts that male mortality from cancer, especially stomach and intestinal cancer, is higher in socially repressive environments (distinguished for example, by poverty, divorces, restricted living quarters). These statistical relationships—possibly related to the higher risks within certain groups of single and economically inactive persons (see Chapter 5)—in no way confirm any causal relationship and do not identify causal factors. However, they indicate the importance of considering psychosocial factors (which can have an hereditary element) when attempting to clarify causes of cancer, besides the chemically and physically measurable components of life-style and of the environment, such as diet, tobacco and alcohol consumption or occupational exposures.

6.5 Infections, inflammations, etc.

Cancer diseases in general are not spread by infection. Viruses and bacteria may, however, contribute in various ways to an increased cancer risk, and may in certain cases be actual causal factors.

The role played by so-called cancer viruses (oncoviruses) has been touched upon in Chapter 3. These viruses act as transporters or activators of 'cancer genes' (oncogenes) or as stabilizers of their products. It seems probable that in humans this phenomenon is the starting mechanism for those types of cancer which increase rapidly in patients treated with immuno-suppressive drugs or who suffer from a congenital lack of T lymphocytes (which attack and destroy cells infected by viruses: see Möller and Möller, 1975). These types of cancer include, in particular, certain lymphomas, which constitute a few per cent of the total incidence. Cancer of the naso-pharynx (in Sweden some 50 cases per year) also seems to have a viral aetiology in many cases.

The possible significance of a herpes virus in the occurrence of cervical cancer (in all some 550 cases per year in Sweden) has already been mentioned (Section 6.4). Evidence supporting a role of infection in this disease, as in the case of cancer of the penis (some 60 cases per year in Sweden), is supplied by the highly elevated risk of cervical cancer for wives of men who later develop cancer of the penis.

It could also be surmised that the development of a tumour is furthered by infection in a more indirect fashion. This could take place as damage to tissues which leads to reparative growth, in principle a promotive effect (see Section 3.4). Such a mechanism has been discussed in connection with the role played by the jaundice virus (hepatitis B) in the development of cancer of the liver, in which the mycotoxin aflatoxin is one likely initiator. Similar modifying (co-carcinogenic) effects of infections could also be envisaged for other tumour diseases. Thus a viral or bacterial infection of the lungs may contribute to the risk of lung cancer. A relationship between previous tuberculosis and lung cancer has been demonstrated (see Holmberg and Ehrenber, 1984). Viral infections of the lungs and chronic bacterial bronchitis, aggravated by cigarette smoking and by air pollutants such as nitrogen dioxide (NO_2), might contribute to the higher lung cancer risk in urban areas. Well-known relationships exist between cancer and chronic inflammations, infections and reparative states, for example ulcerative colitis, chronic sinus and middle ear inflammations, chronic ulcers and fistula, and scarring after burns.

Doll and Peto (1981) have suggested as 'a very uncertain best estimate', that about 10 per cent of the total cancer mortality in the USA depends on infections of various kinds. Considering that a large proportion of the cases of cervical cancer are probably caused by viral infections, it appears that at least some 2 per cent of the total cancer incidence in Sweden can be assigned to infections and other factors mentioned here, but the true figure could be substantially higher.

6.6 General air pollution in urban areas

In urban areas, in particular the big cities, the levels of pollutants from the combustion of fossil fuels, and to varying degrees from industrial activity, are higher than in rural areas. For many years this has been considered to be one of the reasons for the elevated incidence of lung cancer and certain other tumourous diseases and mortality from them in the large cities, as observed in many countries.

Since urban and rural areas differ with respect to other important cancer risk factors, such as smoking, dietary habits and occupational exposures, it is difficult to verify effects of general air pollution.

The fact that air pollution in Sweden consists of a large number of mutagenic and cancer-initiating substances (EHE 1977; Holmberg and Ahlborg, 1983) implies—if the dose–response curves are assumed to be linear—that this pollution is responsible for an increased cancer risk. The fundamental question in connection with planning preventive measures thus concerns the *magnitude* of this risk increase. Various approaches to answering this question have been summarized by Ehrenberg and Törnqvist (1984), and have also been touched upon in Section 4.4.5 in connection with the effects of benzo[a]pyrene and other polycyclic aromatic hydrocarbons. The complexity of the matter means that epidemiological studies must be complemented by risk estimates based on exposure levels, as in the case of passive smoking.

LUNG CANCER
Epidemiological studies from various countries over the last two decades do not provide an unequivocal answer to the question of *whether* general air pollution contributes to an increased cancer risk in urban areas. In certain studies, statistical evidence for a direct risk increase has been obtained, but in other studies an urban-factor effect is obtained only as a reinforcement of the smoking-dependent (and possibly occupation-dependent) risk. In yet other studies, no excess

risk at all can be detected when due consideration is given to differences between urban and rural areas in smoking habits and occupational exposures. In some studies, as discussed by Törnqvist (1984) correlations between the levels of specific pollutants and mortality from lung cancer and certain other tumourous diseases have been detected, but in these studies proper consideration was not given to variations in smoking habits and other living habits, which in turn are correlated with the levels of air pollution.

Taken together these results seem to indicate, but not to prove, a certain risk contribution from urban air pollutants. However, the statistical methods are extremely insensitive (see Section 6.7). It should also be added that the effects of general air pollution include contributions from tobacco smoke in the environment and cannot easily be separated from this contribution.

An international Task Group meeting in Stockholm in 1977 (Cederlöf et al., 1978) concluded: 'Combustion products of fossil fuels in ambient air, probably acting together with cigarette smoke, have been responsible for cases of lung cancer in large urban areas, the numbers produced being of the order of 5–10 cases per 100 000 males per year (European standard population)'. A later meeting (Holmberg and Ahlborg, 1983) 'reaffirmed' the estimates made by the 1977 group, 'in spite of a great deal of uncertainty in the epidemiological evidence' and 'found no reason to substantially change the [previous] numerical estimate'.

Doll and Peto, in their survey of causes of cancer in the USA (1981), also stated: 'these crude estimates probably provide the best basis for the formation of policy' with regard to cancer prevention.

Significant statistical relationships of cancer incidence with the degree of urbanization and with socio-economic variables characterizing larger urban areas and big cities in Sweden have been found, after due consideration has been taken of diagnostic routines and the proportion of regular smokers, as referred to in Chapter 5. These variables expressing urban characteristics stand for several important factors with regard to incidence, no doubt, for example, certain distinguishing features of the smoking-habit pattern. No variables reflecting air pollution levels were available in that investigation. The results obtained concerning factors other than smoking (see Ehrenberg and Ekman, 1984) cannot, however, be considered as inconsistent with the above assessment of lung cancer risk due to general air pollution, especially if the uncertainty of this assessment is taken into account.

OTHER FORMS OF TUMOUR

Most carcinogens which enter the body are distributed systemically and can thus lead to an increased cancer risk in organs other than the lung.

The Swedish study mentioned in Chapter 5 indicates an association between urbanization and a big-city environment and increased incidence for all cancers taken together as well as for specific types of cancer (besides lung cancer). This risk increase is without doubt mainly due to causes other than air pollution. In the absence of variables adequately reflecting the levels of such pollution, the risk contribution from this latter factor must be estimated by other means. A couple of approaches in this context are presented by Ehrenberg and Törnqvist (1984). One approach is that of assuming that the ratio between the total cancer risk and the lung cancer risk is the same for general air pollution as for tobacco smoking, namely about 3. This figure is to some extent consistent with epidemiological observations. Another method of computing the risk from general air pollution in urban areas would be to make risk estimates for specific components and then add up the risks. However, the basic data for such a treatment of the problem are lacking. Estimates in Section 4.4.5 above indicate that ethylene, mainly from automobile exhausts, might be responsible for up to 10 per cent of the total estimated cancer risk attributed to air pollutants and, furthermore, that benzo[a]pyrene and unsubstituted polycyclic aromatic hydrocarbons probably cannot be responsible for more than a fraction of a per cent and a few per cent respectively of this risk. A large number of common pollutants which are active mutagens in screening tests (see Holmberg and Ahlborg 1983), are to be found in urban air, however, but quantitative data which could be used for risk estimates for these agents are lacking. Important components in this context are aliphatic and aromatic carbonyl compounds as well as products formed from oxides of nitrogen in the air (nitroarenes, nitroalkenes) and in the body (nitrosamines, see Törnqvist (1984)). The possibility of locally higher levels of precipitated pollutants in foodstuffs, leading to further cancer incidence variations between urban and rural areas, should not be rejected (see Section 4.4 above).

RISK ESTIMATION: SUMMARY
The number of lung cancer cases per year in Sweden due to general air pollution may be estimated as approximately 100 cases, with an uncertainty of at least a factor of 2. The total cancer incidence due to such causes is more difficult to evaluate, but should fall in the interval of roughly 100–1000 cases per year, according to all reasonable assumptions. This presupposes that approximately one-fifth of the Swedish population is subjected to the exposures typical of European urban areas, and that the risk is about the same for men and women.

6.7 Factors in the working environment

The question of how many cancer cases should be ascribed to factors in the work environment in Sweden, in particular occupational exposures, does not have a straightforward answer, in spite of the number of detailed studies of many specific exposure situations. It is difficult to isolate occupationally induced cancer as a specific category. How, for example, should lip and skin cancer induced by ultraviolet light be classified among those working out of doors? How should cancer ascribed to higher tobacco and alcohol consumption in occupations associated with extensive entertaining be interpreted?

For example, Fox and Adelstein (1978) have shown that differences in lung cancer incidence between various occupational groups are mainly due to differences in smoking habits. Certain occupational exposures such as from roasting kiln work, mining work (radon daughters) and asbestos have been analysed with respect to the aetiological role played by the exposure in question and its interaction above all with smoking habits (see Section 4.6). The case-control method used here does not, however, directly generate any data from which the number of cases per year due to the respective exposures may be calculated.

Another difficulty is the insensitivity of the epidemiological methods; in practice only relatively high risks (excess risks of 50 to 100 per cent corresponding to relative risks of 1.5–2.0) can be detected with statistical significance. In all probability lower risks are much more prevalent in occupational environments, so that many diagnosed cancer cases will not be considered as occupationally caused.

However, an estimate of the order of magnitude of the occupationally caused cancer cases in Sweden has been made as follows. It is known that there exists a considerable excess risk for cancer in certain industries, such as the mining industry, the rubber industry, roasting kiln work and chemical laboratory work. However, only a few tens of new cancer cases each year can be attributed to exposures in investigated, specific work environment situations.

In a preliminary analysis of the Cancer-Environment Registry, for the years 1961–73 (Einhorn et al., 1980) the ratios between the number of observed and expected cancer cases for combinations of occupational group and type of cancer were calculated. Only combinations showing a risk ratio greater than 2 or statistically significantly greater than 1.5 were included. When adding together the differences between the numbers of observed and of expected cases, which may be said to provide a rough estimate of the magnitude of the excess risk, some 100 new cases of cancer per year are found in Sweden in the occupational groups thus affected. (This figure is consistent with data recently presented by Malker and Weiner (1984).) This figure may be too high since it includes possible cancer cases caused by living habits and exposures other than those occurring occupationally; the Registry data do not contain information in this respect. On the other hand, the figure probably represents a gross underestimate of the true number of cancer cases due to occupational causes, partly because of what has been said concerning the epidemiological method, and partly because of the relatively limited follow-up period (13 years).

An upper limit for the cancer risk attributable to occupational exposure can be imagined if it is assumed that all persons with any potential exposure in their work are at the same risk as an occupational group with an extremely high exposure to carcinogenic substances. A suitable extreme risk for this purpose (Malker, 1982) is the observed excess risk for cancer among chimney sweeps. Proceeding from the analysis of Hogstedt et al. (1983) of the same type of occupational exposure, and taking into due consideration the fact that this analysis is limited to mortality, a rough estimate of the number of cases (morbidity) yields a figure of between 1000 and 4000 cases, i.e. of the order of magnitude of 2000 cancer cases per year. This is a theoretical upper limit, since the mean exposure load in various occupations is actually much lower.

Overall, therefore, the annual number of occupationally induced cancer cases in Sweden seems likely to lie between 100 (an underestimate) and 2000 (an overestimate), a reasonable figure being about 500 cases per year, or approximately 2 per cent of all cancer cases. Occupationally induced cases of cancer seem to be five times more prevalent among men than among women.

This estimate for Sweden constitutes a likely value for exposures during the 1960s and early 1970s. Due to great improvements in standards of cleanliness at places of work during the 1970s and 1980s, with reduction of the exposure levels of known carcinogens, the cancer risk associated with present exposure conditions could be a good deal lower.

The aim of this chapter has been to discuss factors underlying *the total number of cancer cases*. In such a context occupation seems to play a smaller role than is often thought. However, much attention should be paid to the working environment with regard to specific risk groups. Excess risks shown in certain studies have often been considered to be unacceptable (see Chapter 7). In many cases such excess risks have been reduced by measures aimed either at eliminating an identified causal factor such as vinyl chloride—or at generally reducing exposures. As concerns the counteracting of high *individual risks*, the work environment is an important target for preventive measures. A prerequisite is a clearer picture concerning risk groups. It is also important that better facilities should be made available for assessing the number of cases of occupationally induced cancer, and its relation to occupational exposures. This will require improvements in information systems and in epidemiological monitoring.

6.8 Consumer products

The modern individual uses a wide variety of products such as detergents, cosmetics, toiletries, paints, solvents, pesticides in the home and garden, plastic articles, electrical materials, impregnated fabrics and so on. This results in potential exposure to thousands of chemical substances, and if impurities from the manufacturing processes are included, probably to tens of thousands of substances. The actual exposure varies considerably, however. As well as accidental intake, for example through the dissolution of heavy metals from badly made containers into foodstuffs, certain substances can penetrate the skin and some products give off particles into the air or gaseous substances which can be inhaled. For most consumer products, however, the potential for exposure to chemical substances seems in practice to be small. There are exceptions of course, for example in cosmetics and solvents and also with certain products which are normally handled in an occupational setting, according to proper regulations, which are often not observed in domestic circumstances. The risk to the individual nevertheless still seems to be small, provided that the exposure is limited. However, deficiencies in available information on the composition of consumer products and on the way in which these products are used make it impossible to rule out altogether any occurrence of high individual risks.

Any estimate of the total number of cancer cases attributable to consumer products must be very uncertain. Where risk contributions are additive, even small individual exposures without any practical bearing on the risk for the person concerned could contribute non-negligibly to the total cancer incidence if large groups in the population are exposed. Some known or suspected carcinogenic components previously used in solvents, hair-colouring compounds and pesticides have been restricted or banned, and toxic monomers such as vinyl chloride in plastic products are now regulated. The present state of knowledge is nevertheless insufficient to exclude the possibility that certain consumer products or product groups contribute unacceptably to cancer risks. Doll and Peto (1981) have attributed a 'nominal less than 1% of all current cancer deaths' in the USA to 'industrial products' which should correspond to 'consumer products' in this chapter. They point out at the same time, however, that 'there is too much ignorance for complacency to be justified'.

The contribution from consumer articles to the total cancer incidence in Sweden is likewise thought to be small. However, the Cancer

Committee otherwise adheres to the opinion of Doll and Peto. Efforts thus need to be made to obtain better information on the chemical composition of consumer products and possibilities of harmful exposures from them. The risk contribution from ionizing radiation in consumer products must, however, be considered to be so small that it presents no problem (see Section 6.9).

6.9 Physical factors

6.9.1 Ionizing radiation

Estimated risks attributable to ionizing radiation from various sources in Sweden have also been discussed in Section 4.5.2 against the background of a review of collective doses by the Swedish National Institute of Radiation Protection (NIRP). These risk contributions can be classified into specific risk areas according to the subdivisions in this chapter. The calculated numbers of ionization injuries, mainly cancer deaths, have been presented in Table 4.19. It should be noted that the table gives estimates of *future* effects of the *present* exposure levels.

FACTORS IN THE WORKING ENVIRONMENT (Section 6.7)
The largest contribution here has been occupational exposure in mining (Table 4.19, category 9). However, improvements in the miners' environment during the last decade have led to a considerable reduction in the expected number of cancer cases (to about two cases per year). Quite well-recorded doses of radiation in other areas of activity, namely research and education (category 12), industrial work (category 11) and health care (categories 13, 15, 17, 19 and 21), lead to a risk estimate which in total corresponds to less than one expected case of cancer per year.

CONSUMER PRODUCTS (Section 6.8)
Consumer products (Table 4.19 category 10) are associated with a totally negligible risk (less than one case in 10 years).

IATROGENIC FACTORS (Section 6.10)

Other Risk Areas

Activities which give a risk contribution to the population in general include mainly the *testing of nuclear weapons* (Table 4.19, category 6)

48with about two cases per year, and *atomic energy production* (category 4), which appears to be associated with a negligibly small number of cases per year in Sweden.

Much of the exposure to radiation from natural sources cannot be prevented. This *background radiation* includes cosmic radiation (category 1), radiation from bedrock (category 3 and a small part of 7 and 8), as well as radiation from natural radioactive materials in the body (category 2). The total risk contribution from these could amount to about 150 deaths from cancer per year. A further, man-made contribution to the collective dose of natural alpha and gamma radiation is above all due to the building techniques used for the construction of houses (the main part of categories 7 and 8). *Gamma radiation in buildings* is thought to induce some 80 cases per year, and *alpha radiation from radon daughters* will induce between 100 and 1000 cases per year in the future (see Section 4.5.2).

Altogether, ionizing radiation, excluding that from radon daughters in houses, is calculated to induce somewhat more than 300 deaths from cancer per year in Sweden (or about 600 new cases of a cancer disease), corresponding to about 2 per cent of the incidence. More than a third of these cases may be assumed to be caused by diagnostic medical examinations (see Section 6.10). The additional risk contribution from radon daughters in houses applies to lung cancer, which means practically equal incidence and mortality rates.

The cancer cases which have here been attributed to ionizing radiation are assumed to be induced almost exclusively at such low dose levels that the radiation has only an initiator effect. These cases will thus sometimes also be included among cancer cases attributed to causal factors with promoter effects.

6.9.2 Ultraviolet light

There are strong indications that the ultraviolet component of sunlight (particularly UV-B) is a predominant aetiological factor for various types of skin cancer and also contributes to the lip cancer incidence (see Section 4.5.3).

Regarding skin cancer, the aetiology is most evident in connection with squamous cancer and basal cell cancer. Since the latter form is not recorded in the Swedish Cancer Registry, it is not included in the total incidence figures. For malignant melanoma too, sunlight cannot be eliminated as a major causal factor, in particular in connection with intermittent intensive sunbathing. It appears that approximately 1500 cases of cancer per year (excluding basal cell cancer) may be attributed to the effect of sunlight.

6.10 Iatrogenic factors

Health disorders attributable to 'iatrogenic factors' are those due to medical activities such as X-ray and isotope *examination* (ionizing radiation) and *treatment* with ionizing radiation, ultraviolet radiation and drugs (including medicinal products not connected with illness).

Medical procedures are based on a risk–benefit appraisal towards the patient. Iatrogenically increased cancer risks cannot be completely avoided even under optimal conditions, apart from those risks which may be due to malpractice including unnecessarily large risks in cases where appropriate alternative methods of examination or treatment are available.

It is theoretically estimated that somewhat more than 100 deaths from cancer per year result from X-ray and isotope diagnosis (Table 4.19, categories 14, 18 and 20), corresponding to about 0.5 per cent of the cases occurring annually in Sweden. As pointed out earlier (Section 4.5.2) this is probably an overestimate since it has not been taken into consideration that a large number of examinations concern patients with grave illnesses and a short expected survival time. Although there is a potential for a certain lowering of the collective risk through technical improvements, the usually small risk to the individual should be weighed against the usually great advantage of an appropriate diagnosis. A corresponding risk–benefit evaluation applies to radiation treatment of patients (Table 4.19, category 16). These are mainly cancer patients who receive relatively high doses. Although the collective dose is considerable, a collective risk figure is clearly not relevant in this context, and is not given in table 4.19.

Similarly, all drugs may cause side-effects and their use presupposes striking a balance between the beneficial effects of the medicine and the risk of side-effects. A number of drugs associated with the induction of cancers have been extensively discussed in Section 4.4.5. Available data do not allow assessment of how much the use of drugs has contributed to the total Swedish cancer incidence, nor whether such cases could have been avoided.

Doll and Peto (1981) have estimated that iatrogenic factors are responsible for about 1 per cent (0.5–3 per cent) of the total number of cancer deaths in the USA, of which approximately one half may be attributed to ionizing radiation. There is no reason to believe that this figure is higher in Sweden.

6.11 Conclusions

The number of cancer cases per year in Sweden and the proportions of this incidence attributable to various categories of causes reflecting living habits and other factors in the environment, as subdivided in the previous sections of Chapter 6, are summarized in Table 6.1. In addition to this, the influence of hereditary factors, as mentioned in Chapter 2, is to be noted.

> It is important to remember that the figures given in the Table 6.1 are of greatly varying reliability. The role played by tobacco smoking is fairly clear. Some other figures are rough estimates and are, therefore, much less certain. This is, for example, the case with dietary factors, sexual habits and general air pollution in urban areas.

Due to interactive effects the proportions attributed to various causal categories are not simply additive, as in the case of independent units. For example, some of the cases ascribed to sexual habits and the reproductive pattern probably also fall into the category of dietary habits, in particular a high intake of fat and/or associated dietary factors. Similarly some of the cases ascribed to tobacco smoking, occupational factors and ionizing radiation will also be counted among other causal categories. Thus if all separate causal factors were known, the sum of all proportions of the total incidence ascribed to them would substantially exceed 100 per cent.

The proportions given in Table 6.1 add up to about 65–70 per cent of the total incidence, which is considerably less than the sum (over 90 per cent) of 'explainable' proportions estimated in the study of variations between Swedish municipalities referred to in Chapter 5. The low total reflects caution on the part of the Cancer Committee. This is partly due to a need for further evaluation of error possibilities and uncertainty intervals in the calculation of 'explainable' proportions but more because of incomplete knowledge about which causal factors underlie the observed variations. It is, for example, possible that far more than 10 000 cancer cases annually should be attributed to dietary factors, but likewise it cannot be ignored that this figure may be grossly inflated and that future research will pinpoint other, as yet unidentified, quantitatively important factors related to living circumstances. The role that may be played by such factors is only denoted by a question mark in the table under the title 'Other living habits—possible unknown factors'. A similar degree of uncertainty concerns the role played by infections, inflammations and the like, which may be underestimated.

Some of the estimates have been qualified with intervals for uncertainty or by other comments in the text, which allow a rough estimate to be made of their maximal aggregate importance in the total cancer incidence. Thus about 15 per cent, and at most about 20 per cent, of the cancer cases in Sweden have tobacco smoking as a causal factor (Section 6.2). This figure rests to a large extent on adequate epidemiological data and is fairly reliable. Corresponding evaluations of general air pollution (Section 6.6), occupational factors (Section 6.7), consumer products (Section 6.7), physical factors (Section 6.9) and iatrogenic factors (Section 6.10) indicate that the individual risk contributions from each to the total incidence is rather insignificant; aggregated they only attain somewhat more than 10 per cent. In the absence of interaction between different causal factors, the total causal proportion from the factors listed would amount to 25 per cent to 30 per cent of all cancer cases and the actual proportion might be less. At any rate there is considerable space left for other explanatory factors. According to the list, these have to do with living habits (such as diet) including infections, etc., in addition to hereditary factors.

The presentation in Table 6.1 both illustrates the deficiencies in the present state of our knowledge—with indications of needs for further research—and at the same time constitutes a summary of the basis for discussions of preventive measures.

Apart from tobacco smoking, radiation and certain factors in the working environment, little is known about the specific initiators which are assumed to cause the induction of tumours, e.g. the majority of the tumours which have been ascribed to dietary and other living habit factors.

Table 6.1 deals with *collective* risks in the sense of the total number of cases of cancer per year in the population as a whole. However, where a collective risk is small because only a few people are affected by a certain exposure, the *individual* risk may still be unacceptably high.

Table 6.1 An attempt to estimate the number of cancer cases in Sweden attributable to living habits and various other environmental factors.

Section in Chapter 6		Proportion of the total incidence in Sweden (%)	Cases per year[a] (approximate)	Comments
6.2	Tobacco smoking[b]	~15 (12–20)	5500 (4500–7500)	The figure is quite reliable since it is based to a large extent on adequate exposure data. This factor is responsible for 75–80% of the lung cancer cases and for about 10% of other cancer cases.
6.3	Dietary factors[c]	~30 (±?)	10 000 (±?)	The figure is uncertain, see text.
6.4	Other living habits:			
	sexual habits and fertility pattern	~10 (±?)	3500 (±?)	The total is uncertain; for certain forms of cancer the causal relationships are well documented
	possible unknown factors	?	?	
6.5	Infections, flammations, etc.	>2	?	2% corresponds to c 600 cases. The basis is uncertain; the figure could be much higher.
6.6	General air[d] pollution	~1	100–1000	
6.7	Occupational factors	~2 (±?)	500 (±?)	The figure is uncertain, see text. Probable value for the 1960s and early 1970s. Proportion of men taken to be about 5 times higher than of women.
6.8	Consumer articles	<1?	Probably few cases	Extremely uncertain basis.
6.9	Physical factors ionizing radiation except	~2[e]	600[e]	The figure is based on principles for calculations in radiological protection.

	radon in houses			About one-third of the cases may be classified as iatrogenic.
	radon in houses	<1?	100[f] ?	The figure is uncertain. Only lung cancer cases.
	UV radiation	~5[g] (± ?)	1500 (± ?)	The magnitude of the figure seems to be fairly reliable.
6.10	Iatrogenic factors	~1 ?	?	The total effect of iatrogenic factors is uncertain.

These figures are not simply additive. Due to interaction effects one and the same cancer case might be assigned to more than one causal category. The table nevertheless provides means for approximating the relative importance to the various presumpted causal factors. Most of the figures are uncertain, but they represent the 'best possible estimate' at the present state of scientific knowledge.

a Somewhat more than 30 000 cancer cases annually (1979), [*viz.*] about the present incidence is the figure used as a point of departure. The investigations upon which the estimates are based refer to incidences at present or in the recent past, and may thus be ascribed to causal factors prevalent years or decades ago.

b Based on data concerning smokers. The figure is not appreciably affected by a risk contribution from *passive smoking*. No basis exists for estimating the risk contribution from *snuff* and *chewing tobacco*.

c In addition to this, there is *alcohol*, assumed to account for about 500 (at most 1000) cases annually, to a large extent in interaction with smoking.

d Based on information concerning urban conditions.

e The figure actually refers to future cases of cancer attributable to present exposure. The total exposure does not however seem to have varied to any major extent during the past decades.

f The emphasis in the text is on *future* cases of cancer, for which the figure of 300 (100–1000 cases) is thought probable.

g Basal cell cancer not included.

Part II
Prerequisites and measures for reducing the harmful effects of cancer diseases

Part II

7
Strategy of cancer prevention—possibilities and aims

7.1 General prerequisites

In cancer diseases, body cells lose their ability to control their growth. The idea of preventing induction of cancer diseases is based on the assumption that such diseases are to a large extent caused by factors which can be influenced. A large proportion of cancer cases in all probability have a causal factor in the environment (in a wide sense of this word), that is, in personal life-style and other environmental factors. It is possible to indicate roughly several such major causal areas. Although the specific causal factors within these areas are so far seldom known, it is certain that many of these factors in the environment or related to life-style are ones that are open to influence.

It is not possible to predict unambiguously the effect of preventive measures. The incidence of certain forms of cancer could certainly be decreased, but other forms might show an increase because other existing combinations of environmental and hereditary factors would become of greater relative significance. Further, competing causes of diseases and death should be considered, particularly among older people. However, all evidence speaks in favour of the possibility of reducing the total cancer incidence, although one cannot say how far. In a few cases the causal correlation between a certain factor and a specific form of cancer is so clear that the result can be predicted with great certainty; for example, the number of lung cancer cases among men in Sweden would have been only about one sixth of today's number (about 250 cases per year instead of over 1600) if there had been no tobacco smoking. For other cancer diseases or suspected causal factors it is usually more difficult or impossible to express in numerical terms the expected positive effect of a certain change.

A strategy for cancer prevention with measures against relevant environmental factors should be supplemented with measures for promotion of natural protective mechanisms in the body against cancer induction. This field to a large extent remains at the research level, although it now seems probable that, for example, the normal diet contains chemical substances with an anti-carcinogenic effect. The qualitative and quantitative importance of this for human cancer and for defined populations is still not clear. For the future, great expectations can be placed on research within this field. It is not, however, possible to predict when or even if scientific breakthroughs can be expected that would make possible an increase in the capacity of the human body to resist development of a cancer disease, nor to what extent hereditary disposition to cancer development or susceptibility to carcinogenic agents may be open to modification.

The best possibilities for improved cancer prevention lie in the future, with certain exceptions where there is already good knowledge about causal correlations. Progress will depend on continued intensive research work.

7.2 The concept of cancer prevention. Main aims of the strategy

'Cancer prevention' must not be understood to imply that total prevention will ever be possible. The aim is for *risks* of cancer to be *reduced* and for those cases of a cancer disease which do nevertheless occur to appear later in life than they would have done otherwise.

As mentioned above, the cancer pattern (the distribution of cases by different forms of cancer and by age groups and sex) as well as the total number of cancer cases is also dependent on 'competing' causes of death, particularly since the average age at diagnosis of a cancer disease is comparatively high (see Chapter 2). If the mortality in, for example, cardiovascular diseases should increase, the number of cancer cases and the cancer mortality would decrease. Inversely, the number of cancer cases will increase if other causes of death decrease.

A quantitative estimate of the effect of cancer-preventive measures is feasible only for populations (in the sense of defined groups of persons). The success of cancer prevention in terms of risk reduction can be measured through a decrease in the population's age-standardized cancer incidence between two points of time. The effect could be expressed as an increased average life-span for the population concerned, other factors influencing the life-span being taken into consideration. As regards the individual, the effect of preventive measures cannot be gauged; irrespective of whether or not the person in question develops a cancer disease, this fact cannot with complete certainty be associated with the presence or absence of particular living habits or other environmental factors (except in rare cases with a known hereditary component leading to cancer). So for an individual it is not possible to go beyond—at best—a good calculation of the reduction in risk following certain measures aiming at cancer prevention.

The concept of risk is thus central to cancer prevention, as with other disorders where phases of events are not predictable and the biological damage seen is a chance (or stochastic) effect. This follows from the theories of mechanisms of cancer induction (see Chapter 3).

> A carcinogenic substance has the *property* of being able to cause cancer under certain conditions. The *risk* to an individual of developing cancer from exposure to such a substance is the probability of his being afflicted with a cancer disease. This depends on chance, on the magnitude of the exposure (the higher the exposure, the higher the risk) and on congenital or acquired susceptibility to the carcinogenic agent. The effect of chance (as in a lottery) means, for example, that not all smokers with the same cigarette consumption and with the same biological susceptibility will develop cancer.

In certain cases the individual risk may be high, for example where there is a specific exposure to a carcinogenic agent in the work environment. If the number of such exposed individuals is small, preventive measures will have little effect on the total cancer incidence. In so far as one is dealing with factors which exert their effects by chance and where each risk contribution thus increases the probability for tumour development, the concepts of collective dose and collective risk will be applicable in the population concerned. (All doses to exposed individuals in the population are added and the importance of this collective dose, expressed as the number of cancer cases, is estimated according to a set pattern by reading off a dose–response curve.) If the individual risk following exposure to such an agent is low but the exposed population large, the collective risk could be important or in any case not negligible; its significance for the total cancer incidence must then be considered (see also Section 7.5.2).

The Cancer Committee here uses the term 'cancer prevention' as a comprehensive concept both for reduction of individual risks—irrespective of the number of individuals concerned—and, where applicable, for reduction of collective risks and of effects on the total numerical cancer incidence.

The main part of the Committee's investigation has been aimed at a survey of large causal areas, which have widespread factors which could conceivably be of considerable quantitative importance to cancer incidence as a whole. In many cases the specific factors are not yet known and proposals within the strategy might be to recommend research. One major aim in the strategy should be to reduce the total figures for cancer incidence where these causal areas become the target.

The other major approach is to consider risk factors from the individual's point of view. Unacceptable individual risks should be identified and dealt with adequately. This applies mainly to specific causal factors, for example a particular chemical substance. One target in such a strategy will therefore be the various societal 'mechanisms' such as the areas of responsibility and organization of official agencies, and also the particular methods of achieving this aim of risk reduction.

The immediate problems are those concerning present populations and their disease development and health risks. However, the possibility of damage to future generations must also be considered. Such damage could arise through different exposures of today's parent generation (including possible effects on the fetus via exposure of the mother); data allowing an estimate of the magnitude of such effects are not yet available. To try to limit delayed exposures to persistent carcinogenic chemical substances or such exposures from emissions or from radioactive waste with substances of long half-life must also be part of the strategy.

7.3 A special strategy for cancer only?

Should or can the risk of cancer induction be isolated from other risks? Should or can societal mechanisms and resources for cancer prevention be separated from what is needed to counteract other types of health risk? What are general features in the promotion of good health and in the prevention of health and environmental risks, and what are specific to cancer prevention?

Cancer diseases form one part of the population's overall disease pattern, and measures to prevent cancer must be seen in this larger picture, to avoid introducing risks of other health damage from cancer-preventive measures.

Cancer-causing factors, or factors suspected of increasing the risk of development of such a disease, at the same time often entail other health risks. Many conditions of life generate ill health and cancer diseases can be caused by phenomena touching several sectors of society.

Conceivable practical forms of health-promoting action, of risk management, of developing new knowledge, as well as demands on decision mechanisms and resources usually imply that an integrated approach is necessary. With respect to measures aiming at cancer prevention, the strategic principle therefore ought to be to *start* from broadly aimed functions, such as the existing general policy, known plans, current activities, existing organizations, and laws and regulations already in force, and try to determine how well these will also contribute to cancer prevention. When applicable, one should then *supplement* these means with what is specifically needed in order to prevent cancer to a greater extent or in a better way than before.

The comprehensive type of analysis indicated above has not been undertaken in this report. In discussing prevention of cancer diseases, the Cancer Committee has in principle taken as its starting point the cancer risks, and identified or recommended a number of desirable measures, some of which form part of a larger structure or fit in with aims broader than pure cancer prevention. Much of what concerns policy issues in such a discussion tends to be of a universal nature and also touches upon general principles within society about people's rights and obligations. The more limited objectives and ambitions of the Committee to concentrate on cancer prevention mean that descriptions and analytical reasoning within more general areas, such as the demands on statutory risk control of physical and chemical agents, will of necessity be rather superficial.

7.4 Components of the strategy

7.4.1 Extent—general viewpoints

Major components

A conclusion of the picture of current knowledge that has emerged in previous parts of this report is that the cancer-prevention strategy should encompass both *known risks* or risk areas and *unknown or insufficiently known risks*. It involves both specific measures directly or indirectly aiming at cancer prevention and continued accretions to our general understanding of the disease and other relevant knowledge. The feedback of information about effects of measures taken on the disease pattern or on other observable clinical parameters is also important. The relations between certain elements according to Figure 7.1 (see also Figure 7.3) also indicate a continuous process, with increasing knowledge which in its turn should influence the real preventive measures. The *time perspective* is therefore part of the strategy, with planning and realization of definable measures in the short-term perspective and, in the longer term, a readiness for action in the face of different conceivable situations, and especially new knowledge.

Cancer: causes and prevention

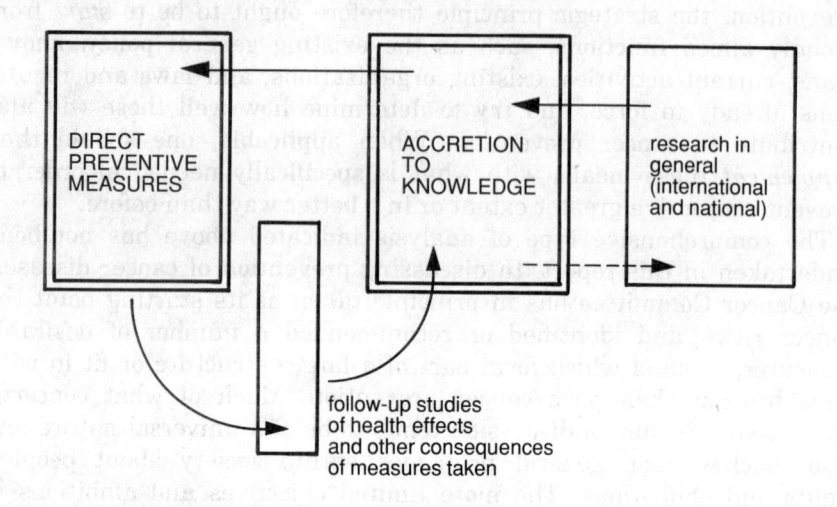

Figure 7.1 The extent of the strategy—some major components.

Adding to the general knowledge base must be done through research at both the international and the national levels. Information systems for demographic studies and epidemiologic monitoring are important in the study of cancer diseases and are discussed in Chapter 8. Research into cancer and measures to prevent it are dealt with in Chapter 15. Special research projects to clarify risks or to follow up measures taken are mentioned in some other contexts later, for example in Chapter 10.

Follow-up studies of various effects as indicated in Figure 7.1 are of particular importance if the measures imply radical changes. Apart from illuminating, as far as possible, to what extent the desired effects have been achieved, such studies should also aim at monitoring undesired side-effects and at otherwise increasing knowledge, so as to allow the programme of preventive measures to be made more effective.

Measures aiming at prevention can be seen either as direct or as indirect measures, as developed and exemplified below. However, the borderline between these two categories is not always distinct.

DIRECT MEASURES AIMING AT PREVENTION

Direct measures for disease prevention could be changes made by an individual concerning his own living habits or measures taken by an enterprise to reduce exposure to carcinogenic agents, for example through substitution for such substances in products, through choice of different process techniques or introduction of better emission control. Measures intended to lead to changed behaviour by another party can also be included in the group of measures directly aiming at prevention. Various forms of health education, as discussed in Chapter 9, are thus one part of the direct measures. Another part is the statutory control of health and environmental risks from chemical and physical agents (Chapter 11), by which a responsible authority could inform those concerned about a certain risk or regulate the exposure through bans or other restrictions. One might thus say that certain implementations of the law, rather than the law itself—unless it is very detailed, which is unusual in this context under Swedish conditions—mean direct disease-preventive measures through risk reduction.

INDIRECT MEASURES
A number of very different factors or circumstances are prerequisites for, or could otherwise influence, taking effective direct measures of cancer prevention. Improvements in this field could thus be called indirect measures for better prevention.

Some such factors are identified below, all of which also need to be seen in a wider context than cancer prevention. In only a few cases have they been dealt with in more detail later in this report and certain improvements have been recommended. However, the Committee wants to make it clear that a long-term strategy of cancer prevention must include close surveillance of all these factors and their development with regard to the aims of this strategy.

Institutional and *organizational circumstances* at different levels should thus, for example, be considered. Discussions will follow in Chapter 11 on relations between certain central government agencies and in Chapter 16 on the possibilities for the government, through the ministers concerned, to be kept informed of scientific progress as well as new needs and continuing work on disease prevention. In Chapter 15 the organization of research is touched upon. The *resources available* to the responsible authorities and other organizations are obviously of great importance to their activities, but so is the quality of work, which is influenced by the staff's competence and the recruiting policy, internal work routines and planning, and so on.

Public opinion and the moulders of opinion have an influence on the knowledge and values of members of the general public and of decision-makers, and so affect their behaviour and the measures they will take. Public opinion could facilitate or—from the point of view of risks—render a proper resource allocation more difficult, it could influence the results of health education, have an impact on the internal policy of businesses, and so on. Both the possibilities of an independent public opinion and the relations and mutual trust between different parties, in particular in the process of risk control, are strongly dependent on *information*, its availability and quality. The mass media in particular have here an important but difficult task of spreading correct and balanced information. This is elaborated on in Chapter 12.

In certain cases *economic incentives* for industry and individuals must be considered to be of great importance, for example how the economic responsibility of industry appears in such cases as rule breaking and/or having caused health damage. Here the Cancer Committee has limited itself to pointing out the significance of an economic incentive to the individual in connection with certain living habits (for example, raising the price of tobacco products to discourage consumption, in Section 10.1; pricing is also mentioned in connection with dietary habits in Section 10.2).

Laws with obligations, prohibitions and possible punitive sanctions remain important instruments in all risk management. Besides regulations that are direct measures taken to reduce a risk, for example from a specific carcinogenic agent, the significance of the general legislative basis in a country should be recognized. One might in this context want to look at a number of non-specific regulations both within and outside the sphere of laws with health-protective aims.

Certain phenomena associated with the application of legislation also deserve attention, since they can indirectly influence the efficiency of cancer prevention. They include, for example, the *decision-making process* and how the parties concerned are able to participate in this process (through institutionalized procedures for obtaining comments on draft decisions or through other means; the matter of free access to information versus secrecy). *Decision principles* including a *risk philosophy* are very important according to the Committee, which has developed this theme further with regard to cancer risks (see Section 7.5 and Chapter 11 in particular). Another factor is the material on which a decision taken by a responsible authority rests (the *decision base*). How comprehensive is this in the sense that matters such as alternative measures, consequences and conflicting interests have been illuminated? The actual availability to the general public of relevant information from the decision base should also be specially considered by the decision-maker (see Chapter 11).

Strategy for whom?

There are *public bodies* with responsibility for disease-preventive measures and risk management at different levels in Sweden. The Swedish government and, when applicable, parliament should take decisions on overall matters of principle, point out the major direction of activities and establish the general targets. Several central control agencies (see Chapter 11) will then be responsible for the implementation of existing regulations, for information within their respective sectors, and for taking the initiative in certain cases to improve knowledge on specified problems or to amend the regulations. Regional and local supervisory agencies in risk management have their own defined areas of responsibility. The county councils have a responsibility for disease-preventive measures according to the Health Care Act (see Chapter 14). The strategies of the public bodies concerned with health promotion or risk management should also more specifically consider cancer prevention when applicable.

Commercial enterprises which produce goods or carry out activities that may influence other people's health positively or negatively should as far as possible also include cancer-preventive aspects in their business strategies. Swedish legislation in force is very clear about risk management placing a fundamental legal responsibility on the enterprises. However, prevailing attitudes within enterprises strongly influence the actual exercise of these responsibilities, for it is important to follow not only the letter of the law but also its spirit.

The components of the strategy as indicated previously also show that *individuals* are concerned not only as mere targets of activities directed towards them but in a more active way. Besides a person being able to govern his or her own life-style to a varying extent, he or she could try to influence decisions on rights and obligations in society and on resource allocations through political parties, trade unions and voluntary organizations in the health and environmental protection field. It is important here that the strategies developed by various organizations such as these should rest as far as possible on the same basis of knowledge as those of other parties participating in cancer prevention.

Individual scientists or groups of scientists and *research-financing institutions* are other vital parties, since the direction of their respective research strategies might lead to new knowledge that could make improved cancer prevention possible.

An important matter, which can influence the results of the work, is how different participants perceive their roles in risk management and in other health-promoting measures. However, this has not been dealt with by the Committee in detail beyond what is said in Chapter 12 about the role of information for interaction and mutual trust in the process of risk control (*see also* Söderbaum, 1984a)

7.4.2 Risk areas and quantitatively important causal factors

Considering cancer prevention with the view of forming a strategy, one could look at the risk areas described in Figure 7.2a and distinguish between people's living habits (irrespective of whether there is an exposure or not) and exposures (usually involuntary) to potential carcinogens, which the individual has little chance of avoiding.

Mainly involuntary exposures	Living habits including mainly voluntary exposures
Examples: occupational exposures, background radiation, food contaminants, environmental tobacco smoke	*Examples*: the use of tobacco and alcohol, inappropriate dietary habits, deficient sexual hygiene, careless sunbathing

This diagram does not reflect conditions of magnitude.

Figure 7.2a Types of cancer risk areas and causal factors

There is a mutual dependence between education, economy, social and cultural patterns and personal life-style, profession or employment. In cancer prevention, this association with the general conditions of life must be taken into consideration, in particular where changes in individual living habits are being considered.

Besides life-style and other environmental factors, genetic (hereditary) factors play a role in cancer risk. In extreme—but very rare—cases of family-linked cancer nearly all members of a family who have the critical set-up of genes are afflicted. As with many forms of cancer, including the most frequent ones, genetic inheritance modifies an individual's capability, for example to metabolize a procarcinogen to a chemically reactive final carcinogen, to repair DNA-damage or to mobilize the immune defence. This leads to a genetically caused variation in susceptibility to carcinogenic agents. On the basis of today's limited scientific knowledge, one cannot assess the importance of genetic factors or base any strategic deliberations on them. In the longer term, it may become possible to determine variations in susceptibility to different carcinogenic factors. This might in turn make possible individually directed preventive measures concerning various living habits, as a supplement to general measures.

The requirements and feasibility of direct preventive measures are obviously not the same in the two main categories in Figure 7.2a namely involuntary exposures and life-style. In the former case those taking the risk and those benefitting from the risk-creating activity are usually not the same. A cost–benefit or risk–benefit analysis—a concept which here should be used in a broad and not simply a monetary sense—can be complicated (see Section 7.5).

Certain living habits are easier to change than others. Just to provide available scientific information to those concerned about both risks and expected positive health effects connected with certain living habits is a minimum requirement, which can be placed on the responsible public bodies. A further step is health education proper, which is an active process of instruction, specially designed for the purpose and directly aimed at making target groups change their attitudes and behaviour. In this category are also measures which by other means make it harder for the individual to keep up a specific risk-creating behaviour. There is an ethical question here that requires continuous attention and debate, namely how much persuasion or outright compulsion one is entitled to use to make individuals change their health-damaging living habits, as long as these habits do not hurt anyone else.

Based on the estimates in Chapter 6 of the importance of different causal factors for cancer cases in Sweden, the Cancer Committee has, in Figure 7.2b, more closely defined the *risk areas and causal factors* which should be included in the strategy and where preventive measures or continued research or both are called for. For the estimated number of cases the reader is referred to Table 6.1 and the accompanying text. It can be seen that the predominant so-called environmental factors behind the total cancer disease pattern are those correlated to living habits.

Three major causal areas are tobacco smoking, dietary factors and other living habits, mainly sexual habits and fertility pattern. Ultra-violet-radiation through sunlight and intentional, intensive sun-bathing also contribute to the cancer incidence. Research must be directed towards clarifying the importance of different dietary factors in particular.

General air pollution, factors in the work environment, consumer products, radon in buildings and iatrogenic factors have so far probably contributed relatively little to the total cancer incidence; in certain cases however, the individual risk may have been high. Data are to a great extent lacking for a reliable assessment of the type and extent of involuntary exposures in Swedish society and hence also of their importance for future cancer incidence. There have certainly been improvements in recent years through a combination of better scientific understanding, improved statutory risk control and certain non-specific exposure restrictions (leading to a general reduction of exposures) both in the work environment and in the general environment. This does not preclude the possibility of new risks being introduced in the meantime or arising later; they should then if possible be counteracted at an early stage. For the future, the need remains for good systems for monitoring and control with regard to both cancer risks and other health risks, and research on early biological warning systems is therefore essential.

The matter of special *risk groups* should also be considered. In the context of total cancer incidence this has been partly illuminated already, through the identification of different risk areas or causal

Figure 7.2b Specified cancer risk areas/casual factors

Note: The three step scale of scope for improvement can only give a rough idea of realistic possibilities of cancer prevention. A component in most cases consists of greatly differing factors, some of which might be totally eliminated while others are maybe almost non-influenceable.

For quantitative importance, see section	COMPONENT	Scope for improvement	Comments
6.2	tobacco smoking: smokers' own tobacco use	xxx	Ought practically to cease in the long-term perspective. Further, see section 10.1
6.2	environmental tobacco smoke	xxx	It should be feasible to rapidly achieve more reductions of involuntary exposure. Further, see section 10.1 (and 10.5)
6.3	use of alcohol	xx	Present societal alcohol policy aims at a reduction but not elimination of the use of alcohol. Further, see section 10.2
6.3	excess and deficiency of different dietary components; food preparation habits, methods of preservation and other factors such as food contaminants	xx	Dietary habits can be modified. The feasibilities greatly vary of influencing such dietary factors as imply an involuntary exposure. Further, see section 10.2 and chapter 11
6.4	sexual habits and fertility pattern	x	Here, especially sexual hygiene can be improved
6.5	infections, inflammations, etc.	x	Difficult to influence more at present (except sexual hygiene, cf. above). Further research might lead to the identification of risk groups
6.6	general air pollution	xx	Mainly urban areas are concerned. The composition and extent of pollutants present in ambient air can be improved for example, through measures concerning traffic emissions and heating of dwellings. Certain specific pollutants may, in a long or short-term perspective, be totally eliminated – if and when their risks have been illuminated adequately. Further, see section 10.3 (and 10.5) as well as chapter 11

For quantitative importance, see section	COMPONENT	Scope for improvement	Comments
6.7	factors in the working environment	xx	Exposure to specific agents can, in a long or short-term perspective, often be totally eliminated – if and when their risks have been illuminated adequately. Further, see chapter 11
6.8	consumer articles	xx	Exposure to specific agents can, in a long or short-term perspective, often be totally eliminated – if and when their risks have been illuminated adequately. Further, see chapter 11
6.9	ionizing radiation: background radiation	–	The background radiation is unavoidable
	radon in dwelling units	xx	Radon concentrations in dwelling units can be reduced but not totally eliminated. Further, see section 10.4
	other	x	Applies mainly to trans-frontier pollution. Swedish emissions from energy production could in principle be reduced
6.9	UV-radiation	xx	Excessive sunbathing can be reduced
6.10	iatrogenic factors incl. radiation	x	Medical diagnosis and treatment is based on risk-benefit evaluation for the individual. Iatrogenically increased cancer risks can never be totally eliminated.

(The graph is not meant to reflect conditions of magnitude.)

factors and their likely quantitative importance. In an overall strategy for cancer prevention one ought to take the risk areas as a starting point and then, within each such area, attempt to find, on the basis of continuous surveys of actual living habits and exposures, those special groups towards whom preventive measures should be directed. One cannot take for granted that the composition of risk groups is constant. Certain cancer diseases are linked to the reproductive functions and therefore afflict mainly or exclusively one sex, such as cancer of the prostate in men and cancer of the breast in women. Apart from this there is nothing indicating that living conditions in general in Sweden show differences between men and women that could be a starting point for general cancer-preventive measures. Within limited risk areas, however, differences might now and then appear. As mentioned earlier, there have, for example, been considerable variations over time in smoking habits between men and women. Occupational exposures to carcinogenic agents can also vary (see Section 6.7). It is important to locate individuals or small groups with high individual risks. Living habits and/or conditions of exposure for these people probably differ greatly from the average.

7.5 Special policy issues

7.5.1 Importance of a risk policy

All human life and activity is connected with risks one way or the other. Certain risks can be reduced or totally eliminated; others must be lived with. As has been stressed earlier, this also holds true for cancer risks. The fact that a person falls ill with cancer is the result of a number of events, none of which on its own could cause a cancer disease, but which together and under suitable genetic circumstances lead to a cancer disease. In this multi-stage process in the body at least some step is a random ('stochastic') event. Here the risk is the mean probability that an individual will develop a certain disease. Risk in the context of cancer prevention is always a projection into the future, in contrast to cancer risk as it is measured, retrospectively, by way of incidence or mortality numbers.

Cancer risks ought both to be judged as such and to be seen in a wider context. The latter is of special weight since many decisions actually are a *choice between different risks,* a fact to which attention is not always paid.

Each decision to take or to abstain from taking a direct measure aiming at cancer prevention always implies some sort of risk evaluation, explicitly or implicitly. It is particularly important that those public bodies responsible for different sectors, where their decisions affect other people, form and openly state a policy for risk evaluation and risk control, as an integrated part of the overall strategy which they will apply to their activities within the framework of current legislation.

The mere construction of a policy statement means (a) that those processes that take place within an organization before and during decision making become visible and easier to keep apart, (b) that current practices must be summarized, analysed and if necessary reconsidered. The latter also means that all difficult major questions which may appear in individual cases must be discussed in a generalized way at one and the same time and that judgements of principle must be made with as wide a scope as possible.

Naturally, an articulated risk policy does not exclude decisions on a case-by-case basis, which is prescribed for many areas in current Swedish legislation. The handling of individual cases ought rather to be considerably facilitated, and special care will automatically be given to preparing the information base for decisions where there are indications of the need to deviate from the general policy.

A risk policy cannot be static. It should be continuously reviewed and revised as new knowledge, changes of values or other circumstances make it desirable. A risk policy should also be developed in close contact with all the various parties concerned. An open debate on policy matters should be one of the means of gaining an increased understanding and acceptance by large parts of the general public of risk reasonings, and a wider insight into possibilities and limitations where risk management and disease prevention is concerned.

With the exception of radiation protection, approaches towards an explicit risk policy within the cancer sphere seem so far to have been fairly limited in Sweden. Very likely, one main reason for this is the often doubtful scientific basis for identifying risk factors and the difficulties of quantifying the degree of risk to human beings at different exposure levels or doses. To a great extent, one seems still to have to rely on rather crude principles for a risk policy. As knowledge about the induction and causes of cancer diseases grows, it will become possible to refine this policy.

At the same time, an intensified policy discussion may help to lead to scientific break-throughs, by addressing relevant questions to the scientific community and by allocating resources to specific scientific fields.

In addition to this, it is essential to press for improvement and use of other components of the risk management process than the medical/ scientific ones, such as cost–benefit analyses (in a broad meaning of this concept), as described in Section 7.5.2.

It is natural that a risk policy should grow from the diverse experience of the different central agencies and other bodies concerned. In a long-term perspective, the target should be a consistent approach to comparable matters such as evaluations of scientific material as a basis for risk estimates and how risk contributions from different sources should be regarded. This does not necessarily mean that a harmonization of direct control measures over all sectors is possible or even desirable.

7.5.2 Components of a risk policy

Discussion based on a model for risk management

There are nowadays several models in the international literature illustrating risk analyses (or risk assessments) of various kinds and the entire 'risk management' process. Often used is O'Riordan's model (Figure 7.3). This model refers to control of environmental factors such as physical and chemical agents against which man (or the environment) should be protected. It may also be usable to illustrate the process of assessing living habits and their importance as cancer risk factors, although the risk evaluation and direct risk control measures in such cases should also take matters such as personal freedom into consideration.

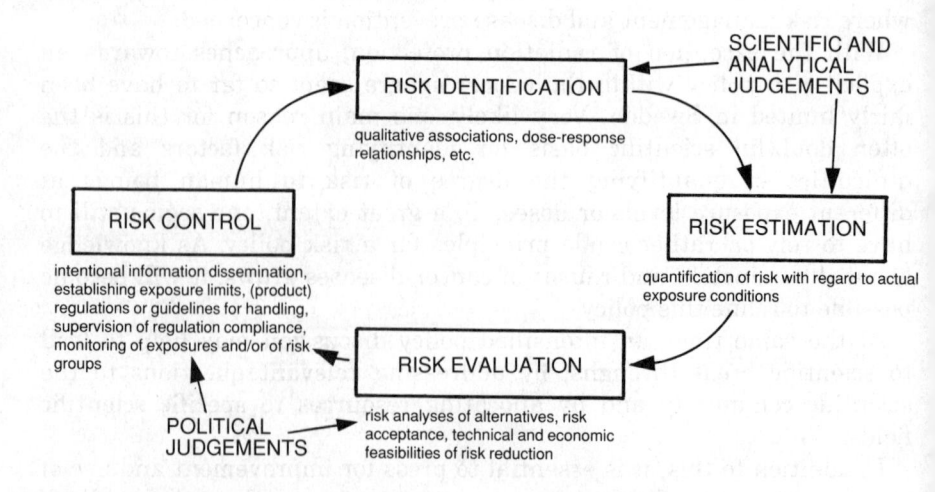

Figure 7.3 Environmental risk management functions with regard to cancer risks. Based on O'Riordan (1979).

It is essential to make a clear distinction between scientific judgements on the one side and social and political judgements on the other (Figure 7.3). Scientific data are still often incomplete and seldom give clear-cut answers about the size of cancer risks or even about causal correlations. Scientific judgements ought not to attempt to take into account administrative principles or what may be legally, economically or in other respects feasible by way of limiting risks. Such considerations enter into the next phase, the risk evaluation, which is very closely related to the question of choice of specific risk control measures. However, scientific judgement as a function in risk management should provide a basis—in an administrative context—for decisions to act or not to act at a certain point with regard to risk reduction or other health-promoting measures. The demands on those experts who participate in the risk-management process to take a position ('on the best scientific grounds') must therefore be stringent even though the scientific material is often inadequate.

Medical and scientific contributions to risk assessment are also needed to assess correctly the uncertainty of the size of an identified risk or of an unconfirmed but probable risk. Scientific principles must be applied to matters in the risk evaluation phase; for example, the clarification of risk perception and risk acceptance often requires contributions from psychologists and other scientists as considered below. The cost–benefit analysis, which is very much a matter of a systems analysis approach, also requires scientific input.

Direct control measures to protect human health are usually required long before all questions about the carcinogenicity of a certain factor have been completely answered. It is part of the scientific and analytical judgements in the processes of risk identification and risk estimation to review critically the value of available data from a scientific point of view. The next phase, the risk evaluation, then includes the question of how much proof is necessary to justify taking action in a particular situation.

At the request of the Cancer Committee, an extensive expert document has been produced (Nilsson and Ehrenberg, 1984), dealing in more detail with the scientific interpretation and use of different types of data in risk assessments, including statistical aspects. Among other things, such a document can provide certain guidance both for the layman and for the specialist outside his own discipline. With regard to its primary task of presenting a major cancer prevention strategy, the Committee has found it to be sufficient, in this context, to point out a few factors only.

Human epidemiological studies are really the only means of providing complete 'proof' of human carcinogenicity. *Animal carcinogens* (in tests according to good scientific practice) must also be considered, although such agents do not necessarily represent an increased carcinogenic risk when man is exposed. It will in many cases never be feasible to decide by epidemiological methods whether, and if so to what extent, an animal carcinogen presents a risk to man at realistic doses. The most common models for animal tests, as in international standards for the introduction of new chemicals, imply tests of substances one by one and are in principle based on the idea that the substance tested functions as a so-called complete carcinogen at the high doses usually applied in the test. Should this not be the case, as with factors which (in the animals) would give an increased cancer risk only through, for example, a promotive mechanism or a modifying (co-carcinogen) mechanism, it is not certain that those risk properties will also show up as an effect in the common tests. Nor are there any other general or standardized methods to identify such risk factors.

Certain short-term tests of *mutagenic activity* (and/or transformation or damage of the genetic material) have shown a good or relatively good correlation with carcinogenic activity in *qualitative* terms. A well-chosen battery of short-term tests (such as the Ames test) could therefore, if positive, indicate that the agent tested would also show carcinogenesis in animal tests, and would, in addition, give an indication of a possible mechanism of action. Short-term tests are mainly used as supplementary information when other data are insufficient.

In an ideal case, the scientific judgement will result in a quantification of risk at actual exposure levels for human populations and/or exposed individuals, expressed in a way suitable for comparisons between different risk areas, for example n cancer cases in 100 000 person–years (i.e. a risk of $n \times 10^{-5}$).

Where radiation protection is concerned, there is an internationally accepted scientific practice on the use of risk coefficients for different types of ionizing radiation (though not for radon alpha radiation) when quantifying risks (see Section 4.5). These risk coefficients are based on epidemiological data. The risk coefficient implies more than one concept that differs from traditional toxicological thinking. Thus there is a need to express doses of different types of ionizing radiation in the same unit which allows for the biological effectiveness. The dose contributions or risk contributions are treated as additive with regard, for example, to the cancer-initiating effect of radiation. This also applies to addition of contributions over time; one speaks about dose commitment and risk commitment respectively. Assuming dose-response relationships to be linear, collective doses can be calculated by multiplying the average individual dose by the size of the affected population, and from a collective dose—for instance related to a particular source—the corresponding collective risk is obtained through multiplying by the risk coefficient. A source-related collective risk may be expressed as the expected number of cancer deaths. In the case of widely spread risk factors, for instance a cancer initiator in food-stuffs, the large size of the population concerned could lead to a considerable collective risk even when the individual risk is considered negligibly low. In radiation protection there is likewise an internationally accepted policy for risk evaluation. The difficulties are much greater for other agents or living conditions which may be associated with increased cancer risks. Only in rare cases do we have human data with a dose–response relationship which makes a satisfactory risk quantification possible.

Risk evaluation is also complicated because the concept of risk has essentially qualitative aspects. Individual persons *perceive risks differently*, even when the statistical magnitude of the risks is exactly the same. Interesting insights into risk perception have begun to appear in recent years.

People tend to consider a generally occurring risk as lower than it actually is and, therefore, less necessary to counteract. On the other hand we easily overestimate a rare risk which, objectively seen, may be smaller. Natural risks (earthquakes, background radiation, etc.) are in principle regarded as inescapable and the risk levels thus as acceptable. Cancer diseases are not self-evidently a natural risk in the sense that they cannot at least to some extent be prevented. We tend to underestimate a risk that is far away in time and geography even if it is great, but we react strongly to a risk close at hand even if it is small, in general. We also regard a voluntary risk as being less necessary to counteract than an involuntary risk. It is considered unethical deliberately to expose others to a risk, particularly if the consequences are serious. With regard to matters concerning us personally we also weigh risk against benefit more or less consciously, even if both variables are extremely difficult to quantify. The methods and theories for systematic risk–benefit evaluation generally have very great in-built uncertainties.

A rank ordering of regulatory actions will depend on, among other things, how one measures the value of cost and benefit, risks to be seen as one of the cost components in this context. There exists no obvious system for such a rank ordering. Several non-comparable determinations play a role here. Risks that are more or less forced on people have to be balanced against the benefits, but sometimes one group bears the risk and another receives the benefits. Risks connected with one type of job should be seen in the context of possible risks connected with alternative employment. Decisions also tend to include more judgements on the concept of 'quality of life'.

An example where the balance between different risk-reducing measures cannot simply be referred to relations between cost and effect, even within closely related areas, is the regulation of road traffic as compared to the safety levels for prevention of air traffic accidents. One could say that, in Sweden, society accepts about 700 deaths per year from road accidents, but would not tolerate such high mortality in air traffic accidents. This example also illustrates differences of risk perception between a voluntary and an involuntary risk and emphasizes that risks involving many victims at the same time are perceived as being more serious than ones with the same number spread over a long period of time. As regards cancer, there are seldom large clusters of cases. Society has also—at least so far—accepted the several thousand cancer deaths per year resulting from tobacco smoking but would never accept fatal accidents in the working environment even remotely to the same extent (*all* occupationally caused accidental deaths in Sweden nowadays amount to about 100 cases per annum).

In spite of the difficulties mentioned here, it is important to retain the idea of cost–benefit analysis (maybe under some other suitable name) as an all-embracing concept of a process, where monetary and non-monetary values should be defined and presented in such a way as to enable decision-makers to see *where* the conflicts lie.

The traditional cost–benefit analysis where all factors are given a monetary value entails arbitrary judgements of, for example, the value of an increased average life-span in different age groups. A more common approach is cost-effectiveness analysis where the cost in monetary terms of measures taken (and possibly of other so-called sacrifices) is weighed against an effect as such (expressed as, for example, an increased average life-span or, somewhat misleadingly, as 'the number of human lives saved'). This type of analysis may have a certain value in cases where the expected effect can be quantified or—in retrospect—when comparing costs of actual effects. However, as already mentioned, this ought not to be the only part of a cost–benefit analysis in this context. A number of methods have been suggested for structuring—at the societal level—the information needed for decisions in risk management. They may be classified according to degree of aggregation or disaggregation (keeping apart) of effects with respect to type, time periods and affected individuals or other interested parties (Söderbaum, 1984b). According to the Committee one should, as a major principle, strive for a disaggregation of the information (with extreme aggregation or 'reduction', information losses will appear).

The scope for cancer prevention is too heterogeneous to render it possible—with reasonable resource inputs—to produce a comprehensive, experience-related basis for further and more advanced discussions on the two last steps in risk management, namely risk evaluations and direct control measures. However, as a supplementary background to the recommendations given later in this report, some case studies have been made.

Four of these studies (Westermark, 1984b) refer to industrial activities with ethylene oxide, vinyl chloride, arsenic, and polycyclic aromatic hydrocarbon emissions in aluminium production respectively. The number of studies is too small for wide-ranging conclusions to be reached with regard to a risk-management strategy. There are also great differences between the cases. However, the author was able to draw certain general conclusions, such as the existence of a fairly good, and improving, knowledge of the health effects of industrial activities and a willingness to discuss and to take measures to reduce risks—as part of the 'power-play' between the parties concerned, such as the company management, trade union(s), authorities, scientists and media. Further, he has found a widely spread acknowledgement of the need for quantitative measurements describing human exposure to hazardous agents and, importantly, an ambition to reduce the probability of new cancer cases as a result of a given activity to no more than the occasional case. The 'economy of actions taken' has also been addressed in these studies, including a cost–effectiveness analysis; this will be referred to later in this chapter.

A fifth case study (Ericsson, 1984) is of a different type and attempts to illustrate the possibilities and economics of substituting other products for asbestos for certain uses. This turned out to be difficult because of a lack of good data. For some uses, however, substitution meant little or no remaining cost increase or even an economic advantage. Repair or demolition of buildings containing asbestos, used, for example, as insulation in boiler-rooms or for fire protection, remains a special problem both from a practical and an economic point of view.

In the next section, the established radiation protection philosophy (which to a major extent concerns cancer risks specifically) will be mentioned and comparison will be made with other cancer risk factors, in particular chemical substances in the environment. However, for the known major causal factors of present cancer incidence that are connected with our living habits, good models and comparisons are lacking with respect to risk evaluation and control measures.

Discussion based on the principles for radiation protection

The International Commission on Radiological Protection (ICRP) has presented three major guiding principles for protective work. These may be summarized as follows:

(1) All activities leading to exposure to ionizing radiation must be justifiable, with benefits greater than the drawbacks.
(2) No individual shall be exposed to unacceptably high risks.
(3) All risks shall (besides principle (2)) be reduced through protective

measures as far as possible with regard to social consequences and costs: the so-called ALARA principle ('as low as reasonably achievable').

Principle (2) reflects the demands of individual-related protection and may lead to the competent authorities establishing general *limits of exposure* if the risk sources are new, and to the setting of levels where protective measures are to be taken, if the sources already exist. Principles (1) and (3) are directly source related.

Ehrenberg, (1984b) and Lindell (1984) have provided more details as well as discussions on the radiation protection model from a wider perspective.

The ICRP has made certain recommendations about exposure limits both for people employed in radiological work and for individual members of the public (though excluding medical diagnoses and treatment). Through comparisons with certain other professions regarded as having a high safety standard, with a yearly risk of accidental death of less than 10^{-4}, the ICRP has drawn the conclusion that this is usually perceived as acceptable and thus applicable also to radiation workers, unless the risk cannot be further reduced through use of the ALARA principle. Through a comparison with generally accepted risks in daily life, the Commission has similarly concluded that risks of the magnitude of 10^{-6}–10^{-5} per annum would probably be acceptable to individual members of the public. When establishing the recommended exposure dose limits that correspond to these risks, one assumes a linear dose–response relationship for stochastic effects. It should be stressed, however, that one reaches these 'acceptable' levels of risk through a combination of the ALARA principle with the use of the recommended dose limits.

The ALARA principle is of particular interest and is beginning to be discussed outside the sphere of radiation protection. It should not be mistaken for a somewhat related principle which one sometimes has to apply in the implementation of other legislation on health and environmental protection, namely to ignore principles (1) and (2) above and try directly to reduce a risk or an environmental disturbance without first quantifying this risk and establishing acceptable risk levels.

The question has been raised as to just how far one should pursue radiation protection. Is it reasonable to protect individuals over and above what the recommended exposure limit implies? Is it meaningful to supplement the individual-related protection with a source-related protection? Within the radiation protection sphere it has been agreed that this is the case. A well-defined risk source for ionizing radiation with an expected average of eight deaths per annum means an individual yearly death risk of 10^{-6} in Sweden, usually a negligible risk from the individual's point of view. If, on the other hand, even these eight cases can be eliminated by means of a 'reasonable contribution', most people would probably support this. This judgement on what is reasonable must then include a number of both monetary and non-monetary components in the cost–benefit analysis, as suggested earlier. Within radiation protection in the industrialized countries one counts on a 'willingness to pay' of the order of US$20 000 per man-sievert for radiation dose reduction, which roughly corresponds to US$1 million per premature death avoidable through such a dose decrease.

It ought to be stressed that the sum mentioned of US$1 million per case has not resulted from any ethical values but is a figure that has emerged from studying actual measures taken. In fact society is often willing to spend very large sums for saving identifiable human lives. The limited resources in society, instead, set a limit to more generally formulated ambitions of protection.

In the case studies mentioned above, undertaken as a background for the work of the Cancer Committee, the costs of measures taken turned out to be of the order of magnitude of US$2 million 'per life saved' according to the calculation method used—in as far as the protective effect from the measures taken was considered reasonably quantifiable. A mitigating factor is that a change of industrial processes or substitutes of materials in products sometimes influences the economics of a business in a positive way, for example in the case of asbestos mentioned earlier.

The costs of measures for cancer prevention obviously cannot be generalized since the types of measure are very different. As regards the large risk areas connected with life-style, for example, even a considerable increase in concentrated health education efforts would mean relatively small costs per case where a cancer disease can be avoided or postponed.

With respect to comparable, controllable risks in the environment (primarily ionizing radiation and chemical substances with stochastic effects), efforts should be made to devise consistent principles of safety and protection—unless the risk perception in certain cases does not appear to be essentially different. In principle, total individual as well as total collective risks of cancer ought to be estimated and limited rather than risks from individual components in the risk array. Radiation protection has taken one step in that direction through source-related assessments. With regard to several other risk areas, such a conceivable idea for the future would require new or in any case supplementary legislation and totally different administrative routines and ways of thinking.

However, the great differences existing between radiation protection and control of chemical cancer risks must be stressed with regard to present scientific knowledge and to practicalities. As concerns chemical factors, one is still far from being able to make total risk estimates through the addition of all conceivable risk contributions. The sources are to a large extent unknown and risk quantification is difficult even for known sources. Under these circumstances one will have to work for the foreseeable future using the principles underlying the present legislation and with the use of other methods, mainly through rank-ordering of measures, try to optimize the employment of available resources.

The multifactorial origin of the cancer diseases should also be borne in mind. An acceptance of this principle implies rejection of the principle of 'one cause—one disease'. It means that measures could be directed against either one or other of several interacting causal factors in order for the same effect to be achieved. Here, too, scientific knowledge is fragmentary. To a large extent it is not known how different factors interact, which factors may be unspecific promoters, and so on. It is generally not possible to make any particularly sophisticated assessments, and measures ought, therefore, to be deployed on all fronts against factors entailing an increased cancer risk irrespective of whether these are initiators, promoters or co-carcinogens.

Although all evidence suggests that cancer diseases are multifactorial in nature, it has, nevertheless, been normal to regulate the exposure to specific factors one by one, in parallel with more general measures against exposure. This is true internationally and for factors like ionizing radiation, individual chemicals in the work environment and food additives. There is no reason to change this state of affairs; on the contrary, given today's knowledge, it is probably the most effective way of reducing risks. This statement also includes allowance for the fact that measures against possible cancer risks are often the same as or integrated in measures with wider aims in the protection of human health and the environment.

A couple more aspects on the matter of optimizing resources in risk management should be pointed out.

Where dose–response data are available for a cancer risk in man, one could theoretically calculate the expected risk at a low exposure through extrapolation from an observed risk related to a high exposure. As a basis for regulating sources not only of ionizing radiation but also of chemical substances, one should use the theory of a *linear dose-response relationship* (in the low dose area) unless available data clearly indicate the existence of a 'threshold dose' for effect. A linear dose-response relationship means that no exposure level or dose is a 'safe' risk level. This does not preclude that a dose, at least in theory, may be so low that one cannot demonstrate an excess cancer frequency as compared to a control group. The assumption of a linear dose–

response relationship ought to be used also to determine whether a certain factor lacks quantitative importance from the point of view of risk at actually occurring exposures.

In practice, a regulation of cancer initiators according to a linear model is a pragmatic way of acting against exposures, where such factors as analytical techniques, economic and technological criteria will be decisive. The question of linearity in the low-dose area also has an ethical and a health-policy aspect. To work according to the philosophy of the linear model as regards measures of risk control thus in all circumstances, leads to a factual reduction of the cancer risks (Rall, 1978). Were regulatory measures instead to be based on the assumption that a threshold really exists for effect, fewer short-term economic losses will appear. This latter way of working might on the other hand lead to a result where no cancer prevention at all is achieved—if the dose–response relationship for initiators is indeed linear in the low dose area.

Carcinogenic factors vary considerably in strength, which combined with actual exposure determines the size of the risk. To tackle small as well as large cancer risks—without any system for the ordering of priorities—might mean a misallocation of resources where cancer preventive measures are not optimized.

A so-called *de minimis* principle, applied for instance by a regulatory agency, would mean no resources directed towards measures against the smallest risks (which thus, at least in a short-term perspective, would be considered acceptable) but a concentration of efforts on known or suspected risk factors entailing higher risks for individuals or populations. Correctly applied, such a principle ought to be combinable with the ALARA principle that even small risks should be further reduced towards zero when this is feasible without difficulty. It is not possible in this latter context to be absolutely consistent, something which also follows from the situation that many presently unknown cancer risks might be so small that they will not be found by current methods.

When an agent is qualitatively characterized as a carcinogen, the great difficulty, however, lies in assessing the carcinogenic potency, although the exposure analysis sometimes also offers problems in the risk estimation. In cases where there are only animal data, 'translation' to man is extremely difficult. The differences between species can be great; there are examples where these differences have amounted to several orders of magnitude. On the other hand, there are also data on a few chemical agents where one has a good correlation between results in animal tests and human data. Extrapolations of animal data to man are based on the idea that there is a greater probability of being right than wrong; this can be a practical policy in risk evaluation but is not science in a true sense, unless other available chemical and toxicological data clearly support such an extrapolation. With increasing understanding of species differences and with knowledge of target doses in DNA (for initiators), the uncertainties could be reduced. Another pragmatic but less far-reaching approach is to try to rank-order one's actions according to information on *relative carcinogenic potency*—in so far as comparable test data exist which allow potency expressed in similar units.

Attempts at graduating risks might on the other hand lead to suboptimization if they are not properly applied. Thus lack of possibilities to counteract a risk factor within one area must not lead to other factors within the same or other risk areas being unregulated either, if such regulation is feasible. Even if society abstains from regulating tobacco smoking, it cannot abstain from regulating, for example, industrial emissions, when applicable.

It should be added here that there are also other ways of risk management and of rank-ordering of control measures, which mean an approach to the problems from technical–economic or purely administrative points of departure with, for example, surveys of different branches of industry and with as far-reaching preventive measures as are considered technically and administratively feasible at the points where risks prevail— without attempts at any ordering of these risks, in particular where the scientific basis of risk assessment is uncertain.

Within the work environment, the risk management policy has been expressed as two general principles with the aim of eliminating or minimizing exposure and thus minimizing the cancer risks as far as possible (here summarized from the relevant ILO convention (1974); this convention is binding for Sweden):

(a) All measures shall be taken to substitute non-carcinogenic substances or less hazardous substances for carcinogenic substances.
(b) The number of exposed persons shall be reduced as far as possible and the exposure level and exposure time shall be reduced to a minimum.

In a scientific discussion (ILO, 1977) on the problems mentioned, it is stated that 'from a practical point of view, exposure to an experimental carcinogen should be kept as close to zero as possible in the occupational environment, irrespective of dose level in the test system, animal species, tumour site, type or frequency'.

To sum up, the principle of minimizing exposure to chemical carcinogens should apply also within other areas of risk management than the working environment—taking into consideration possibilities for the grading of risks and for establishing threshold doses in certain cases for substances which do not bind to DNA.

8
Information systems relating to cancer and cancer risks

8.1 Different information systems and their utilization

8.1.1 Published literature

Every year about 50 000 scientific papers are published concerning cancer, as well as many from closely related fields. Active collection and utilization of the literature and literature data-bases is necessary to follow this mass of results. This is facilitated by the fact that a number of international abstract journals and data-bases are available. Several cancer research organizations also contribute by condensing and reviewing results from different specialist areas.

A problem is that the results of many investigations carried out by national bodies do not get published. This is frequently the case as regards chemical analysis data from the environment or from products on the market, social conditions and living habits as well as investigations with regard to occupational hygiene.

Of great importance are national and international contacts between research workers and government agencies, for example, through conferences and congresses of different kinds. A number of cancer research organizations and scientific societies play an important role here, in particular the International Agency for Research on Cancer (IARC) and the International Union against Cancer (Union Internationale Centre le Cancer, UICC).

8.1.2 Population-based information systems

One part of the work on the prevention of cancer diseases is the study of the pattern of different cancer types in the population. As the causes of cancer diseases are to a great extent unknown, the work must be focused on identifying risk groups and clarifying their environment and living conditions.

Several decades may pass between a certain exposure and the appearance of a cancer disease and retrospective investigations about conditions long ago are often difficult and unreliable. Therefore, prospective investigations are necessary where one can follow the health and exposure of the individuals in certain groups over decades. This needs systematic efforts to improve the quality and acquisition of data.

Other prerequisites for epidemiological monitoring and research will be dealt with later in this chapter, as well as questions concerning international co-operation on population-based studies.

8.2 Prerequisites for population-based studies

8.2.1 General remarks about registers ('files')

Methods for epidemiological research

In order to collect knowledge about the occurrence, causes and effects of a disease in a population, information systems containing data about the diseased persons as well as other individuals in the population are needed.

In most countries, *causes of death* have been recorded for a long time and this has been of great value for the study of cancer diseases. These registers indicate the cases where a cancer disease is the actual cause of death. For this reason many countries over the last few decades have introduced *cancer registers*, that is *incidence registers* based on reports of all new cases of cancer. In some countries the registers have been limited to certain geographical areas (e.g. USA, Japan, West Germany and Poland) while in others, for example the Nordic countries, cover all cases. Countries with cause-of-death and cancer registers usually publish annual statistical reports, while summaries from the registers of the different countries are published at longer intervals through international organizations (WHO (World Health Organization), IARC, UICC).

Through these registers, and with access to demographic data, the mortality and incidence of different cancer diseases can be studied in different age groups, time periods and geographical areas. Differences between regions can sometimes give clues as to causes. Such clues can also be detected through a combination of information from registers on causes of death and on new cancer cases with other types of data recorded for the same individuals. One example of this is the Swedish Cancer–Environment Registry (see Chapter 5), where the Cancer Registry data have been supplemented with information about, for example, occupation from a population census some years ago.

Another way of getting clues about aetiology is to study correlations between cancer incidence, cancer mortality and some average environmental data in different populations (e.g. dietary habits, smoking, alcohol consumption). Some different aspects of using disease and cause-of-death information from registers and data bases were discussed in Chapter 5.

More detailed knowledge about the nature of the risk factors can be obtained though analytical epidemiological investigations where an attempt is made to define the individual's relationship to the suspected risk factors. These analytical studies are usually of two kinds, namely cohort studies and case-control studies. In a *cohort study* a group of individuals with a defined exposure is followed. Within the group the number of cases of the disease (or other biological changes) one wants to study is recorded and compared with what is found in a corresponding group of non-exposed persons. In *case-control studies* one starts with a number of cases of the disease and maps suspected causal factors for both this group and the control group which does not have the disease for an analysis of differences between the groups. For analytical epidemiological studies, access to data of good quality is essential. The registers are needed in, for example, cohort studies in order to find persons with cancer diseases and persons who have died of a cancer disease, and to calculate the expected number of cases of cancer in the population. Registers are also of great value for case-control studies in order to select suitable cases.

Obviously such studies have limitations in trying to find and identify the causes of disease. They cannot produce anything more than correlations expressed in statistical terms. Other common aetiological factors of cancer disease, such as smoking, must be controlled in an investigation so that they do not become confounding. If, however, several epidemiological investigations point in the same direction, and especially if experimental data support these findings, it is often possible to clarify the real cause–effect relationships with acceptable scientific reliability.

Registers which include diagnosed diseases or other biological changes as well as causes of death can be called 'effect registers'. Existing registers that contain possible causal factors have rarely been established specifically with the aim of facilitating studies of the relationship between causes and effects. Such 'causal' data-base factors are usually indirect and they can be found in connection with ordinary demographic information, for example occupation, or they are factors that can be linked to whole populations, for example data characterizing different types of domicile. Moreover, exposure registers of physical and chemical agents are of great interest, although few such registers exist in Sweden. Registers with hard data are in principle available only for agents, of which the risks are already well known. As well as in epidemiological studies, information about exposure is necessary for estimating the risk in different populations from suspected hazardous agents in a risk management system (see Chapter 11).

Through studies of the population, there should also be a possibility of tracing the causal relationship between cancer and other diseases such as infectious diseases. Other patient related registers in the health care sector, besides the Cancer Registry, are thus of importance also for aetiological studies.

In order to study how hereditary factors influence the frequency of different diseases including cancer diseases, data about family relationships are necessary. In Sweden information about parents is recorded manually in church registers.[1] The so-called Medical Birth Register gives the relationship between child and mother. In the general Population Registers (held by each county administration), as well as in a central service register (SPAR), information about parents and children is linked but only until the children are 18 years old. The Swedish Twin Register, which started during the 1960s and is run by the National Institute of Environmental Medicine, is an important resource in studies of those questions where genetic factors can be kept partly under control. The observation time has until recently been too short to allow studies of tumour diseases but the Twin Register is now becoming adequate. It also offers a wider use in cancer epidemiological studies, especially because certain data are continuously being collected about the individual's personal living conditions and other environmental factors.

The usefulness of different register data is often determined by the possibility of linking different systems together. The linkages are sometimes difficult because the data are not directly compatible (e.g. definitions of terms may differ) and also the linkages are often planned and carried out long after the initial computer routines in the registers have been established. This means that specific transfer routines must be constructed. Linking usually means that a new register must be created. Whether such a register is then also kept as a special register and perhaps updated, like the Cancer–Environment Registry, will partly depend on the expected interest in using the register in the future. There is certainly a need for increased recording of environmental data which could easily be linked to various registers with medical information.

The different kinds of data in aetiological studies must be related to the same population or to the same individual through a personal numerical identification. Aetiological studies on an individual level usually mean that only a manual 'linkage' is possible as information about exposure is usually especially hard to find and very rarely recorded in computer systems. An interesting illustration of the problems but also of the possibilities of doing retrospective epidemiological studies, when the cause of the disease can be related to a specific type of exposure, is given in what is known as the Rönnskär study (Wall and Taube, 1983), which has been briefly outlined in Section 4.4.5. For cancer studies, where the time between exposure and disease is long, it is essential that the relevant information relating to exposure is preserved for decades.

Information systems for health care

National cause-of-death and cancer registers are the backbone of an information system about cancer. Information about the individuals in such registers must be restricted to a few variables. In order to allow more detailed and reliable registration of information concerning cancer diseases, the Swedish National Board of Health and Welfare recommended, as long ago as 1974 (see Chapter 14), regional cancer recording in connection with the now six regional hospital oncological centres. Using further data from local medical registers and registers of histopathological data, and through the collection of information in connection with treatment programmes for different cancer diseases and controlled clinical studies, more detailed data-bases on cancer emerge.

Since the early 1960s there has also been in Sweden manual registration of all visits in in-patient and out-patient care. In addition to this, most of the in-patient care is registered in data-bases, including the diagnoses.

Of special interest here is the development work carried out in the Stockholm County Council area to produce a computer-based information system for health and medical care covering the total population in the county. Administrative and medical information has been integrated in a system that has been built up through updating via terminals in the different ward units. The system also allows searching of all individual-based information through a terminal. The data-base covers *all* residents within the council area and is updated from the (general) Population Register so that it also holds information about the addresses of the individuals. The medical information has been collected since 1971 and contains details of in-patient care including diagnoses, operations, X-ray examinations, etc. For parts of the area, similar medical information related to out-patient visits is also registered.

A data-base of this type, containing demographic and medical data from both in-patient and out-patient care, facilitates, among other things, epidemiological studies and allows continuous follow-up of the different diseases.

Since 1984 it has been mandatory for all Swedish county councils to keep a patient data-base with information about state of health, diseases and treatment given. The content should be at least a minimal defined and agreed data set. The county councils have also been given a more direct responsibility for preventive measures, and need for that purpose, among other things, to analyse the relationships between environment and health.

A copy of the patient data-base minimum data set must be made available for a national data-base for the social sector, to be used for planning purposes. The information there excludes individual identification. This 'planning data-base' also includes information from other sources.

Descriptions of certain registers

As mentioned in Section 5.1.2, four registers are of special importance for cancer epidemiology work in Sweden. These are the present Cancer Registry, the Cause-of-Death Registry and the two registers resulting from combination of certain data, namely the Cancer–Environment Registry and the Mortality–Environment Registry. An overall description of the first three of these registers has been published (Swenson, 1984). The descriptions include details about the acquisition, the variables and the quality of the data. Corresponding information about demographic registers of various kinds is available from Statistics Sweden.

The Committee's assessments

Modern computer technology has increased the possibilities for building up efficient information systems useful for epidemiological studies. Sweden, like the other Nordic countries, has excellent possibilities in this field because of its social structure, the availability of good demographic data and the national personal identification system, a socialized health care system and very good facilities for collecting data about morbidity and mortality related to other valid information.

The Cancer Registry and the Cause-of-Death Registry are the key elements in an information system about cancer, and are described in more detail in Sections 8.2.2 and 8.2.3, respectively.

Patient data should be recorded in a uniform way, irrespective of where they are generated. The main responsibility here rests with the county councils, which should consider the requirements for comparing information. A certain co-ordination must be aimed at, not only for routine use but also for special investigations and in activities such as industrial health services. A uniform registration of certain patient information facilitates not only the retrieval of information on the patient's previous medical examinations and treatment, but also epidemiological investigations. Thus, for example, population cohorts with different living habits or exposures can more easily be followed for health effects in general as opposed to what has so far been the rule, namely, only studying a single, predefined effect.

From the epidemiological viewpoint, certain general population-related information ought to be readily available. From this point of view the present computer-based registers in Sweden function well. However, there are difficulties concerning obtaining peoples' previous addresses as well as information on parent–child relationships.

Information about addresses may be needed to trace information about a person's previous diseases, different exposures etc. Information on family relationships is needed for medical research in studying the importance of hereditary factors in different diseases, including cancer. Under Swedish conditions, better availability of these types of data ought to become possible simply through a change of routines for clearing out data from the computer-based population registers.

For epidemiological studies, individual-related information about certain known cancer-aetiological factors, especially smoking, is of great importance because these factors influence the possibility of detecting other risk factors. Extensive collection of information concerning personal life-style, such as smoking habits, for example through enquiries to large population groups, may be very difficult, since people tend to resent such questions. However, experience from New Zealand (Foster, 1980) indicates that this approach can work.

There are also possibilities available in primary care for collecting information about individual patients. Such information is usually available today in an unstructured form in the medical records and is impossible to use without the help of computers. One can see a trend towards more uniform recording of patient data, including some information on environment and living conditions.

Census information, such as particulars about occupation, has been used in epidemiological research work and has also been merged with information about cancer diseases and causes of death. In Sweden, such information has been collected through written enquiries to all households, lately every fifth year. For some time there has been discussion about abolishing this procedure in favour of linking information from existing registers. Opinions differ as to how data obtained through the two procedures compare. From an epidemiological point of view it is important that those indirect environmental descriptors which were collected through the regular censuses should not disappear. There is also a need to make such data more easily available for research purposes.

Registers and information systems with information about individuals have many different objectives. Even under normal conditions in a country, such data-bases can be looked upon as a threat to personal privacy. There is a clear need for individual-related registers with detailed information about diseases, environmental factors, and so on. At the same time, the question of privacy must be looked at very carefully. This issue was taken up very early in Swedish legislation especially through the Data Act of 1973. The general debate more recently also shows that there is great public concern about the generation and storage of individual-related information. However, it is necessary once again to stress that registers with such information are very valuable tools for deriving better understanding of the aetiology, prevention and treatment of cancer and other diseases.

8.2.2 Cancer registration

A central cancer register and regional cancer registers

The Swedish Cancer Registry started in 1958 in order to make possible the compilation of reliable statistics on new cancer cases. The National Board of Health and Welfare is responsible for the Registry. Registration is based upon legislation which makes it mandatory for physicians to report new cases of cancer, cancer-related diseases and certain pre-cancerous lesions. The objectives of the Registry are:

(*a*) to form a basis for presenting information on incidence of types of cancer — this is done mainly through an annual publication with numerical information (*Cancer Incidence in Sweden*);
(*b*) to create a basis for epidemiological and other medical research by providing a service to research workers.

In each of the health care regions in Sweden there is an oncological centre for co-ordinating various functions of cancer care in the region (see Chapter 14). Among other things these centres also carry out regional recording of cancer cases. Regional cancer registries have been in operation for the last few years in Umeå, Stockholm and Lund, and others have recently been started in Uppsala, Gothenburg and Linköping. The regional cancer registries in Umeå, Stockholm and Lund have been supplemented retrospectively and now hold complete data back to 1958. Systems for the registration of data from various treatment-programmes have also been developed at the regional registries. These may include more detailed information about certain cancer diseases, for example concerning environmental factors, patients' disease history, their treatment and the clinical development of the disease.

The Committee's assessments

All the information now recorded in the Cancer Registry must continue to be collected in the future and must be available for computer usage. The obligation to report new cases should be with the responsible physician, as is the case today.

There is already an established routine for physicians to send information on all new cases to the regional registries, which then take responsibility for the primary data treatment including certain quality control, coding and computerization. This also makes it possible to transfer (in computerized form) such data as are required directly to the central Cancer Registry of the National Board of Health and Welfare.

The Committee recommends a continued development of the regional cancer registries. These regional registries should, on a routine basis, update their files with the same type of information as the central Cancer Registry contains at present, with the addition of any other information that the oncological centre in the respective region considers to be of value.

The regional registers are also of value for epidemiological and clinical research, and can provide a good service to research workers.

This model of division of labour between the central and regional levels has many advantages. An oncological centre needs continuously to monitor the cancer morbidity in the region. The supplementing or clarification which is often required for information in the case reports, as well as ensuring data quality in general, is facilitated by the close contacts between a regional centre and the limited number of reporting hospitals. The central Registry thus relieved of many of its previous tasks can now concentrate on those matters which are of special importance to a central unit with information on a nationwide basis, especially certain data analyses.

From now on, the central unit ought to be better able to give *priority to the use of the information system* and to concentrate its work on statistical analyses and presentations, epidemiological studies, service to research workers and contacts with other registries both in and outside Sweden. The need for staff at the central Registry has switched from coding personnel to personnel with statistical and epidemiological competence. However, it is desirable, according to the Cancer Committee, also to set down formally some requirements to promote the full use of a register that is comparatively expensive to keep updated. Individual researchers working on their own initiative should be provided with better facilities to use the registry data. The Board of Health and Welfare should be given a clearer responsibility than before for both of these issues. The Committee suggests that the Board—as responsible for the central Cancer Registry—must, within 18 months after a calendar year, publish descriptive national cancer statistics for that year of the same type as has previously been found in *Cancer Incidence in Sweden*. (This requires that the inevitable delay in registering primary data should not exceed 12 months; due to lack of resources this time lag was for many years much longer.) The Board should also be formally responsible for a 'watch-dog' function and identify needs for more detailed analyses of the material with regard to problems that arise in society. It is of special importance that the Registry can give signals when there are unexpected changes in the statistics. Assistance to scientists who wish to use the Registry should include help in linking this information with data from other registries. There must also be good co-ordination between the central Registry and the regional registers.

An advisory group should be attached to the central Registry to deal with questions such as co-ordination and the setting of priorities between projects where researchers need to use Registry data. Harmonizing the coding and registration routines must be shared with the regional cancer registries.

High data quality must be guaranteed through quality control at the regional registries. Some quality control is needed at the central Registry as well. This should include studies of uniformity and quality in the coding and recording routines, on a random sampling basis. Since formally independent organizations are responsible for different parts of the registration, legal consequences of this should be looked into.

8.2.3 Registration of causes of death

The central Cause-of-Death Registry

At Statistics Sweden (previously named the Central Bureau of Statistics) causes of death have been recorded for a very long time. Such statistics have been produced since the middle of the eighteenth century. Since 1911, cause-of-death statistics related to broad diagnosis groups have been available and, since 1951, more specific statistics that allow, for example, studies of mortality for individual cancer diseases. The registration today is based upon medical information in the death certificates sent to Statistics Sweden through the church registers. The death certificates are checked manually and, if necessary, any information that is missing is collected and added. The Registry objectives are:

(*a*) to give annual statistics of deaths by cause, sex, age, etc.;
(*b*) to build up an individual-related register of deceased persons for research purposes.

In addition to research on mortality and morbidity, the register should be usable in studies concerning health effects of different working environments and other environmental factors.

The quality of the death certificate and the coding of the causes of death are of great importance. Therefore, there are both manual as well as computer quality controls but there are still some problems. These are mainly the coding of the diagnoses and the choice of which of the diagnoses was the main cause of death in an often complex disease picture where the reporting physician may not have made himself clear.

The Committee's assessments

For cancer research a registration of causes of death as well as of total mortality and cancer mortality is a necessary complement to the registration of cancer diseases. The Swedish Cause-of-Death Registry covers a considerable time span in the past and can be compared with similar registries in other countries. Access to individual-related information about date and cause of death is important too for other reasons. Reliable information about the date of death can be transferred to other individual-related registries. The survival time for cancer patients can be calculated regardless of the cause of death. The registration of causes of death also makes it possible to compare cancer diseases with other diseases, which is of great importance in many epidemiological studies.

There is a need, however, for measures to be taken to increase the data quality. One reason for problems with the quality is that the death certificate has to be produced within a short time after death. Another is the lack within Statistics Sweden of resources for certain check-up routines and of enough medical personnel for classification and coding.

The layout of the Swedish death certificate form is based on the recommendations from WHO. This form is old fashioned and there is a need for a modernized version, more in agreement with other forms used in the health-care field. The death certificate should not be designed for use as, for example, evidence in a trial, but only as a certificate of the physician's view as to the cause of death.

In a longer-term perspective it may be possible to completely change the present routines of reporting. Besides providing information for medical statistics, the death certificate has, according to existing laws, a function in proving that there is nothing to prevent interment. So-called preliminary death certificates are accepted for that purpose but must in such cases be followed by 'supplementary' death certificates. Suggestions have already been made in favour of splitting the two functions, so that the first allows interment and the second provides more detailed medical information which can be delivered directly for registration of the cause of death. The Committee recommends that this question should be further investigated without delay. Concerning the coding, there is a need for medical supervision, which should include evaluation of information from cancer registries and patient data-bases, to be obtained through more 'linkage' between files. New routines for using *all* the available information are thus needed.

The present structure of government agency responsibilities should also be considered in this context. The Cause-of-Death Registry obviously forms an important part of the general registration of diseases. Therefore there is a need to bring about a co-ordination of certain responsibilities, namely the medical part of the central recording of causes of death, with other recording within the health care sector. The National Board of Health and Welfare, which rules on systems of medical classifications and which is already responsible for several medical registers is considered to be the natural responsible authority. The advantages of having this Board take over part of the duty from Statistics Sweden – though not necessarily the Cause-of-Death Registry as such – are several. The knowledge concerning medical classification could be better used in the actual coding work, and expert inputs in this area could be concentrated and therefore more readily used for further development and in training of staff and supervision. The quality of the information in the Cause-of-Death Registry should thus be improved.

Such a re-organization should also facilitate an exchange of information between the Cause-of-Death Registry, and the registers for cancer and other diseases. The reliability of coding of the cause of death in cancer cases should be much improved by access to up-to-date information in the Cancer Registry during the coding of the cause of death. This should raise the quality of the statistics on mortality within the cancer field and give more reliable results in studies on survival from cancer diseases seeing that deaths even from other diseases than cancer could be taken into consideration.

The Committee also proposes the inclusion in the Cancer Registry of information from death certificates of cases not previously registered but which have cancer as one of the causes of death. This is already done in the other Nordic cancer registers.

Division of labour with regard to non-medical data registration and other functions connected with the Cause-of-Death Registry may be regarded as a mere practical problem, to be solved jointly by Statistics Sweden and the Board of Health and Welfare. Statistical presentations concerning the causes of death have, however, long been a part of the so-called official statistics where the responsibility for production rests with Statistics Sweden according to governmental policy. In addition to this, and in line with its views on the use of the central Cancer Registry Data, the Cancer Committee considers that the Board of Health and Welfare should have some responsibility for also encouraging the use of the information about causes of death with respect to the perceived needs within the health care sector.

8.3 Epidemiological monitoring

Epidemiological monitoring implies systematic collection and analysis of information in order to observe differences for different health variables in a population and try to find out if these can be linked to living habits or other environmental factors. Information about cancer incidence and death from cancer plays an important role in such epidemiological surveillance. It is essential to be on the look-out for special risk groups, taking into account environment and living conditions. Information that is routinely produced in monitoring systems may be connected with some kind of alarm function that signals abnormal changes.

Further research is necessary and the development of true 'systems for epidemiological monitoring' must be seen in a long-term perspective. Population-based long-term research programmes in the form of prospective studies directed towards specific issues are an important complement to more routine work.

Current activities and previous propositions

The question of systems for epidemiological surveillance has been brought up by several committees of the Swedish Government in the last decade, with recommendations both in general and in specific terms. It has also been discussed in the Swedish Parliament and in the Nordic Council, an assembly of Scandinavian parliamentarians.

The central and regional cancer registries already provide a tool for investigations and surveys of public health and of the influence of environmental factors on human health. Given a wider concept of a monitoring system, other existing subsystems are the Registry of Congenital Malformations, the Registry of Infectious Diseases and the Registry of Pharmaceutical Side-Effects.

The existing registration of work injuries can also be seen as a part of surveillance systems. Other special systems for monitoring of ill health caused by occupational environments are being developed by the National Board of Occupational Safety and Health, at clinics of occupational medicine and within industrial medical services.

The county of Älvsborg provides an example of a system being developed for epidemiological surveillance at a county as well as a municipality level. This system now gives a warning signal according to different criteria when defined population groups show differences in existing patterns of death. The system is to be supplemented with disease data from in-patient care.

Possible effects of industrial plants on the health of the local population are being investigated in various places. One extensive such project concerns Stenungsund, in the West of Sweden, which has a petrochemical industry.

One government committee looking into the siting of heavy industry suggested some years ago that an epidemiological surveillance system concerning health impacts with a possible bearing on physical and chemical causal factors influencing health should be established in each county. The former Council of Environmental Information considered a systematic monitoring approach at the national level to be needed in any case, in order to obtain better knowledge of the effects of industrial pollutants and other environmental factors.

Certain organizational changes of later dates and new legislation such as the Health Care Act 1982 have led to an increased and better defined responsibility of the county councils for the health status of their populations. Special groups responsible for environmental hygiene are envisaged (i.e. units for 'community medicine'); such groups or functions have so far developed in different ways in the various counties. As far as cancer diseases are concerned, several of the regional oncological centres are already examining environmental medical problems through cancer epidemiological studies.

Finally, a special project run by the National Institute of Environmental Medicine should be mentioned. The aim is to try to define guidelines for a stepwise development of epidemiological monitoring systems within the counties as well as for the central agencies. Two different concepts are involved. One is a general system where several types of health and environmental conditions are being followed with regard to the whole population. This would allow only rather broad division of categories and its early-warning capability would often be limited. The other concept implies specific surveillance systems where selected groups or selected factors are studied, with higher precision in the correlation analyses.

Further, specimen banks have been considered, with systematically collected reference samples such as biological material from human beings, animals and plants, food, etc. Such material can later be used for different studies both of agents already known today and of environmentally occurring toxic substances not yet noted. Certain limited human specimen banks exist already in Sweden. In an international context, the IARC has made an extensive inventory of such banks. Biological specimen banks also form a part of the Swedish programme for monitoring of the natural environment, and certain fauna and flora material has been banked for a long time.

Special conditions pertaining to cancer diseases

The cornerstones of the epidemiological monitoring of cancer diseases are the registers concerning the incidence of cancer and the cause of death due to cancer. By continuous analysis of these registers it is possible to detect changing patterns. There are some difficulties, however, in connection with this kind of epidemiological surveillance.

As for other diseases, one such difficulty is of a statistical nature. Changes in incidence for small groups of the population often have a statistical uncertainty that in practice makes it difficult to detect risk changes smaller than around 50 per cent, or even 100 per cent. It is therefore possible that statistically significant increases in incidence constitute only the 'tips of icebergs', the largest parts of which are contained in a 'background incidence from causes unknown'. This is a limitation in the use of the registers mentioned above for generating hypotheses about cause–effect relationships; the data as such do not permit identification of cancer-causing factors. Experience has shown that such factors are usually detected by clinical observations with subsequent analytical epidemiological studies or through experimental studies, and this is likely to remain the case in the future. The registers are, nevertheless, very important tools for epidemiological studies of the cohort and case–control types.

Another difficulty is the long time between exposure to a factor and start of the tumour disease. Only in exceptional cases can life-style factors or exposures be retrospectively described in that one can identify specific causal factors. The limited effectiveness of epidemiological work makes it urgent to find early-warning indicators of increased cancer risk using other clinical information than actual cancer diseases in individuals or populations. Ehrenberg (1984) has discussed the value of collecting certain data on humans at the population level or individual level as a supplement to epidemiological studies with regard to morbidity or mortality. The possible end points fall into three categories, namely

(a) disturbances in reproduction,
(b) genetic disturbances and
(c) biological and chemical changes in tissue.

One question is of course how relevant these observations are to a cancer risk. All are measuring something which is not itself cancer but which with varying degrees of certainty can be related to stages in the development of cancer. Even if the relevance of a studied parameter should be high, such an early-warning system as discussed here cannot indicate the *number* of possible cancer cases in the future. Instead, the scientific principle behind these observations is that one should be able to measure the cancer-initiating potential from, among other things, factors in the environment of the individuals studied. There is no corresponding theoretical basis for early-warning systems with regard to other types of carcinogen that act as promoters or as co-carcinogens.

With the exception of the Registry of Congenital Malformations, none of the clinical data referred to by Ehrenberg is collected routinely or on a large scale in Sweden. However, the importance of several of these methods is likely to increase in the future, after further development. The question of biological early-warning systems is also the subject of scientific work in both Sweden and other countries. A couple of methods which have been noted especially in recent years are so-called sister chromatid exchanges (SCE) in human cells after exposure to a genotoxic agent and chemically quantifiable adducts to DNA (or to an amino acid) which are usually measured in blood samples. The latency period here is very short and conceivable, and specific causal factors are therefore easier to find. In addition, the latter method implies a possibility of chemical identification of the active agent.

The Committee's assessments

GENERAL TRENDS. DIVISION OF TASKS AND OF RESPONSIBILITY

There is at present a movement towards introduction of epidemiological monitoring systems in Sweden. Several factors are promoting this trend, such as the increased responsibility for the health of the population given to county councils through new legislation, proposals from various governmental committees, and on-going work to characterize and to record both environmental conditions and health effects.

It is important that this development of epidemiological surveillance should continue, but this is only one of several means of elucidating causes of disease.

Epidemiological monitoring with regard to cancer diseases should not be isolated from other issues in connection with medical surveillance. A few general observations will therefore be made.

The lowest organizational level for a health-monitoring system in Sweden is probably a county, although the municipalities should be encouraged to participate in mapping of potential risk factors. It could also be important – not least for register and data-base studies of the type reported in Chapter 5 – to be able to refer environmental variables as well as health effect data in a monitoring system to smaller units such as municipalities or parishes.

The county councils seem to be the most appropriate organizations to be responsible for epidemiological monitoring. For many questions, regional co-operation between several counties is necessary. Within the field of cancer a regional organization already exists in the oncological centres with regional cancer registries, which through their responsibility for regional registration and the compiling of statistics form a natural part of a epidemiological surveillance system.

A system for epidemiological monitoring also needs resources on the national level. The National Board of Health and Welfare here has an overall responsibility for following up environmental factors' effects on the health of the population. This requires co-ordination of data acquisition and a review of the material. Better scientific and technical possibilities for creating an epidemiological surveillance system will place increasing demands on this Board.

Other central government agencies such as the National Environmental Protection Board, the National Food Administration, the National Board of Occupational Safety and Health and the National Institute of Radiation Protection have to some extent their own needs for systems for continuous supervision of the influence of different environmental factors on people's health. In order to optimize the use of resources, these needs should as far as possible be met within one integrated monitoring system. It is natural that the National Board of Health and Welfare should try to co-ordinate the different interests.

A very special resource on the central level is the National Institute of Environmental Medicine, which has responsibility for collecting and presenting material concerning the physical environment for health impact assessments. The Institute also has to carry out research on physical and chemical environmental factors.

From an organizational point of view two questions arise, firstly, the co-operation between the county and regional levels and the national level and, secondly, the distribution of responsibility between the different public bodies at the national level.

At the county level, it would seem natural for the county councils to co-operate both with organizations within their own area, especially local authorities and industrial health services, and with other county councils in the same region. The latter is essential not least with regard to cancer diseases.

The responsibility of the National Board of Health and Welfare is to stimulate and co-ordinate activities which can form part of an epidemiological monitoring system for the whole country. The administrative and co-ordinating responsibility must rest directly with the Board as do initiatives and recommendations concerning disease-preventive measures. The operative part of a monitoring system on a national level could be handled by the National Institute of Environmental Medicine, e.g. developing a model for data registration and analysis, follow-up and research in conjunction with the use of information from the decentralized systems. The Institute ought to plan, co-ordinate and carry out training of all the different categories of personnel participating in field work.

Close co-operation is necessary between the National Board of Health and Welfare, the National Institute of Environmental Medicine, university institutions with oncological, oncotoxicological or epidemiological research, oncological centres, county council 'community medicine units' and also the clinics of occupational medicine and the Research Department[2] within the National Board of Occupational Safety and Health (the two latter institutions also being an important resource with regard to research in environmental medicine). A great deal of the work with primary data treatment and subsequent analyses as well as the development of early warning systems are in fact research tasks. Besides co-operation between various scientific institutions, there is thus also a need for special efforts by the research-funding organizations.

COMPONENTS IN AN EPIDEMIOLOGICAL MONITORING SYSTEM
Information about diseases and the causes of death and other patient-related information ('register information') will remain the basis for epidemiological monitoring.

Data on exposure to potential risk factors and quantifiable information about people's living habits are of great value for investigations of causes of cancer diseases. Retrospective studies referring to conditions long ago are often difficult to perform; when documentation is lacking, estimates of the size of such factors become very uncertain. One of the aid functions in a surveillance system should therefore be to collect data on certain factors for prospective studies. This is no easy matter and requires inputs from many parties in society, both public and private, and from scientific groups as well as from people voluntarily participating in research projects. Recording data on life-style factors is an especially sensitive issue considering the individual's right to privacy and secrecy of data obtained.

A matter of detail, but an urgent one, concerns routines for clearing out existing data related to exposures, for example from municipality and industry archives. Some of this information may be valuable for epidemiological investigations and ought not to be destroyed.

Human specimen banks may serve as a useful tool for validating previous exposures to environmental factors. Such banks could be built up for example in connection with specific prospective studies. It is further recommended that the feasibility be investigated of setting up a general 'reference bank' of, for example, blood samples, in co-operation with the county councils, in such a way that the bank becomes statistically representative from various points of view.

The National Institute of Environmental Medicine should be commissioned to present a plan, according to the ideas above, for improving information and documentation of factors which may have a role in the induction of diseases such as cancer.

Later in this report there is a discussion on improving exposure data generation through the statutory risk control process (section 11.2) and on prospective studies of health effects of smoking and different dietary habits (Sections 10.1 and 10.2), which must include a prospectively designed collection of data on the occurrence of such factors.

Specified aims or performance requirements for an epidemiological monitoring system cannot be given here and now. Generally speaking, one such performance function is to follow variations in known risks and risk factors, among other things through monitoring of special risk groups in the population.

Another important function is to give indications of previously unknown risk factors. In spite of the usually long latency time for cancer, traditional epidemiological surveillance may well provide information on probable causal factors leading to important preventive measures, although a number of disease cases or deaths must have already occurred, as a prerequisite. However, early-warning systems are highly desirable in order to initiate preventive measures as early as possible. Supplementary systems of this kind build on the principle of a genotoxic effect where the frequency of manifest damage such as a hereditary disease or a disturbance in the fertility pattern is measured or where changes at the cellular level in human systems are determined in effect/no-effect studies or measured for size. However, the relevance of these types of observation for cancer initiation needs to be further explored.

In Sweden, support should be given in particular to continued and expanded studies of chemical dosimetry with determination of adducts to proteins or DNA (see Chapter 15). General scientific developments with respect to methods for early warning of cancer risks must be closely followed as well. More pilot activities using such methods ought to be initiated by the National Institute of Environmental Medicine and carried out in close co-operation with the scientific groups concerned.

NEED FOR RESOURCES

Good epidemiological surveillance which includes cancer risks needs considerable resources distributed among several parties. A major share of this work rests with the county councils, who therefore need to find the resources to carry out the task. Another part, namely the cost of running the central Cancer Registry, including the compiling of statistics from the data recorded, must be a responsibility of the government. Many of the information components for a monitoring system are wholly or partly generated in activities with other primary aims, such as patient information about hospital patients, the environment, etc. It is therefore impossible to give a total picture of the need for resources for an epidemiological monitoring system. Since this can only be built up step by step, the rate of development will also influence the annual resource needs.

At the national level the Cancer Committee's recommendations imply that the National Board of Health and Welfare and the National Institute of Environmental Medicine should allocate special resources for the tasks mentioned here. Some of these, such as the development of new parts of an epidemiological monitoring system and certain scientific analyses of the information, will no doubt require additional resources for the Institute. The primary responsibility for specifying the resource needs for the two agencies mentioned here should rest with the Board of Health and Welfare in conjunction with its annual budget requests to the Government.

More extensive data collection in the future for an epidemiological monitoring system will also open up new possibilities for research in general, from different research budgets. One must therefore presume that more resources will then be allocated to the use of data from epidemiological surveillance by funding organizations of both basic and applied research. It may also be envisaged that some such bodies will be supporting large projects going over several years. (Again, it should rest with the research-funding bodies themselves to judge their resource needs in this context; see also Chapter 15.)

BUILDING UP KNOWLEDGE

A prerequisite for epidemiological monitoring, as for population studies in general in the health care field, is a good build-up of knowledge. Sweden has long been behind several other countries when it comes to research education in epidemiology for physicians and statisticians and access to well-trained epidemiologists. Activity in this area has increased over the last few years. In 1982 epidemiology was given high priority by the Government. This is not enough. According to the Committee, resources for training in epidemiology must be allocated in the universities. This, in conjunction with research and the increasing demands for help from society, ought to stimulate young researchers in both medicine and the social sciences. In particular, scientists in the mathematical–statistical field should be able to make a valuable contribution to epidemiology.

A decentralization of certain activities might also stimulate epidemiological research. Instead of the collection and treatment of medical data being among the activities centred upon large, national databases, such work should, as far as possible, be done within bodies that have a more direct responsibility for health and medical care, such as oncological centres.

Another important matter with regard to building up knowledge is the development of and access to methods and resources such as registers of different kinds. The general development of methods is a natural part of the research work carried out by the universities. When it comes to physical resources, such as the Cancer Registry, the Committee presumes that funds will be made available both from the

Government and from the county councils. Bodies distributing research funds should also be prepared to allocate money for unconventional purposes such as scholarships for training abroad or for building up registries when resources are urgently needed. Permanent needs, however, should be met with permanent funding. Besides activities running according to long-range planning, such permanent resources ought also to cover funding requirements for a reasonably large input of research and development.

8.4 International co-operation

Existing activities

The Nordic countries co-operate in the Nordic Medico Statistical Committee (NOMESCO). This group is a permanent working party under the Committee on Health and Social Affairs (the Nordic Council of Ministers), and its work has so far concentrated on issues of methodology, some of which are of importance for the registration of cancer incidence.

The cancer societies in the different Nordic countries are also linked in the Nordic Cancer Union. This body arranges annual symposia for people from the different Nordic cancer registries. At these meetings the results from the different co-operative projects are reported and new projects are initiated.

The pooled material from all the Nordic countries gives great advantages, especially in the study of rare diseases, through analyses that can be based on a population of about 20 million. One example is a co-operative study of exposure among patients with nasal cancer.

In the epidemiological field, the IARC in Lyons has, in several respects, a co-ordinating role. In co-operation with other research institutions in different countries many epidemiological projects have been initiated and completed. The IARC also produces a summary of information from all the cancer registries around the world called *Cancer Incidence in Five Continents*. Similar summaries from registries of causes of death are published by the WHO.

Cancer registries all over the world are represented in the International Association of Cancer Registries, which has a secretariat located at the IARC. Voluntary cancer organizations, which usually have prevention and research as their main goals, co-operate through the international organization UICC.

The Committee's assessments

More active co-operation between the Swedish Cancer Registry and registries in the other Nordic countries would be desirable. This is necessary both for the development of new methods in registration and epidemiology and also for joint use of the material.

The Nordic Council has recommended the Nordic Council of Ministers to produce guidelines for national epidemiological warning systems and to initiate closer co-operation for the exchange of knowledge and experience concerning scientific and practical methods. This involves the recording both of exposure to different factors in the environment and of the state of health of the population. Systematic and standardized collection of data on the level and duration of exposure to different pre-specified factors is needed as well as exploratory studies in other directions. The proposed warning system will otherwise only facilitate the measurement of the magnitude of already known risk factors rather than helping to discover new and unknown risks.

First and foremost, national activities must be strengthened, but at the same time all possibilities should be used to introduce similar routines in all Nordic countries for those parts of the national warning systems not yet developed. Further development of the work within the Nordic Cancer Union and the Nordic cancer registries should also be seen as a very important part of Nordic co-operation.

8.5 The Committee's summarized assessments

General aspects

This chapter has discussed information systems based on the population data and the prerequisites for epidemiological studies.

Any work aiming at cancer prevention requires continuous epidemiological monitoring of the disease pattern in the population and its changes over time. Population-based long-term research programmes, especially prospective studies with reference to specific questions are very important and complement more routine activities.

Modern computer technology has greatly enhanced the opportunities for building up effective information systems for these purposes. Sweden, like the other Nordic countries, has excellent prospects for carrying out continuous epidemiological studies of cancer diseases as well as of other, especially chronic, diseases or disturbances in the state of public health. Sweden has access to good demographic data, by virtue of, for example, the personal identification system and a health care system for the most part administered by public bodies, and is therefore well placed to contribute through epidemiological work to international knowledge about different diseases and their causes.

In order to supply the expertise required for the increased efforts in epidemiology, improved and more widespread education, especially postgraduate, in this subject is necessary.

Scientific methodology and resource needs such as data-files of different kinds or fully developed information systems are to a great extent common to the whole of the health care and disease prevention field. The Committee's assessments in this chapter have therefore, to a great extent, the nature of descriptions and discussions of epidemiological requirements in general. Added to this are assessments of specific conditions as regards cancer diseases, monitoring of cancer risks and the possibility of clarifying the causes of cancer.

To some extent this concerns well established activities including the registration of national demographic data and the registration of all cases of cancer. Other important elements, such as patient databases, are under development. Activities envisaged to follow some time in the future include methods and routines for early-warning within a more comprehensive system for epidemiological monitoring.

The general Population Registers in Sweden contain basic demographic information, most of which is easily accessible. With regard to epidemiological research needs, it is recommended, however, that more of the data once recorded be kept in the computer files and not removed at later stages. This is particularly important for data on child–parent relationships and on a person's previous address(es).

Known cancer-aetiological factors such as smoking are generally confounding in epidemiological studies. The feasibility of obtaining and recording information on a large scale about smoking habits, on an individual basis, should be investigated.

It is expected that some kind of 'patient data-bases' will soon be in operation in all health care areas in Sweden. The Stockholm County Council has developed computer-based information systems covering *all* residents within the Council area. Such a source of information with both demographic and medical data facilitates epidemiological studies and provides direct possibilities for continuously relating different diseases to different parameters. Patient data should be recorded in such a way that comparisons are possible. This holds for medical treatment and examinations in all county council services as well as outside, for example in industrial health services and within special research projects.

Two special registries

In addition to population registers with general demographic data, accurate information about all cancer diseases and about all deaths related to cancer is most important for cancer epidemiology.

As a minimum, all information on new cancer cases now being recorded in the central Cancer Registry should continue to be collected in the future and should be available for computer usage. There should be continued development of regional cancer registries at the oncological centres in the six health regions. All of these centres have now begun to record all new cancer cases in their respective regions, and this information is subsequently transferred to the central Cancer Registry at the National Board of Health and Welfare. This procedure will give the central Registry more time for co-ordination (checking the quality and uniformity of source data) and development of analytical activities. Publication of the annual statistics should take no longer than 18 months.

The resource needs should be met by the county councils and by the state through allocation of funds to the Board of Health and Welfare. As problems are identified by the Board which require special cancer epidemiological studies, supplementary funding will have to be sought.

The Cancer Registry does not include data about survival time. The Cause-of-Death Registry is therefore a necessary complement to cancer research. This also allows analysis of interacting and competing causes of death. The main source of the information here is the death certificate received from a doctor.

The quality of the medical information in the Cause-of-Death Registry should be improved. There is a need to change present routines for notifying a person's death and its cause; the administrative and legal function of the death certificates should if possible be separated from its medical function. With respect to the coding phase, more medical supervision is needed, also utilizing existing information from the Cancer Registry and other health data files. Co-ordination of at least the medical responsibilities should be brought about. It is therefore recommended that this responsibility within the Cause-of-Death Registry should be transferred to the National Board of Health and Welfare, while the administrative function could remain with Statistics Sweden. The latter would continue to produce official statistics on the causes of death.

Epidemiological monitoring

In epidemiological monitoring, health information is collected systematically and analysed with the aim of observing any discrepancy from normal values for different variables within the population in order to see if this can be linked to living habits or other environmental factors. Such an activity could include the monitoring of special risk groups. Information produced may be linked to some kind of alarm system notifying abnormal changes.

Also for epidemiological activities outside a surveillance system, data components, competence and functions in the system may be of importance. A monitoring system must be able to react to non-planned incidence such as a cluster of disease cases of a certain kind in a specific geographical area or in some special occupation.

Systematic collection and analysis of information about cancer incidence and causes of death should be seen as components of a wider system for epidemiological monitoring. This increases the possibilities for improving basic monitoring routines as well as of carrying out analyses and research activities initiated outside the scope of programmes already planned. As regards cancer diseases, the latter have been of crucial importance for the building up of knowledge. Epidemiological monitoring concerning cancer diseases should therefore not be seen separately from other questions about epidemiological surveillance.

Information about diseases and the causes of death and other patient-related information from the health care system constitutes the traditional basis for epidemiological monitoring. The need for co-operation and co-ordination of this type of data alone justifies a systems analysis approach, which will also help in the consideration of other components required for the system. The development of epidemiological monitoring should therefore include measures towards better documentation concerning exposure to potential risk factors and other quantifiable information about people's living habits. Retrospective investigations are often difficult today due to the limited information available, so it is important that data should be collected for future use and that prospective research work be encouraged. Specimen banks, for example, of human blood samples, can be valuable in investigations of earlier exposures.

In view of the long latency period between exposure and the appearance of the disease for most types of cancer, epidemiological studies of cancer diseases should be supplemented by the monitoring of other clinical parameters which may be related to early steps in the development of cancer, as an early warning. Active efforts must be made to encourage research and development work in this area.

The 1982 Swedish Health Care Act places an increasing responsibility on the county councils for the health and well-being of the population. It is therefore natural that the responsibility for the development of epidemiological monitoring should rest with the county councils to a large extent. From their activities the councils can best contribute in the gathering of health information on the population, while information on environmental exposures ought to be collected mainly from municipal authorities, industrial enterprises and other sources, with whom a county council should therefore seek to establish co-operation.

The most suitable steering body at the county level for a health monitoring system would be the county council's special unit for community medicine. When two or more councils need to co-operate, for example to increase the population size in an epidemiological analysis, existing inter-council liaison groups should assist. As regards cancer epidemiology in a monitoring system, the oncological centres will be of great importance for the work, both within a council area and the health care region as a whole.

At a national level, the National Board of Health and Welfare has the responsibility for this monitoring; general planning of epidemiological surveillance and, especially, co-ordination of different demands on basic evaluation material are central tasks. Several other central government agencies also have to some extent their own needs for systems for continuous supervision of the influence of different environmental factors on people's health. These needs should as far as possible be met within one integrated monitoring system, co-ordinated by the National Board of Health and Welfare.

The National Institute of Environmental Medicine constitutes a very special resource in this context. The Institute has a duty to collect and present material concerning the physical environment for health impact assessments. It has recently investigated matters concerning epidemiological monitoring systems and it is natural that the Institute will also be engaged for the operative parts of the responsibility that formally rests with the Board of Health and Welfare.

A good epidemiological monitoring system will continue to require a considerable expansion of resources, the costs of which should be covered by the county councils and the state. Besides support for research through the separate research-funding organizations, government involvement includes general co-ordination and planning, as stated above, as well as support for the central Cancer Registry.

Finally, it is important to emphasize that this is only the beginning as far as monitoring systems are concerned. Much work is needed to develop good methodology and these activities must be viewed in a long-term perspective.

International co-operation

It ought to be re-emphasized that Sweden must be considered to have certain responsibilities in the field of epidemiology. Both purely national activities and participation in international research work will contribute to our general knowledge. Co-operation should be sought with other countries, especially the Nordic countries, and with international bodies such as the IARC.

More co-operation between the Swedish Cancer Registry and the cancer registries in the other Nordic countries is important. This means the development of methods for data processing and analysis and cancer epidemiology as well as more effective use of the material through combination of data from several registries. The Nordic population can be used as a basis for epidemiological studies, as it has the advantage of being a population with fairly uniform living conditions.

Note

1   The National Church of Sweden keeps population registers of all citizens irrespective of church membership. [*Ed. note.*]
2   Now an independent body: the National Institute of Occupational Health. [*Ed. note.*]

9
Health education as a component of disease prevention

9.1 Introduction

9.1.1 Some starting points and delimitations

The previous chapter dealt with information systems as a prerequisite for monitoring the disease pattern within a country. This, together with the international scientific literature, constitutes one of the bases for assembling new knowledge. Such information contributes to an understanding of the need for disease prevention measures.

It is clear from earlier chapters that a large proportion of cancer cases are related to our living habits, such as the consumption of tobacco and alcohol, unsuitable eating habits, deficient sexual hygiene and excessive sunbathing. Changes in habits within these areas could probably reduce the incidence of cancer significantly. Health education with a view to influencing peoples' attitudes and changing their behaviour is therefore a central instrument in cancer prevention work. However, changing ingrained living patterns is a slow process.

Although the significance of living habits can generally be established, the precise causal factors behind current cancer patterns and cancer incidence are still often incompletely known. Health education and the opportunities for reducing the incidence of cancer as a result of influencing living habits should therefore also be seen strategically in a long-term perspective. As more detailed knowledge emerges, the importance of health education will also increase, so plans should allow flexibility to take into account possible future improved understanding.

The aim of health education at present with regard to the cancer diseases can take its point of departure from the state of knowledge given in this report. In certain cases, for example on the question of tobacco smoking, the state of knowledge is good: the role of tobacco smoking in the occurrence of a series of cancer diseases is well authenticated and can be quantified with relatively high certainty. Smokers also exhibit an excess mortality of certain other diseases. It is thus possible to estimate the likely effect in society of, for example, a total ban on smoking. It is also possible on an individual basis to state the size of the risk and the risk reduction, at least approximately, and to illustrate it for the individual. In other cases it is, as stated previously, still difficult to quantify the effects of changed living habits, even where individual causal factors are known with a high degree of certainty. Also several causal factors must as a rule work together for a cancer disease to occur at all. All this makes even rough estimation of the size of expected effects of individual measures difficult.

Certain ethical and practical socio-economic questions arise here. To what extent should changes in attitude and life-style be striven for when the magnitude of the effect cannot be foreseen with certainty? There is no general answer to this question. Every situation must be judged separately. There is, however, good justification for informing the public about measures which the individual can take without wider social changes, to reduce either certain or probable cancer risks. The principle 'avoid what can be avoided' can be related to, for example, tobacco smoking, excessive consumption of alcohol, high fat consumption, unnecessarily high temperatures when cooking, severe sunning of unpigmented skin and deficient sexual hygiene. Avoiding several of the above factors also lead to a wider disease prevention than that relating solely to cancer. In reality, at least, the main part of this message has long constituted the core of health education, although primarily for reasons other than possible cancer risks.

This argument can be advanced one stage further. Changes in habits can be encouraged if they will do no harm. In other words, if certain measures, looked at broadly, are not considered capable of entailing any damage to health and can be carried out by the individual relatively easily, full scientific demonstration of efficacy need not be demanded before advice can be given to the public. It will then be a matter of *how* the information is structured. It must be honest and not promise anything which does not hold good. At the same time it must clearly show that those who are ultimately responsible for the content of the message, for example, a specific working group or organization, consider that it is sensible to follow the advice if one wishes to improve one's own health and reduce one's own health risks.

Chapter 10 looks more deeply into the importance of health education for a few causal spheres (tobacco use and eating habits) and, especially concerning eating habits, develops certain views on the actual message to be given in health education.

The term 'health education' is often given different meanings in different contexts. Here it is taken to mean primarily information which is aimed at individuals or groups of individuals with a view to influencing attitudes and life-style, to promote the health of the persons concerned. There is naturally no definite limitation against information which has no specific objective quoted, such as simple supply of knowledge, or news information. More sensational forms of information dissemination, for example a 'hard-hitting' news item on television about some health risk, would probably have powerful repercussions on peoples' attitudes—irrespective of whether the information was strictly correct or not. From a planning aspect, however, when it is a matter of contributions from public bodies, it may be appropriate to keep to health education in a more well-defined sense. However, cancer questions, like those of many other diseases, are complex and difficult to explain in a satisfactory manner in a health education programme, and it may be useful to supplement this with a supply of purely factual scientific information. Information matters generally, including the roles of research workers and mass media in the dissemination of information, the quality of the information, and so on, are dealt with in Chapter 12.

Health education is included as just one feature in the social strategy for improved public health. In fact, to accommodate practical provisions for the individual to use health-promoting knowledge, it may be necessary to introduce related measures at the community level which lie outside the individual's sphere of influence. This has already been touched upon in Chapter 7. Practical examples of such measures, intended to support changed living habits, are given in Chapter 10. In Chapter 16 a comprehensive view on the question of different measures which can result in improved public health is discussed.

9.1.2 Health education aimed at preventing cancer—a part of general health education

Should cancer-preventing health education constitute a separate sphere, in which the education is concentrated on living habits that entail cancer risks? Or should general health-promoting education also include a cancer-preventing element?

There are several reasons for integrating cancer questions into other health-promoting educational activities. One fundamental reason is that one and the same external factor or habit often has importance as regards the occurrence of completely different diseases or has an adverse effect on the well-being or condition as a whole. This applies to, for example, tobacco smoking, the use of alcohol and certain eating habits. A combined description of such disease-related factors will therefore give more information and will be many times more effective than one which focuses only on cancer questions.

Another reason is that cancer diseases probably seem more threatening than do other diseases. This fear is paradoxically to be found behind many peoples' resistance to taking in information about how the risks of getting cancer can be reduced. The fear of cancer screens off the information. Integrated education about the importance of various living habits for health as a whole may circumvent this screen and be more effective.

Another experience is that health education should have a mainly positive impact in order to gain a hearing. Health education which concentrates its message on those risks of disease which the individual runs as a result of some habit which he or she enjoys will find it more difficult to get a hearing than education which mainly stresses the opportunity of improvements in health and well-being. For this reason it is often better to avoid health education aimed at any specific disease.

What has been said here does not of course preclude efforts by special bodies, such as, for example, the Swedish Cancer Society. Such inputs constitute a valuable supplement to more generally directed health education.

Taken as a whole, the nature of cancer diseases and their mode of occurrence may certainly sometimes justify more specific efforts within the framework of general health education. Particular national situations may need to be picked out, for example an increased lung cancer risk due to indoor radon in conjunction with tobacco smoking (see Section 10.4). Explanations are also required as to why everyone does not get cancer, even though they are exposed to carcinogenic factors.

Because the occurrence of cancer is regarded as a result of interaction between at least two events, of which at least the initiation (see Chapter 3) is a chance (stochastic) phenomenon, *risk* becomes the central concept—and the risk of tumour occurrence increases with increasing dose of a carcinogenic factor. The magnitude of a risk is a statistical measure and is an expression of the likelihood that something will occur, such as occurrence of a specific disease in a person for given exposure conditions (see Chapter 7). Many people find this difficult to grasp. It is therefore important to try, in conjunction with health education, to describe the risk concept and relate quantifiable cancer risks from specific causal factors, such as tobacco smoking, to other risks which the individual is prepared to take or not take.

Against a background of what has been said here, the Cancer Committee has looked at health education principally from a general viewpoint. To a large extent this has relevance also for cancer prevention work. There is no room for really thorough analysis. Sections 9.2–9.5 below should rather be seen as a compilation of information from different quarters, stating trends, objectives, existing or conceivable contributors, resources, and certain problem identifications. In the last section (9.6) the Committee summarizes its own assessments.

9.2 Some future aspects of general health education

This section is based on two recent reports from a project, 'Health Services in the 1990s', run by the Swedish Ministry of Health and Social Affairs' Health and Medical Care Committee. This project took as one of its points of departure that the work of health and medical care must emanate from an aggressive health policy approach. Health education is seen here as an important means of achieving the aims of a health policy. In this section some topics from this project which have relevance for health education are covered.

In one of the reports (HS '90 Group, 1981a), it is stated that the health policy efforts in Swedish society with more emphasis on health education coincide with the World Health Organization's (WHO) overall formulations on health education as an important part of health work. It is assumed that a general raising of the level of knowledge could result in changed attitudes and improved behaviour from the health point of view.

Among the tasks of health education are:

(a) to increase private individuals' and whole groups' factual knowledge;
(b) to give guidance for private individuals' conduct;
(c) to develop an increased health consciousness;
(d) to clarify the direct relationship between matters of health and social and environmental conditions.

Health education can never be seen as an isolated medical question. The information must be related to the social and cultural patterns which characterize the environment in which the individual lives. Information must also be aimed at politicians, decision-makers and others who design the environment in the long and the short term.

Even though the interaction between knowledge, attitudes and behaviour is unclear, health education programmes should include information to try to influence peoples' attitudes towards and interest in health questions, as well as giving realistic instructions as to how habits should be changed (HS '90 Group, 1981b). However, one is usually dealing with deep-rooted habits which were perhaps formed in early childhood and reinforced in contacts with other people, as is seen in our eating habits, as well as our alcohol and smoking behaviour.

According to the group responsible for the project 'Health Services in

Health education as a component of disease prevention

the 1990s', further work in this project ought to be directed towards solving methodological problems in health policy planning and towards drawing up a concrete action programme which provides for measures aimed at the individual and at influencing society as a whole. The action programme is expected to form a basis for society's combined efforts to reduce health risks. It should be directed towards certain serious problem areas, among these the cancer diseases.

The starting point for health education should be that health education must:

(a) be integrated as a natural part of, preferably, primary care;
(b) take place in close collaboration with, for example, schools, occupational health services and voluntary organizations;
(c) preferably be directed towards specific risk groups, such as children, juveniles, certain immigrant groups and pregnant women.

The project group mentioned above also suggests that one should illuminate how trial activities and methods development could be stimulated, locally, regionally and at national level, with regard to efforts aimed at the individual to encourage a healthier life-style.

9.3 Distribution of responsibility and resources among bodies with present health education duties

9.3.1 Role of the authorities

Many authorities and organizations in Sweden supply information on health questions. In certain cases the information is combined with recommendations for healthier living habits, which can include a cancer-preventing effect. On the question of governmental obligations or efforts it can be said, however, that the major part of the information constitutes the supplying of pure knowledge about physical or chemical health risks, which are controlled by special legislation and therefore touches upon the individual's life-style to a limited extent only. Actual health education under the auspices of public bodies has grown alongside statutory risk control, gaining in status in recent years and receiving increased attention from decision-makers.

In Sweden the Government began to interest itself in health education during the 1940s, when the Board of Health started a more organized health education programme. The work mainly concerned information about venereal diseases, tuberculosis and dental health care. In 1958 a health education delegation was added to the Board. Following various organizational changes, a special office for health education was set up in 1981 within the National Board of Health and

Welfare, allocated to the section for preventive work and planning. At the same time, the responsibility for alcohol education was transferred to the office for alcoholic and narcotic matters.

An obvious shift from a central governmental level to the county councils on matters of health education has been taking place over the years. In the bill (Parliament session 1979/80, No.6) which dealt with the organization of the National Board of Health and Welfare and in the bill (Parliament session 1981/2, No. 97), which later led to the Health Care Act, the Government and Parliament pronounced that health education should be the task primarily of the county councils.

Health education is now characterized by increasing co-operation within and between the levels of different social bodies and organizations. Firstly, county councils are co-operating with government bodies—and here mainly with the National Board of Health and Welfare. Secondly, the Government and county councils are both co-operating at different levels with organizations which work at national, regional and local levels. County councils' health education is in many cases being developed towards a broad co-operation at local level between non-official organizations, county council and local municipal bodies.

In the following section an account is given of the role distribution between county councils and governmental authorities.

The role of county councils

Health education for an individual, for example in a doctor–patient relationship, is the overriding factor in the established preventive work within medical care.

Health education and health advice to private individuals and specific target groups in the community as a step in an outwardly directed, aggressive medical-care policy will be an increasingly important task for county councils. In the Swedish national budget for 1982/3, the county councils' overall responsibility for health education is stated and it is pointed out that it is the county council which is best placed to carry out health education in the field. Health education will be organized firstly through council staff, and secondly through co-operation with appropriate bodies at the regional and local level, for which county councils take the initiative.

County councils' individually directed preventive measures include

(a) information and health education;
(b) other measures for preventing the occurrence of disease;
(c) investigatory work directed towards diseases or their preliminary stages.

According to the Swedish Parliament and Government, health education and other individually directed preventive work is mainly a task for primary care. Information and health education is, however, expected to be included in all forms of health and medical care. Health and medical care staff therefore need to be prepared and motivated for this task.

Good efficiency in county councils' preventive measures presupposes that the aim of these measures is related to the health situation in the respective county council area. The councillors therefore require knowledge of those health problems which predominate within that area. Well-structured information systems and functional sociomedical or environmental-medical units here constitute prerequisites for successful preventive work.

Each county council is now responsible for developing environmental medical knowledge within its medical care area and for disseminating knowledge to various interested parties. In most county councils there is a health unit with separate resources intended for direction of health-education efforts. As far as cancer diseases are concerned, cooperation within larger areas than that of a county council (the 'health service regions') should be especially emphasized. Oncological centres, of which there is one in each such region, should thus according to the National Board of Health and Welfare advise county councils on the drawing up of guidelines for the prevention of cancer (see Section 14.1).

The total input to health education by county councils is difficult to calculate, since this is given within the framework of mother and child health care as well as health and medical care generally.

The role of governmental bodies

The Government's duties in health education are primarily laid upon the National Board of Health and Welfare (NBHW) which bears the ultimate responsibility for necessary central initiative within this sphere.

The task of the NBHW within health education is to set priorities on the basis of its own work and national and international experience of health risks and health-promoting measures, with regard to important areas for health education work and to provide county councils with information as a basis for their work. The NBHW has the task of encouraging and helping medical care officers' efforts in health education and of spreading knowledge and experience—for example through training and the production of educational material. The Board should also have a comprehensive outlook on health education in Sweden and should follow up developments and promote evaluations of actions in this field, as far as possible. The NBHW role in health education has predominantly the character of development work. According to the previously mentioned national budget for 1982/3, particularly urgent tasks in which the NBHW should assist county councils are abortion prevention, information about the harmful effects of using tobacco, and information about health-promotion diet and exercise habits. The NBHW also has a co-ordinating function within health education. The NBHW's role and contributions should be regarded as particularly important during the current build-up period of health education activities.

Health education also concerns other central government agencies to varying degrees. Thus, pertinent food matters require co-operation between the NBHW and the National Food Administration. The National Board of Education has an important task at the level of, for example, the roles of schools in health training. Information about special health risks and how these can be avoided is also produced by the National Road Safety Office and the Board for Consumer Policies. Other national authorities with responsibility for control of particular risks or risk areas are: the Board of Occupational Safety and Health, the National Institute of Radiation Protection and the National Environmental Protection Board. Regional state supervisory bodies, such as the Labour Inspectorate and the county administrations, are also involved. Even though these authorities hardly carry out health education in the more limited sense, they sometimes provide resources or channels for general or specific health education.

The NBHW was allocated approximately 4.4 million Sw.Kr (about US$600 000) for health education for the financial year 1983–4. Of this approximately 55 per cent constitutes grants to organizations which run health education. The grant to the NBHW's health education programme has been reduced annually since the financial year 1982–3, but the cuts must be seen against the background of the shift in the work from government to county councils.

9.3.2 Co-operating parties at the local, regional or other levels

It has been pointed out above that in the current phase of development in health education there is a strong movement to widen the circle of co-operating parties. The message of health education is more effective if it reaches people in different environments and contexts. Co-operation between the parties is therefore essential for effective work and for consistency in the contents of health education.

The importance of collaboration and co-ordination in health work is stressed in the new aggressive health and medical care policy. This applies to collaboration between health education representatives of county councils and other professional care and aid providers, for example the local municipal social service. There should also be collaboration between official public health education and the layman level in various voluntary organizations and the like. It is important that collaboration is not built up solely at the central level. Co-operation at local and regional levels is of fundamental importance.

By means of health education, knowledge is spread about the often considerable opportunities for individuals to influence their own state of health. So health education information must be matched in both content and form to the social context in which people live. Health education should be channelled so that it meets people in various contexts of their everyday life. Individuals must be able to relate health education to their own environment and day-to-day habits; there should be a consistency between message, life situation and opportunity to change life-style. Here, schools, companys' health services and popular movements have an important task to fulfil. One might mention, for example, sports groups, the temperance movement and other organizations which operate with specific health objectives (for example, reduced use of tobacco), as well as associations which more generally work for good health and environment. Many organizations of this type receive contributions from the Government or county councils.

ASSOCIATIONS AND OTHER NON-OFFICIAL ORGANIZATIONS
These often have well-developed channels for carrying a specific message and frequently operate at both national, regional and local levels. These channels can be used for information relating to health risks which will reach the individual in a familiar environment and context. In these associations there is a general knowledge of conditions in the field, which is valuable when designing health education work. Collaboration between public bodies and voluntary organizations has in many cases proved successful in Sweden.

Within the funds allocated to health education by the NBHW currently (1984) just over 2 million Sw.kr (about US$300 000) are contributions to non-official organizations. The largest recipient is the National Smoking and Health Association (NTS), whose work is of central importance in cancer prevention. Several organizations also receive in total a considerable contribution from county councils. The economic value of private organizations' combined total efforts within health education cannot be estimated, but they are significant.

The information dissemination activity of the *Swedish Cancer Society* is of particular interest. The Society's information concerns four areas:

(a) preventive work;
(b) early diagnosis;

(c) information for the public, patients and their relatives, and nursing staff about cancer research, the symptons of cancer diseases, diagnosis and treatment as well as rehabilitation;
(d) information about the Swedish Cancer Society.

In the health education context, the preventive information is particularly interesting, and the Society has given priority to information work specifically touching on the harmful effects of tobacco. The Society stresses the desirability of collaboration with other organizations, to increase the effectiveness of their information work aimed at preventing cancer. Also included in the Society's efforts to limit the harmful effects of cancer diseases is information aimed at the early diagnosis of breast and cervical cancers.

The Society receives an annual state grant of 3 million Sw.kr (US$450 000), though not only for its information work (see Table 15.1). The main task of the Society is to collect funds to support cancer research.

Organized Protection at Work
In *the work environment* in Sweden, obligatory mechanisms for health protection and risk prevention of each workplace also provide several channels for general health education for people in employment. So far this seems to have been utilized to only a limited extent.

Occupational Health Services
In Sweden these services have a vast knowledge of diseases and other health problems related to the individual's physical and social working environment. Within an overall view of man's different environments and life-styles and their combined importance for health, inputs from the occupational health services will probably increase in importance in the future.

Schools and Play Schools
These also play a major role in health education. Health education will be much more effective in contributing to reducing cancer risks if habits can be influenced from an early stage in life. Consequently, cooperation with schools and play schools in matters of health education is of great significance. The National Board of Education stresses that efforts in a programme for health training should be based on local conditions, and that this training should take place in collaboration with, for example, parents' associations and municipal bodies. Health education is not an actual subject in school but should be integrated in the school's daily instruction and other work.

MUNICIPAL ADMINISTRATIONS

These constitute important collaborating parties within health education at the local level. The Social Service Law states the local government's responsibility for working preventively and in collaboration with other official bodies, and with private organizations. Particularly stressed is the importance of preventing and counteracting the abuse of alcohol and other agents that can lead to addiction or dependence. Both the municipal social service and the local recreation administration should here be seen as collaborating parties for primary health care provided by the county councils. Contributions when planning health education at the local level should also be expected from the municipal environmental and health protection authorities.

INDUSTRY

This has invested some resources in information about healthy eating habits, and certain insurance companies have produced health information for distribution to the public and to their policy-holders.

THE MASS MEDIA

The media play two, sometimes overlapping, roles. The first is that the mass media is used, in accordance with current regulations, to promulgate messages by means of advertisements in the press, and to spread official messages on television. The latter, however, has so far been little used for pure health education.

The other role is the mass media's own information-dissemination by means of press, radio and television with articles, interviews, news and feature programmes, including training programmes for schools. Experience shows that it can often be difficult to establish collaboration here in pure health education objectives, since the judgements of the mass media of what is newsworthy and of general interest may differ from those of the bodies responsible for health education.

Health information from such a wide circle of actual and potential collaborating parties can be full of contradictions. This is the price which must be paid for the positive fact that so many parties, including the mass media, are involved. This sometimes confusing situation emphasizes the importance of an effective, soundly based and credible health education policy in the public sector to counterbalance media reports of 'one day wonders'.

9.4 County councils' health education at present—an activity in the making

Health education as part of an aggressive health policy and an instrument to achieve the objectives set (see Section 9.2) is a relatively new activity. It has been developed in Sweden in various forms largely since the 1960s. Not until the introduction of the new Health Care Act, in which the county councils have been given responsibility for preventive work, has this type of work generally come to be recognized as a specific activity in the work of county councils. All county councils now carry out some form of planned health education.

Health education is on the whole in an early stage of development, in which county councils are feeling their way forward in matters of direction, extent, methods, target groups and aims. The forms of preventive work and health education vary not merely from county council to county council, but also from one primary care area to another within a county council. There is thus no uniform model for health education in Sweden, though certain county councils which systematically developed their own health education programmes in many respects stood as models for others where the work began later. In the question of funds for health education the differences are also very great.

Common to the work as a whole is that the main emphasis is on the areas given priority by the National Board of Health and Welfare, namely alcohol, tobacco, sexual behaviour and cohabiting, and food.

In certain county councils attempts have been made to relate health education and other preventive work specifically to the current health situation in the county. For example, in Skaraborg County Council the health situation is surveyed systematically and presented in the form of municipal state-of-health 'diagnoses'. With such a point of departure it will be natural to define the aims of the health education operationally, that is, in terms of the identified health problems or risk factors which one wishes to influence. Setting such aims also provides the prerequisite for evaluating the effect of the efforts and consequently for further development.

To some extent the direction of health education can be influenced by the existence of a unit for environmental hygiene ('community medicine') in the county council administration. These units, anticipated by Parliament when transferring certain governmental duties to the county councils, are intended to play an important role in health education. They are, however, largely at the development stage and have—where they exist at all—varying aims and degrees of organization. This means that the split of roles between those responsible for health education within a county council and a community medicine unit can easily become blurred if both parties find themselves in an early stage of development.

9.5 Strategic questions for health education—limitations and possibilities

Traditional health education is supposed to operate in accordance with the following sequence:

Health education → Health knowledge → Attitudes in health matters → Changed habits → Better health

This sequence may not always be followed through, because of various limitations. When increased knowledge does not result in the intended changes in attitudes and habits, the causes may be found in *individual* physiological, psychological or social conditions. But the limitation may also be due to *structures in society* including pre-conditions in the physical and social environments.

9.5.1 Can we count on health education to have effects?

An important question is whether there is any experience of results directly related to health education.

The difficulties of measuring the effectiveness of health education are considerable. One reason for this is that health education is most frequently only one activity among many in a preventive project and it is therefore difficult to measure the effect of *one* component in a combined effort.

The evaluation is made easier, as stated above, if the activity can be related to specified aims. When it comes to cancer diseases, due to the long latency period, effects on health will not be measured until far into the future.

The effects of health education can instead be related to objectives other than health and/or reduced incidence of disease in a target group. Two types of objective can be described: firstly, so-called activity objectives, secondly, so-called condition objectives. Activity objectives are taken to be certain activities which should be achieved—for example, establishment of anti-smoking groups at a place of work or a measurable change in some eating habit. A condition objective is taken to mean that a certain level of knowledge or a certain attitude must be achieved by means of health education (Qvarnström *et al.*, 1980).

Health education is long term, and expected health effects from altered living patterns will often not become obvious until many years later. During such long periods of time, other changes in society will occur which further complicate the assessment of health education effects. Nevertheless, it has been possible to show that health education very probably constitutes an important part in successful preventive work. A few examples are quoted here.

One large-scale example of results of preventive measures is that 15–20 million people stopped smoking in the USA during the latter 1960s. This has been related to the fact that, firstly, programmes against tobacco smoking—in contrast to tobacco advertisements—were transmitted on television and, secondly, doctors involved themselves and discussed smoking habits with their patients (NTS, 1970).

A Swedish example of successful preventive work within another field is the resource input on abortion-prevention efforts in connection with the abortion law which came into force in 1975. In this case teenagers are the main target group for broad training and education efforts in matters of sexuality and cohabiting, which were developed by the National Board of Health and Welfare in the so-called Gotland project—today further extended to a large number of county councils and municipalities. The abortion frequency in the 15–19 year-old age group decreased by a quarter during the period 1975–82. Concentration on the teenagers in this context stems from the assumption that early-established living patterns tend to be retained throughout life. The methodology in the work is based on co-ordination of advice on contraceptives, training and education efforts, and on developing collaboration between different professional groups which meet young people in various life situations (report of the Abortion Committee, (1983)).

An example of how one can favourably influence the health situation is the North Karelia project in Finland of 1972–7. The project's background was that the region was considered to have the world's highest death rate from ischaemic heart disease. Health education was carried out by means of broad collaboration between health and medical-care groups, social welfare bodies, schools, voluntary organizations and the mass media, with the primary aim of influencing smoking and eating habits. To this end, the tracing and treatment of high blood pressure was included in the project. The health education received practical support, in that the authority responsible for the project, through local arrangements with, for example, dairies and butchers, made foodstuffs available with products less rich in fat. During a 10-year period nearly half of the men who previously smoked stopped, and the average serum cholesterol level among the population decreased by 12 per cent (Puska 1983; Puska *et al.*, 1981; Puska *et al.*, 1983). During the period 1969–79 deaths from cardiovascular complaints decreased by 24 per cent among middle-aged men and by 51 per cent among women (Salonen *et al.*, 1983).

In Sweden the Government began to take measures against smoking in the mid-1960s. During the 1970s the previously continuous trend of an increasing proportion of regular smokers among men was broken, and the curves go downwards. The trend among women has been different, and the proportion of regular smokers of cigarettes is now greater than among men. Even though a small average reduction seems to have taken place in womens' smoking habits during very recent years, remarkable differences remain; for example, young women smoke about twice as much as young men.

Health education has played an important part in these examples. The conclusion may be drawn that preventive work can yield favourable results and that health education constitutes an important component in this work.

The trend towards decreasing smoking among men indicates that health education does have an effect. The fact that almost one third of of the adult population continue to be regular smokers and that the proportion of younger women who smoke is very high suggests that, nevertheless, there are certain limitations to the effectiveness of the knowledge and health awareness imparted. Almost every schoolchild and every adult must by now be conscious of the harmful effects of smoking tobacco. If knowledge were the decisive factor in our actions, it would be reasonable to assume that no one in Sweden would be smoking today.

9.5.2 Some factors which limit the effects of information

Among factors which limit the possibility of influencing people by means of disseminating information is the fact that human actions are by no means controlled only by objective knowledge. Equally important are standards, attitudes and specific living conditions in the social and physical environment, as well as individual psychological and biological needs and processes. Health education which aims to change living habits must therefore be based on an overall perspective of human behaviour, where these different aspects are taken into account.

Health education, including cancer-preventive education, comprises provision of information which will help individuals to assess which risks they should avoid and which risks they are prepared to take. It is important to remember that people, in their assessment of risks, often take considerable health risks despite available and well understood knowledge. Furthermore, certain health risks which the individual consciously takes are linked to various forms of physiological dependence. Another factor to be reckoned with is that differences in people's elementary knowledge can of course affect their ability to convert information supplied into a proper understanding.

Other risks which people take in relation to cancer diseases are less obvious and are linked to the fact that there is still a lack of clear knowledge about the induction and causes of cancer. The information about different risks which is specifically disseminated through the mass media is therefore often so full of contradictions that individuals become resigned and shut themselves off from actual health education giving clearer, more objective and factual information. In addition to this there is a certain weariness in the face of the quantity of information which comes from different quarters and the difficulty of deciding what information is relevant. The uncertainty relating to the causes of disease is unavoidable, but resistance to taking in relevant information poses a problem in health education.

There is a widespread fear of cancer diseases, which means that people consciously or unconsciously shield themselves from information about cancer risks by means of psychological defences of a denying, suppressive or repressive nature. A common attitude, which constitutes a barrier to many peoples' receptiveness to health education, is the perception that it is not meaningful to try to avoid cancer risks through their living habits, since death is after all unavoidable and cancer is often associated with death. It is important to work against this attitude by means of health education. This applies especially to young people who as a result of health-endangering habits established at an early age may risk considerably shortening their life-span.

The chances of health education having an influence seem to be surprisingly small among certain groups. One such group is young women with regard to their smoking habits. Making health education methods more effective requires that this limitation should be better understood.

9.5.3 Some factors which contribute to the effectiveness of information

Although the factors just described may lead to a certain resignation about the possibility of influencing the health of individuals, it may be in order to point out that the will to live and the instinct of self-preservation are powerful forces, and that people to a large extent do pay attention to relevant risk information which comes to hand. This requires, however, that the information be put over in a psychologically adequate manner and that conditions in a person's environment are such as to allow them to act in accordance with the information.

Exactly what constitutes a psychologically adequate method of transmitting information is decided to a large degree by the aim of the information and the target group. Even if the whole population is the actual target group for health education, it is often necessary to pick out more specific target groups, to which the design and content of the health education message can be matched, to make it more likely for the information actually to reach people. The choice of target groups in health education can be made using various criteria—for example, risk groups subject to special exposure or groups in which there is a higher than normal level of environment-related health disturbances of a certain type, often within certain age groups. A clear idea of the intended result in the target group will help in adapting the message's content and form to that group. Experience shows that health education reaches people with a good education most easily. Adapting health education to different target groups should improve the possibilities of also reaching other categories of people. This approach helps in deciding not only the actual message, but also which channels and forms of communication should be selected, at what times, and in what circumstances the information should be supplied.

Health education aims to increase a health consciousness which will form the basis of lifelong healthy behaviour. How health education is to retain relevance for the individual's requirements over the different phases of life and environments will therefore be important in the planning of health education. Since the *timing* of the presentation of information is just as critical as its form, in its ability to influence people, health education should, for example, be available to us when we find ourselves at a cross-roads in life and have a chance to test our living habits, such as, when we leave home, start a family or lose a spouse. This underlines the need for collaboration between those representing health education and other bodies which influence people's everyday environment, such as occupational health services, schools, and voluntary associations.

Health education is carried out both in the form of general campaigns aimed at the public at large, and information aimed at individuals or groups of individuals. Health education only in the form of a general campaign has not proved to have a deep and long-lasting influence. General campaigns have, however, proved to have an effect as a means of intensifying concern and 'raising the temperature' in a continuous activity. The best health education is that which is disseminated from person to person in a specific situation and on the basis of a specific problem; health education is about an interaction between the sender and the receiver of the information. Health education must always be given in the right context and be seen in relation to the recipient's physical and social situation.

Bearing in mind that standards and attitudes in people's immediate environment have great significance for their life-style, in several different projects information strategies on health matters other than those indicated in the simple, sequential diagram at the beginning of Section 9.5 were tried. Thus the information was aimed not only at the individuals in the primary target group, but also at people important to them in their immediate environment. In addition, the significance of local opinion-formers was taken into consideration, since information given by a person who is at the centre of attention (for example, a leading figure in sports), on whom other individuals seek to model themselves, is taken seriously. These projects also drew on the experience that people who are themselves in any way active with respect to processes for influencing attitudes, etc., find it easier to take in and identify themselves with a message's content than people who receive the same message passively.

An example of a project which was based on these assumptions is the previously mentioned North Karelia project. Smoking and eating habits were influenced by the project, and a favourable change in the medical status of the region's population regarding cardiovascular complaints was noted.

This strategy for health education differs from what has been customary, in the degree of activity among the recipients, and also in the efforts made to base the information firmly in the recipients' immediate environment.

9.5.4 Some ethical questions

All social information which aims to influence peoples' attitudes, standards and living habits is linked to ethical questions. The questions touch, for instance, on society's right to try to influence peoples' life-style and standards for health promotion, the right to give information about health risks which the recipient can only partially influence, the right to give information on health matters where science can still only give probable cause–effect connections, and the right to give information on anxiety-provoking matters. The ethical questions also touch on methods for influencing attitudes.

Another important ethical problem, but of a different type, is the fact that general recommendations on, for example, diet, which are judged to be useful at group level, are in certain cases unsuitable or even harmful for a particular individual with a special constitution or complaint.

A point of departure for general health education is that people need and are entitled to knowledge which can benefit their health. The health educators' most important aim should be to help people gain a deeper understanding of matters concerning their health, so that they can independently reach wise decisions affecting their living habits. In this respect health education differs from manipulative methods which aim at changing the individual's habits unconsciously. This respect for personal integrity implies a respect for peoples' rights to take health risks, despite the relevant information.

In the public's right to knowledge lies also a responsibility of society, through active health education, to supply information about measures which probably—if not with scientific certainty—can reduce the risk of disease or otherwise promote health (see Section 9.1.1). It must also be assumed in such situations that the measures are fairly easy to carry out, with the individual sacrifice being relatively modest in relation to the potential gain.

One question which touches on the scientific basis of disease causation is the following. Health education, not least regarding cancer risks, may create anxiety among those who do not wish, or are unable on their own, to follow advice about changing living habits. Much depends on *how* the message is presented and its timing, as well as on what help society (or voluntary organizations) can give the individual at the same time. Anyone who develops cancer may suffer anguish and guilt towards relatives for having brought the disease on himself as a result of ignoring health education and other information about cancer risk factors. It is important therefore to explain that it is not possible to decide unequivocally in any individual case what caused the cancer, and that risk assessments relating to, for example, tobacco smoking, or unsuitable diet, are based on 'group statistical' correlations. Individual differences between people should also be stressed. This does not, however, apply only to cancer diseases, but to many other sometimes fatal complaints such as cardiovascular diseases.

9.6 Summary assessment of the Cancer Committee

General conditions

In Swedish society major resources are concentrated, by the public system and popular movements as well as by other voluntary organizations, to promote health and prevent ill health through various activities.

Since the total incidence of cancer in Sweden is largely related to life-style, the Cancer Committee sees health education which aims to alter living habits as a central instrument in cancer prevention.

Although the importance of life-style can be established to a large degree, it must be emphasized that the precise causal factors behind present cancer patterns and cancer incidence are still not fully known. As more detailed knowledge comes to light, the importance of health education will also increase. It is therefore important to plan for flexibility in this work.

Health education with the aim of preventing cancer will to a large extent be a part of health education for reducing other health risks as well. It is important, in planning general health education activities, that where appropriate, the possibility of influencing certain forms of cancer should also be considered.

Special questions about health education and its effects

Public health education about cancer risks should be designed and given in such a way that it does not cause mental stress. It would be unfortunate if cancer came to be regarded as a self-inflicted disease. The Committee, therefore, wishes to point out the importance of not simplifying information given to the public to the extent that it becomes misleading. Collaboration between, for example, cancer research workers and journalists or other information-presenters should be such as to ensure that the public learns about the complex character of the cancer risk. This requires sound knowledge on the part of all those contributing (see also Chapter 12).

Training in matters of health education should be introduced for people whose profession involves informing others about health risks and health-promoting measures, for example in medical care. Opportunities also should be provided for voluntary workers to receive training in this field.

For health education to be effective, suitable conditions must exist to allow the public to carry out the specific changes in life-style required in order to reduce cancer risks. Creating such conditions requires suitable political attitudes and decisions, as well as the individual's conscious choice of habits, rather than medical measures.

One of the great difficulties with information about cancer risks is that the recipient, because of the fear of cancer diseases, can unconsciously screen off the message. If the information is fragmented or inconsistent, this further aggravates the difficulty for the recipient in absorbing the information. This is a reason for co-operation between various parties active in health education and a reason why they should have suitable educational literature available adapted to activities at the different levels where health education is carried out.

The ethical aspects of health education should be kept in mind, for example when and how information about probable but not proven health risks should be supplied and what are suitable and admissible methods for society to influence individuals' attitudes and life-styles.

Organizational questions

According to current legislation the overall responsibility for health education in Sweden lies with the county councils. These councils are therefore assumed to be responsible for planning, organizing and carrying out health education. Governmental authorities and primarily the NBHW are assumed to support this work in various ways. Collaboration between public and voluntary efforts is necessary in order to obtain the best results from health education.

In line with the intentions of the Health Care Act, there has for some years been an obvious shift from central governmental level to county councils in the responsibility for health education under public auspices. County councils' health education is an activity under development, in which, by and large, county councils are testing the way forward in matters of the aim, scope and methods of health education. Especially during this stage there is a great need within county councils for the NBHW's support in the form of assistance with training, the passing on of experience, development of methods and dissemination of facts. Where cancer diseases are specifically concerned, collaboration within the health service regions should be stressed, and oncological centres should, according to the NBHW, advise county councils on the drawing up of guidelines for the prevention of cancer (see Section 14.1).

During the build-up phase now going on in county councils as they take over responsibility for preventive efforts, a broadening of the circle of collaborating parties is important, to reach out with health education via different channels. Effective forms of collaboration need to be developed between health education representatives in county councils and other professional providers of care and aid, as well as between official public health education workers and the layman in various voluntary organizations. At the local level, county councils should try to co-operate with, for example, schools, occupational health services, industry, and various municipal administrations. Contributions towards health education, at the local level, should be expected from, for example, the municipal environmental protection and health protection authorities against a background of these bodies' legal responsibilities. Within county councils it must be assumed that the community medical units will assume an important co-responsibility in matters of health education's content, priority allocation, and so on.

In Sweden the national service system, which involves the majority of men of military service age, ought to be able to fill an important role in matters relating to smoking and alcohol habits, as well as in following up school training regarding sexual hygiene and cohabitation.

It is important also to co-ordinate as far as possible at a central level the activities of everyone involved within the areas given priority. Where governmental funds are involved, the NBHW should take the necessary initiative, whether it is a matter of directing funds from the Board's allocation to other organizations and where the Board thus has formal control, or a matter of using other funds. In certain cases this could mean an increased requirement for the organizations affected to co-operate in that area which relates to government funds. One example here is the Government's contribution to the Swedish Cancer Society, which is used to a certain extent for health education relating to the risk of development of cancer, especially the dangers of tobacco smoking. Action against the use of tobacco has been given priority in the NBHW's health education programmes as well and is also supported by means of governmental contributions to, for example, the National Smoking and Health Association. In Chapter 10 the Cancer Committee returns to the question of increased efforts against smoking. The Swedish Cancer Society should also have an important role to play in planning future health education, in collaboration with the NBHW, not just in matters of field activities. As a result of its strong link with active cancer research, the Society has a good view of the research front and of recent scientific advances. This is helpful in discussions on such matters as revising the content of health education and allocating priorities. In this way the knowledge which exists in the Society can obtain wider dissemination. The Cancer Committee also wishes to stress the Society's broad approach when it comes to information in the sphere of cancer diseases, from preventive measures and early diagnosis to rehabilitation of patients.

The Committee has not examined in any detail the choice of the most suitable media for carrying out health education. The mass media's importance as an information channel must, however, be emphasized, and two forms of collaboration with broadcasting services will be touched on here—firstly, the broadcasting of official information and, secondly, the role of programmes.

As concerns 'official information' issued by means of radio and television in accordance with the Radio Act [1], it would be desirable for the broadcasting authorities to agree to more health education being included in this category. The relevant official bodies should disseminate factually based information of importance for public health. Brief information given through the media should help to focus attention on and support continuing long-term activities in health education at the field level and should be planned in consultations between the broadcasting company and the responsible societal bodies.

As far as programmes are concerned, there are several examples of active television programme inputs on matters of health education from countries with broadcasting rules similar to those of Sweden. One example is the British Broadcasting Corporation (BBC) which, through its education department, has made eye-catching and repeated contributions in conjunction with anti-smoking campaigns in UK. During 1984 the BBC also transmitted five programmes in a series specifically aimed at cancer prevention. The introductory programme, featuring the well-known research workers Doll and Peto, dealt with possibilities for avoiding cancer, whereas the following three programmes dealt with smoking, cancer risks in working life and the environment, and the connection between diet and cancer. The final programme dealt with methods of early diagnosis and treatment options.

Another example is the previously mentioned North Karelia project, in which Finnish Television played an important part through a nation-wide transmission of 10 programmes which were aimed at influencing smoking and eating habits (Puska et al., 1981). In both these examples very good viewing figures were recorded, which means that the programmes appealed both to those who watched out of general interest and those who were particularly interested in this type of programme.

Against this background, the Cancer Committee proposes that in the first instance the National Board of Health and Welfare and the Swedish Broadcasting Corporation (or the programme companies within this organization) should jointly study, firstly, how the authorities concerned could use radio and television more extensively for health education and, secondly, the ways in which a programme company could take the initiative for increased programme contributions which would help to expand interest and knowledge and change attitudes in matters of health-promoting life-style and known health risks.

Scientific co-operation

Various authorities and other groups in Sweden have already indicated the need for interdisciplinary contributions in designing and carrying out health education dealing with general health risks. According to the Cancer Commission this should also take place in the specific area of cancer risks. Developing practical methods of health education aimed at altering life-style requires research on how attitudes may be influenced and on the processes of information transfer.

Health education relating to cancer risks must be evaluated firstly from the aspect of its information content, form and distribution, and secondly from the point of view of how it coincides with the recipient's realistic chances of acting in accordance with the information. The NBHW should take the initiative for an overall discussion with the parties engaged in health education, to highlight difficulties and problems encountered in evaluating health education activities.

Support with scientific backing on various health risks, especially from the NBHW and oncological centres, to different bodies concerned with health education at a practical level is important. So also are central and regional contributions in following up the effects of different measures, especially their long-term effects on the population's general health (see Chapters 7, 8 and 15).

Since this involves dealing with, among other things, pure research aimed at producing new and reliable knowledge about health risks and health-protecting measures, collaboration with the research world within the university sector as well as the research councils should follow naturally.

Notes

1   The rules for public service broadcasting in Sweden are set down in the Radio Act and in the agreements between the four programme companies (the Swedish Radio Company, the Swedish Local Radio Company, the Swedish Television Company and the Swedish Educational Broadcasting Company) which are parts of the Swedish Broadcasting Corporation.

According to the Radio Act, the programme companies alone decide what to transmit. According to the agreements commercials are not allowed. Also according to the agreements the Radio Company, the Local Radio Company and the Television Company transmit 'official information' (mainly on the rights and responsibilities of the citizens), but still at the discretion of the broadcasting company concerned. Some instructions on how to minimize certain risks, for example that of drowning, have also been broadcast in this category. On television this is being done mainly through a programme item called the 'notice-board'. [Ed. note.]

10
Special measures in certain risk areas

10.1 Tobacco use and tobacco products

10.1.1 General background

Cancer risks due to tobacco use, etc.

The deleterious effects of tobacco use were not shown until the 1950s, long after the extensive spread of its use in large parts of the world.

The harmful *biological effects* of tobacco smoking are above all due to the following factors:

(a) the toxic substance nicotine, which has several effects on the body, including a stimulating action creating a physiological dependence that increases the habit-forming nature of smoking;
(b) carcinogenic and/or irritating components in the smoke associated with several forms of cancer as well as various smoking-induced annoyance reactions and also chronic bronchitis and emphysema;
(c) carbon monoxide, also a component of smoke, which does not cause cancer but which does seem to contribute to the excess mortality rates of smokers from cardiovascular diseases.

Section 4.2 has dealt in depth with the risks from tobacco use, in particular smoking, concentrating on *cancer risks* but also underlining the obvious excess in *mortality from other diseases* which is characteristic for smokers.

Tobacco smoking is the largest single identified cause of cancer in Sweden. It induces about one in every six cancer cases (approximately 5500 annually) partly in interaction with other factors. This means that on average some 15 per cent of all cancer cases among men and women would not have occurred if there had been no smoking; with a range of uncertainty between 12 and 20 per cent, this implies between 4500 and 7500 cases.

The differences between males and females are still considerable and are due to wide variations in past smoking habits. The Cancer Committee has estimated that about one out of every four cancer cases among men and some 7 per cent of cancer cases among women can be attributed to tobacco smoking. During the last 15 years there has been an obvious change in the pattern of smoking, with the average consumption decreasing among men and increasing among women. Tobacco smoking is more common in older men, while in women the younger above all, are smokers. If smoking habits remain at present levels, we can expect an increasing number of smoking-associated diseases and deaths among women when the high-smoking age groups reach ages where the harmful effects of tobacco are generally manifested.

Table 4.6 shows estimates of the number of different forms of cancer cases in Sweden caused by tobacco smoking in 1979. There is scientifically overwhelming proof that tobacco smoking is by far the dominant causal factor of male lung cancer. Other tumour sites with high likelihood of association with tobacco smoking are the lip, oral cavity and pharynx, oesophagus and larynx (all having direct exposure to smoke) but also the pancreas, urinary tract and kidney and, among women, probably also the cervix. The proportions of cases which can be ascribed to tobacco smoking of course varies. It is suspected that there may in fact be an association between some fraction of other malignant tumour diseases and tobacco smoking which is not normally recognized. There is, however, no proof of a causal relationship.

Lung cancer due to tobacco smoking is the cancer risk most widely studied in the world. As tobacco smoke contains both initiators and factors with promoter capability it can be the sole cause of this type of cancer. Moreover, factors in the smoke can combine with other factors such as exposure in the work environment to radon daughters, arsenic or asbestos, to mention only a few.

The lung cancer risk shows an obvious dose dependence which can be illustrated by the relation between relative risk and number of cigarettes per day. This dose dependence is also shown by the decreased risk among those smoking cigarettes with filters and/or low tar content, by the increasing risk with increasing depth of inhalation and by a relation to the lifetime dose, i.e. the number of years of smoking.

It has been argued that cigar- and pipe-smokers run a lower risk of lung cancer than cigarette smokers. This seems to be the case only if the smoke is less often inhaled. Even non-smoked tobacco products, namely snuff and chewing tobacco, carry a certain cancer risk, although it has not been possible to estimate its magnitude. The form of cancer mainly associated with the use of such products is cancer of the oral cavity, but this is not common.

Most discussion of hazards related to tobacco smoking as well as of the available scientific data have been concerned with the risk to the smoker. So-called passive smoking or secondary smoking, meaning involuntary exposure to 'environmental tobacco smoke', is attracting increasing attention. Further, possible health hazards to the fetus and to future generations have to be considered, although information is more uncertain in this field.

Passive smoking clearly does carry a certain increase in cancer risk. Data that would permit an estimate of the *size of this risk* are at present inadequate. The total number of cancer cases caused by tobacco smoking as assessed from the smoking population is not influenced a great deal by the risk contribution from passive smoking, which seems to be rather low. The risk to the individual of course varies with the exposure conditions and should generally be low, although in certain extreme cases it could be substantial, as in rooms where many persons are smoking during a long period of time. The number of passively exposed persons is, however, high and special groups among them, like children, are not easily able to avoid exposure.

In conclusion, tobacco use, in particular tobacco smoking, is an extremely serious health problem and constitutes the largest single identified cause of cancer. The risk to the smoker is so great that import and sales of tobacco products in Sweden would not be allowed if medical considerations alone were to govern. Passive smoking too influences health and constitutes a certain cancer risk. Here an ethical problem arises as well, since we are dealing with an exposure which is in principle involuntary.

Previous action

The World Health Organization (WHO) has on many occasions over recent decades recommended that its member countries take initiatives to combat tobacco smoking. The recommendations have been further developed and made more specific in the expert report published by the WHO in 1975, *Smoking and its Effects on Health*. The WHO has stated that no other preventive action can contribute more to improved health than the control of tobacco smoking. The need for such measures has been recognized in many countries.

In 1973 the Swedish National Board of Health and Welfare presented the 'Tobacco report', prepared by a specially convened expert group. The report proposed a number of measures, the ultimate goal of which was to decrease cigarette consumption to the extent that no consequences for public health should be detectable. In practical terms this meant a reduction to the consumption level of the 1920s.

Resources for anti-smoking information were subsequently increased. Further, another expert committee was established to look into advertising of tobacco (and alcohol) and, in 1977, warning text and declaration of certain smoke components on tobacco products became compulsory by law. Certain restrictions on the marketing of tobacco products came into force 2 years later.

Also in 1977, the Swedish Government set up a 'Tobacco Committee', with the task of developing a programme aimed at reducing tobacco consumption and counteracting its harmful effects. The Tabacco Committee's report (TC, 1981) proposed a number of measures which included:

(a) a law prohibiting smoking in public places;
(b) wider limitations in the marketing of tobacco products (to achieve identical rules for marketing alcohol and tobacco);
(c) a stronger programme of information about the harmful effects of tobacco;
(d) special educational measures for health personnel;
(e) establishment of more 'smoking cessation' clinics;
(f) increased efforts for research, in particular social and behavioural research.

The proposal to ban smoking in public places was made because of the dangers from passive smoking. It was criticized on the grounds of unenforceability and because of the difficulty of defining what would constitute a 'public place'. The Government did not initiate legislation on this point but instead instructed the relevant national agencies to draw up recommendations on limitation of smoking in workplaces and premises to which the public has access. Such recommendations were issued in 1983, their aim being that no person contrary to his/her will should be subjected to discomfort or health risks in places where both smokers and non-smokers have a right or an obligation to be present together. A non-smoking environment should be considered the normal situation, and the desire of a smoker to smoke should be secondary to the non-smokers' right to a smoke-free environment. The Swedish National Board of Health and Welfare launched a major campaign to promote smoke-free environments.

The Government turned down the Tobacco Committee's proposal for stricter marketing restrictions for tobacco. Other measures that have been suggested but not yet adopted in Sweden include a total ban on tobacco advertising, and a special fee to cover costs of a central campaign of information about tobacco's harmful effects. In discussing these matters, however, Parliament was not satisfied with the situation and asked the Government to continue systematic efforts to bring down the tobacco consumption (Parliament session 1983/4).

10.1.2 Tobacco smoking must decrease

Possibilities to evaluate the effects of measures taken so far

The ultimate objective is a decrease in the health damage and mortality caused by tobacco use.

There is generally a *long latency period for the development of cancer*. The increase in lung cancer (the most thoroughly studied form of cancer related to tobacco smoking) has paralleled the increase in smoking; in particular the risk of lung cancer is higher for those who start smoking early in life. This has been shown in a UK study (see Figure 5.5). Similarly, a rise in the number of lung cancer cases among Swedish women and, up to 1977, among men is clearly related to the growing proportion of smokers in the population.

However, it is important to underline that *the health risks rapidly decrease* when tobacco smoking decreases. For instance, the risk of developing lung cancer is already substantially reduced within a few years after smoking has ceased, even for people who have been smoking over a long period. Summarized in Figure 4.9 are a number of international reports which indicated that the excess risk for lung cancer death was reduced to half only 2–3 years after the cessation of smoking. The excess risk is obviously decreasing far more rapidly than the average time needed to develop the disease.

Chapter 5 reviewed the time trends for lung cancer incidence and mortality and also described estimates of future development of this disease. The lung cancer incidence among Swedish males decreased by some 10 per cent during the latter 1970s (see Figure 4.8). There is good reason to relate this change to the much lower quantity of cigarettes smoked by men since its peak in 1969 (see Figure 4.5). A certain increase in lung cancer incidence among males has, however, been observed since 1980. A change to different types of cigarette might have contributed to the health improvement first registered. The changed age distribution among smokers tends to counteract the effect of reduced numbers of smokers, so without that change in age distribution the decrease in lung cancer would have been larger. The lung cancer incidence decreased earlier among males in Stockholm, which might indicate that changes in life-style are most rapid in cities.

The lung cancer incidence in Sweden is still high among males and remains about four times higher than among females, probably due to previous differences in smoking habits. The total lung cancer incidence among women does not show signs of a decrease. On the contrary, as mentioned earlier, a serious increase in lung cancer incidence can be expected to continue among women (as well as increases in other smoking-related diseases) as a consequence of their present smoking habits. Already the lung cancer incidence among women aged 40–49 years is as high now as it was among males in that age category some 15–20 years earlier.

Smoking habits and changes in them can be easily measured and provide a basis for projections of future health effects. Trends in smoking habits have been described in Section 4.2.4.

In Sweden, almost one-third of the adult population are *daily regular smokers*. Women have overtaken men as cigarette smokers. In the younger age categories females smoke almost twice as frequently as males. In recent years, since the recognition of the health effects of tobacco smoking, men have decreased their smoking, though a substantial increase has been observed in snuff taking, in particular among younger men. Increased snuff taking causes some concern partly because the cancer risks associated with snuff taking have not been well studied, and partly because it creates a nicotine dependence which can lead to smoking. Tobacco consumption by women, principally of cigarettes, has on average stayed level for several years, although with substantial differences between different age groups. There may have been some decline in the average proportion of regular smokers among women during 1980–2. During the 1970s, smoking declined among schoolchildren, although the proportion of smokers among schoolchildren is still alarmingly high, with more than 20 per cent of boys and some 35 per cent of girls as smokers in the 15–16 year age group. However, the number of smokers in the 12–13 year age group has been cut to half during the 1970s (Table 4.2).

The average daily consumption among cigarette smokers seems to have been fairly stable for a long time at about 13–14 cigarettes per day. On the other hand, cigarettes sold today weigh less and also contain less tar than before, which decreases exposure to cancer-causing agents. A decrease in nicotine content of cigarettes sold today may be compensated by either more cigarettes and/or 'more effective' smoking of such low nicotine cigarettes. If this happens, the advantages of the new types of cigarette may to some extent be negated.

It is difficult to relate variations in smoking habits to specific measures taken with the aim of changing those habits. Nor is it known whether the general debate and the presentation in the media of scientific results about health hazards from smoking have contributed to these changes. However, there are indications that smoking habits in the population really can be changed. The switch to low-tar cigarettes is an example. It does seem likely that better understanding of the detrimental effects of tobacco has contributed to the major decrease in tobacco smoking, particularly among younger males. There are also differences in smoking habits between different socio-economic groups (educational level, occupation, type of living area), as described in Section 4.2.4. Cigarette smoking has decreased among well-educated men and women, but not so much among the less educated, in particular among women. The differences in smoking habits between different social strata seem to have been less pronounced in the 1960s. Changes in the smoking habits of schoolchildren can certainly be attributed to special measures aimed at them. Such measures are particularly important to stop so many children starting to smoke at an early age.

A general change in attitude to environmental tobacco smoke has been evident in Sweden in recent years. Both smokers and non-smokers seem to prefer non-smoking environments in public transport, in rooms for common use, etc.

The trends are not unequivocal with regard to future smoking habits. Even among groups which earlier showed an encouraging trend towards decreased smoking, there may now have been a halt in this trend, or even a tendency towards an increase. Nor has anyone been able to explain properly why certain other groups have increased their tobacco consumption substantially over the last few years.

An important question is why people smoke at all. Knowledge of mechanisms that control smoking behaviour and the starting of smoking will provide a basis both for evaluating measures already adopted and for improving programmes to discourage smoking.

Why do people smoke?

The question 'why do people smoke?' is not simple to answer. Starting to smoke seems to be related to social and personality-related circumstances. A 'social breaking in' has generally taken place during the adolescent years when appreciation by friends and their attitudes are of particular importance. Further, the products are easily accessible, they are frequently glorified in the media and, last but not least, the daily use of tobacco has been and is still generally accepted in society, although certain changes have taken place during recent years.

The smoking habits of children often resemble those of their parents. The attitude towards smoking at home and to what extent parents accept children's smoking could obviously be of great importance.

For many who have tried to smoke tobacco either as a child or as an adult the experience stops after a trial. Others continue and frequently develop smoking habits that become difficult to break. A dependence has been established which, at least among habitual smokers, can be classified as an abuse comparable to that seen with alcohol and narcotics, with physiological, psychological and social circumstances combining to perpetuate the dependence. The mental dependence is considered to be due to the effect of the nicotine on the central nervous system (CNS). Many smokers report that they are stimulated by smoking and can concentrate better, although the opposite effect has been reported by others who use smoking as a tranquilizer. (Both effects are compatible with the mechanisms by which nicotine acts.) In these ways tobacco smoking is found by the smoker to provide support and protection during otherwise psychologically stressful situations. Data showing development of tolerance towards tobacco smoke and development of physical withdrawal symptoms in its absence indicate that the dependence is also physiological. Stopping smoking is easier when combined with chewing nicotine gum which indicates that nicotine is involved in the dependence process (Fagerström, 1981).

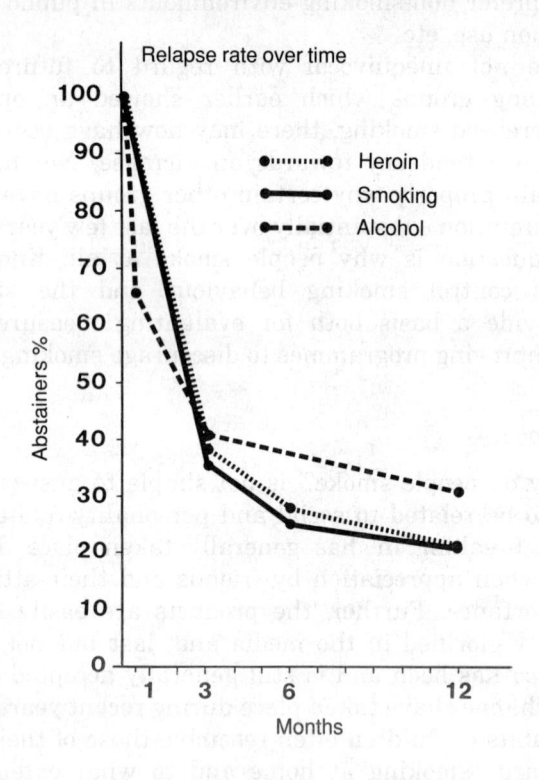

Figure 10.1 Relapse frequency in treatment programmes against certain dependence-forming drugs.
From Hunt *et al.* (1971).

Although there are important differences between addiction to different substances, and although the social damage from smoking is very different to those caused by alcohol and narcotics, certain similarities can be seen between addiction to tobacco smoking and to other drug dependence. Figure 10.1 (based on some 80 studies of which most refer to smoking) illustrates the similar frequencies of relapse between the three types of dependence. It shows that 1 year after stopping smoking, only 20 per cent of the subjects were still non-smokers. Such studies of smoking cessation have only been performed on people within treatment programmes for smoking cessation; there are no studies on relapse frequencies among people who stop smoking by themselves. The change over time in smoking pattern and in different groups of people in various countries shows, however, that many people are capable of stopping smoking. Only a small fraction of those are likely to have participated in special individually oriented programmes for smoking cessation. It is not known how much other forms of support and help by health personnel, family members and fellow workers have contributed. By 1982, in Sweden, there were about 1.3 million persons who had stopped smoking, of whom almost half a million had stopped smoking in the period 1976–81.

Although the majority of behavioural science literature on smoking deals with ways of stopping smoking, we still do not know which factors effectively contribute to the smoker's successful cessation. To a large extent this is due to the very complex character of the tobacco smoking habit which demands an extraordinarily careful design of scientific studies. Accordingly there is a great need for interdisciplinary research into these questions. In future studies experts from the behavioural sciences, medicine and sociology should cooperate in the assessment and evaluation of effects of different measures taken.

Conclusions. Proposed intensified health education, etc.

Continued, powerful attempts need to be made aiming at a considerable reduction in tobacco consumption.

Further research is required into what measures can influence people's desire and ability to stop smoking, but this cannot be used as an argument for not adopting any measures now.

In spite of much good work by public and voluntary organizations, the need for measures against tobacco use to reduce the health risks seems to lack adequate understanding and support in Sweden. It is, therefore, not only a question of resources; there is a need for a general awakening to the dangers, among both smokers and non-smokers. It should be impossible for a modern society to accept the health hazards and damage that tobacco smoking clearly leads to. There is a need for a thorough change in attitude towards smoking as a national problem and for a clear statement of intent, not least from politicians and decision-makers at all levels, with two main goals:

(a) tobacco use should decrease to a level as close to total abolition as practically possible;

(b) the attitude to tobacco use should be changed so that consumption does not increase again once such a level has been achieved.

There is no longer any need to come up with new proposals for what should be done but rather to argue again with all the power of scientifically based health risk assessments that actions must be taken and that powerful measures have now to be directed against tobacco smoking. Even if previous information on the various health risks has not resulted in the necessary recognition of tobacco use as a national problem, the growing scientific evidence of recent years should help to bring about a real changeover provided it becomes widely known. With special regard to cancer risks it seems likely that a large number of people are still not aware that:

(a) the number of cancer cases that can be associated with tobacco smoking is of the magnitude that the Cancer Committee estimate shows in this report;
(b) cancer from passive smoking is a risk that cannot be dismissed on scientific grounds;
(c) the cancer incidence in the years ahead among certain groups with a high proportion of smokers, particularly young women, will continue to increase drastically unless their smoking habits are profoundly changed.

One of the most fundamental prerequisites for success in changing smoking patterns is a wider understanding about the hazards among all members of society. Health education and other measures that can encourage and help people to stop smoking should accordingly be intensified as discussed in detail in Chapter 9. Health education can of course also be an important factor in combating the start of tobacco use. In relation to what has been said about the spread of tobacco use in different age groups and social strata, it is specially important that information, like other measures, should be tailored to the specific target groups. Certain living conditions may make it more difficult for some persons to change a detrimental habit if it is experienced as positive.

In health care, regular smokers with a high consumption of tobacco should be seen medically as high-risk cases. Physicians should routinely inform smokers about the detrimental effects of tobacco and help them give up smoking. Health personnel should be given better education about smoking, more support in trying to reduce their own smoking and better practical opportunities in the course of their work to inform and help others who are smokers and even to prevent the starting of smoking. Personnel in nursery schools, teachers, persons in different voluntary organizations etc. should be taught and given advice about how to set a good example without smoking and how to encourage people individually and in groups to stop smoking. In certain difficult cases, specific medical support and treatment of withdrawal symptoms might be needed. Existing special smoking cessation clinics within the health care system might be given further importance, in particular through research on methodology. Otherwise, tobacco smoking is such a major problem that it ought to be integrated into practically every kind of activity within the health care sector.

Possible measures to prevent children from taking up smoking and for dealing with problems of passive smoking are covered in the next two sections.

Special programme with the aim of preventing children and adolescents from starting smoking

The most effective form of change to achieve a decrease in the total smoking in a long-term perspective must be to decrease the number of people who start smoking. Measures specially directed towards preventing children and adolescents from starting smoking should accordingly be given high priority.

A programme of anti-smoking health education in schools can be especially valuable. Youth organizations should be encouraged to work against smoking and to prohibit it during their activities. Wider-ranging anti-smoking measures which also affect the young, and even adults who refuse to give up smoking, can help to create a non-smoking environment for their children or other young people at home, in schools, at work and in social activities.

Considerable resources should be directed towards this goal,— besides certain activities already in operation in Sweden—and some central co-ordination of the use of these resources is essential, even when some measures are taken on a purely local basis. Such co-ordination will also help in planning for evaluation of the effectiveness of the whole programme. Indeed, the programme should be organized in such a way as to permit sound scientific studies of its performance.

An annual budget of 5–10 million Sw.kr (about US$1 million) is perceived as a minimum for the programme during an initial period of at least 5 years. The financing ought to be shared between several parties: the county councils (as directly responsible for the health care of the population), certain governmental agencies, and voluntary organizations including the Swedish Cancer Society.

Exposure to environmental tobacco smoke

Less smoking overall will automatically result in less exposure of non-smokers to tobacco smoke in the environment (passive smoking).

Conversely, social norms or regulations which limit smoking in places where other people have to be present would in practical terms probably also lead to a decrease in total smoking, as smokers find difficulties in finding somewhere where smoking is accepted.

Although the risk to the individual from passive smoking is generally low, it is related to the conditions of exposure and increases if people are exposed for a very long time. Other health hazards from environmental tobacco smoke exist too (see section 4.5). It should, therefore, no longer be left to the individual smoker to decide where he or she will smoke.

The continuing changes in attitude towards tobacco smoke in the general environment, among both smokers and non-smokers, have contributed to a decrease in passive smoking in many situations. Further measures to reduce this problem should have one basic goal: *that no one should be exposed against his or her will to tobacco smoke in the environment*. The means of attaining that goal depend above all on what is suitable and practical in any particular situation.

Legislation has drawbacks because it has clearly to define the localities in which it shall be applied; this in turn implies that in other localities it is *not* applicable, which carries a risk that voluntary measures in those localities might be delayed. Legislation also requires effective enforcement, which could necessitate a disproportionate allocation of resources for reducing health hazards. 'General advice' by a governmental agency (the *formal* alternative in Sweden to legislation) can be used more flexibly because it can deal with all the different kinds of localities where people spend their time and because it can respond more quickly to changes in attitudes against environmental tobacco smoke as an air pollutant. It can also include practical advice concerning matters such as ventilation conditions. On the other hand there are drawbacks such as the lower status and the lack of sanctions. The present approach in Sweden is to depend upon voluntary procedures which may well be the quickest way of attaining the goal just mentioned. One precondition of this approach, however, is that the relevant advice must be well propagated and understood and that the health authorities must have the resources to disseminate such advice effectively and to stimulate compliance. Further measures including new legislation will have to be considered if it turns out that:

(a) certain groups of people are particularly exposed to environmental tobacco smoke in public place;
(b) change is particularly slow for certain types of localities and people in these are involuntarily and seriously exposed to environmental tobacco smoke; or
(c) new scientific data call for a more rapid cut in the amount of environmental tobacco smoke.

Of especial importance is the provision of smoke-free environments for children. This is relevant not only for the development of their own smoking habits later in life but also because children cannot easily avoid exposure to environmental tobacco smoke by themselves. Furthermore, pregnant women certainly should not smoke, due to the risk of various kinds of damage (though probably not mainly cancer) to the fetus (see Section 4.2.5.).

An active price policy for tobacco products

It is reasonable to assume that the price of tobacco products is a factor that does influence their consumption. In most countries a major part of the price of tobacco products consists of taxes. Society can accordingly influence the price of tobacco more directly than that of most other consumer goods.

In Sweden and in some other countries, taxation and accordingly pricing of alcoholic drinks is used as an instrument to limit their consumption. The principle in Sweden is to adjust continuously the price of alcoholic products in line with general price inflation. The same should be done for tobacco. This should go for all kinds of tobacco products, whether for smoking or otherwise (snuff and chewing tobacco).

During the 1970s the price of cigarettes in Sweden increased more slowly than consumer prices in general (Figure 10.2).

Before that, the proportion of smokers started to fall from a peak around 1969–70 when the price of cigarettes was in real terms higher than at any other time in the last 25 years. Of course, it is not possible to draw any definite conclusion from this, since smoking habits are influenced by so many other factors, such as health education.

The price of tobacco ought never to be allowed to fall in real terms (after allowing for inflation) if smoking is to be discouraged. An immediate return, in Sweden, to the higher relative price of 1970 would also be desirable.

Another suggestion that has received attention is for a differential tax structure between strong and weak cigarettes. However, there is a danger in this that it might encourage smoking of the lower-tar and nicotine types rather than discourage smoking in general. Therefore the Cancer Committee has not included this suggestion among its recommendations.

10.1.3 Legal control of tobacco products

Among measures to decrease health risks associated with tobacco use, the main emphasis must be on different ways to decrease smoking itself. However, there are also good reasons for looking at the different

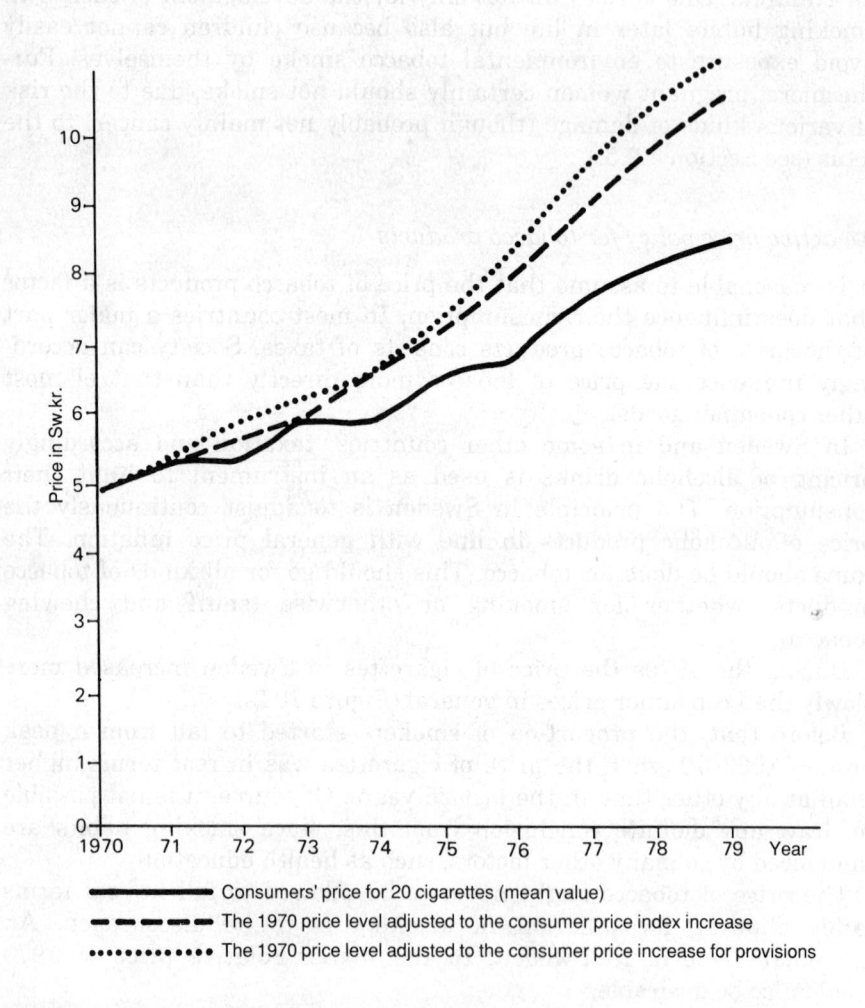

Figure 10.2 The price of cigarettes during the 1970s.
From TC (1981).

products separately. Various sets of rules and/or voluntary agreements controlling the compositions of the tobacco products exist in certain countries.

Brands of cigarettes differ from each other in the exposure to carcinogenic agents that they cause with identical ways of smoking. The differences can depend on differences in chemical composition of the tobacco leaf, pesticide residues, the drying process, additives, ways of filling with tobacco, the filter, etc. Reports from the US Surgeon

General (1979, 1981) have listed different methods for decreasing the toxic activity of cigarette smoke.

Most of the harmful substances found in mainstream and in side stream smoke from a tobacco product are formed by the combustion process itself. By various modifications of the product, the amount of tar which the smoker inhales in relation to the amount of nicotine has been reduced in several cigarette brands. However, such changes cannot be carried on indefinitely if the smoker is still to get his supply of the much wanted nicotine. Therefore the 'totally harmless' cigarette is a practical impossibility. Nevertheless, product development should be encouraged with regard even to small risk reductions, and the matter of additives and their effects ought to be a formal responsibility of one or more government agencies. Regulations for the control of composition of tobacco products need to be examined from the points of view of effectiveness and enforceabilty.

Legal restrictions on the *use* of tobacco products (e.g. smoking in certain localities) should not, however, be linked to legislation about product control. A general basic principle ought to be that tobacco products should be subject to at least the same degree of control as other biologically active chemical substances or products. In practice there is a wide difference between what current Swedish regulations demand from producers or importers of chemical products hazardous to health or the environment and those who produce or import cigarettes and other tobacco products meant for smoking.

Tobacco products in Sweden, have to carry a warning and a declaration of content indicating the level of carbon monoxide, tar and nicotine in cigarettes (measured by prescribed methods). Snuff and chewing tobacco are considered as food products within the meaning of the legislation on food safety and can thus be controlled with regard to health hazards associated with both naturally occurring and added substances. Within this framework, the occurrence of certain cancer-producing agents in such products is already being studied (see Section 4.2.4).

Tobacco products ought to be treated without exception as products dangerous to human health and the environment, and therefore should be covered by laws dealing with such hazardous consumer products. There can be difficulty in defining which products fall within the scope of which specific law. The food legislation should be quite adequate to control snuff and chewing tobacco. But tobacco products for smoking are at present excluded in Sweden from most of the laws controlling particular classes of product. One solution would be to broaden the food legislation to cover all tobacco products, however 'consumed'. Another would be to extend the limited laws on tobacco labelling, so as to incorporate requirements for notification and control of the composition of the products. A third alternative would be to remove the exclusions from the hazardous products legislation and treat tobacco products in the same way as any other dangerous material.

The authorities appropriate to exercise the control would depend on which legislative approach was adopted. It seems clear that the national health authorities must have an important role, both in applying expertise in chemical and toxicological evaluation of hazardous materials and in integrating such control work with the other aspects of the health effects of tobacco.

The present state of knowledge indicates that we are here dealing more with an important matter of principle (namely to have legislation covering all chemically hazardous products) than with health problems to which radical solutions can be immediately applied through product legislation. A beginning could be to require notification of all tobacco products on the market and any new ones introduced. This could also facilitate the financing procedure, since the Committee recommends that the cost of the new control system should be borne by the producers and importers of tobacco products. The manufacturer's control of certain substances in tobacco smoke from the different products is important and should of course continue. However, it should be supplemented by testing carried out by the controlling agency and analyses conducted on its behalf. This does not necessarily mean that new national specialist resources should be developed, if the analysis can be performed by competent laboratories elsewhere that are independent of the tobacco industry.

10.1.4 Monitoring the effects of anti-smoking programmes and other studies

There should be a continuous follow-up of smoking habits and changes in them and of the health effects related to tobacco smoking. This should be done as part of a continuous programme of epidemiological monitoring (see Chapter 8) with recording and analysis of data, particularly those likely to have a bearing on cancer risks. Existing activities such as the regular studies of smoking habits performed by the NTS (National Smoking and Health Association) could be included as a part of the monitoring if this is considered suitable.

The general change in smoking habits can probably only seldom be related to specific previous measures taken against tobacco use, though general trends that appear for smoking habits and health effects should give guidance in the design of different measures to be taken by society. Special types of follow-up have to be applied to evaluate the effect on smoking habits, attitudes etc. of the total or separate parts of action programmes, sometimes combined with pure research on methodology (see also Chapter 9). Different socio-economic groups and special risk groups of other types should be monitored. The smoking habits of children and adolescents should be documented within the proposed special programme to prevent children and adolescents from starting to smoke, with the help of the education authorities. This should also lead to a proposal for how such a documentation should be performed in a more continuous fashion in order to become included as a component in an epidemiological monitoring in the long-term perspective.

Information on the individual level about certain known cancer aetiological factors, in particular smoking habits, is important for epidemiological studies because such factors may otherwise be 'confounding' and reduce the scientific opportunities of identifying other health risk factors. In Chapter 8, a couple of ways to improve the information base in this respect have been discussed. Another approach to individual related data would be a continuation of the basic study on the smoking habits among Swedes performed in 1963, which was described in Section 4.2 and Chapter 5. The 1963 questionnaire study involved a representative sample of 55 000 Swedes (men and women) in the age group 18–69 years (SCB, 1965) on the initiative of the tobacco company Svenska Tobaks AB. A follow-up survey of the smoking habits was carried out in 1969, and causes of death during the 10-year period up to 1973 have been studied (Cederlöf *et al.*, 1975), providing the data that have been used here to characterize Swedish municipalities with regard to frequency of smokers and for the estimation of lung cancer risk among non-smokers.

The data are recorded on a personal number basis and include information usable for characterizing, for example, geographical areas and socio-economic and occupational groups with regard to smoking habits. They also probably provide the best available basis to establish the associations in Sweden between smoking habits and different diseases and the causes of death. The results obtained for lung cancer incidence are of fundamental importance for the estimation of cancer risk due to radon daughter exposure in houses (Section 10.4) and to exposure to general air pollution in urban areas (Section 10.3).

Another 10-year follow-up of the same sample with regard to causes of death would be highly desirable, as it would give much more definite conclusions than the analysis from the first 10-year period during which relatively few cases of cancer had time to occur in the interesting groups, and the influence of urban factors upon mortality among non-smokers could not be estimated.

As far as passive smoking is concerned there is a need for continued research to provide more precise estimates of risks than has so far been possible (Section 4.2.5). Actual exposures to environmental tobacco smoke should be measured and related to smoking habits in different sections of society and different environments. Further chemical or biological analyses should be carried out to establish the effects of special measures taken to decrease the involuntary exposure to environmental tobacco smoke. Completely separate spaces for smokers and non-smokers would obviously provide good protection against involuntary exposure to environmental tobacco smoke, but in other cases, only measurements can determine what effect has been achieved, if any. The question of indoor air quality is, however, not only one of environmental tobacco smoke and the whole issue is dealt with in more depth in Section 10.5.

10.1.5 Future development

Against the background of the extraordinarily serious health problems related to tobacco smoking, it is reasonable to hope that, in the long term, public awareness of the detrimental effects of tobacco will become so widespread that the present changes in attitude against smoking will accelerate. With active measures to decrease smoking and increased pressure from non-smokers against involuntary exposures to smoke, it should be realistic to expect that within a couple of decades smoking could more or less cease to exist. Any other development in a modern society, with the resources available, should be regarded as a failure.

10.2 Diet and dietary habits

10.2.1 Points of departure

The supply of nutrients and water are essential conditions for human life, and malnutrition can cause special deficiency diseases. Both malnutrition as a result of either overeating or undernourishment and harmful components in the diet can cause or aggravate other diseases. It is now well established that diet plays a role also in relation to cancer diseases, but detailed knowledge is still only fragmentary.

Diet is not a uniform concept. Even very restricted diets can have a varying and complex composition. Physical properties vary too, which might influence the breakdown, absorption and time for passage through the gut.

The major groups of substances that supply the body with energy are proteins, lipids and carbohydrates, which in turn are composed of a large number of components or chemical building blocks. Some of these, such as amino acids and fatty acids, are considered essential for special processes in the body or for building up parts of the cells of the body. Other chemically quite different substances are needed for similar purposes, but only in very small amounts, and are known as trace substances, which include certain metals and vitamins. Some of these may be deleterious to health if taken in large doses.

In addition to these nutrients in the diet, both vegetable and animal material can contain harmful natural substances. Further, raw materials for food production and foods ready for consumption can become contaminated by substances produced by micro-organisms. Other possible sources of contamination are pesticides and components in packing materials. Chemical reactions of naturally occurring compounds or additives during cooking can also generate new substances with carcinogenic properties.

Yet another group of food components are the 'additives'. When chemical substances such as preservatives are to be purposely added to foods, the positive effects of reducing what may be a health hazard from a micro-organism have to be weighed against possible health hazards from the additive itself.

The role of water both in food production and for drinking is also relevant. Environmental conditions at the source as well as the purification process in the waterworks (to combat bacterial pollutants) and the condition of the pipe system can all influence the chemical quality of drinking water.

During the normal metabolism in the body, chemically reactive intermediate products are formed which could in theory act as cancer initiators. Little is at present known about the possible role of such substances in the genesis of cancer.

Individual differences between people—which certainly do play a role in both cancer and other diseases—may be particularly significant for diet. Complicated chemical processes are involved in which the different components of food act as sources of metabolic energy after several transformation steps or are used to build up the components of the body itself.

The question of a relationship between diet and cancer was for a long time concerned mainly with whether single chemical substances, generally in low concentrations as contaminants due to human activities or additives, could carry an increased risk of cancer. In addition, it has become clear that agents produced by certain micro-organisms, in particular the aflatoxins (a type of mould toxin) are very strong experimental carcinogens. Lately, attention has also begun to turn to nutrients in the diet and the question of the importance of the overall composition of the diet —in other words our dietary habits. There are strong indications that inappropriate dietary habits contribute to cancer and that there are also substances in the diet that have a certain protective effect.

For a more comprehensive review of these questions, reference is made to the previous text, especially to Chapters 4 and 6. An extremely comprehensive literature survey with a thorough overview and evaluation is the US report *Diet, Nutrition, and Cancer*, mentioned in Section 4.3 (US National Research Council, 1982) and produced on the initiative of the National Cancer Institute in the USA. The same topic was discussed at a small international conference held in Sweden in 1981 (NFA, 1981).

Epidemiological and experimental studies have together convincingly shown that the diet has great importance for the total cancer incidence, but detailed knowledge so far does not permit accurate quantification. It appears that about one-third of the total cancer incidence in Sweden could be the result of dietary factors (see Chapter 6). This corresponds to roughly 10 000 cases per year, though this number has a considerable margin of uncertainty. This does not mean that diet is the only contributing environmental factor in these cases; usually one or several other factors are likely to have contributed or been necessary for the development of the cancer.

From a preventive point of view, it is important to try to identify what aspects of the diet can be influenced. This must itself build upon knowledge of the importance of different dietary components or habits for development of or protection against cancer diseases. This knowledge is still fragmentary, and has been summarized in Sections 4.3 and 4.4.

With respect to individual dietary components, conclusions on their quantitative influence on cancer incidence must be very cautious, so far. In Chapter 6 high fat intake and/or associated dietary factors were assumed to be a factor in some 5000 cancer cases annually in Sweden.

A medical reason for reducing fat intake has existed for a long time, particularly in relation to cardiovascular diseases. For cancer there are statistical correlations between high fat intake in the diet and several different forms of cancer and, in addition, certain dose–response relationships have been observed (see Section 4.3). It seems reasonably certain that a high fat intake, and/or dietary factors associated with it, plays a substantial role in the incidence of intestinal cancer and breast cancer. It is even possible that this factor is the most important of all environmental factors for these two forms of cancer, which have increased in Sweden, even taking changes in the age distribution into account. Several other forms of cancer have to various degrees been related to the same factor. The statement is supported by the fact that epidemiological as well as animal experimental data point in the same direction. Further, a number of biologically conceivable mechanisms have been proposed for the effect of fat in the body, of which some have received support in biological experiments. It cannot be excluded that different forms of fat have different biological effects, perhaps in association with the composition of the diet besides the fat and the magnitude of the total energy intake. It is therefore essential to find out what fat components and other associated dietary factors imply an increased cancer risk.

In earlier chapters, examples have been given of specific substances in food which can contribute to cancer risks. But, in general, the quantification of such single risk contributions for diet-related cancer cases is still difficult to make. It has to be assumed that what counts is the sum of the effects of what may be a large number of components, naturally occurring, deliberately added or formed by contamination or in preparation of food. The result of deficiency in the diet of possible protective substances against cancer would show up in the statistics as 'more' cancer cases and can accordingly not in principle be separated from other risk factors (causal agents).

Although we might be dealing with a large number of specific risk factors which individually give a comparatively small risk contribution to the total share of diet in cancer incidence, some specific components or groups of components could well turn out to be of greater importance than others. Pesticide residues and additives subject to regulatory testing, as well as drinking water, appear not to play a major role in cancer disease in Sweden. The consumption of alcohol (ethanol) may also be considered in this context, although as a general health problem it is more often referred to as an abuse matter than as a dietary habit. Alcohol has been considered to contribute to perhaps 500 (maximum 1000) cancer cases annually.

Clearly, relationships between diet and cancer are complicated and still poorly understood, but the same goes for the relation between diet and a number of other diseases or effects on health as well. The relation between diet and health from a preventive point of view has until recently attracted remarkably limited research interest all over the world, apart from the nowadays classical deficiency diseases. The major problem in large parts of the world, particularly the developing countries, is the lack of available food, but to a certain extent also the presence of harmful substances in food and beverages. In the developed countries—even with a good supply of nutritive substances and good quality control, at least in principle—there still remain considerable problems, particularly with poor dietary habits. The increase in cardiovascular diseases is probably related to high fat intake and overweight, and here research has made good progress in analysing the risks and benefits from different kinds of fat. This single example shows that with regard to diet, as in many other circumstances, there are wider perspectives within which the cancer diseases must be examined. Measures taken must be optimized within a comprehensive view of health and well-being.

10.2.2 The importance of research on diet for cancer prevention

Research on diet is one of the most important areas in order to increase available knowledge for future cancer prevention.

Diet is probably the environmental factor with which man is in most intimate contact but so far it has largely been neglected from the genotoxic point of view in Sweden. Other equally or more significant aspects of the importance of diet for development of cancer diseases concern different direct or indirect mechanisms of action like influence on the hormonal balance in the body, increased secretion of certain metabolites, influence on the composition and function of the bacterial flora etc. In this context the major nutritional components of the diet are especially discussed. Besides fat, protein intake has been a particular subject of scientific discussions. The possible protective action of certain components of the diet against development of cancer diseases offers an extremely important research field.

Epidemiological investigations are necessary to study associations between environmental factors, in this case diet, and cancer. Long-term programmes with prospective studies of specific relationships should be an important complement to epidemiological monitoring on a routine basis (see Chapters 8 and 15).

The Nordic countries have a particularly suitable socio-political system for such studies to be carried out, as was pointed out in Chapter 8. On the other hand, there can be problems if a studied population is very homogeneous with respect to the variable being studied. If, for instance, the dietary habits are very similar, no statistical association with a disease will be detected even if one does exist. This is an important factor to consider when planning epidemiological studies on diet. In studies of the effects on health of measures taken (see Section 10.2.7) to change the diet over a period of time in a (sufficiently large) group of people, a comparison must be made with a control group in which the dietary habits have changed less, so that possible differences in disease patterns will stand out.

In general the dietary habits of the Swedish population are poorly known. Total food consumption or rather the amount of food available (including waste) is documented in broad figures but the data are not detailed enough to show real variations in consumption betweeen different groups in the population. Studies on food intake need to be conducted more systematically and much more widely than before and the methodology should be brought to the fore, including measures to build up scientific competence in this field. Intensified research to find biological markers for different components of the diet is especially urgent. This could permit more reliable information about dietary intake than hitherto and/or be a cheaper way of getting the relevant data.

For large prospective epidemiological studies of the influence of diet on health, in particular effects like cancer that require a long observation time, good solutions to the methodological problems concerning dietary data become crucial. A special grant has been given in Sweden for the study of these problems, the results of which are expected to influence primarily a major 15 year survey initiated recently and covering some 40 000 persons in the city of Malmö, on the importance of diet and other factors for the origin and development of cancer. This study is being planned in co-operation with the International Agency for Research on Cancer (IARC).

10.2.3 Control of hazardous substances in food

In Sweden, legal control of harmful substances in food applies to marketed food, restaurants and similar outlets but not to food produced privately for one's own use. The legislation makes it possible to control additives, residual amounts of foreign substances, microorganisms and, of course, natural components if they are believed to constitute a health hazard. Water which can be used for food production, in cooking and as drinking water is also included in the legislation, but not water from private wells.

A special category of additives comprises substances intended to increase the nutritive value of the diet, like supplements added in order to protect against different deficiency diseases or other diseases. The law on food in this case serves not only as an instrument *against* harmful factors in the diet but also *for* the introduction of better food in some cases, in that it authorizes the responsible regulatory agency, the National Food Administration, to stipulate 'enrichment' of food.

The control through legislation of harmful substances in food does not differ in principle from other forms of risk control, be it against development of cancer or other health hazards from chemical or physical agents. Chapter 11 looks at the public control machinery including questions such as the responsibility of the producer, testing of chemical substances, availability of exposure data, principles for setting priorities and follow-up of the effectiveness of the measures taken.

Many questions about the role of diet in cancer aetiology seem to lie at the borderline between ordinary legislative risk control and research on the roles of specific components. It is essential that the National Food Administration should have sufficient opportunity to participate actively in scientific work in this area.

In the following, harmful substances will be considered briefly in a context formally outside the food legislation (which does not apply within the home). The *aim* should be the same as for food which is marketed or commercially offered to others, namely to limit possible risks as far as possible (see Chapter 7). The *means* will mainly be general health education or specially directed information about specific risks.

Recommendations to avoid eating or limiting the intake of liver from certain kinds of fish or fish from lakes 'black-listed' because of high mercury contamination may serve as examples of information given to the general public in order to reduce health risks from hazardous substances in food. These official recommendations from the National Food Administration seem to be fairly widely known. There are other examples, however, where policy as well as practical advice aimed at members of the general public have been presented in a much less conspicuous way, and not always as official advice but rather as a staff member's own views. This is illustrated by a comprehensive article in an agency publication series on a number of ways to reduce one's exposure to N-nitroso compounds, which are potent animal carcinogens (Slorach, 1981). It would seem that this type of information deserves more effort towards wide distribution. Admittedly it is often difficult to decide when the scientific evidence about a potential risk, like the probability of occurrence or formation of a hazardous substance in food, is sufficiently clear to give reason for far-reaching measures like a health education campaign with realistic prospects of actually reaching a large number of people (see also Chapter 9). It may be even more difficult when going from special risk situations like pike with increased mercury levels to situations related to human habits and attitudes. This might (in addition to the general composition of the diet) also concern the ways of preparing and storing food in the home. Such risk aspects should be paid more attention in the future in both research and health education.

The national authorities for health and for food need to co-operate closely in matters of informing the public, as well as on issues relating to investigations on food quality and nutritional value from a general health perspective. It would seem natural that the duty for informing the public about potential health risks from hazardous compounds in food should rest with the agency which has the best knowledge about the relevant problem; this would normally be the authority for food. At the field level, it is expected that health education will be considerably expanded in future years, involving more input from regional and local bodies (see Chapter 9). With respect to diet, the central agencies for health and food should be jointly responsible for the 'vertical contacts' and provide a factual base for health education carried out by others, whether with the aim of reducing exposure to specific hazardous components (see above) or of improving dietary habits in general (see Section 10.2.5).

10.2.4 Alcohol habits and alcohol policy

The health and social consequences in society of the present pattern of alcohol consumption are quite devastating. In this wider perspective, the cancer risks associated with alcohol might be considered of less importance. As a single risk factor for the cancer incidence, however, alcohol plays a non-negligible role.

Alcohol is a contributory cause of several forms of cancer. In many cases there is probably a joint action between tobacco smoking and alcohol. In other cases there is reason to believe that ethyl alcohol acts as a carcinogen or co-carcinogen together with other factors. Epidemiologically observed differences between risks with different alcohol-containing drinks are probably related to other specific components derived from either the raw materials or the production processes. The data on human cancer point especially to a correlation with *high* alcohol consumption, though the total alcohol intake has frequently been difficult to assess in these studies. The magnitude of the cancer risk among 'moderate drinkers' is not yet certain but it seems to be small.

The largest intake of alcohol obviously comes through products meant to be drunk, and which constitute food in the meaning of food legislation. Illegal production of alcohol-containing beverages occurs, as well as abuse of alcohol-containing products meant for other purposes. Ethyl alcohol as a risk factor to health is primarily controlled through measures beyond the food legislation.

In Sweden the dangers of alcohol consumption have received attention for several centuries, but the problem still cannot be considered to be under control. Public policy towards alcohol is continuously under debate. Although the impact of alcohol on the development of cancer is now much clearer, it does not seem to call for any special control policy. This is not to say that the cancer risks should be ignored; they should indeed be included in other health education programmes dealing with the health hazards of alcohol (see Chapter 9).

10.2.5 Dietary habits and diet recommendations

Certain recommendations on diet have existed for many years in many countries. In this area there is also international co-operation, for example within the WHO and between the Nordic countries. Originally the work was directed towards indicating levels of intake of certain nutritive components desirable to meet physiological needs 'nutritive recommendations'. The need for changes in the diet for other health reasons is a matter of more recent concern. In the developed countries the 'dietary goal' is a concept with a broader and more practical basis than nutritional physiology data and it aims to decrease the risk for a number of diseases related to luxurious living (Bruce, 1981).

It seems appropriate to label at least certain forms of cancer as diseases related to luxurious living, although the multiple causal factors of these diseases must again be underlined and the causes of a particular cancer disease in individual cases might relate to quite different conditions.

However, quite different diseases, primarily cardiovascular diseases, led WHO experts, for instance, to recommend a limitation of the total fat intake to 30 per cent of the energy intake. In Great Britain a group report (NACNE, 1983) makes the same statement, and also recommends an increased fibre intake when discussing colorectal disorders. The US report *Diet, Nutrition and Cancer* (US National Research Council 1982) is the most comprehensive review of dietary aspects of cancer diseases and has also made some provisional diet guidelines directly aiming at cancer prevention, considering the conditions in the USA. Most of the suggestions should, however, be applicable to other western developed countries; these include a recommended decrease of fat intake, greater emphasis on fruit, vegetables and whole grain products in the daily diet, and moderate drinking.

During the twentieth century, Swedish food consumption has undergone substantial changes, while large differences may have existed between different socio-economic groups. Since the 1920s, consumption of fruit, fruit juice and vegetables has increased while potato and milk consumption has decreased. Meat consumption increased markedly from the beginning of the 1960s while fish and shellfish products have not changed much during a 60-year period. The consumption of fat seems to have tripled (counted from the beginning of the century to 1970) but nowadays it has decreased somewhat from a peak around the year 1960. The average total fat intake for almost 30 years has been at a high level in Sweden, at around 40 per cent of the energy intake. The fat intake calculated in grams per person per day has, however, fluctuated and was, for instance, lower in the late 1960s and early 1970s, with an estimated minimum in 1972 of 115 g per person per day, which by 1982 had risen to 123 g (NAMB, 1984).

In Sweden during the 1970s, a special expert group under the National Board of Health and Welfare studied questions of diet and physical activity as a basis for health education. In several publications it pointed out among other things the importance of overweight, total fat intake and the proportion of polyunsaturated fats for cardiovascular diseases. Recommendations were made that fat should constitute no more than 35 per cent of the total energy supply and included practical advice on how this could be achieved. Some increase in consumption was proposed for fruit and vegetables including potatoes and root crops, fish, non-fatty dairy products, blood-based food products and bread and other grain products.

The traditional type of official recommendations of daily intake of certain nutritive food components was first issued in Sweden decades ago. The present (1981) recommendations from the National Food Administration are designed to form a basis for planning a diet which both satisfies the primary nutritional needs of the body and also provides what is required to ensure general good health and to avoid diet-related diseases. A basic principle is that the diet should contain plenty of variety. The desired division is given for the components needed to supply energy (proteins, fat and carbohydrates) as well as recommendations for the intake of certain vitamins and minerals. Fat ought not to exceed 35 per cent of the energy requirement but should at the same time not fall below 25 per cent according to the National Food Administration. Guidelines for the ratio between polyunsaturated and saturated fatty acids are given, as well as for the intake of essential fatty acids.

It should be noted that the Swedish dietary recommendations just described were drawn up at a time when there was little scientific information on the relevance of the diet for cancer.

Expert judgements on dietary habits have been presented lately in another context as well. In the course of a critical review of present national agricultural policy, including industrial food production, among other things a group was established to especially review the diet–health relationships in this context (DHG, 1984). Again, some changes in the average food intake were said to be desirable. According to this group, the total fat intake ought to be decreased by 5 'energy per cent' until 1990 and then continue to decrease until fat becomes responsible for only about 30 per cent of energy intake by the year 2000. Without otherwise taking up the cancer issue, the group indicates that ongoing research will show what the impact of a reduced fat intake might be for a decrease in risk of occurrence of certain forms of cancer.

The Cancer Committee has given careful thought to the issue of dietary recommendation. It is not reasonable to give such recommendations from the point of view of a limited question like one single disease or group of diseases. The conclusions that can be drawn scientifically about dietary habits which would be desirable in relation to cancer are, however, well in line with the main direction of present Swedish recommendations. These may therefore be qualified in at least one major respect: as matters now stand a reduction of the total fat intake should be given first priority.

In further deliberation, the distinction between recommendations that may be given to the individual and what may constitute a health policy goal for society in general should be stressed.

For the planning of meals in the home and in institutional kitchens, in order to achieve a well-balanced diet for the *individual*, the official recommendations remain the basis. It may be recalled that these include the figure of between 35 and 25 per cent for fat as an energy source (this applies to healthy adults and children above 3 years of age). There is now a proposal by the Cancer Committee to go in the direction of the lower of these two values (25 per cent), providing that the diet satisfies all requirements in other respects. The desired substantial reduction in fat intake must not—in the individual case—lead to a shortage of other nutrients for any reason. It is of particular importance that persons with very high fat intake should reduce their fat consumption.

Since some fat intake is essential for the functions of life, the total fat intake cannot be reduced too far without jeopardizing the energy supply. Many persons either have a present energy intake much higher than the amount they 'burn up' in terms of physical activity and individual metabolism, or are already overweight. In the individual case it may well be that a reduced fat intake ought not to be compensated with other energy-supplying nutrients, unless there is a corresponding increase in physical exercise. Frequently in such cases not only the fat but also the sugar intake is too high compared to the desired intake of other products. It is accordingly important that the comprehensive aspect of diet is emphasized, particularly in health education through all possible channels. Where a reduced fat intake is to be compensated for, under Swedish conditions this ought to be done mainly through an increased intake of grain products and potatoes and preferably also root vegetables.

The long-term *national goal* for societal measures (see Section 10.2.6) should be that the *total fat consumption* is gradually reduced to an average below 30 per cent of the energy intake with an initial, partial goal during the next decade of a reduction to 35 per cent from the present almost 40 per cent.

Among possible protective substances in the diet, the scientific discussions have covered, among others, dietary fibre, vitamin A or its 'precursors' like B-carotene, ascorbic acid (vitamin C), vitamin E and the element selenium (see Section 4.3.4). The positive data available mainly refer to the total diet composition and not single components. It must, therefore, suffice to underline the importance of large food groups, like cereal products, fruit and vegetables. Further, the diet should be varied, so as to ensure that scarcer nutrients are obtained in adequate supply from suitable sources; for example, selenium is a necessary trace element found especially in fish and shellfish. From the point of view of cancer prevention, the basis is not yet strong enough to allow recommendations of specific substances to be used as supplements to a varied diet or added to foodstuffs, but this does not exclude that other reasons for enrichment of foods might exist.

The amount of known or potential carcinogens (characterized as genotoxic substances) should be kept as low as possible in the diet. In part this is a matter for legislative food control rather than for the single individual. However, as far as substances formed during storage, curing or cooking are concerned (Section 4.3.3) the risk of formation of potentially cancer-causing substances at high temperatures means that unnecessarily high temperatures should be avoided in preparation of food, particularly in frying and grilling.

A brief summary of the Cancer Committee's dietary recommendations follows, principally with Swedish conditions in mind.

A reduction of the total fat intake appears to be most urgent at the present time. A probable favourable effect on the incidence of at least certain cancer diseases can be expected to add to other expected benefits, not least with regard to cardiovascular diseases. The planning of diets, adjusted for individual needs, should go towards achieving the lower values given in existing official Swedish recommendations for fat intake (between 35 and 25 per cent of the energy supply); in particular, persons whose fat intake is extremely high should reduce it. The national goal should be to bring down the total fat consumption to an average below 30 per cent of the total energy supply.

Other aspects of the diet are that it should be varied. The importance of fruit and vegetables as well as cereal products should be especially pointed out.

10.2.6 Prerequisites for changes of dietary habits

Dietary habits are a part of people's cultural and social patterns and thus are difficult to change.[1] Certain obvious changes in the food consumption have, however, taken place in Sweden during the last few decades, although little is known about the distribution of such changes over different population groups.

The increasing affluence of society, which means that people can satisfy their hunger easily, also tends to lead to deterioration of the diet in several nutritional respects. If real incomes increase in the future, we have to expect that the consumption with unchanged preferences in households will change towards increased fat intake.

First of all the aim should be to create permanent *changes in attitudes* to dietary habits in the direction stated in the previous section. Health education will be the method of choice (see Chapter 9). Changes in attitudes and possibilities for people to alter their dietary habits can also be facilitated in other ways, such as ensuring that *suitable products are available* on the market, and adjusting the *price structure*.

Good dietary habits are formed in early life. The diet, attitudes and habits of children, not only at home, but also in day care homes and in school canteens are therefore of great importance. Adults too take many of their meals outside their homes. Although positive changes can be noticed in several places through increased availability of vegetables, 'campaign weeks' for a diet of high food value, etc., many restaurants are criticized for boring and fatty food. Large catering facilities, like school kitchens and works canteens, can be reached by specifically targeted information, and continuous education of all members of the public could be encouraged by activities from the health promoting agencies in society.

The supply of products on the market (through the producers of food), the availability (through the distribution network), the demand and prices are all linked together. The price systems should at least not act against encouraging better dietary habits. To some extent a price policy that built in differentiation of consumer prices based on public health principles would probably lead to positive results for dietary habits. However, it is extremely difficult to see how such a price differentiation could be made.

The pricing policy for agricultural products that has been used in Sweden since the 1940s has not included health considerations. Furthermore, several product groups are outside this price regulation system. If price regulation is to be used at all as part of a food policy, then the health aspects ought to be given equal weight with the other goals of that policy. (The same applies, for that matter, to consumer subsidies, which do not exist in Sweden any longer (except for milk) but where, in the past, some were criticized by experts in nutritional physiology for having been adopted without regard to health considerations.) The achievement of desired price relations between different kinds of food products has been mentioned in this context (NAMB, 1984), although its feasibility has not been studied. This idea is based on surcharges *and* subsidies: surcharges on the sale of high-fat products to finance subsidies for other types of products whose consumption one would like to increase.

Product development in both primary production and the food processing industry should be stimulated in different ways. Grants for technical and biological research and development could be one route. Another might be the use of price differentials when new and nutritionally interesting products have been found. It might, for instance, be beneficial to increase the price difference between standard milk and less fatty milk and to achieve a similar price shift for cheese; in the latter case a product development towards lean types of hard cheese with a fuller flavour is urgent (DHG, 1984), not least in view of the high cheese consumption in Sweden. The food legislation has a place in this discussion, especially because it allows the responsible agency to set standards for certain common products (maximal as well as minimal amounts of specified components) which means that new nutritional aspects can influence changes in these standards. The legislation also gives opportunities for improving the declaration of content by means of labelling, which in turn should improve the consumer's chances of selecting food products according to dietary recommendations.

10.2.7 Effects of changing diet

What effect could be expected in terms of cancer diseases if the average fat intake were decreased by about a quarter from today's intake? There certainly would be some effect on the cancer pattern. All the evidence suggests that there would be a decrease in the total cancer incidence as well and at the same time a number of other diseases would be reduced or else be influenced in a favourable way. On the other hand it is hard to make any numerical estimations for single forms of cancer (see Section 6.3). Part of the effect of a changed diet as described will not show up until a very long time has passed. This is also the case, wherever applicable, for positive effects of an increased intake of likely protective substances in the food. If there were to be an obvious decrease of the cancer incidence as a result of reduced fat intake, it should, however, be possible to recognize this within a more limited time, maybe 5–10 years, as a high fat intake is believed to act mainly as a promoter in cancer induction.

The net effect might also be influenced by the way the energy shortfall is compensated for and how the changes vary across the population (it is not likely that this will be uniform). Although we have good reason to expect positive health effects, unexpected side-effects cannot be excluded in advance.

With all possible measures for cancer prevention follow-up studies are essential (Chapter 7). They are particularly important when the measures taken are profound. They are also important in for example, dietary habits and their relevance to health, where the scientific basis for change is incomplete but where actions still are considered urgent.

The first obvious task is to establish whether real changes do take place in dietary habits. Follow-up studies are then needed to monitor health effects (see also Chapters 8 and 15). Planning and execution of these epidemiological studies should constitute an integral part of the strategy for action from the start. In this way the influence of dietary habits and different components of the diet on the occurrence of various forms of cancer over time and on the total cancer incidence should be illustrated. It is important that the studies should be planned in such a way as to permit the investigation of possible effects upon other diet-related diseases at the same time. In order to gain a complete picture of the social consequences of the measures adopted, it would also be valuable to study economic or other effects on the food production system.

It is difficult to assess the economic consequences of dietary changes to individual households and to national production and trade, particularly agriculture and the food industry. Moderate changes of dietary habits by the individual, including reduction of the total fat intake by a few percentage units and a certain increase in intake of other products such as cereals, would not imply cost increases to Swedish households. After some time the agricultural production would probably adjust itself towards the national consumption pattern. Based on the present national agriculture policy and price regulations (1983), a reduced demand for certain agricultural products as discussed by the Cancer Committee would imply a considerable drop of income in the agricultural sector on a long-term perspective, according to expert judgement obtained (NAMB, 1984). Price aspects as well as other food policy matters are at present being reconsidered in Sweden.

10.3 General Air Pollution

10.3.1 Background and general considerations

A person inhales about 20 m^3 air per 24 hours, and carcinogenic or otherwise harmful substances in the air constitute a potential health hazard. Inhaled air pollutants may have a local effect on the lungs and airways and/or effects on other organs in the body as substances are spread via the blood and lymphatic routes.

Many factors affect the air quality in built-up areas, including exhaust from traffic, domestic heating and other energy production, industrial processes, waste incineration and so on. In addition to this general air pollution, many people suffer further exposure to substances in the air at their workplaces from processes or products used there. The cancer risks from such occupational exposures have been discussed in Section 6.7.

In Section 4.4 examples have been given of levels of air pollution for substances of interest from the point of view of cancer. Available information of this kind is extremely limited and its representativeness often dubious. In a few cases, it is clear that the average individual dose through inhalation of a particular substance is up to several multiples of 10 higher in the work environment, although estimated contributions to collective doses for the total or parts of the population may be greatest from the general environment (Tables 4.17 and 4.18).

Airborne substances that are not rapidly broken down reach soil or water and human exposure can result from eating products thus contaminated. The highest levels are generated mainly near industrial establishments, in urban settlements or close to roads carrying heavy traffic. The total population dose of individual substances emitted as air pollutants can be larger from polluted food than from inhaled air, although the absolute figure may still be low (see the entry for benzo[a]pyrene in Table 4.18).

The increasing acidification of soil and water is another risk factor, which is mainly caused by oxidation products of sulphur and nitrogen in rainfall and dry deposition. This effect is caused by both close and distant sources. The acidification can cause metals with toxic properties to become dissolved from sediment etc. Available data on metal concentrations in water give no reason to suggest that cancer risks will have increased so far (see Section 4.3.6) but the development has to be monitored. If the acidification causes increased uptake of toxic products by plants or animals destined for human consumption, there may be further risks to health.

Much of the general air pollution in urban areas today is due to motor vehicles. The contribution from energy production in permanent installations varies depending on distance, and on the construction, type of fuel, etc., of the installation.

With respect to detrimental health or environmental effects, one and the same probable causal factor may originate from more than one type of source. As a rule it is difficult to differentiate between such potential sources by means of chemical or epidemiological methods.

Particles containing polyaromatic hydrocarbons or their biologically active transformation products, or gaseous agents of possible relevance for cancer risks in the urban environment like unsaturated hydrocarbons and nitrogen oxides, are formed in all combustion of organic material, although motor vehicles are probably the most important source. Other substances are almost specific for one source, such as lead from lead-containing fuel and sulphur oxides from combustion of oil and coal.

In Section 6.6, an estimate of the importance of general air pollutants for the number of cancer cases in Sweden has been presented. The fact that the air pollutants include a large number of mutagenic and cancer initiating agents means—if the dose-response relationships are presumed to be linear—that these air pollutants do cause an increased cancer risk. The question is the magnitude of this risk.

It is primarily the *lung cancer* risk in urban areas that has been scientifically studied although results have been rather contradictory. Taken together they suggest a certain risk contribution from urban air pollutants but are not sufficient to prove it. However, the statistical methods are by nature very insensitive. In this case the effects of general air pollution also include contributions from tobacco smoke in the environment which are not easily separated.

At two international meetings of scientists in Stockholm (1977 and 1982) the conclusion was that 'combustion products of fossil fuels in ambient air, probably acting together with cigarette smoke, have been responsible for cases of lung cancer in large urban areas, the numbers produced being of the order of 5–10 cases per 100 000 males per year (European standard population)'. In spite of the large uncertainty in this estimate it probably constitutes the best basis available for risk estimation and risk policy. In addition there are the risks of *other forms of cancer*, but in this case the data are even more limited.

The Cancer Committee has estimated that the total number of cancer cases (men and women) in Sweden caused by general air pollution in urban areas falls within the range of roughly 100–1000 cases per year. The average risk in the whole of Sweden for cancer from general air pollution in urban areas will, therefore, be around 1–10 per 100 000 person years. If it is assumed for simplicity that only the quarter of the population which lives in cities is so exposed (and that all members of this population are exposed to the same degree), the cancer risk in the exposed population becomes four times higher. It is probable that many people will regard this as a low and acceptable *personal risk* compared to their judgement of the corresponding benefits. However, particularly because we are largely dealing with involuntary exposure (see Chapter 7), this risk is high enough to warrant a discussion on means to reduce general air pollution. The large *total number of cancer cases* that might be caused by air pollution also justify preventive measures to be taken wherever technically and economically feasible.

Plans for measures against air pollution should not be based only on the above estimate of cancer risk. Other risks to the health and the environment have been in the foreground for a long time. In taking decisions on such matters as choice of energy systems, all risks, and possibilities for their reduction, need to be considered for all kinds of energy sources and through all the processes involved, including any air pollutants generated.

In an attempt to reduce their dependency on oil, many countries have increased their coal consumption. In Sweden the central agency responsible for energy supply the National Power Administration (NPA, 1983) reported on health and other environmental problems connected with the use of coal and how they could be reduced. Energy production in stationary installations by combustion of fossil fuels (oil and to a lesser degree coal) is responsible for a high proportion of the total amount of the general air pollutants in Sweden. This includes pollutants passing over the frontiers from other countries, mainly sulphur and nitrogen pollutants and certain toxic heavy metals. One aspect of increased health risks is a delayed exposure to genotoxic and often hazardous substances, for example through the food chain via air pollution but also from coal ash maybe generations later. Another aspect is the effect of direct exposure to air pollutants generated in this context, where the uncertainty about the role of NO_x emission for cancer risks may be mentioned (Törnqvist, 1984). Increased use of coal will lead to increased emission of nitrogen unless very efficient technology for reduction of such emissions is used. In 1984 the Swedish Parliament concurred with a government proposal on guidelines for the use of coal to 1990, so far implying only a 'cautious interduction' with a limited use level per year.[2] In this report, the Cancer Committee generally concludes that combustion of organic material (oil, coal, peat, wood, etc.) always produces pollutants including potential carcinogens. In accordance with the policy recommended (Chapter 7) emissions from all combustion processes should be reduced as far as possible.

The air pollution problem caused by vehicle exhausts has been studied in Sweden by a special government appointed committee, which reported in 1983. The measures proposed by this committee to combat exhaust pollution are outlined in the following section.

10.3.2 Car exhausts

The Car Exhausts (C Ex) Committee, according to the terms of reference, based its proposals on a comprehensive view of both health and environmental risks (C Ex Committee, 1983). Later in the same year the Committee strengthened its recommendations for measures to reduce exhaust pollution, with reference to the rapid changes in informational development on the European scene.

The C Ex Committee proposed (*a*) an action programme with regard to Sweden and (*b*) that discussions be initiated to achieve as wide an international agreement as possible on such an action programme.

The major proposals concerned:

(*a*) the fuel;
(*b*) emission limits for light vehicles;
(*c*) emission limits for heavy vehicles;
(*d*) air quality criteria;
(*e*) local authority actions;
(*f*) continued research and development.

It was thus recommended that unleaded petrol (maximum lead level, 0.013 gl^{-1}) should be introduced in parallel with leaded petrol, so that each station with two pumps or more should supply unleaded petrol; the petrol tax should be somewhat reduced for unleaded petrol.

Stricter requirements for exhaust cleaning with regard to light vehicles were initially to follow two parallel lines. As an obligatory minimum, new requirements decided in another European country (quoted as 'Switzerland –87'), but then not yet in practical application, should apply to petrol-driven cars from the 1988 year model, according to this proposal. The more far-reaching federal demands in the USA (quoted as 'US–83') for both petrol-driven and other passenger cars should be acknowledged simultaneously to make certification, delivery and purchase of such cars legal in Sweden. The special vehicle taxes should be differentiated to stimulate purchase of cars meeting the US–83 demands. Another recommendation was to extend the car manufacturer's responsibility for vehicle performance with respect to emission limits. For heavy vehicles, the major recommendation was to introduce the corresponding 1983 federal US requirements as obligatory in Sweden. Guidelines for air quality should be issued with concentration limits for carbon monoxide, nitrogen dioxide and ozone. Locally, municipal authorities should be supported, through guidelines, in their efforts to reduce discomfort and other disturbances from the traffic. For the same purpose they should also be given a legal right to impose special fees on motor vehicle traffic.

The main reason why the Car Exhausts Committee did not consider it feasible to introduce the US requirements as obligatory for light vehicles immediately, was that they—in contrast with the proposed requirements for Switzerland—necessitate advanced catalytic exhaust cleaning on cars, which in turn requires unleaded fuel. It would be essential that unleaded fuel should become available in neighbouring countries at the same time.

It turned out later that several of these countries were already discussing the introduction of unleaded fuel alongside leaded fuel. The committee responsible therefore modified its original proposal and said it should be feasible without much delay to make the US–83 requirements mandatory in Sweden on all petrol-driven cars with a maximum loaded weight not exceeding 3500 kg.[3]

It is difficult to compare the effects of different possible exhaust cleaning requirements, among other things because the test procedures differ considerably, but Table 10.1 shows estimates of the release of certain regulated pollutants from petrol-driven cars under different exhaust control regimes relative to the levels from new cars under existing Swedish requirements (1984), all values referring to tests according to the latter (A10) regulations.

The total emissions from petrol-driven cars will change quite slowly even if we assume that all new such cars after 1988 would have catalytic exhaust cleaning, as the cars presently in use will be only slowly replaced. Table 10.2 shows the estimated effects on car exhaust pollution in city centres that might be achieved by the year 2000 compared to the situation in 1980.

Table 10.1 Relative emissions (%) per petrol-driven car according to different car exhaust(s) requirements estimated for A10 tests[a]

Regulations[b]	New cars (6400 km)			Used cars (80 000 km)		
	Carbon monoxide	Hydrocarbons	Nitrogen oxides	Carbon monoxide	Hydrocarbons	Nitrogen oxides
A10 (present Swedish)[c]	100	100	100	145	150	115
ECE 15/04[d]	115	140	150	155	195	155
US-83[e]	30	20	25	75	65	60
Switzerland–87[f]	40	40	60	95	95	85

[a] For reference see the NEPB (1981).
[b] Information in notes below pertains to the situation in the early 1980s and more stringent rules are generally in force. [*Ed. note.*]
[c] From the 1976 car models the following emission limits are in force (A10 tests) in Sweden for petrol-driven cars of a maximum loaded weight up to 2500 kg and a cylinder volume of at least 0.8 litre:
  carbon monoxide (max.) 24.2 g km^{-1};
  hydrocarbons (max.) 2.1 g km^{-1};
  nitrogen oxides (max.) 1.9 g km^{-1}.
  Stringent conformity of production test schemes apply.
[d] Proposed requirements for the EEC. Emission limits relate to a test regime very different from the A10 and vary with vehicle weight.
[e] From the 1983 car models the following emission limits (according to US 83 test procedures) apply in the USA for passenger cars of a maximum loaded weight up to 2720 kg (6000 lb), irrespective of fuel:
  carbon monoxide 2.1 g km^{-1} (3.4 g mile^{-1});
  hydrocarbons 0.25 g km^{-1} (0.41 g mile^{-1});
  nitrogen oxides 0.62 g km^{-1} (1.0 g mile^{-1});
  particulates 0.37 g km^{-1} (0.6 g mile^{-1}).
[f] Proposed requirements for Switzerland. Initially based on the same requirements as the present Swedish ones, they imply the following reduced emission limits:
  carbon monoxide 9.3 g km^{-1};
  hydrocarbons 0.9 g km^{-1};
  nitrogen oxides 1.2 g km^{-1}.
From the C Ex Committee (1983).

The actual differences in total pollutant concentrations (at street level) from the concentrations according to the different emission control requirements will be less than indicated above if it is presumed that contributions from heavy duty diesel vehicles and stationary sources do not change much.

The C Ex Committee also presented some calculations of the costs of introducing new rules for exhaust control in Sweden, compared to present regulations in that country. Petrol consumption would be, for example, between 3 and 5 per cent less with the proposed regulations for the EEC (ECE 15/04) and anything between 9 per cent less and 2 per cent more with the US–83 requirements. In the latter case the cost of unleaded fuel has to be added and often also the cost of an increased petrol consumption by about 3 per cent because the unleaded fuel used has a lower octane number. However, petrol consumption on average was not noticeably affected by the US–83 requirements. Production costs, i.e. manufacturing of components, would be slightly less with the ECE 15/04 requirements but would increase with the US–83 stipulations by about 3000 Sw.Kr (1981 costs; equivalent to about US$600 for that same year).

Table 10.2 Estimated effects of different exhaust requirements for petrol-driven cars under practical driving conditions (in city centres). The table shows changes in emissions (per cent), at 0°C, from an 'average' car in the year 2000 compared with 1980. See also notes for Table 10.1.

Regulations	Carbon monoxide	Nitrogen oxides
A10 (present Swedish)	−35	−10
Switzerland 87	−55	−25
US 83	−70	−65

From the National Environmental Protection Board, in the NIEM (1983).

The health aspects were investigated separately by the National Institute of Environmental Medicine (NIEM 1983). This study deals with:

(a) substances which affect mainly the respiratory system (sulphur-oxides and particles, nitrogen oxides, ozone and other oxidants);
(b) substances in car exhausts which cause systemic toxic effects (carbon monoxide and lead);
(c) cancer risks;
(d) annoyance reactions (these already become relevant before demonstrable medical effects appear);[4]

The Institute points out that recommended values for environmental air quality (air quality criteria) are built up from the lowest adverse effect levels that often are unreliable and with very small safety margins. These air quality criteria have frequently not taken into account tendencies to possible effects at very low concentrations which indeed have not been verified in other studies but not rejected either, nor possible interactive effects between different factors such as individual chemical substances.

In urban communities there is excess morbidity in several diseases, including chronic bronchitis. Even if this excess morbidity can be explained by other factors such as tobacco smoking, there are indications that air pollution plays a role which may be substantial though it cannot be accurately quantified. Urban air certainly contains a number of substances that are mutagenic and/or carcinogenic, which according to the Institute might at least in part explain the finding in epidemiological studies that lung cancer is more common in urban than in rural areas. The Institute also draws special attention to the results from studies performed in Sweden of annoyance reactions which show that 'today's situation must be considered as clearly alarming'. High frequencies of annoyance have been registered and their relation to car exhaust seems to be beyond doubt. The results of the annoyance studies also suggest that substantial groups of sensitive persons suffer far more than average and indicate that the air pollution might aggravate some respiratory tract symptoms even if clinical tests have not shown any association between these effects and air pollutants.

The risk of cancer is only one of several health aspects of general air pollutants, in particular those originating from traffic. However, since matters concerning cancer risks and prevention are the task of the Cancer Committee, the proposals made by the C Ex Committee will be examined in that particular context in the following.

The National Institute of Environmental Medicine had not attempted to quantify the *total* cancer risk connection with general air pollution in urban areas. Neither the Institute nor the C Ex Committee has therefore tried to estimate the impact on the cancer incidence of the proposed measures to reduce exposure to car exhausts, a caution which seems highly justified.

Test runs have been carried out with differently equipped cars and with different types of fuel, during which various chemical components in the exhaust were quantitatively analysed. In addition, the mutagenic activity of substances (mainly particles) in the exhaust has been studied in short-term tests. These reports allow some conclusions to be drawn regarding possible consequences of changed composition of car exhaust. As the number of cars tested is small, it is the trend in the changes that is significant rather than the numerical values.

It is of particular interest to look at the result of the comparison between a petrol-driven passenger car equipped for Swedish exhaust regulations (A10) and using fuel of the type currently available (1984), and a car equipped for US exhaust requirements (US-83) with a so-called three-way catalyst and lambda-probe (closed loop) driven on unleaded fuel. As the idea behind catalytic exhaust cleaning is to increase combustion of the exhaust products from the work of the engine, there is reason to expect a considerable decrease of the exhaust components that are emitted from petrol-driven cars today. (The ultimate products from combustion of organic material from fossil fuels are ideally carbon dioxide and water, while nitrogen-containing compounds are transformed into nitrogen.)

The *chemical analyses* from the test drive show, with one exception (acetaldehyde), a large reduction in the levels of all analytically determined components, many of which are substances important from a cancer viewpoint, like hydrocarbons (unspecified), nitrogen oxides and polycyclic aromatic hydrocarbons. Also, specific hydrocarbons like ethylene and benzene decrease radically with catalytic exhaust cleaning. The mutagenic and carcinogenic activity which to a varying degree is associated with such substances should, therefore, decrease substantially in the exhaust if the US exhaust cleaning norms for petrol-driven cars are introduced. The *mutagenicity tests* with quantative comparisons indicate the same, but a warning should be given against drawing more general conclusions on differences in risk size, for example to man, based on these tests only. Taking all information into consideration it seems reasonable to assume, however, that a changeover to catalytic exhaust cleaning will in fact mean a decrease of the risk of human gentic damage and cancer, although this is not scientifically proven.

Petrol and diesel exhausts contain mutagenic or carcinogenic substances in both particulate and gasous phases. Calculated per kilometre, diesel cars emit more 'mutagenic activity' (as calculated in Ames test) in the particulate phase than petrol-driven cars without catalytic cleaning, which in turn emit more than petrol-driven cars with catalytic cleaning. The contribution of the gaseous phase to the total mutagenic activity is lower for diesel cars than for petrol-driven cars. As there are different substances that cause the mutagenic activity studied in diesel and petrol exhausts, more exact comparisons between the two types of fuel are difficult to make. Epidemiological studies on garage and railway workers exposed to diesel exhausts have not shown any excess cancer of the respiratory tract. These studies have major methodological shortcomings; they provide in any case no support for the idea that such exposure is associated with any serious cancer risk. Epidemiological and animal experimental studies are beginning to shed light upon the carcinogenic effects of diesel exhaust compared to other sources of air pollution, but they are quite limited and cannot serve as a basis for risk assessments (see Ehrenberg and Törnqvist, 1984; NIEM, 1983).

In evaluating different scenarios for the exhaust situation in urban areas, the C Ex Committee assumed that the share of the traffic workload and emissions of diesel-driven vehicles are largely the same as today. This is because none of the future norms proposed above implies any substantial change in the exhaust emissions from diesel-driven vehicles. In the US, stricter norms for emissions from diesel vehicles are being discussed (1984) which might in the long run mean a reduction of these emissions.

In Sweden, a first step towards reducing the lead content in petrol was taken about 15 years ago. The matter of continued reduction and the introduction of unleaded fuel (diesel fuel is not leaded) is related to the introduction of catalytic exhaust cleaning on new cars but should also be looked at separately. A significant proportion of existing car models could be run on unleaded fuel without adjustment of the engines. If drivers were to change over to such fuel, the total exposure to different lead-components would decrease somewhat further (genotoxic halogenic compounds, which are put in with the lead additive as so-called scavengers, would also disappear from the fuel). The health effects that can be caused by lead are serious (as summarized in NIEM (1983). Mostly these effects are other than cancer but the risk of tumour induction in humans cannot be excluded. There is every reason to reduce exposure to lead via petrol as far as possible, even though the contribution of this source to the total body burden of lead cannot be quantified.

With reference to its general considerations in Section 10.3.1, the further discussion on several health aspects in this Section, and on other large-scale environmental effects, not least of nitrogen oxides from the traffic, the *Cancer Committee's own conclusion* is to support, in principle, the proposals summarized above.

This means, among other things, that the most efficient possible method for exhaust cleaning (catalytic cleaning convertion) on cars should be introduced as soon as possible in order to comply with regulations matching the requirements in the USA. The technology is tested and experience exists of what these requirements entail. Cars with that kind of equipment can only run on unleaded fuel, which is another advantage from the health point of view. Also, unleaded fuel should be available and used wherever technically feasible for existing car models.

Diesel driven vehicles are hardly affected by the proposals. The role of diesel use for different health hazards needs to be examined as well as the improvement of diesel technology to decrease the emissions.

If the proposals on car exhausts are put into effect, cancer risks can be expected to be reduced considerably. However, the scientific basis is lacking to calculate the magnitude of an expected effect. Continued research is urgently needed into the mutagenic and carcinogenic effects of different exhaust components and of their chemical or photochemical reaction products, in particular to quantify the risks. As far as possible, effects of measures taken to decrease emissions should be monitored by quantitative epidemiological studies of different health—and annoyance reactions.

10.4 Radon in houses

10.4.1 Uncertainty in risk assessment

Radon is one of several elements in the disintegration chain of uranium, and therefore exists naturally in the earth's crust. It is a gas, but disintegrates rapidly into other non-gaseous elements (radon daughters) [5] which further disintegrate until a stable product is formed (an isotope of lead) (see Section 4.5, Box 4). The risks are mainly associated with the alpha radiation which is emitted when an atom is transformed into the next substance in the chain. (A certain risk contribution in houses is also due to the gamma radiation from building materials.)

Like other forms of ionizing radiation, alpha radiation leads to a cancer risk in people exposed in a way that permits the radiation to reach the genetic material (DNA) in cells which are able to divide. Radon-daughter inhalation leads to increased risk of lung cancer if the so-called basal cells are 'hit'. The short range of alpha radiation (about twice the diameter of the cell) leads to great difficulty in estimating the dose received by the relevant cells at a given level of exposure during a certain time. For this reason, risk assessments have to be based on epidemiological data for associations between radon daughter levels in air and lung cancer incidence. In this respect the radon risk problem differs from other radiation risk situations where the risks are calculated from estimates of radiation dose using accepted risk coefficients for doses in different organs. The association between radon exposure level and lung cancer incidence has so far been determined with satisfactory certainty only for certain mining populations.

Naturally occurring radiation from radon in the outdoor environment forms part of the unavoidable background radiation. The level of radon outdoors is low irrespective of the character of the ground. However, during recent decades it has been increasingly noticed that the radon levels indoors could be substantially elevated. Building material, above all gas concrete based on shale, in combination with bad ventilation, was for a long time considered to be the main cause of the increased levels of radon that were being measured. The production of this gas concrete was discontinued in 1975. As late as in the beginning of 1981, however, it became obvious that a flow of radon from the soil can play a more important role than previously realized. At that time houses with extremely high radon levels had been found, which could not be explained by the building material alone. The properties of the ground, the method of construction and the ventilation indoors all influence the level of radon in the indoor air. The highest levels have been identified in basements and ground floors in houses.

Measurements of indoor radon levels have also been made in some other countries. The average levels in Sweden and also in Finland are rather high although certain results from other countries have also shown high values; however, Denmark, with different geological conditions, shows low values.

In assessing the risks as in other similar cases, the biological effects of the agent concerned, in this case alpha radiation, and the magnitude of the exposure have to be taken into account. Further, special attention needs to be given to any trends in the change of exposure levels, not least due to a lower air turnover indoors.

With regard to actual exposure levels, there is uncertainty concerning:

(a) The representativity of the measurements (which can be influenced by, for example, the ventilation conditions) and to some extent also concerning the accuracy of the measuring methods.
(b) Transformation of measured values of radon into radon daughter values, which give a better measure of the amount of alpha-emitting material that could be inhaled. As a general rule, the levels of radon daughters are given as 0.5 × the radon level, but this relation varies, depending, for instance, on the dust conditions and tissue doses in those cell layers in the lungs where the cell division takes place (see above).

Radon daughter levels in a recent statistical sample of Swedish houses averaged 53 Bq/m^{-3} indoor air. Previous measurements indicate that the average radon daughter level has increased during recent decades but the comparability of the measurements (for instance choice of houses) is uncertain. However, it seems likely that the levels really have increased, due to the use of new building materials, different construction methods and/or decreased ventilation. It is difficult to determine the exact magnitude of the increase; an increase by a factor of around 3 (2–4) compared with the 1950s seems plausible. It must be expected that the cancer risks will have increased due to this and that the number of radon-associated lung cancers will therefore increase in the future.

Section 4.5 examined different estimates of the size of the lung cancer risk from radon in houses, the risk assessment for Swedish exposure conditions being made by the National Institute of Radiation Protection (NIRP).

The NIRP estimates that the radon exposure in Swedish buildings today may in the future cause some 1100 cases of lung cancer annually, with an uncertainty factor of 3 either way. This gives a range of 300–3000 cases. For the reasons mentioned above the uncertainty is probably even greater than suggested.

As yet there is no satisfactory way of making a risk estimate in this context. Epidemiological studies on miners show clearly enough that radon exposure can cause lung cancer in man and there is no reason to doubt that the same will be true for radon exposure in houses. The essential question is therefore not *whether* radon in houses constitutes a risk but *how large* that risk is. Some uncertainty in extrapolating from the miners' data relates to whether, in moving from high to low exposures, there is simple proportionality between dose and response (a linear dose–response relationship); most evidence supports such an extrapolation for alpha radiation. Much greater uncertainty lies in the quantitative risk assessment itself for miners and in the fact that respiratory physiology conditions, the particle concentration in the air and exposure in mines to other carcinogens than radon may influence the risk. Also, tobacco smoke, which is the dominant cause of lung cancer, may influence the risk assessment. If tobacco smoking and radon exposure do act together synergistically (which some studies on miners suggest (see Figure 4.12)), the same radon exposure level might cause a low risk in a non-smoker but a much higher risk in a smoker.

With reference to its considerations given in Section 4.5 the Cancer Committee is of the opinion that the lower limit of the risk interval suggested by NIRP (about 300 lung cancer cases annually in the future—at present radon daughter concentrations in indoor air in houses) appears more realistic than the estimate of 1100 cases annually and the value could be as low as 100 cases per year. Thus the expected number of new cases per year might be around 300 with a factor of 3, giving a range of some 100–1000 cases. On the other hand, as long as a risk assessment cannot be based on sufficiently extensive epidemiological studies of the association between cancer incidence and levels of radon daughters in homes it is not possible from a scientific point of view to assert that the true risk is really lower than that calculated by NIRP.

The only way to improve on this estimate will be to carry out an epidemiological study of radon levels and lung cancer incidence, and this will be discussed in the next section. Meanwhile, however, it seems clear that radon in buildings does constitute a health problem which could be serious, and it is therefore necessary to decide straight away what measures should be taken during the period before the results from such a study become available. The basis for these measures will have to be the relatively unreliable existing data and the risk assessments made from these data.

10.4.2 Epidemiological study of the association between lung cancer and radon

Epidemiological pilot studies have been carried out in Sweden aiming at illustrating how comprehensive epidemiological studies could demonstrate an association between exposure to radon daughters in houses and lung cancer (unpublished material reported by the Radon Committeee (1983), see Section 10.4.3). Different methods for data collection were considered, as well as the size of study needed simply in order to establish whether or not an association exists. A comprehensive epidemiological study concerning lung cancer needs to take into account a large number of factors both separately and in interaction. Such interactive effects require far more extensive statistical data in the studies done so far.

The Cancer Committee is of the opinion that it is urgent to try to estimate, by means of a well-planned epidemiological study, the magnitude of the cancer risk due to radon in Swedish houses. It is not expected that epidemiological studies in other countries will lead within a reasonable time to new research results which would be transferable to Swedish conditions.

The association between radon exposures and lung cancer risks could be examined by means of so-called ecological studies in which the relation between the average radon concentrations in different geographical areas such as municipalities and lung cancer incidence is studied. Studies of that type might have some value as supplementary indication and might allow estimation of an upper level of the magnitude of the risk. On the other hand such a study can never unequivocally show a causal association. For that purpose analytical epidemiological studies with exposure data linked to individuals are needed. The only realistic possibility at present seems to be case–control studies, in which exposure conditions for a number of lung cancer patients are compared with those of control persons without lung cancer. This opinion is shared by a US expert group which has been working for the US Environmental Protection Agency (Rasmussen et al., 1981). A cohort study (a study where the starting point is the exposed individuals) would need to include hundreds of thousands or even millions of persons to give a clear-cut result. To define such a group (cohort) retrospectively, and to survey the radon exposures, smoking habits and occupational exposures, etc., seems impossible. For Swedish conditions this does not preclude, however, that certain register studies might be of value, and this point will be touched upon again later.

The model for a case–control study that is considered most suitable would use questionnaires to collect data about cases and controls concerning their home addresses, types of houses, smoking habits, occupations and jobs held (including job locations) for a long time (perhaps 30 years) (longitudinal data). Both the weight as evidence and the statistical power of such a study will gain from the inclusion of a large number of variables. Conditions related to passive smoking should also be looked into. The study should be carried out for males and females separately, as conditions might be different with regard to time spent in the home, active and passive smoking, occupational exposure and so on. Information about the individuals' radon exposure has to be collected by other methods, mainly by the measurement of radon concentrations in the buildings.

A major difficulty in radon epidemiological studies is the retrospective determination of radon exposures. Not only is measurement of present levels technically difficult and expensive but changes in ventilation habits, ventilation systems and building construction methods may have changed the radon concentrations substantially. However, there is almost universal opinion that you have to use specific measurement data, which in practical terms means using present radon levels to try to estimate past radon exposures. It might also be possible to estimate indirectly the indoor radon concentration using data about building types and possibly the underground radon levels, which would simplify the calculation of exposures, but this needs to be further studied (see the discussion below about a possible register study).

The sample size needed in a case-control study depends of course on a number of factors, such as how accurately the radon exposures and other aetiological factors related to lung cancer (especially smoking) can be measured, what level of risk increase the study aims to detect statistically and the exactness with which the size of the risk coefficient is to be determined. In the above mentioned US report, 4500 cases and 4500 controls were proposed as a suitable number for detecting a 10 per cent increase in risk. The cost of such a study was estimated at US$9 million and the study was supposed to be completed within 9 years. Since indoor radon concentrations in Sweden are higher than in the USA it is possible that a Swedish study with the same goals would not need such a large sample. To demonstrate a difference in risk of some 50 per cent between the exposure categories—more of a qualitative than a quantitative level of ambition—would probably require some 500 cases, and 1000 controls (Radon Committee, 1983).

However, such a study, with its limited goal, may be seen only as a first attempt. As for the rest the Cancer Committee has not wanted to determine the precise requirements for a radon epidemiological study in Sweden; the discussion in Box 1 might provide some guidelines, though.

There are good reasons for developing and carrying out the study step by step, if necessary modifying the plans in the light of early experience and results. The analysis could be improved by histological classification of the lung cancer cases. All this will also influence the actual cost of the study. It is not possible at present to make a detailed cost assessment for an epidemiological study on radon of sufficient size. A sum in the region of 10 million Sw. kr (US$1.5 million) seems to be realistic as a maximum amount for a meaningful study and is not

Box 1

In order to establish the aims and detailed plans for a study recommended by the Cancer Committee on elevated on lung cancer risks from indoor radon—or for any other comparable study—it is essential to understand what is meant by 'the demonstration of' a certain excess risk due to a certain exposure. Two factors will determine the planning, in particular with regard to the size of the material that is needed:

(a) the real magnitude of the excess risk is not known;
(b) the smallest excess in risk that the study should be capable of detecting has to be decided—after considerations especially of the need for comprehensive cancer preventive measures if the risk is found to be higher than this detection limit.

Bearing these points in mind, if it is felt necessary to detect at least some 200 radon-related lung cancer cases per year throughout the Swedish population, this would correspond to some 10 per cent of the present number of just over 2000 cases per year (in 1979). As the present exposure levels may be 2–4 times higher than when the present lung cancer cases were initiated, 200 cases today correspond to a future incidence of some 600 cases per year. This may be compared with the estimate by the NIRP that the true number in the future will be between 300 and 3000 cases annually due to radon in houses.

The 'statistical power', defined as the probability of detecting this increase in risk with a given level of significance, will increase with the size of the sample. Both the level of significance aimed at and the statistical power required must be decided in relation to the importance of the risk factor in society.

If a statistical power of 90 per cent and significance level of 5 per cent are chosen, the size of the sample needed can be calculated (provided there are no major confounding factors or uncertainties in the measurement of exposure). What these values imply, if the true excess risk is 10 per cent, is the following. Due to random variation in the sampling, there will be a 90 per cent chance (which is the statistical power) of being able to conclude that the excess risk is greater than zero. If you are lucky you may get a quite good estimate (from the point of view of risk protection) of the size of the risk, for example 10 per cent (with a confidence interval of 5–15 per cent) or 15 per cent (with a confidence interval of 10–20 per cent). But you may instead determine it as 5 per cent (with the lower confidence limit close to 0 per cent and the upper

> around 10 per cent (in which case additional studies might be considered necessary to estimate more precisely the size of the excess risk)).
>
> It should be emphasized that a statistical power of 90 per cent is rather low for an important question like this. It means that the likelihood is as high as 10 per cent (100 per cent–90 per cent) that the study will 'miss' a real 10 per cent excess risk, which means that it will be unable to detect that it is higher than zero (e.g., because values of some 3 per cent with a confidence interval of −2 to +8 per cent will turn up). Even a 5 per cent significance is weak: it implies that you are ready to draw a conclusion that a real risk exists with a likelihood of one in 20 even if in reality it is zero or close to zero. The values mentioned here for statistical degree of certainty and level of significance are, however, considered good enough for a first attempt.
>
> If the true excess risk were considerably higher, it could be detected with a smaller sample, which is an important reason to do a stepwise study. This is an accepted statistical method which should be applied, in particular, with very large and expensive studies. Two basic requirements for such a stepwise study should be mentioned: firstly, the statistical analyses have to be made in size-predetermined sub-samples, as parts of the expected total material; secondly, the study has to be planned to ensure that the sub-samples examined in the different steps are taken at random from the expected total material. If these requirements are not met the rules for significance estimation cease to be valid.

unreasonable taking into consideration the great health and political impact and the importance for the national economy. The study would probably require around 4–7 years.

In addition to the recommended case-control study, it should in principle be possible to perform aggregated analyses from existing registers, although the information with regard to exposure at the individual level is rather limited. It would have to be based on knowledge of how radon exposure varies with different characteristics of houses (see NIRP, 1984; Radon Committee, 1983). The mathematical-statistical background for such studies has been examined by Ehrenberg and Ekman (1983), who also discuss how the studies should be carried out—a register study can be designed as a (retrospective-prospective) cohort study or a case–control study. Studies of this kind can cover a large population and a long time span at relatively low cost.

It is important that the whole investigation of radon risks should be integrated, though different institutions or teams may be responsible for different parts of the work. The project includes several interdisciplinary problems, and expertise in many different areas is needed in addition to epidemiological experience. Besides oncological aspects and questions about radiological measurement, building technology biological/technical aspects on other possible cancer-causing or interacting variables (than radon) and calculations of a complicated mathematical–statistical nature will be involved. As we are dealing here with an environmental health risk of general importance the most obvious solution is to suggest the National Institute of Environmental Medicine as the formally responsible agency. Another alternative could be the Council for the Planning and Co-ordination of Research (e.g. see Section 15.2.3).

No project of this size should be started without a guarantee that it can also be completed. This means that the total calculated maximum sum must be available—if it turns out to be needed. This requires a political decision on whether it is considered urgent to try to eliminate the present uncertainty regarding the magnitude of the cancer risk in Sweden caused by radon in houses. If the answer is yes, a suitable agency should be nominated by the Government to carry out the study following the guidelines given here.

10.4.3 The proposals for measures given by the Radon Committee

In 1979 the Swedish government initiated a special investigation of measures needed to reduce radiation risks in buildings. In its final report (Radon Committee, 1983), this investigative group reviewed the sources of radon and gamma radiation in houses (from the ground, building materials and subsoil water), described methods and results of measuring levels of radon and discussed the possible construction and ventilation techniques that could lead to lower radon levels. The main recommendations were that:

(a) A level where measures are needed shall be 400 Bqm^{-3} for the radon daughter threshold in existing houses; however, such an 'action level' should not be regarded as a hygienic threshold limit value and no threshold limit values are suggested below the level of 400 Bqm^{-3}, with reference to the policy in radiation protection that the radon daughter level shall always be as low as practically and economically feasible.

(b) Adequate measures to reduce exposure must be taken in houses with levels above 400 Bqm^{-3} within 5 years (and if radon daughter concentrations are above 1000 Bqm^{-3}, within 2 years); the municipalities have the responsibility of identifying houses with radon daughter concentrations above 400 Bqm^{-3}.

(c) An individual, through the municipality, should be made the offer of having the radon daughter concentration measured in his or her house (this would promote private initiatives beside municipality programmes for identifying high-risk buildings) at cost price.

(d) Owners of houses should, as at present, be given the opportunity of special loans to finance measures against radon in existing houses where the radon daughter concentration is above the action level.

(e) Consideration shall be given to radon from the ground when building new houses according to recommendations by the National Board of Physical Planning and Building which is expected to lead to average radon daughter concentrations in new houses substantially lower than 100 Bqm^{-3}.

(f) The contributions from new building material to the indoor radon daughter concentrations must be kept at an acceptable level; this could be achieved through certain already established rules, with so-called gamma and radium indices.

The Radon Committee especially underlines the importance of good ventilation. The Swedish building norm of 0.5 air changes per hour is, in fact, frequently not achieved at the present time.

The cost estimates for the proposed measures are of necessity far from exact. The major cost will be for measures in existing houses where radon daughter concentrations are above 400 Bqm^{-3} (about 40 000 houses), in total some 500 million Sw.kr (about US$75 million), which in principle will fall upon the owners of the houses. The possibilities for loans with support from the society would according to the Cancer Committee, not appreciably affect the partition of costs. The cost to municipalities of identifying houses with high radon daughter levels is estimated to be between 20 and 40 million Sw.kr (US$3 and 6 million) (the cost of examining *all* houses would be almost 2 billion Sw.kr (US$300 million)). The costs of protective measures against radon from the ground for new houses is estimated to be around 25 million Sw.kr (US$3.8 million) annually.

The measures can be divided into those for new houses and those for existing houses. A reasonable goal would be for all *new houses* to be constructed in such a way that radon daughter concentrations will be below the present Swedish average value. Requirements to ensure that radon leakage from the ground is being considered at building and that new building materials meet certain standards, referred to by the Radon Committee, may be regarded as acceptable at present for practical reasons although they do not guarantee a low radon concentration in an individual case. However, on the basis of tests carried out on 70 houses, these measures could well lead to a dramatic improvement, on an average basis. The reductions in radon levels in new houses should be monitored by the relevant authority. This 'action level' seems to have been based mainly on the risks of damage to the lung function at high doses of radiation and should provide a good safety margin in that respect. However, the Radon Committee also points out that the largest risks of cancer to an individual could also be counteracted by measures taken in houses with the highest levels. This is an important statement. Even down at the 'action level', the individual risk of lung cancer in the future may still far exceed what is otherwise accepted in radiation protection. A calculation based on the NIRP figure of about 1100 future cancer cases would yield a risk of about 100 per 100 000 person–years at 400 Bqm^{-3}, based on a population of 8 million exposed to radon daughters at an average level of 53 Bqm^{-3}. This is 10 times higher than what in some cases has been considered as an acceptable risk in the occupational environment and several multiples of 10 higher than what is being aimed at in Sweden as protection of the general population against radiation risks (see Section 7.5.2). If all radon daughter levels in Swedish houses above 400 Bqm^{-3} were reduced to that level this would mean—as a theoretical example of a calculation—that roughly 165 lung cancer cases will be avoided annually (the calculation is again based on the NIRP figure of 1100 future cancer cases and on figures for exposure distribution presented in the Radon Committee report). The cost would be about 3 million Sw.kr (US$450 000) per case if only 1 year is considered. More correctly, when presuming that the effect of a technical measure taken to reduce exposure will remain for a number of years, for example 30 years which may be the remaining life time of the house, the cost per case will be around 100 000 Sw.kr (US$15 000). If the risk is lower, the number of cancer cases prevented will be lower also and the cost per case will be higher, towards 300 000 Sw.kr (US$45 000) per case or more based on the risk figures discussed by the Cancer Committee in Section 10.4.1. Some examples of costs for avoiding a premature death due to radiation or exposure to chemicals have also been given in Chapter 7. These were of the order of magnitude of 5–10 million Sw.kr (US$750 000–1.5 million). Although the total costs of reducing high level exposures to indoor radon according to the recommendations by the Radon Committee may seem high, there is nothing saying that they are not justified when the full picture of personal risks is being considered.

For the purpose of improving and better understanding a strategy to reduce risks from radon, some further elaborations on the personal risk in relation to the collective risk may be indicated.

With regard to the cancer risks, the total contribution to the collective dose is largest from the many houses with radon daughter concentrations below 400 Bqm^{-3}. Only some 15 per cent of the risk contribution comes from houses with levels above this figure (about 1 per cent of the total number of houses). Considering the individual risk—regardless of its absolute size—it is clearly urgent that the measures are taken 'from the top', in other words that the highest individual risks should be the first to be reduced. The procedure proposed by the Radon Committee, with mandatory measures above a certain level, is consistent with this view. On the other hand it is not obvious what level for measures is the most suitable, considering the present uncertainty in the cancer risks regardless of whether we are talking about individual risks or population risks. It must be possible to discuss lower levels than those proposed by the Radon Committee as well, especially when the high risks as assessed by the NIRP are taken into consideration. The general principle of radiation protection, of aiming to achieve as low a concentration as practically and economically feasible, should be followed. Time, however, may be another important factor to consider.

The epidemiological study recommended by the Cancer Committee on the magnitude of the radon risks is estimated to require some 4–7 years. The Radon Committee recommended that the identification of houses with radon daughter concentrations above 400 Bqm^{-3} and technical changes in these houses to reduce exposure ought to be made within a 5-year period. Considering the practical difficulties in this connection it is, according to the Cancer Committee, hardly realistic to believe that much more can be done during that time period, at the end of which it should be possible to make a new risk assessment. As we are dealing here with supposedly mandatory measures, the demands on the private-house owner (and on the municipalities) have to be reasonable as well.

If at present the lowest level for *mandatory* measures were to remain at 400 Bqm^{-3}, then there is even more reason to underline that this is an administrative level (which should in no way be taken as a 'safety limit' as far as cancer is concerned), and to *encourage* in all possible ways *voluntary measures* below that level.

It should also be remembered that the level of 400 Bqm^{-3} is not one above which the cancer risk from radon is very large and below which the risk rapidly decreases. On the contrary, it has to be assumed that the type of risk that we are dealing with here decreases linearly with dose. It is the rate of that decrease (the slope of the line) which is not known and which determines the magnitude of the risk at any radon level. Indeed, measures should be taken in houses with radon daughter concentrations below 400 Bqm^{-3} wherever practically and economically feasible. This would lead to a decrease in both individual and collective risks.

It should be made easier, e.g. by means of improved loan facilities, for any house owner to take measures to decrease radon daughter levels even when these are already below the level for mandatory actions. Measures that improve ventilation will also, in general, decrease the exposure to pollution in indoor air. Smoking is another factor in this context. The risk estimates made for radon-induced cancer apply to populations with present smoking habits. There is much evidence of an interaction so that the lung cancer risk from radon exposure is substantially increased for smokers. A reduction in smoking would in this case also decrease the cancer risks due to radon.

The distribution of radon levels in existing houses means that more than half of the contribution to the total population dose (some 60 per cent) derives from houses with radon daughter levels below 100 Bqm^{-3}. Should the need arise, it may well turn out to be very difficult, for practical reasons, to influence substantially the collective dose through stricter regulations in the future, at least until a good deal of today's buildings have been renewed. Therefore, the presumed new risk assessment to be made when more scientific information becomes available will mainly be useful for possible considerations of better protection of the individual, for example by lowering the level for mandatory measures in existing buildings to represent an 'acceptable' personal risk—although the collective risk may in such a case remain 'too high'. A large part of the total population dose will under all circumstances in practical terms only be reduced by a generally better ventilation of houses, in combination with well-tailored suitable requirements for new houses.

A brief summary follows to conclude this section. The Cancer Committee supports the proposals by the Radon Committee outlined above as a minimum measure under present circumstances. In addition, the feasibility should be explored of making it easier for house owners, who so wish; to lower the concentration of radon daughters in their homes to below the proposed level of 400 Bq m^{-3}.

10.5 Indoor air pollution

10.5.1 Background

Human beings spend a high proportion of the 24 hours of each day indoors, predominantly in their homes. In Sweden, on average 88–94 per cent of the time is spent indoors and only 4 per cent outdoors (the remaining time is spent in different forms of transport).

This section deals mainly with general aspects of the indoor environment. (Air pollution in an indoor work environment due to products or processes related to that work constitutes a special area of risk which is dealt with elsewhere, although certain aspects are common with what is said here.) During recent years special risk factors in indoor air as well as the indoor environment as such have become subject to health hazard concern. This goes for air in homes, in office buildings, in day-care homes and so on. Exposure to radon daughters from construction material and from radon emanating from the ground, leakage of chemical compounds like formaldehyde from construction materials and passive smoking are examples of special factors of interest from the point of view of cancer risks.

The quality of the indoor air used to be seen as dependent purely on the composition of the air outside (apart from the transpiration from people in the building). However, air pollutants from sources within the building are nowadays gaining more importance. This is enhanced by modern construction methods which, for instance, aim at energy savings by reducing ventilation and increasing draughtproofing in houses. Sources of pollution indoors, such as combustion of different kinds, furniture and other fittings, and human activities, can cause higher concentrations of air pollutants indoors than outdoors, especially when ventilation is poor. In addition, incorrect ventilation can help to spread air pollutants, including infectious agents, from one part of a building to another.

It is particularly important to establish whether indoor air pollution is increasing because of energy-saving measures in construction or renovation of houses. The much higher levels of radon that now occur in houses than previously are believed to be in part related to poorer exchange of air, although other factors may have played far greater roles.

Several air pollutants have been dealt with in previous sections as far as carcinogenic properties and risks are concerned. The scientific basis of the risks from radon in houses has been discussed in Section 4.5.2 and environmental tobacco smoke in Section 4.2.5. The occurrence, properties and effects of certain chemical substances have been described in Section 4.4 (for example formaldehyde and asbestos), and some other substances have been discussed here in relation to their occurrence in outdoor air. However, a scientific basis for more mapping of known or potential carcinogens in different indoor environments and information about actual exposures have only recently appeared in the international scientific literature.

Continuous or repeated exposure to indoor pollutants could arise from three further sources. These sources are (a) indoor combustion processes such as food preparation and heating by open fires, (b) release of volatile substances, other than formaldehyde, from construction materials or fittings and (c) mould formation. The types of mould likely to occur in indoor environments under different conditions are not fully known, nor do they seem to have been studied with respect to carcinogenic properties, if any, of substances emitted into the air. However, some mycotoxins found in other circumstances have strong carcinogenic properties for example the aflatoxins.

The total exposure of different populations to indoor air pollutants and possible interactive effects between such pollutants (see Section

4.6) are other topics needing investigation, since at present little or no information exists.

If pollutants are released into the air faster than they are eliminated through ventilation and by absorption onto surfaces, objects, persons, etc., their concentrations will increase. Sealing of houses increases this pollutant enrichment unless forced ventilation is installed. The degree of ionization of the air and the general content of particles ('dust') influence the concentrations of individual pollutants.

It is not possible to evaluate comprehensively the importance of indoor air for the total cancer incidence. There is nothing in the data so far available indicating that such air pollution has had a major impact, although obvious risks may have existed in rare special cases (such as severe examples of passive smoking). Future trends are even more difficult to predict and it is unsatisfactory that basic knowledge is so incomplete, besides the uncertainty already mentioned with regard to health risks (lung cancer) from present levels of radon in Swedish houses.

In international scientific circles, interest in questions of the quality of indoor air has increased. One example is a recently convened conference in Stockholm (Indoor Air '84).[6] At that conference the importance of the kind of issues raised in this chapter was stressed. Overall strategies to deal with indoor air pollutants, seen in a public health perspective, have been called for (for example by Spengler and Sexton (1983)). In Sweden the responsibility for risk prevention measures and for future research within this area is spread between a number of bodies. At the national level the National Board of Health and Welfare has the general responsibility for air quality in homes and different kinds of indoor premise. The National Environmental Protection Board deals with (mainly) outdoor air pollutants. The National Board of Occupational Safety and Health is the central agency responsible for implementing the legislation for protection of people in the work place, which also covers air pollutants from sources other than the work itself. The National Institute of Radiation Protection has taken several initiatives to investigate the occurrence and risks from indoor radon although natural radiation sources do not seem to be covered by present legislation on radiation protection[7]. The National Board of Physical Planning and Building issues standards for building and for building material by which certain emissions and concentrations of indoor air pollutants may be affected although a low annual increase in building volume (about 1 per cent in the period 1980–1983) means that the environmental conditions in today's houses will govern the indoor air quality for the population in general for many years to come. Finally, building material considered to give rise to health risks due to their chemical composition may be regulated by the Products Control Board.

There are very few official guide lines for indoor air quality (hygienic limit values) in Sweden but, besides those, the Board of Health and Welfare has published information on indoor radon and given authoritative advice on measures against mould. A task force including external experts is at present studying air quality problems at daycare centres, on behalf of the Board.

The National Institute of Environmental Medicine is an important active organization and national resource in this context. Health protection in homes is one of the research lines given high priority by the Institute for the 1980s, with a multidisciplinary approach in co-operation with, among others, the Royal Institute of Technology in Stockholm. The Institute of Environmental Medicine also takes part in international co-operation concerning indoor environmental problems, for example through the WHO and the International Energy Agency (IEA). Other Swedish sectional organizations researching in this area are the National Bacteriological Laboratory and the National Institute for Building Research. Ongoing work with regard to the occupational environment, such as ventilation technology, may in some cases have a future impact in this particular area as well.

Among research-funding organizations, the Council for Building Research has a special programme for health protection in buildings. No research council or the equivalent in the medical and natural science areas (see Chapter 15) is at present running a programme related to health in the indoor environment.

10.5.2 Considerations by the Cancer Committee

Questions related to indoor air pollution cut across the classification of risk areas and causal factors as outlined in Chapter 6. Full attention could not, therefore, be paid to every possible aspect of cancer risks and indoor air pollution.

Besides the general air pollutants, the occurrence of which is greatest in urban areas (for measures to reduce risks see Section 10.3), radon daughters in houses (Section 10.4) and environmental tobacco smoke (Section 10.1) there are certain other sources in indoor environments which should be further examined for possible cancer risks, although these risks are likely to be small. In general, ill health and discomfort due to indoor air quality problems cannot be explained by simple causal associations. As a single substance cannot be held responsible, methods describing the total overall air pollution pattern and its effects on the human being, including cancer hazards, are needed.

Some of the health problems which seem to be associated with the indoor atmosphere have probably increased during the last 10–20 years. Some problems may have existed earlier but not been observed as clearly as now. Other problems are obviously related to modern building techniques, including energy saving measures and modern building materials. In particular the hazards of restricting exchange of indoor air should be emphasized.

The question of health hazards, including cancer, related to pollution of the indoor environment is thus very complex. It calls for co-operation between different national regulatory agencies. Many parts of the overall problem can probably be dealt with individually. However, most of the problems need to be looked at within a comprehensive framework. More knowledge is needed about what risk groups there are in the population, what measures against the emission sources can be taken today and in the future and what medically relevant functional demands can be made on buildings.

As far as cancer is concerned, the top priority should be to improve the scientific basis for an assessment of the magnitude of the risks from present radon daughter exposure in Sweden by means of the epidemiological study proposed in Section 10.4. In addition, the question of health risks related to air pollution in houses must be allocated sufficient attention and resources and be dealt with not only in terms of single substances or other risk factors, but also from a comprehensive perspective. This is valid for research and other development measures as well as administrative approaches. Comprehensive efforts in the form of a programme directed towards, among other things, cancer risk in the indoor environment, in particular housing, should accordingly be added to the research and control measures directed at specific agents.

Future work should build on activities already structured, and there does not seem to be a need to change the distribution of responsibilities between the public agencies, in spite of the many parties involved, but the National Board of Health and Welfare should attempt to co-ordinate the efforts further and also, at least briefly, specify which issues require an input from the scientific community during the years to come. More funding than at present will be needed, which in turn will require that more research councils should support research in this area.

With regard to administrative measures, co-ordinated efforts are urgently needed against air pollution. Whenever applicable, air quality criteria (concentration limits) concerning outdoor air pollution should also take into account possible concentrations of the same substances in indoor air. Administrative measures of a technical nature in building standards, etc., which are not specifically linked to any legislation in the health or environmental protection area, should be encouraged through close co-operation between scientists and the government agencies concerned and, whenever necessary, in the form of a specific research and development agreement with the corresponding partner on the health side. A voluntary co-ordination in the form of the programme proposed in this report could be one way.

Measures against indoor air pollution caused either by building construction methods or materials, or by human activities should primarily be directed towards controlling the sources so as to reduce their emissions of pollutants. This could be achieved either by means of regulations based on available legislation like the one governing environmentally and health-hazardous products, through health education (chapter 9) and other information about risks associated with different procedures, materials, etc., or through advice aimed at voluntary decrease of exposure. One such example of the latter is the official advice to decrease tobacco smoking in certain localities in order to avoid subjecting other people to passive smoking (Section 10.1).

In some cases threshold values for agents in public places or other jointly occupied buildings and in the home can supplement other measures which aim at decreasing health hazards. (Compare with the discussion in Section 10.4 on a radon daughter level of 400 Bq/m^{-3} as a 'level for action'.) It is too early to judge whether a similar administrative procedure can be applied more widely or only in certain exceptional cases as hitherto.

NOTES

1. The report 'Food products and meals—different ways to reduce fat consumption' (Lindvall, 1984) shows that certain changes in the diet do not need to imply far-reaching changes in the traditional Swedish plain food.
2. In the early 1980s, after a referendum on nuclear power, the Parliament had decided to allow an extension of the number of existing reactors to 12 but at the same time setting a deadline for their operations namely to the year 2010. [*Ed. note.*]
3. No EEC country has yet (1989) introduced the US–83 car emission limits as obligatory. Unleaded petrol has, however, now been introduced in all European countries, although in some areas it may be hard to find. In Sweden, some but not all of the proposals cited have led to action, the main being a new law stipulating the US–83 emission limits for all new petrol-driven passenger cars from the 1989 models. Already over 60 per cent of the 1988 models sold are adapted to these requirements. [*Ed. note.*]
4. An international symposium has defined annoyance or disturbance reactions as 'a feeling of displeasure associated with any agent or condition believed to affect adversely an individual or a group' (Lindvall, T. and Radford, E., 1973, Measurement of annoyance due to exposure to environmental factors. The 4th Karolinska Institute Symposium on Environmental Health, *Environ. Res.* 6.1–36.) The definition has varied between different studies, though. In

this study, commissioned by the C Ex Committee, the aims were:
   (a) to describe the annoyance due to car exhausts subjectively felt by the studied population in different types of urban environment;
   (b) to quantify the annoyance of persons expected to be especially sensitive to air pollution, for example those with chronic respiratory diseases. [*Ed. note*].
5   The term 'radon' is often used for 'radon daughters' unless a distinction is needed.
6   The conference proceedings are now available in six volumes from the Swedish Council for Building Research, Stockholm. [*Ed. note*].
7   The new Radiation Protection Act of 1988, covering both ionizing and non-ionizing radiation such as UV-lights, makes no exception for natural radiation sources. However, indoor air quality regulations, for example with respect to radon, are still to be based on other acts concerning public health protection in general, planning and building, the work environment, etc. [*Ed. note*.]

11
Risk management in the legal context

11.1 Introduction

Legislation, along with the creation of authorities responsible for control and implementation, constitutes one of the mechanisms by which society acts to reduce health hazards so as to limit the incidence of diseases and other health impairment.

This chapter, therefore, aims at supplementing parts of the general strategy for cancer prevention laid out in Chapter 7.

Statutory risk control in Sweden involves central regulatory agencies as well as regional (governmental) and local (municipal) authorities who carry the main burden of surveillance to enforce compliance with the regulations (referred to as 'supervision' in the following). Besides giving advice, a 'supervisory body' can sometimes further specify the conditions for a 'risky activity', prohibit further operations under threat of a monetary penalty (which in case of non-compliance can be imposed only by a court of law) or refer a matter of presumed violation of the law to the public prosecutor—depending on what is stipulated in the relevant piece of legislation.

In the context of control of exposure to carcinogenic physical or chemical agents, the most important laws in Sweden are the Work Environment Act, the Environment Protection Act, the Public Health Protection Act, the Radiation Protection Act, the Act on Products Hazardous to Health and to the Environment, the Food Act, the Drug Ordinance, and a number of implementation regulations issued by the Government, or in some cases by the appropriate authorities, as well as guidelines for implementing various rules and regulations. References to these Acts in this chapter should be taken to also include amendments and ordinances issued pursuant to the Act itself.

It is the nature of things that these statutes, created at different times and for different purposes, are not uniform. Also, when very little diversity in form can be perceived between certain regulations, the judicial philosophy which forms the basis of these laws may give emphasis to different aspects in their implementation. However, the major statutes in the field of risk management share certain basic principles, and the issues which, in particular, confront the central authorities seem to a large extent to be common.

Some brief information concerning the legal areas involved will give sufficient background for the subsequent discussion.

The *Work Environment Act* (SFS 1977:1160–1171)[1] provides the legal basis for ensuring acceptable conditions at the workplace. Substances which may constitute health hazards or cause accidents may be used only under conditions which afford adequate safety. The employer has the responsibility for providing information on the risks associated with the work. The importer or manufacturer of a hazardous substance is obliged to take adequate measures to prevent any risks which are associated with its intended use. Packages and containers must be labelled. The Board of Occupational Safety and Health may stipulate conditions for the use of a hazardous substance. Further, the law empowers this agency to issue limit values for occupational hygiene as well as other rules for the handling of chemical substances or for a certain type of work.

The Board of Occupational Safety and Health constitutes the central government agency and implementing body given the task of issuing detailed regulations, following and supervising the Labour Inspectorate, as well as giving advance authorization of certain types of technical equipment. At the local level the Labour Inspectorate is vested with the responsibility of exercising control and providing guidance at the workplace. The Inspectorate constitutes a national system consisting of some 20 separate, fairly independent bodies.

The *Environment Protection Act* (SFS 1969:387) regulates what it describes as 'activities hazardous to the environment' associated with permanent installations (emissions and other forms of inconvenience from motor vehicles are dealt with in a different fashion—see Section 10.3). Certain kinds of activity are defined which require a permit ('franchise') from the National Franchise Board for Environment Protection or, if the potential environmental risk is of a lower order of magnitude, from the County Administrative Board. In these permits the competent authority may include special requirements, e.g. for the emission of carcinogens. It is the duty of the applicant to provide sufficient information so that the authority may assess risks to human health and to the environment.

The Franchise Board takes its decision after having heard the parties concerned in a court-like procedure (see Chapter 12) including the National Environmental Protection Board as special advocate for adequate risk management and the County Administrative Board which is also a supervisory body in this context. Municipal bodies are usually also represented; some municipalities have formally taken over supervisory duties within their own areas from the respective (governmental) County Administrative Boards.

The main purpose of the *Public Health Protection Act* (SFS 1982:1080) is to prevent or eliminate 'sanitary inconveniences'. A sanitary inconvenience is defined as 'any disturbance which may be deleterious to human health and which is not to be regarded as insignificant or of a temporary nature'. Each municipality is responsible for the protection of public health within its area, and the public health legislation can be regarded as a complement to other statutes covering the protection of human health and the environment.

In addition to the objects traditionally regulated in this context (such as sanitary requirements for buildings, sewage systems, water quality in public baths, measures against vermin, bacterial pollution, etc.), cancer hazards may come to the fore, for example in connection with air pollution in urban areas or indoors. The existence of a sanitary inconvenience may force the proprietor of a building to take certain actions in order to remove the cause.

In each municipality an Environmental and Health Protection Authority is responsible for local supervision and may issue formal notices or injunctions required for enforcing the law. Within the county, supervision is carried out by the County Administrative Board. Central supervision is shared between the National Board of Health and Welfare and the National Environmental Protection Board. The National Board of Health and Welfare has to consider conditions pertaining to the indoor environment like the presence of pollutants in indoor air, while the National Environmental Protection Board deals with other issues such as outdoor air pollutants, water supplies, utilization of sewage sludge, etc. These two central authorities can issue general guidelines, e.g. to define the concept of sanitary inconvenience, but are not empowered to issue binding regulations in this context.

The *Radiation Protection Act* (SFS 1958:110) regulates radiological work. This includes work with a radioactive substance, work involving X-ray equipment or any other technical device for the generation of ionizing radiations, as well as work in a nuclear power plant. Ionizing radiation is defined by the law as 'radiation from radioactive substances, X-rays, and radiations inducing similar biological effects'. These carcinogenic agents have been previously discussed under the heading 'physical factors' in Section 4.5.

Licensing by the National Institute of Radiation Protection of all kinds of radiological work constitutes the basic principle spelled out by this piece of legislation.

Anyone who carries out radiological work must take such precautions as can be reasonably expected in order to prevent radiation damage. The National Institute of Radiation Protection may issue general regulations as well as regulations in an individual case. This agency is also empowered to extend the implementation of the law to other areas than those defined above or to decide on exceptions from the law. Some information concerning current practices in radiation protection work can be found in Section 7.5.2.

Supervision according to this act is carried out by the National Institute of Radiation Protection as well as by specially appointed inspectors, acting under the instruction and guidance of the Institute.

Certain radioactive substances which are utilized, or have been utilized in nuclear power reactors, or which can be converted into fuel for such reactors, also come under the Nuclear Power Act of 1956, which provides for a special control system.

The *Act on Products Hazardous to Health and to the Environment*[2] (SFS 1973:329) covers, with certain exceptions, all products (substances, mixtures, objects, etc.) which 'due to their chemical properties and manner of use are liable to cause injury to man or to the environment'. The act applies to the product *per se* and its use irrespective of where it occurs and thus supplements, for example, the Work Environment Act in the case of products found at the workplace. Since it is hardly feasible to undertake all measures required to prevent or counteract ill health, e.g. a cancer risk caused by a product, without knowing that the product is indeed hazardous, and also in what way, it may be argued that this law, in fact, covers all products. Even though failure of a producer or importer to investigate the composition and properties of one of its products may involve criminal liability only if it can later be proven that the product in question is indeed hazardous to health, the duty to investigate in practice covers a much broader assortment of products. In addition, the competent authority may, in principle, request information about any product whatsoever for the purpose of assessing its hazardous properties. Prohibitions, or other restrictions on certain products, as well as rules for labelling (including warnings of cancer hazards), etc., have been issued on the basis of this Act. Premarketing approval involving decisions on a case-by-case basis has been stipulated for some product categories, notably pesticides.

In most cases the Products Control Board constitutes the central regulatory body, and this agency can classify products as hazardous to health and/or to the environment and may further specify many of the general requirements of the Act, such as how the 'duty to investigate' is to be fulfilled, or issue rules pertaining to the manner of use of all or of special groups of hazardous products. The National Board of Health and Welfare is empowered to direct that a specific substance must not be used as a constituent in cosmetics or in toiletries.

Central supervision to ensure compliance with the Act is exercised by the Board of Occupational Safety and Health, within its field of jurisdiction, and by the national Environmental Protection Board in other areas. In addition, regional local supervision is carried out by the Labour Inspectorate, within the county by the County Administrative Board as well as by the local Environment and Public Health Protection Agency within the municipality.

The *Food Act* (SFS 1971:511) applies to production, sales, serving, and other kinds of handling of products intended for consumption by humans (products regulated by the Drug Ordinance are exempted). The Act does not apply to the handling of foods in individual households (see also Section 10.2.3). The Food Act—the purpose of which is not solely restricted to the control of health hazards—stipulates that marketed foods must not have such a composition that consumption is likely to be harmful. In processing and other handling of foods, precautions should be taken to prevent any contamination and to avoid any foodstuffs becoming unfit for human consumption. Food additives must be approved by the National Food Administration prior to their marketing—unless an exception has been made for a certain type of additive by the same regulatory agency. The National Food Administration can also issue regulations concerning the use of any product, substance or piece of equipment used in the processing of foods to prevent any deleterious effect on a foodstuff and can prohibit or issue regulations for the processing of foods, e.g. placing a limit on the concentration of a particular foreign substance. Further, the Act provides general rules for labelling of foods, including information on the composition of the foodstuff. Anyone importing foods commercially must be registered with the National Food Administration.

The National Food Administration exerts central supervision of the implementation of the Food Act. Within the county the County Administrative Board carries out supervision, and the local Environment and Public Health Protection Authority has this responsibility within the municipality.

The *Drug Ordinance* (SFS 1962:701) is primarily applicable to products for internal or external use and which are intended to prevent, diagnose, alleviate, or cure illness or symptoms of illness. According to this ordinance, a pharmaceutical product must be of a 'fully satisfactory nature' and must not induce during normal use injuries in disproportion to the intended beneficial effect. A standardized drug intended to be marketed in the producer's original package must be submitted for premarketing approval. This approval (called 'registration') implies that the National Board of Health and Welfare has evaluated possible health risks in relation to the benefits. However, medical efficacy always constitutes a primary prerequisite for registration.

Retail trade in pharmaceuticals may only be carried out by the

Apoteksbolaget AB—the state dispensing network. The National Board of Health and Welfare may prescribe special conditions for the dispensing and delivery of pharmaceuticals, for example that certain drugs may be obtained only by a doctor's prescription. The label on a pharmaceutical product must contain complete information on the identities and concentrations of active ingredients as well as certain information about other components. A drug registered for use for certain medical conditions must not be marketed on other indications.

A registered pharmaceutical product should be subjected to further monitoring and control on a regular basis by the National Board of Health and Welfare, not least with regard to unexpected side-effects. The Board also supervises the implementation of the statutes concerned with control of drugs.

Since the *Marketing Practices Act* (SFS 1975:1418) can be utilized for the regulation of carcinogenic agents in certain situations, this piece of legislation deserves mention in this context. The Market Court can rule that a trader must not market a product to the general public if it is deemed to entail risk of personal injury. The Consumer Ombudsman exercises supervision of the compliance with this Act and, besides taking matters to the Market Court, can also settle minor disputes by issuing prohibition injunctions.

As indicated above, the different fields of legislation define to some extent the responsibilities, rights and obligations involving the authorities, industry and other parties. The shared responsibilities between authorities and industry constitute a common fundamental principle which characterizes Swedish legislation in this area. Anyone responsible for an activity which involves exposure of individuals directly to the activity as such, or caused by products which have been manufactured or generated during the activity in question and which involve hazardous physical or chemical agents such as carcinogens, has the primary responsibility for reducing or eliminating any risk which may arise. Such activities or products may in some cases be subjected to advance assessment and approval by the authorities. In this case the applicant has the duty to furnish information adequate for a risk assessment. When approval has been obtained, a more or less clearly defined responsibility remains with industry to follow developments which may have a bearing on any previous risk assessment. The legislation is, further, apparently based on the assumption that industry maintains a certain internal control of its activities and/ or of its products in order to adequately fulfil its legal obligations. Such control is sometimes defined by implementation rules or guidelines for analysis, etc. The responsibilities of the authorities and control measures taken by them thus constitute a necessary complement to, but no substitute for, industry's obligations.

Clearly, great difficulties often arise in attempting to control the extent to which industry fulfils its obligations with respect to the gathering of data and preventing potential risks. This applies especially in the identification of previously unspecified hazards, such as chemical agents which have not been explicitly classified as carcinogens by the competent authority. In the case of radiation protection, as regulated by law, the identity of the carcinogenic agent is, in principle, defined and this regulatory field thus presents a different situation to that of the other types of legislation mentioned here.

Even commercial enterprises which have considerable resources at their disposable may experience difficulties in making a realistic appraisal of the limits of their obligations, and planning and executing their testing activities, literature surveys, etc. This state of affairs is bound to remain as long as the generally formulated rules found in different central statutes ('frame-work legislation') are not defined more precisely, or their intended implementation illustrated in other ways. On the other hand, the process of issuing detailed specifications of industry's obligations must be kept within bounds so as not to water down the fundamental responsibilities vested with industry. The issuing of official lists containing examples of agents which may cause different kinds of risk with respect to health and to the environment should be considered as an expression of this philosophy. One of the principles embodied in current Swedish legislation is that hazardous agents such as carcinogens cannot and should not be specified in an exhaustive manner by the competent authority; otherwise previously unidentified risks would fall outside the jurisdiction of the law. This principle does not exclude the special regulation of certain substances. The National Board of Occupational Safety and Health has in fact issued an extensive list of carcinogens classified into three categories, for each of which specific rules are enforced: a total ban, restriction with possible granting of exemption, and carcinogens with a hygienic limit value (see Section 4.4).

In addition to legislation instituted by Parliament, the executive public bodies involved exert great influence on the policy of risk management embodied in the implementation of the basic laws, which finds its expression in regulations, guidelines and decisions on individual cases promulgated by the Government and by the competent authorities. In the rest of this chapter risk management will be discussed primarily as a public function, but certain viewpoints, e.g. concerning prioritization in risk management, may be of equal validity in the operation of large commercial enterprises.

Substances acting by a 'chemical' mechanism rather than through radiation will be the main focus of discussion. Procedures for the control of ionizing radiations are well established and have been described in Section 7.5.2. The principles developed within the field of radiation protection could serve as a model for the control of other types of hazard in our environment, such as chemical initiators of cancer which produce similar effects to radiation. To a certain extent the views expressed below may, however, also apply to radiation protection work.

11.2 Classification of carcinogens

Risk analysis based on epidemiological and/or experimental data is, as a rule, difficult and requires qualified scientific judgement utilizing all available data on properties and effects of a certain agent. In particular, this is true for the estimation of the level of carcinogenic risk to man (see figure 7.3), in relation to exposure to a specific substance or to a mixture of substances. Consequently, it is of utmost importance that regulatory agencies depending on such estimations as a basis for administrative decisions should have access to highly qualified scientific expertise inside and/or outside the organization.

A carcinogenic substance is characterized by the ability to induce cancer under certain conditions. As a rule, the crucial point is whether the substance can be assumed to possess the same properties under different conditions. This concerns especially how the experimental (usually animal) data should be extrapolated to human populations.

The international co-operation on standardization of test methods which is being carried out under the auspices of the Organization for Economic Co-operation and Development (OECD) is of particular value, primarily because this work increases the chances of chemicals with widespread international use actually being subjected to some kind of testing. As to the interpretation of the results and identification of a need for additional studies, there will remain a demand for scientific evaluation even when generally accepted protocols for testing and for the presentation of results are being followed. This is especially so when—as is often the case—divergent test results have been obtained. The search for biologically plausible explanations for such divergences and the identification of the most relevant facts to be used in the subsequent risk analysis requires considerable expertise and experience.

In the context of the Cancer Committee's work, Nilsson and Ehrenberg (1984) have reviewed a number of experimental testing methods and discussed the kinds of conclusion that can be derived from epidemiological and experimental data with special regard to statistical aspects.

From a purely scientific point of view one usually tries to avoid making sharp distinctions between risk and no-risk, or oversimplified classifications of substances which are liable to lead to misinterpretation. As previously mentioned (Section 4.4.4), the International

Agency for Research on Cancer (IARC) uses three levels in the assessment of the reliability of data related to the toxicological endpoints investigated (carcinogenicity in man or experimental animals as well as mutagenicity studies in a short-term test), namely 'sufficient', 'limited' and 'inadequate' evidence. If human data are not available, the IARC will refrain from making any statements concerning the human carcinogenicity of a substance. But information on humans exists for only a few substances and types of exposure, and the IARC has expressed the opinion that it seems reasonable for practical purposes to regard agents for which 'sufficient evidence' of carcinogenicity in animals exists, as if they presented a carcinogenic risk to man.

Risk management in the legal context represents a special situation. When attempting to define and implement a policy for risk assessment and risk management, criteria have to be developed for when an agent should, in the meaning of the law, be considered as 'a carcinogen' and be treated as carcinogenic to man even if this has not actually been proven (again, the fact that proof of human carcinogenicity is hard to come by should be emphasized). Although we are here concerned with a sliding scale of evidence values for risk indications—both below and above such a 'classification point'— there is a need, partly in order that the risk policy discussed in Section 7.5 can become sufficiently firm, that this type of decision be made for individual substances.

A 'classification' of a substance as carcinogenic will automatically provoke discussions on possible measures for reduction of risks, and raise issues relating to cost–benefit analysis for new products and processes. Even before the minimum data requirements for classification have been satisfied, certain measures—or discussion of such measures, including requests for additional data—may be appropriate. The following example provides another illustration. As pointed out earlier, the information that a certain substance has been proven mutagenic in a short-term test is not, on its own, sufficient for an evaluation of risk for cancer, and cannot result in the substance being classified as a carcinogen, in the sense used here. Further, the number of compounds exhibiting such mutagenic effects is very large, including proven or potential mutagens formed metabolically within the organism. It makes no sense to attempt to formulate a general risk policy for reduction of exposure to all such substances in order to be on the safe side. Since it is difficult now to foresee the consequences in the future of delayed exposures, it should however be possible to make consistent efforts to eliminate contamination of the environment by persistent mutagenic compounds.

Criteria for the classification of carcinogens cannot be established once and for all, but must be subjected to a continual reassessment in the light of changes in the scientific evaluation of cancer risks.

Further, it seems feasible to start with a few generally valid guidelines, which can later be elaborated on the basis of further scientific developments and documented experience in classification of carcinogenic agents. International criteria, both implemented and proposed, for the evaluation of carcinogenicity in regulatory risk management, have been reviewed in connection with this report (Holmberg and Säfwenberg, 1984b).

It is important that identical or similar scientific data are evaluated in the same fashion by all the different agencies involved in risk management within any country. Classifications and other decisions involving the singling out of a carcinogen should, thus, be the same. As regards Sweden, the laws on risk management, referred to earlier in this chapter, do not seem to imply an obstacle to such a policy. A classification is to be referred to 'risk identification' in Figure 7.3. The subsequent steps such as considerations of the size of risk at existing exposure levels (though still part of the scientific judgements), the acceptance of risk, the technical and economic feasibility of introducing various measures to reduce risk, etc., should be kept apart from the issue of classification. The administrative decisions with respect to such measures may then diverge within the different areas of agency jurisdiction, even if the fundamental assessment of the properties of a substance and its classification are identical.

At present, criteria used for classification of carcinogens in Sweden are sparsely documented. However, it is assumed that the accumulated experience within the authorities responsible for the assessment of cancer risks should suffice for 'translating' into criteria and—when so required—harmonizing the policy which, in fact, is implied in decisions which already have been taken. This process of explicitly stating current practice should be a first step, in order to avoid abrupt changes. Whether more steps, involving actual changes, are justified at present is difficult to say. Let it suffice here to briefly mention animal carcinogens, which must obviously also be considered in risk management besides human carcinogens. In this context the use is recommended *inter alia* of the IARC's classification of substances according to the availability of both 'sufficient' and 'limited' evidence (see Section 4.4.4). In pointing also at the latter group the Cancer Committee has indicated a suitable purport with respect to the concept of a carcinogenic agent in the sense of the law. In particular, it is felt that a single carefully conducted and well-documented animal study could be sufficient as a basis for classification of a substance. Further information may then be required in order to make a decision about which specific control measures should be taken.

'Negative' results from an investigation will generally not cancel 'positive' results indicating a potential hazard. Negative results from carefully designed studies may, however, provide upper limits of risk. It is important that negative results should be documented to a much greater extent than is done at present.

The mechanism of action, as far as a plausible one can be proposed, should not be given a decisive role when classifying a carcinogen (see Chapter 3). However, such considerations may influence subsequent decisions concerning control measures. The role of carcinogenic potency in classification is another issue, and a thorny one. If epidemiological data are available, this does not represent much of a problem—very low risks cannot be detected by such methods. At the present time, animal data, which, moreover, usually have been obtained using high doses compared with the levels to which human populations are normally exposed, must be characterized as so unreliable that the risk potency value obtained by extrapolating the experimental data to man may differ considerably—both upward and downward—from the true value. In the future, refined techniques and new knowledge may allow the concept of carcinogenic potency to be more generally taken into consideration in the actual classification process—in particular, if it becomes feasible to relate DNA target doses to cancer risks expressed in relative or even absolute numbers. On scientific grounds, it seems likely that a large number of substances possess a certain, though very low, cancer-initiating effect, provided that these agents do reach the DNA in humans. As new knowledge is acquired, it may be necessary in the future to introduce new limits and criteria for classification in order to obtain a reasonable coverage of risks, seen in the light of those risks which present legislation is designed to protect us from.

It should again be emphasized, however, that the clearest distinctions in risk management will be obtained when the classification of substances as carcinogens is administratively separated from regulatory decision making. Similar thoughts have also been voiced from others; see for example the US National Research Council (1983).

It may be that regulatory measures with regard to a certain substance are not feasible for one reason or another or that exposure may be already kept at a minimum and be satisfactorily controlled, due to other hazards associated with the substance; or the carcinogenic potency (if it can be estimated at all) may be low enough to obviate the need for any particular action under prevailing exposure conditions. A substance for which strong indications of a considerable cancer risk exist may need much more stringent measures and 'sacrifices' than is the case for a less well-documented carcinogen—although minimizing exposure is recommended also in the latter case (see Chapter 7).

11.3 Certain priorities. Resources for testing

Generalities

It is necessary to attempt to formulate a realistic level of ambition for each respective risk management activity, with optimal use of the resources which are available at the time. The rates of publication of new scientific data and of introduction of new substances make anything but a selective follow-up impossible. Data on present exposure levels are also often fragmentary (see Section 4.4).

One of the most important components in the planning of risk management activities must therefore be to determine overall priorities. At all different levels in the administration, decisions should then be made on further norms for priority-setting, on a flexible basis, meaning that there must be a continuous discussion on this matter. Each individual collaborator also needs to be consciously aware that priorities must be set as concerns the daily work. When a matter under consideration is put aside because another question from outside demands attention, for example because of mass-media interest, this should happen only after a deliberate decision. Otherwise, powerful voices from various quarters in society may influence resource allocations to a greater extent than is warranted by factors such as new data or public concern.

Some general principles for ranking regulatory measures have already been discussed in Chapter 7. The general views on priorities expressed here are more directly connected with actual day-to-day work and proceed from the assumption that the available resources will always remain limited in relation to the probable expectations concerning risk control.

Realistic efforts in risk control

The international scientific literature provides the foundation for the aims of risk control. In order to establish priorities as to which agents should be the subject of risk assessment, with possible subsequent control measures, risks must first be identified by qualified scientific experts. Insofar as this has already been done elsewhere, utilization of available material should be given precedence. An approach to the question of priorities should thus be to carry out exposure analysis and risk estimation for known or strongly suspected carcinogenic agents (including products and their methods of handling, industrial processes, and specific emissions) and at the same time to follow up new developments, especially with regard to available risk assessments of good quality.

Even using existing knowledge places demands on resources, and it is not realistic at present to plan extensive national efforts, as part of the process of statutory risk control, to produce new data on the properties and effects of other agents. (Further aspects concerning test resources and the need for international collaboration are considered later in this chapter.) Certain priorities should, however, be set for risk identification with regard to specific environments or specific agents in circumstances where the exposure in individual cases may be considerable and/or where a large number of persons are exposed. In such a case, data concerning the risks ought to be available from the company responsible, or else scientific investigations could be carried out either at that company's expense or with public funds, for example in the case of mixed exposures. In addition, sufficient resources should be allocated for initiating further studies of special national problems or observations which could indicate the existence of as yet undetected risks (see Chapter 8).

In principle, the reasoning above applies to existing chemical substances or risk environments. In addition, new chemicals must be dealt with. It is likely that in Sweden some kind of extended reporting procedure ('notification') for all new chemical substances will come into being in the relatively near future, with the manufacturer or importer being obliged to submit certain data to the responsible authority as a basis for risk assessment. Gradually, at least, some basis for scientific evaluation will then be provided even before the substance is introduced; the risks that may be identified from this information can then be counteracted at an early stage.

Not even extremely far-reaching demands on documentation of new substances can constitute a guarantee against the later occurrence of new risk aspects. Demands for priority of efforts in risk monitoring will follow immediately when a 'new' chemical becomes an 'existing' one, and—it must be stressed again—the changing pattern of exposure should have a major influence on resource allocations. Specifications concerning risk monitoring of individual substances or groups of substances will also more easily be formulated on scientific grounds when certain basic data concerning new substances gradually become available to the responsible authorities. The point of departure will thus improve, in a longer-term perspective, over the present situation, in which for an extremely large number of chemicals, available risk documentation (if any) is of varying quality and is furthermore widely dispersed in the literature.

To specify what basic data should be required is no easy matter. This is also being discussed internationally. Sweden has concurred with a proposal within the OECD concerning new chemicals: the Minimum Premarketing Set of Data (MPD) (OECD, 1982).

Demands for provision of information about potential cancer risks before a substance or product becomes available for use vary considerably depending on the legislation and established practice in its application. The OECD MPD, which in turn is quite similar to the recently enforced requirements for a 'base set' of data upon the notification of new chemicals with the EEC, prescribes tests for mutagenicity but no long-term experiments on mammals for cancer. However, mutagenic properties detected in short-term experiments, together with other toxicological information and subsequent reports concerning actual exposures, could give rise to demands for additional investigations. For specially regulated products, stricter rules may apply, and in Sweden, for example, the regulatory authorities now without exception prescribe cancer tests on pharmaceutical products before official approval (see Section 4.4).

No one country has sufficient resources for tracking down, evaluating and supplementing, within a reasonable period of time, all scientific information required for the risk identification of all chemicals now used in commercial contexts. Only a few existing substances have been fully evaluated with respect to potential cancer risks, and many have been only unevenly evaluated with respect to most other risks. In certain cases, furthermore, specific impurities from the manufacturing process or substances which may be formed in the prescribed use of the product or during environmental transformation or degradation might need evaluation. International co-operation is therefore essential and it can take many forms, from the normal 'spontaneous' collaboration between scientists and research groups in various countries, to formal co-operation within or through various international organizations.

Another part of the OECD's activities in the chemicals field should be recalled here, namely that concerning risk control of existing chemicals. A large number of OECD countries participate in various projects under this heading. One of the approaches has to do with priorities in risk identification of existing chemicals, in principle with regard to all detrimental health and environmental effects. Eventually this should also allow certain agreements between countries for the division of labour. Such international division of labour to generate, within the foreseeable future, better but still summary knowledge about the properties and effects of existing chemicals might be more valuable than attempting to derive in each case unimpeachable scientific results on which to base a definitive risk evaluation.

Certain countries have compiled and made public lists of priorities for their own investigative and testing activities, such as the National Toxicology Program in the USA. This can allow other countries to avoid duplicate work.

Resources for testing

Discussion of testing resources for the assessment of cancer risks cannot be separated from that of available toxicological expertise in general and of financial resources for toxicological research and investigations. Toxicology should here be seen in a broad sense.

Toxicology has long been a rather neglected area, both in Sweden and in many other countries. Toxicologists, both general and specialists within particular disciplines, are needed, but in Sweden the number of researchers with sound scientific qualifications is small, and the educational resources are limited. Any country needs a strong emphasis on toxicology within various faculties if it is not to become entirely dependent on scientific data and evaluations from elsewhere. In order to be able to have access at all to the latest foreign developments, a home independent contribution is often required.

Toxicological research should aim at improvement of test methods for agents with different mechanisms of action in cancer induction and of methods allowing risk quantification. Certain research matters are touched upon briefly in Chapter 15, such as dose measurements in the target organs and target material in the cell. In planning improved testing resources, it is important not to be too tightly bound to specific methods, for example by their being more or less standardized through international recommendations or agreements. A broad national stake in the development of toxicological knowledge should provide the necessary flexibility in terms of basic physical and human resources within suitably qualified research groups for reinforcement to allow testing activities outside their normal programmes to be carried out. This should conform with a plan commissioned by the Swedish National Board of Universities and Colleges (UHA, 1982). According to this plan, toxicological work and competence should be increased gradually, in principle with an integrated approach as concerns training, research and testing. As further stated in the plan, in view of this approach and the experience to be gained from it, the question of whether or not to set up a separate national laboratory for routine testing could be somewhat postponed.

Of particular interest in the present context are the possibilities for carrying out cancer tests on mammals and various tests for genotoxic effects in short-term experiments on lower organisms, cells or tissues. However, the latter cannot replace, but only supplement, animal experiments in the foreseeable future.

Both traditional cancer tests, for example of new chemicals, and more sophisticated dose–response research, presuppose long-term experiments on animals. A frequent test animal for this purpose is the mouse. These tests demand human and physical resources for animal handling, including sufficient experience in pathology for monitoring the animals and assessing biological changes. Also, although there is no difference in principle between working with radiation-induced or chemically induced animal cancer, the differing techniques for exposing the animals or dose administration of the agent under investigation require their own special know-how.

Since available resources for long-term experiments are extremely limited in Sweden (see Chapter 15), it is recommended that this matter —with special regard to cancer testing—be looked into separately during the gradual build-up of toxicological resources in general. The question of resources for short-term tests should also be studied although the situation here is slightly better.

11.4 The availability of exposure data

Exposure data are required:

(a) when a priority order is to be established for control measures, specific investigations or other research tasks with regard to high-volume or widely distributed substances;
(b) when a substance with known properties has been selected for a more precise estimation of the magnitude of the risk for populations affected;
(c) when it is of interest to follow up trends in exposure for substances with known properties, for example in connection with inspections or other forms of surveillance for compliance with the regulations;
(d) as part of epidemiological monitoring systems and for other epidemiological studies (see also Chapter 8).

Section 4.4. presented and analysed available exposure data concerning a large number of carcinogenic or suspected carcinogenic substances, from several central authorities in Sweden. No more far-reaching comparisons of the results can be usefully carried out, since there apparently exist differences between the agencies concerned in their formal and practical means of following up the exposure conditions, and in their working routines. In view of the central role of exposure analysis, it is clear, however, that the availability of exposure data for the future should be generally improved.

Exposure data do not constitute a unified concept. Rather they are a whole set of various pieces of information which directly or indirectly contribute to a clarification of the existence and levels of exposure to chemical substances of potential interest in risk control. In Sections 4.4.2 and 4.4.3 the dispersion of and exposure to chemical substances in the environment is discussed, and also general prerequisites for the determination of exposures, various exposure and dose concepts relating to the uptake by and metabolism in the body, chemical dosimetry, etc. Therefore we do not try to specify in detail here *how* the need for better exposure data is to be met. Such a task rests primarily with the authorities responsible for risk control. Some information sources and desirable approaches for improving exposure information will be mentioned below.

In Sweden there exist data-bases containing information about composition, volume of sales and so on for certain product groups. Registries with, in principle, complete coverage exist for pharmaceuticals, food additives and pesticides as well as certain other chemical products, the latter as part of the general Products Register, mentioned in Section 4.4.4. Recording takes place continuously at each appropriate central authority. Nothing is recorded however as to *where* exposures take place, and how many persons are exposed or to what extent.

'Exposure data' in the form of concentration measurements in various environments or media are mainly recorded only for specific purposes, and in general are not available in integrated registers. However, in some situations information is generated on a more continuous basis. Within the framework of the Environmental Protection Board's special programme for the monitoring of environmental quality, measurements and environmental samples with respect to environmental pollution in certain areas with a low pollutant charge are compiled continuously, to serve as points of reference.

To some extent, data are generated on emissions to air and water of pollutants from factories posing a potential hazard to the environment and therefore subject to licensing requirements. Since the aim of such measurements is enforcement of individually prescribed emission limits rather than production of statistically representative figures, these data rarely provide a good basis for exposure calculations. There is, however, also an increasing interest at the regional and local levels in monitoring environmental quality, and data are being produced on various pollutants in many lakes and waterways. Ambient air quality, as expressed by one or several parameters, is measured in some individual municipalities, but often only as short series of measurements.

The National Board of Occupational Safety and Health compiles certain exposure data, for example on workers' lead exposure, in a separate computerized register. Other occupational measurements are made as part of the activities of the Labour Inspectorate. Some such data are being computerized on a trial basis. Measurements at the workplace are also undertaken upon local initiative.

The National Food Administration runs internal analysis programmes for various contaminants in foodstuffs. Information concerning heavy metals and pesticide residues is computerized.

Where there has been no regular supply of data on which to base exposure calculations, authorities seem often to have used or initiated 'tailor-made' industrial branch inventories, for instance of chemical products in use. Such inventories could provide good indications of activities with potentially hazardous exposures to man or to the environment, but require supplementary data to yield quantitative exposure indications.

A large number of other exposure data recorded for particular research projects and for administrative purposes on a case-by-case basis are often difficult to access. Furthermore, it can be difficult to generalize from such data, which are often incomplete in some respects.

Chapter 4, in particular Section 4.4.6, specified certain areas and means for improving exposure data. The following aspects should also be considered.

In view of the present availability of exposure data, there seems to be above all a need for a more systematic approach. Any kind of comprehensive exposure data network is, however, out of the question. It will still be necessary in the future often to fall back on temporary efforts in specific branches of industry, etc.

Chapter 8 discussed exposure data as part of epidemiological monitoring systems and recommended that the National Institute of Environmental Medicine be commissioned to investigate how to improve recording of factors of special relevance to cancer induction, including the setting up of human sample banks, such as blood banks, for future studies of earlier exposures. Other types of bank could perhaps consist of 'market-basket' samples of foodstuffs and ambient air samples from workplaces and from the general environment. This possibility should be investigated further, primarily by the relevant central agencies responsible for statutory risk control.

As especially concerns the occupational environment, the responsible central agency ought to specify some requirements about exposure-related information to be recorded by employers where there are potentially hazardous exposures. Recommendations pointing in the same direction as those of the Cancer Committee, which follow below, have been issued in connection with ILO Convention (1974).

It would be desirable for personnel registers to be established, containing unique identification of the individual, information concerning duration of employment, and an occupational code and/or data which would allow the duties of the employee to be linked with specific types of activity, technical process, machine, etc. Since updated registers of personnel are kept for other purposes such as salary accounts, the extra work should be minimal. Taking the period of latency for cancer diseases into account, such personnel registers should be stored for a considerable time, and ought to be moved for some kind of central storage to help epidemiological investigative studies, in case a company goes out of business.

Beyond this, it is difficult to define in a general sense reasonable demands on companies as concerns recording of exposures. In certain cases there is, in Sweden, an obligation to carry out air sampling for specified substances or to take biological samples. As a first additional step one might contemplate requirements for cataloguing chemical products in use, at any rate any which are used in manufacturing processes or the like. Even in this case, it would be a matter of using rather simple notation on purchase invoices or other paperwork, and the information could be stored in a similar way to the personnel data.

Stipulations for systematic recording of exposure levels or dose levels by analysis of air, biological samples, etc., could gradually be extended to further substances and/or branches of industry. This will require a close co-operation between the central agency and the field organization, i.e. the Labour Inspectorate. Furthermore, one can assume that the growing system of special occupational health services for the individual companies will produce more mapping of risk groups and their various exposures. With due consideration for personal privacy, such information should where possible be stored for future investigations.

Concerning the general environment, statistically representative data need to be obtained to a greater extent in order to allow direct or indirect evaluation of current exposures, in particular in urban environments.

Monitoring of air quality in urban areas by means of concentration measurements should be carried out more systematically than hitherto and with greater continuity. Individual municipalities have an important role to play here, and general guidelines from the Environmental Protection Board would undoubtedly facilitate their efforts. Furthermore, it should be a challenge to the research community to identify suitable and practically analysable indicator substances for various types of mixed emission. Attempts to 'characterize biologically' mixed discharges (into water), through simple systems of measurements of certain effect parameters in aquatic organisms, as a first step in the identification and quantification of risk substances should be developed further so that comparisons between different samples become scientifically more informative. In the case of mixed emissions to the air, both the particulate and the gaseous phases have to be considered; the latter has hitherto often been disregarded, because of difficulties in obtaining good samples. The system of individual control programmes in Sweden for discharges from plants posing a potential environmental hazard should be developed further, with increasing emphasis on specific substances (in addition to traditional endpoints such as particulate matter and biological oxygen demand (BOD) and chemical oxygen demand (COD), not least when information concerning the manufacturing process indicates that emissions of genotoxic substances may occur.

Exposure to certain air pollutants in the indoor environment has been treated in various parts of Chapter 10. Only further research can show what the future needs will be for monitoring exposures in the home.

Evaluation of exposure to foreign substances in foodstuffs should be improved, mainly through more chemical analyses. Under Swedish conditions, this means supplementing present routines of analysis directed towards 'hot spots' with samples that are statistically representative of the consumption, in particular for the purpose of calculating the total population load of, for example, genotoxic substances. Also, the total number of substances followed in the food monitoring programmes should be increased, through expanded searches followed by concentration determinations as the case may be. It seems perfectly possible to raise today's level of ambition considerably, if the municipal authorities responsible for inspection and control of compliance with the food laws were to increase their taking of samples for chemical analysis according to plans worked out in co-operation with the National Food Administration. As for the economic burden involved, one should bear in mind that the Food Administration may also prescribe that all costs of sampling and analysis be carried by the party subject to the inspection.

The product registries as they are now run by the authorities can to a certain extent also provide indirect information on exposures. Their value is obviously entirely dependent on the degree of coverage and the nature of the contents of the registry. Wherever meaningful, the use of existing product registries should be part of an integrated approach to follow current exposures, with a view to further reasonable priority ordering of control measures.

11.5 Risk evaluation and risk control measures

The documentation of decisions

Using the terminology of Figure 7.3 for the various functions in risk management, risk evaluation is the immediate precursor to decisions concerning direct measures for risk containment. Initial risk estimations based on medical and scientific data and judgements are supplemented with other information and deliberations concerning risk–benefit assessment, technical and economic possibilities for risk reduction, and so on. At this stage there will usually be a formal decision whether or not to take certain measures, which must be documented.

On the other hand, it seems that the documentation of the grounds for decision could vary in different respects. Even in cases when the material is complete, it may be difficult to comprehend.

It is of great importance that the authorities should account for their decisions as openly as possible, within the framework of existing regulations. As is discussed further in Chapter 12, most or even all documents in a case that are filed by a public authority in Sweden should usually be made available on request. In spite of this, there is a need for special initiatives to help members of the general public find out the reasons behind a decision made on risk control. The decisions should be documented in an easily understood form, with summaries of the risk estimations, cost–benefit analyses and other considerations which influenced each decision. As a clearer policy of risk evaluation and control measures evolves, it is particularly important that the motives for any deviations from this policy or for more difficult decisions in its application should be well documented. The goal should be to publish as much of the documentation as possible, at least in matters of wide concern or of fundamental significance.

The proposed simplification of the supporting documents should not imply that the judicial grounds for possible appeals should be changed, since the parties obviously must be able to invoke all available material. The kind of documentation discussed here is ideally a summary of a problem area or a case for the benefit of the decision-maker as a 'good memorandum', which after possible addition of further material from the final deliberations should be adjoined to the original dossier.

It is particularly important that decisions *not* to introduce control measures in any specific case should be clearly documented. This could happen also at earlier stages in the risk management process than after a full 'risk evaluation' (see Figure 7.3), for example if it is judged that no exposure to the agent under consideration can occur, or if all evidence points to the risk from any exposure being so low as to be negligible. Similarly, if agents are to be legally defined as carcinogens or non-carcinogens, all the scientific data upon which the definition was based must be recorded, as must the way in which the data were interpreted. This applies especially to negative decisions, since it is never possible to *prove* non-carcinogenicity.

It is not feasible to also prescribe a reporting procedure for cases where the officer responsible believes that he should examine a certain risk factor, but also that other tasks are more pressing and should therefore take precedence (see Section 11.3). However, in some cases there might be good reasons for making public internal action programmes, prescribed job procedures and the motives for priorities set by the authority.

Design of measures for risk reduction

No general recommendations can be given as to the design of measures for reducing cancer risks, from an administrative point of view. The circumstances will always vary and a pragmatic approach should be taken.

The approach to taking administrative decisions should be 'result oriented' rather than 'law oriented'. That is to say that the administrator should as a rule first set the goals for a risk reduction in a given situation and then find the best means to reach these goals, i.e. identifying the most suitable piece of legislation to be invoked or other measures to be applied.

If the goal according to Chapter 7, simply expressed, is to reduce or minimize exposures, there is often a whole spectrum of partially overlapping, partially complementary potential measures available. Options include straightforward bans or other restrictions by means of general decrees or decrees tied to specific agents, warning labels on products or other means of informing people so that they themselves can reduce their exposure, etc.

When the *individual risk* in connection with existing exposures is not negligible, it is natural that the protection of the individual should first of all be attained by formal restrictions such as special regulations concerning well defined carcinogenic agents. Such regulations may then need to be supplemented with information to the individual, e.g. at the workplace, about how unnecessary exposure can best be avoided.

Moderate or low cancer risks must in some cases be accepted with regard to members of the general public. To the limited extent that it is a matter of risks, which cannot be influenced by the individual, this should also be considered when regulatory measures are taken. If a product is so hazardous that very special risk control measures are called for, it is unacceptable for use by the general public. However, there are products which for the ordinary user entail only negligible cancer risks but which may—under certain conditions— pose higher risks for a few. This could occur in connection with a hobby where the person is exposed for long periods of time or for a person in contact with a product in such a way that exposure to its components is higher than normal; thus the scraping and grinding of paint containing lead chromate can cause much higher exposure and consequent cancer risk than normal use of the paint itself. It may thus be necessary clearly to inform all users so that the individual himself can choose how to reduce his risks, especially in the latter situation. Care must also be taken to tailor-make the information; to say only that the product contains a carcinogen would probably confuse the 'painter' and would not suffice for the 'scraper'.

As with other kinds of risk factor (see Chapter 9 on health education), the intelligibility of information given about cancer risks depends to some extent upon the ability of the recipient to distinguish between the hazardous properties of an agent and its related risks, especially if the induction of cancer is considered as a random (stochastic) effect in the body. There is now a move in many countries to make information on cancer risks obligatory on the product label. This seems to be a reasonable and justified development but there is a great need to inform people about what warning labels mean, so that risks will be neither over- nor under-estimated. One should also bear in mind that difficulties often arise in attempting to assess correctly the magnitude of a risk.

When it is a question of limiting exposure to cancer initiators, which carry negligible individual risk but to which many persons are exposed, formal restrictions, such as limits on concentrations of agents in the atmosphere or in foodstuffs, seem to be the only plausible means in order to reduce a theoretically calculated collective risk.

In the absence of better quality data than are presently available on all the specific risk factors, each of which could contribute to the load on the individual and on population groups, including factors relating to life-style, it is impossible to judge if or how modified individual behavioural patterns could also constitute a component in the statutory risk control aimed at reducing a collective risk. However, in today's situation, there is no doubt that efforts to change attitudes and behaviour should concentrate on factors in areas *not* subject to regulation by law, namely life-style. Such factors contribute extensively not only to the total cancer incidence, but also often to considerable excess risks to the individual.

To what extent is there a need to harmonize administrative practices between national authorities in risk management? Whereas there remains a serious need for unification of practices in the scientific estimation of risks of cancer-inducing agents, this is less obvious when it comes to risk evaluations and decisions on measures for risk control (see Figure 7.3). The prerequisites for risk containment measures can be so different in different areas of risk that completely different approaches are called for. On the other hand, matters of administrative practice and consistency in proceedings with regard to the business community and the public should be discussed with the aim of neutralizing unnecessary differences in attitudes between agencies. As discussed in Section 7.5.2, the long-term goal of harmonizing principles for protection against similarly acting risk factors should also be kept in mind.

In certain respects co-operation between authorities in the administrative area is particularly needed. Where a particular risk factor is found in different environments, a coordinated strategy for risk reduction is clearly required. The same holds for exposure to agents from different sources which act together synergistically in a risk situation or which act together to generate new active agents, for example nitrogen oxides (NO_x) in inhaled air which can lead to the formation of nitrosamines in the body by reaction with amines absorbed, for example, in the diet. In this context, a unified strategy for taking action also presupposes co-operation in the earlier stages of risk management, i.e. in mapping out the potential risk areas and exposures.

In all probability it would be most valuable if co-operation between authorities could also take place in those areas of risk evaluation which include problems of an economic or behavioural science nature. Cost–benefit analysis—in the broad sense—is often primitive and needs to be developed further (see Section 7.5.2). This is, however, a general problem in risk management rather than a problem specifically related to cancer, and it is therefore not examined further here.

Finally, the importance of international co-operation should be emphasized—when it is a matter of general administrative policy for risk control, legislation, measures against trans-boundary pollution, experience gained from various types of measure for exposure containment, etc.

Follow-up of administrative measures for risk containment

The follow-up of administrative measures for risk containment can have two main objectives. One objective is formal and is dependent on the constitution and other legal conditions in a country: to ensure compliance with the new regulations. The other objective is concerned with the effects as such, is often less dependent on national administrative systems, and may coincide with the first objective, but does not always do so.

It goes without saying that the first type of supervision is very important—and not only for enforcing a certain piece of legislation. The individual citizen will have greater confidence in the public bodies and in the measures taken if he can see such control processes in operation.

The primary aim of risk reduction measures is to reduce or eliminate exposures to the factor in question, the actual goal being to improve people's health. At the same time as such measures are being drawn up, plans should be made for monitoring and evaluating the results within a given time, at least with regard to the primary aim. This can involve bringing in other bodies whose co-operation will be needed.

Since measures to reduce the effects of one specific factor on its own will rarely produce dramatic reduction in overall cancer incidence, it is important that the monitoring systems set up should look broadly across the spectrum of measures being taken and different factors involved.

11.6 Organizational aspects

Some of the matters discussed above also justify consideration of how public risk management is organized in Sweden, with special regard to central co-ordination. One such matter is the limited availability of good scientific expertise for cancer risk assessment. Another matter, partly related, concerns criteria for the identification of carcinogenic agents and for estimation of cancer risks. In this context there is also reason to look again at the need for co-operation to improve the efficiency of public risk management as a whole.

Besides the different functions in the risk management process, the objectives of this process must also be considered. The relations between risk areas or risk factors to be controlled and the responsibilities of each agency are of special importance. In Sweden, as in other countries, these sometimes impinge upon each other.

Some of the authorities concerned have research departments within their organizations, besides administrative departments. For Sweden, scientific research and investigative work is carried out in particular by the Board of Occupational Health and Safety.[3] Some agencies have a system of external scientific advisers; these persons cannot always respond to the extent or as quickly as is desirable, due to other full-time engagements. One of the key agencies in cancer risk control, the Products Control Board, has none of these facilities. Several authorities in Sweden seem to need greatly improved basic resources to fall back on, not only in a crisis situation such as a sudden 'alarm' over a new risk causing great public anxiety, but also for their day-to-day work.

There is a need to extend (and also to establish a firm organizational structure for) co-operation, primarily between the relevant public agencies at the central level. This applies particularly to the scientific risk estimations, and would ensure that experience and knowledge are shared.

Although this report deals with carcinogenic agents only, it is reasonable to assume a need for scientific co-operation in the control of other types of risk as well. Besides, it is hard to envisage an efficient co-operation regarding cancer risk assessment without considering matters of quality and interpretation of toxicological data in general. There is in fact a need for a general collaboration across the whole field of scientific evaluation in risk control, with sub-groups for specific questions, of which one would be for cancer risk analysis, since this requires special knowledge and experience.

An institutionalized scientific collaboration between the authorities would facilitate broader and more intensive contacts with the rest of the scientific community. Thus it is important that external scientific experts should also take part in discussions concerning criteria for risk analysis and in specific risk assessments. This is already the case to a certain extent in, for example, the establishment of criteria for agents in the work environment, but such activities could well be amplified. Unnecessary competition between agencies for scientific assistance with regard to similar or even identical problems could be reduced. More efficient use of limited expertise would result.

Increased collaboration between central authorities should also facilitate the division of labour between them, particularly as concerns investigations for risk identification and risk estimation, but also as concerns the planning and execution of tests, etc.

The collaboration should preferably be subdivided into one purely scientific area and one or more for other matters of common interest. A special forum should thus be created where administrative policy could be discussed and compared, where optimal measures for risk reduction in the legal context could be identified in cases where more than one law is applicable, or where results are dependent on concerted action by several agencies.

Since chemical risks are so widely spread, almost any conceivable organizational system for the management of such risks implies the possibility of matters being pushed from one agency to another or of falling between them altogether. The danger of this happening would decrease with determined and well organized co-operation between the authorities concerned. However, it is not suggested that there should be a new 'super-group' authorized to take decisions over the heads of existing agencies. The responsibility and independence of each agency should be maintained.

The areas of co-operation which are outlined here for the authorities may be viewed as a two-dimensional scheme. The work content in one dimension is proposed to include matters concerning risk control as prescribed in the existing legislation, where a number of authorities are 'equals' within their respective areas of responsibility. Here one finds the separate bodies responsible for the working environment, the natural environment, foodstuffs, pharmaceuticals and cosmetic and hygienic products, local sanitary conditions, commercial products hazardous to health or environment, and radiation protection. The work content in the other dimension— with special regard to cancer and other health risks—might be considered to be questions of overall health protection. The latter deal with interrelationships between agents in various environments including the interaction between life-style and factors regulated by law, the load on the individual and on the population as concerns particular risk factors as well as a continuous monitoring of the total cancer incidence and its known or suspected causes, identification of possible loopholes to be closed or other alterations required in the legislation.

To a large extent, the matters discussed here relate directly or indirectly to the control of chemicals in general. Under Swedish conditions, it therefore seems preferable to place a responsibility for organizing and promoting the collaboration between agencies with the Products Control Board, except of matters of overall health. The responsibility for initiating and co-ordinating actions in the latter case should be with the National Board of Health and Welfare, whose statutes in fact already contain such a clause.

The recommended co-operation is mainly oriented towards chemical health and environmental hazards, but should also in relevant cases include questions concerning radiation, in which the National Institute of Radiation Protection should take part. It would be advantageous to continue the discussions concerning the usefulness of the radiation protection policy in other fields as well (see Chapter 7). As concerns radiation protection, there must be a broad network of contacts in the medical/biological field—in addition to close co-operation with the radiobiological institutions directly.

11.7 Overall conclusions

Points of departure

Legislation (and related authority responsibilities and resources) are among the mechanisms by which a country's citizens are to be assured of a reasonable protection against conditions in the environment which raise the cancer risk, primarily against involuntary exposure to carcinogenic or co-carcinogenic physical and chemical agents. Protection of the individual against unacceptable individual hazards must come first but, in accordance with the aims of the preventive strategy, the collective risks must also be considered in relevant situations when shaping and applying the laws, these risks being expressed as the theoretically calculated number of cases of cancer in a certain exposed sub-population or in the whole population.

The cancer risks considered here fall within several areas of jurisdiction regulating health and environmental hazards in various environments or regulating hazards from various activities or products. This legislation provides more exact specifications as to the responsibility of the authorities, companies and individuals concerned. Certain fundamental principles are evident in this legislation as outlined in this chapter, in particular the division of responsibility between authorities and companies. Although the outward appearances seem to differ, this legislation provides ample formal possibilities for the Government and the relevant authorities to bear their part of the responsibility in risk control, by means of bans and other regulations on usage, general advice and special resolutions.

Classification of carcinogens and priorities in risk management

Scientific risk analysis—in particular as concerns the estimation of the magnitude of a potential cancer risk in humans exposed to a specific substance or mixture of substances—is, as a rule, difficult, requiring careful scientific assessments of all available information about the properties and effects of the agents.

From a strictly scientific point of view, it is usually desirable to avoid sharp delimitations of risks or substance classifications without nuances ('black versus white') which might be misunderstood. However, statutory risk control presupposes that certain agents are defined in the legal sense as carcinogens with a risk to humans, although such carcinogenicity is seldom proven. The principles by which such definitions or classifications of 'carcinogens' are made should be further developed, well documented and explained as far as possible to the general public.

It would be advisable to separate the classification of a substance as carcinogenic on the one hand from decisions concerning control measures on the other. This would also mean assessing the scientific weight of the evidence from more than one point of view. The Cancer Committee has recommended that the demands for such a classification, in the legal sense, could be 'moderate', whereas decisions on type and degree of measures to reduce the risk thus pointed out should be influenced more by the strength of the evidence.

It is desirable that scientific data be judged uniformly by the various risk control authorities, which in turn implies a need for unified criteria for the evaluation of substances considered as carcinogenic in a legal sense.

The setting of priorities in risk management is another important aspect. Here one should include the question of optimal use of test resources. Even though the sphere of activity, in particular as concerns chemical agents, would seem to be nearly unlimited, it should not be impossible to manage health risks in such a way that reasonable demands for safety and efficiency are met. However, this requires a careful priority setting in the public sector. The relevant international literature is vast, and intensified international co-operation should be encouraged not only with regard to common guidelines for risk management but also a possible sharing of the workload between countries.

In producing a basis for risk assessments, priority should be given to exposure analysis of already known or strongly suspected carcinogenic agents, rather than comprehensive data collection on the properties and effects of other agents. In addition, certain priorities should be set as concerns resources for risk identification with respect to specific environments or specific agents in situations where exposure in individual cases is thought to be high and/or when large numbers of persons are exposed. Sufficient resources should be allocated to allow more detailed investigations or studies of special national problems or observations suggesting the existence of risks not detected previously. The availability of testing resources for the evaluation of cancer risks is intimately associated with the general build-up of toxicological knowledge and toxicological research and investigative resources. An integrated approach to training, research and testing is required, but it is important to focus on particular sectors of toxicology during the build-up period, such as facilities for long-term cancer tests in animals and also resources for short-term testing.

Exposure data

Exposure data, obtained through direct measurements or extrapolated from data of other kinds (e.g. on inventories of products in use within a certain industrial branch) are required for the purpose of risk management by the authorities and companies as well as in epidemiological research. The availability of data and of procedures generating data is somewhat patchy in Sweden. The authorities' grasp of the overall exposure situation should in many cases also be improved. Above all, there is a need for a systematic approach. Any kind of comprehensive exposure data network is, however, out of the question and in many situations in the future it will still be necessary to fall back on temporary efforts. Section 11.4 outlines various ways of augmenting the availability of exposure data in practice.

Some administrative questions

Decisions by authorities concerning control measures of various kinds should be documented in an easily understood manner with summaries of risk estimations, cost–benefit analyses and other relevant information, so that the documentation includes all data and deliberations which actually have influenced each decision. In particular, the motives for any deviation from the policy of the authority itself, or more difficult decisions based on this policy, should be well documented. Furthermore, considerations that lead to a decision not to take direct risk reduction measures should be particularly carefully recorded. The approach to taking administrative decisions should be result oriented, so that the first goal to be attained is established, and then the legal or other means available and their likely effectiveness in attaining the goal are assessed. If the risk to the individual from an involuntary existing exposure is not negligible, it is evident that the protection of the individual should be attained primarily through formal restrictions such as special regulations concerning well-defined carcinogenic agents. Such regulations may need amplification in the form of information to the individual. The intelligibility of this information to some extent depends upon the ability of the recipient to distinguish between the hazardous properties of an agent and its related risks, in particular if cancer induction is considered as a random (stochastic) effect in the body. Co-operation in risk management, as well as in risk assessment, is needed between central agencies. This should include public bodies working at regional or local levels to supervise the compliance with regulations. A co-ordinated strategy for risk reduction may be needed when, for example, a particular risk factor appears in different environments or when the factors which appear in different environments interact.

International co-operation in matters such as administrative policy and legislation is also important.

An authority taking a decision on risk-reducing measures should at the same time plan for a future follow-up of actual results obtained. Independent of such plans, though possibly partly coinciding, a continuous, wide-scale monitoring of the observance of existing rules is essential, especially in order to promote the confidence of the individual in the control mechanisms of society.

Since co-operation is essential between the various administrative authorities within whose spheres of interest different forms of cancer risk may fall, its organizational structures need to be considered. This applies to the central agencies in particular, whose co-operation should be institutionalized especially as regards scientific risk assessment. This may prove the best way of using the collected scientific knowledge within as well as outside the agencies.

The co-operation might also include the mapping of risk factors and the planning and carrying out of tests and matters of administrative policy. It is important that overall cancer risk problems including lifestyle factors should also be taken up in this context, irrespective of regulatory aspects.

Notes

1 SFS is the Swedish Code of Statutes, available from Liber Förlag. [*Ed. note.*]
2 After investigation by an *ad hoc* governmental committee (main report of the Chemicals Commission 1984) and largely in accor-

dance with its recommendations, the Swedish Parliament has adopted a new act to supersede the 1973 legislation (later issued as the Products Control Act, SFS 1985:426). However, this new act seems to a great extent to build on the principles in the previous one, referred to here.

The Chemicals Inspectorate has superseded the Products Control Board as the central regulatory agency and certain other organizational changes have been made. It is envisaged that the new agency should concentrate on the products as such, their risks and safe handling in general and on importers'/manufacturers' duties, whereas central supervisory agencies will have more power than previously to actually regulate product handling in more specific situations.

In its original report, the Cancer Committee referred especially to this investigation, which was still in progress, as a reason for not discussing in depth what legal instruments, and resources in this context, are required to manage chemical risks including those of carcinogens. [*Ed. note.*]

3   The scientific department of the Board of Occupational Health and Safety was separated and set up as a more independent body in 1987. [*Ed. note.*]

12
Co-operation and mutual trust in risk control—the role of information

12.1 Introduction

The possibility of controlling and preventing risks (as for promoting health in general) in a community depends on a number of conditions and relationships in that community. Legislation, resources for authorities or other organizations, and various research contributions are not the only decisive factors. The interaction between affected parties is also very important. One such party is the individual citizen. Everyone needs to be able to judge fairly well firstly the risks in his own life situation, which are important, for example, in the case of cancer risks, and secondly the risk situation in a wider social perspective. Here the individual citizen has the opportunity of influencing resource distribution, as well as rules about rights and responsibilities in the community through his elected representative in political decision-making gatherings. Those attitudes which are formed by interaction between individuals and organizations of various types are decisive. Opinion-formers in the mass media here play a prominent role. It is important for democracy to counteract the confidence gap which easily opens up when information is sometimes too general or difficult to understand, or too limited to give the public a chance for consideration and comprehension.

This chapter is restricted to a specific matter which relates closely to possibilities for co-operation and trust in risk control—namely access to information in the broad sense. In appropriate sections the question will be discussed from a general point of view regarding the individual's right to information in our society—not only as regards risk control.

The Cancer Committee here chose to discuss the question of access to information by examining certain points, namely statutory availability or secrecy regarding information in Sweden, the information flow, the information offered, as well as the quality and interpretation of the information.

Even with this limited contribution to a number of specific questions regarding information, one is dealing with phenomena which have a far wider relevance than to cancer alone. So the discussion here is relatively superficial, aiming primarily to bring some of these problems to the fore, rather than produce final answers.

Two fairly large governmental reports have recently dealt with the question of information in this context. The investigation concerning information about risks in the work environment (INRA,1982) took up the whole problem of risks in the work environment—from monitoring the development in the understanding of risks and precautions, to training, advising and other information needs, as well as questions relating to the legal and practical opportunities for gaining access to information. Information and other consultative services relating to risks were touched upon, as were, for example, specific technical advisory and communication systems. The mass media's role was generally discussed as was that of periodicals which supply society with information about working environment risks, and opportunities for stimulating research workers into making popular scientific presentations of their experience in important work environment matters. The former Swedish Council of Environment Information (MDN, 1982) gave an account in its main report of, for example, an enquiry including certain project work under the heading Toxicological Information Service. The need for different sorts of information and information levels (unprocessed/processed) relative to the recipient's prior knowledge was explained. Different options for developing further existing literature into a more general information service were discussed. Following the Council's report and the subsequent comments by various interested parties, the Swedish Parliament adopted a governmental proposal to set up a toxicological information service at the Karolinska Institute's library and information centre from July 1982.[1]

12.2 Information—openness and secrecy

Background

It is vital that there is as much openness as possible between the parties concerned with managing risks. The duty of a company, for example, as regards its responsibility to keep itself informed about risks, and in specific cases to inform the authorities, is controlled by legislation. Responsible authorities must ensure that this system of regulation functions. Some difficulties in this area have been touched upon in Chapter 11.

If the public loses confidence in statutory risk control, panic situations may easily arise and pressure be applied to make decisions based on inadequate information. In the long run, such decisions may prove to be unjustified but, meanwhile, the production of a useful product may have been halted. In other cases it may subsequently turn out that public anxiety about a certain activity was justified. In such cases the confidence gap would have widened further, had the hazardous activity continued.

The problem with decisions that must be taken under conditions of uncertainty has been touched upon in Chapter 7. It is necessary, however, to distinguish between, on the one hand, information which was actually available at a specific time or which could have been put forward on scientific grounds, and, on the other hand, information which may come to light long afterwards as a result of new scientific theories and new methods being used. The fact remains, however, that public confidence in risk control in all circumstances will depend very largely on the availability of information.

Legislation

The openness which has long characterised Swedish society has gained an important expression in the Freedom of the Press Act, one of the four constitutional documents of this country. The Act in chapter 2 decrees that 'to further free interchange of opinions and enlightenment of the public, every Swedish national shall have free access to official documents' (including information stored on computer). Seen in an international perspective, the access to information in all matters dealt with by public bodies is very wide. In the same chapter of this constitutional document it is stated that exceptions may be made only for the purposes established therein, and that such exceptions 'shall be scrupulously specified in provisions of a specific act of law ...'. This has been done with the Secrecy Act, the one now in force adopted by Parliament in 1980 (with subsequent amendments).

With regard to the issues discussed in this report the most important of established purposes for secrecy is that the right to study an official document may be restricted if this is necessary to protect 'the personal integrity or the economic conditions of individuals'. In Chapter 8, Paragraph 6 of the Secrecy Act, there is a regulation regarding secrecy for certain governmental authority activities, such as licensing, inspection and support in commerce and industry. In relation to the aim of the activity, secrecy may be prescribed for 'a private subject's business or management conditions, inventions or research results if it can be assumed that the person concerned would suffer loss should the information be disclosed'. Secrecy does, however, require a governmental provision (usually by means of an amendment to further specifications and lists in a special governmental decree, which in this respect supplements the Act), and an exception from this secrecy can be made both generally and if the government in certain cases finds that it would be important for the information to be distributed. *The Secrecy Act does not therefore imply any absolute ban on an authority releasing various details of commercial and industrial circumstances.* A refusal to release assumes that an individual or body (usually the company which the information affects) will suffer damage if the information is released to someone else. The assessment of the risk of damage is the responsibility of the authorities. It is therefore not enough for the entrepreneur to consider that publicity would be detrimental. Let us assume, for example, that a producer of a certain hazardous chemical has not given the obligatory information on the label about which substance(s) render the product harmful, but revealed this to the control agency in a letter. In such a situation there could obviously be no 'protection' through secrecy and the authority concerned would not refuse access to the document or feel inhibited from making it public itself as the case may be. Furthermore, there are listed in the legislation several important situations where the ruling of the authority in a specific case is completely exempt from secrecy.

It is significant that the opportunity to inspect official documents is given in the law as a *right* to the individual, irrespective of whether he is personally involved in the matter. A refusal by the authority concerned to release information can therefore be appealed against, normally to one of the two Administrative Courts of Appeal, and the authority must accordingly give a legally tenable justification for its decision. It should, however, be pointed out that this guarantee can be put to use only if the individual knows of the existence of the pertinent documents.

What can be accessed on the basis of the Freedom of the Press Act is only such information as is *documented* one way or another by an authority, for example, in connection with licensing matters or an inspection. When it comes to working life and conditions at the place of work, there are special regulations, primarily the work environment legislation, which make provision for *requesting* information, primarily from an employer. As concerns, for example, occupational cancer risks, this opens up other ways besides the Freedom of the Press Act. With regard to information needs as expressed by employees and trade unions there has, however, also been some controversy both over responsibilities and procedures according to the work environment legislation and over certain exceptions from the Freedom of the Press Act (see also INRA, 1982).

Even though the protection of secrecy has been deliberately broken in various areas by legislation, the fact undoubtedly remains that much information which is sought both by research workers as well as by opinion-makers, individuals and interest groups cannot be released even by authorities who themselves have access to it. Access to information is important in competitive situations, not least internationally, and increased openness is therefore something which should be aimed at by those representing Sweden at an international level. This has already taken place to a considerable extent.

In addition, a change in international attitudes seems moreover to be occurring with regard to the will to take up these matters. One can quote as an example the fact that EEC countries have, by means of a Council directive (EEC, 1979) 'advance notification relating to new substances', prescribed that industrial and commercial secrecy shall not apply to certain information about a notified substance.

Within the Organization for Economic Co-operation and Development (OECD) these matters have also attracted attention. In 1983 the OECD's highest decision-making body (the Council) adopted two recommendations in this area (OECD 1983a, b). One is similar, but not identical to, the EEC directive. It states that, for example, summaries of risk information (health, safety and environmental data), including precise figures and conclusions, should be regarded as open information in all circumstances, irrespective of the legislation in the respective countries (it is assumed that summaries are made in collaboration with persons providing the information). Opinions can be divided as to whether this goes far enough in the delicate balance between providing incentives to development work in industry and the public's and the research community's right to as much complete information as possible. The recommendation is, however, a good example of a platform from which more work can be done. It should be added that this recommendation (as distinct from the EEC regulations) relates to existing as well as new chemicals.

The second of the two OECD recommendations relates to data submitted to a responsible authority in conjunction with notifications of new chemicals. The OECD requests the member states in such matters to accept 'risk data' only when the person concerned can show that he has the right to make use of this data. This increased protection for a manufacturer against competitors' making use of his perhaps large investment, in the form of tests on a new substance, seems at the same time to contain considerably increased opportunities in the long term for openness as regards data of this sort—and at an international level. With regard to pesticides, this is clearly expressed, for example, in documentation from the UN Food and Agriculture Organization (FAO) in its work to harmonize international requirements for registration of such agents. Statements from the pesticide industry's collaborating body GIFAP (Groupement International des Associations Nationales de Fabricants de Produits Agrochimiques) have pointed out that the protection of secrecy as such is not important to the industry (with the exception of traditional so-called business secrets such as production methods). According to GIFAP, there are thus no objections to public access to the 'health and safety data' which accompany a registration application for a pesticide, so long as this does not include the right to copy such data, i.e. proprietary information.

Although all the detailed rules concerning secrecy in Sweden for certain information have recently been the subject of revision after a long investigation period, this is not an issue to be left to take its own course now. Matters relating to this subject are very complicated, and it is important that both the practical national application as well as the international developments be followed, with the aim of bringing about as much openness as possible.

The INRA committee investigating information matters about risks in the work environment considered that there was a need for some clarification of the Secrecy Act so that 'a request for information which is prompted by the wish to protect life and health' should be 'dealt with more favourably'. In the 1982/83 budget proposal, the Labour Market Minister gave notice that she intended to take up these matters specifically.

What may be described as a test case concerning the limit of Swedish secrecy protection (on the question of documents relating to registering pesticides) is currently (1984) being tried in the Stockholm Administrative Court of Appeal. The authority most involved here, the Products Control Board, has stressed the public's interest in the matter and its own interest in being able to give an open account of the basis for its decision.[2]

As far as pharmaceuticals are concerned, an official Swedish investigation into the monitoring of drug legislation and related matters is considering to what extent secrecy should apply when testing and registering a drug. According to the terms of reference, 'both the manufacturer's need for secrecy as regards, for example, the invention and research results, as well as the community's and the public's legitimate needs for openness should be taken into account'.[3]

In abstaining from further pursuing matters concerning the formulation and application of regulations about publicity and secrecy, the Cancer Committee expresses the following general view. For confidence in risk control and for free research, it is important that access to information held by an authority about possible health risks should in principle be unrestricted, for example in matters relating to data about the presence of specific chemical and physical agents, their properties and effects. Not least by international collaboration, it should become possible to increase the public's access to such information whilst at the same time satisfying companies' legitimate interests in protection against competitors utilizing the asset inherent in the information.

Hearings

Consultation, in which one seeks to reach a 'consensus', i.e. agreement between parties concerned, for example, in a risk assessment or with regard to a proposed measure, is a much used informal, non-institutionalized method of working in Swedish administration. Representatives of different interests discuss the matter together with the authorities and also go through the information available, though not in detail when it comes to items formally designated as secret. Not infrequently a common point of view is reached regarding the pertinent question or risk, and the participants subsequently inform their mandators. As far as the work environment is concerned, procedures in this area have become somewhat more institutionalized.

However, other, less restricted forms of contact between different parties ought also to be tried to a greater extent than hitherto, and then more for an exchange of information than for consultation. Open hearings, where members of the general public also have a chance to put questions to the experts and interested parties present, may be desirable in specific important or controversial situations where different health and environmental risks or potentially dangerous products are concerned.

At least one of the acts with some bearing on the control of cancer risks, namely the Environment Protection Act (see Chapter 11), provides for a procedure which can be regarded as a special form of hearing. Included within the legal procedure for licence examination applicable to certain types of polluting factories and other establishments, there are court-like proceedings. The firm in question has an open 'trial' in which to answer questions from both the licensing board (the Franchise Board for Environment Protection) and from others, for example, the local population.

There are other examples of hearings, alongside what is formally required by the Environment Protection Act. Thus in 1981 the Environmental Advisory Council, which is an advisory body to the Government, held an open discussion about a controversial activity (planned uranium mining), including reports and replies from the firm in question. As indicated above, central control agencies usually restrict themselves to discussions directly with representatives of concerned parties, together or individually. In this area it would perhaps be especially valuable to hold public hearings. Local authorities have sometimes arranged open debates about questionable activities within the municipality, for example, forest spraying with pesticides, where opportunities were given to put questions to the firms involved.

Other legislation in the field of health and environmental protection, such as that concerning various types of product (food, drugs and other chemicals), does not *impose* on the relevant firm the need to produce information during public discussions. There seems however, to be no *impediment* against any questioning in this context. Most frequently it should lie within the interest of the firm in question to collaborate by offering reliable information about its work or its products during such public hearings.

Regarding both hearings and other forms of information dissemination, it is particularly important that competent scientists are given the opportunity to collaborate, and to do so on their own responsibility, irrespective of where and for whom they work. *Questions about openness and secrecy of information in connection with risk assessments will, in the opinion of the Cancer Committee, be meaningful only if an imperative demand for quality is placed on the information supplied, for both primary data and their scientific evaluation.* These questions are considered further below.

12.3 Information supply

International scientific literature

A large amount of information about risks, risk factors and possibilities for counteracting risks is to be found in the international scientific literature. This was touched on in the introduction to Chapter 8 on information systems.

The most respected journals demand a high quality for acceptance of contributions. Once published, scientific reports can be seen, assessed and discussed by other scientists, which is an essential tool for the development of high quality scientific work.

There is also research and investigative work, the results of which may be of practical significance even though they lack great scientific news value. For instance, an institution may, at the behest of an authority, test a series of substances for a specific biological effect, by a known method and without any surprising result. Such investigations are usually reported directly to the commissioner of the work and/or in unpretentious (national) report series—without peer review.

A comprehensive view of the huge amount of information available is facilitated by international review journals within many different fields, for example, biomedicine. Among these some touch on cancer specifically. Using literature *data bases*, both new and previously published reports can be identified and located by means of search words. Review articles of high scientific quality, which summarize the current state of knowledge within certain fields, are to be found in many journals. Certain international journals specialize in scientific news items and review articles.

'Digested' (evaluated) information assumes a special place. In this case a broadly based scientific group may have assessed and weighed up the detailed information available from different sources and studies. Certain organizations operate planned, continuous assessment work of this sort, for example the UN Scientific Committee on the Effects of Atomic Radiation (UNSCEAR), the International Agency for Research on Cancer in Lyons (IARC) and the (World Health Organization) (WHO). The Cancer Committee has used, among others, lists of chemical substances classified by the IARC and NCI as carcinogenic (see Section 4.4). Certain scientific associations collaborate indirectly, in that members make their expertise available by participating in different working groups to make comprehensive evaluations of various data, and risk assessments. As far as Sweden is concerned, continuous work is being carried out (by scientists from the Board of Occupational Safety and Health) on so-called 'health criteria documents' for different materials in the work environment; this is taking place as a Scandinavian collaboration.

Such qualified group assessments (as a rule resulting in a 'scientific consensus') can take place at the instigation of a scientific institution, an industrial branch organization, an authority or other body. As always in interpreting and evaluating scientific data of the type under consideration here, one must presume that the result will depend on those taking part. However, special conferences, to which prominent scientists are called to discuss and, to a greater or lesser extent, evaluate scientific documents about some relevant matter, are a natural way of seeking to improve quality and objectivity in decision making. Such work normally results in written reports without restrictions on secrecy. Several such conferences within the Committee's field of interest have been held in Sweden in recent years (one on dietary factors and cancer, 1981, see Section 10.2.1, and two conferences on general air pollution in 1977 and 1982, see Section 6.6).

Here one is dealing with fully 'open' information which in theory is available to all, although it is sometimes difficult in practice to gain access to it.

Information transmission

The usability of the scientific information available, for example, in cancer prevention, depends on whether the information can be transmitted to concerned parties and individuals in a comprehensible form, without being distorted on the way.

In the first place it is individual scientists who, each in their own specialist field, try to follow what happens at the frontiers of knowledge. The access of other interested parties to information will as a rule depend on an intermediate stage where the information is interpreted, summarized or processed in some way. Governmental authorities, the larger firms and branch organizations in industry and commerce and other organizations, for example, within the trade union movement, to a certain extent run their own research or keep up to date with new literature using competent specialists. Such organizations also usually need contacts with outside scientists as well as different types of information services.

The Cancer Committee has recommended (Chapter 11) increasing the amount of formal co-operation between some central authorities with control responsibilities in the field of health and environmental protection. This action was justified partly by the fact that any collaboration would improve opportunities for procuring the necessary information for the authorities by monitoring the scientific literature. Systems which improve the chances of the Government itself following developments within particular relevant spheres are discussed in Chapter 16.

The needs of individuals or common-interest organizations for information about causes of cancer, chances of cancer prevention, etc., can be grouped roughly into the following types of information, which partially overlap: (a) news; (b) information in the event of an emergency; (c) specially processed information within different (often fairly large) factual spheres; and (d) information in the form of health education, aimed at influencing peoples' attitudes and behaviour.

There ought to be many different sources and channels of information in a country, even at the risk of the information contradicting itself or even becoming erroneous in subjects such as cancer which are difficult to grasp from a scientific or an emotional standpoint. This risk must be counteracted, but in ways other than by limiting the number of information channels.

As a component in the task of disease prevention, health education assumes a special position (see Chapter 9). Other forms of factual information mentioned above will also influence peoples' willingness to change from an unhealthy life-style, or otherwise, to avoid risks and can, therefore, be seen as important additions to planned health education.

Mass media (press, radio and television) are today the commonest sources of information about the majority of risks, including that of cancer. The mass media's importance in this respect, both for employees and, particularly, for small firms was highlighted in the report referred to earlier in this chapter (INRA, 1982).

From the community's side, attempts are being made to make complex information more accessible and comprehensible. Governmental authorities in Sweden have recommended systematic development and a trial project to supply more information about research results. In recent years the State has increasingly supported and initiated the spread of popular scientific information. The Swedish

Council for the Planning and Co-ordination of Research stated in 1981 that it had 'in a successful manner interacted with and even contributed towards an increasing interest in scientific information, also among the mass media, and contributed towards an increased consciousness of the significance of research matters in general'. Periodicals supported by government funds, such as *Källa* (*'Source'*) and *Forskning och Framsteg* (*'Science and Progress'*) distribute popularly presented scientific information. It is, however, in the nature of things that individual fields of research cannot be given continuous coverage in such a periodical. Children and young people constitute special target groups, and national funds to the said Council have been increased for helping to disseminate research information to them.

Certain authorities issue their own journals or other news and information sheets. Central governmental agencies, which hold control and inspection data concerning, for example, cancer risks, should present simplified information in an attractive manner, within their respective spheres of responsibility. Naturally, representatives of these bodies must also contribute information and comments in 'alarm situations', even if it is the mass media which really decide what information will reach the public. Such recommendations constitute nothing new. When certain guidelines were adopted in 1971 by the Swedish Parliament and Government for public information activities, this meant that information dissemination should be seen as an integrated part of the authorities' work. For bodies responsible for risk control and supervision, this means primarily making information available to the citizens about their rights and obligations.

Several scientific libraries in Sweden maintain services supplying information from international literature data bases and other sources. Of special interest in this connection is the Toxicological Information Service within the Karolinska Institute's library and information centre (see Section 12.1). According to the original intention endorsed by Parliament, such a service should include both literature monitoring and reference to information sources in the form of books, reports, journal articles, data bases, individuals and so on. In the Committee's view, this has indeed increased the possibilities for interested parties to obtain help with information in relation to, for example, cancer risks or specific chemical risk factors. Both experimental and epidemiological information is included in the service. Experience will show how far this information centre can go in processing scientific information to meet the user's need. This could become a question of cost.

It was felt by some members of the Cancer Committee that there might exist a more general requirement for 'news services'—in particular relating to scientific reports—which may be related to the occurrence of cancer and to practical possibilities for reducing risks of cancer. However, since the actual need was difficult to judge, no specific recommendation along these lines was put forward. It was also stressed that those bodies which are active in the information or publishing spheres also have sufficiently close contact with users that they can anticipate requirements and try to satisfy them as they arise.

In conclusion there is good reason to recall once again the great importance of the mass media as regards the spread of information alongside contributions from authorities and research workers, for keeping the public informed. This applies both to news and review articles or radio and television programmes on fairly large problem areas. It is important that both the mass media and the higher education authorities (see below) assume their responsibilities in this context. Firstly, access is needed to well-informed journalists or other experts for monitoring the research front. Secondly, a policy for the media is needed as regards their scope, direction and aim in connection with information concerning risks, so that it is not solely directed into alarmist or other dramatic news items. Efforts to explain scientific problems and to provide information about research do occur to some extent in the Swedish mass media and deserve to be supported. Compared to information presented about topical events, information concerning basic medical and biological research is minimal, in spite of the latter being of such importance for our health and living conditions as human beings. The mass media ought to try to help the general public to understand and assess critically, for example, a complicated (or simplified!) debate about risks in a critical situation, by encouraging a basic general knowledge among the public. The Committee considers it important that the mass media should provide more complete information in the important areas discussed here, since they are, in principle, best suited to telling the public about it.

12.4 Quality of information

Background

Wise application of reliable scientific data is obviously a necessary requirement for an effective health and environmental protection policy which includes cancer prevention measures. For this reason, the tendency, which sometimes occurs in public debate, to belittle the importance of such research results is disturbing.

Like many other biological questions, the causes of cancer and cancer risks can rarely be explained with absolute certainty, even by means of the best research, but nevertheless they can be illustrated and assessed with a greater or lesser degree of scientific certainty. To demand 100 per cent accuracy in such situations is as foolish as to disregard totally the importance of research results as the primary basis of risk control. The interpretation of scientific data thus becomes one of the key issues.

The understanding of the significance of scientific data presumes that it has been disseminated correctly, and interpreted with maximum objectivity and in a way which can be understood by the respective target groups. The quality of the information depends both on the scientists themselves (the primary informers) and on the journalists and other professional informers—and, in addition, on the actual communication processes in between. Any communication which is coloured by mistrust and polarization usually produces poor understanding in return. The conditions vary, depending on the informer's own prior knowledge and occupational role. Specialist press journalists work under rather different conditions than do 'news journalists'. In particular the latter often lack basic knowledge in the medical or natural science fields. The research worker who presents his own work generally has a more limited task and is in a different situation to the decision-makers or officials who have to use all the available, but often still incomplete, scientific material in a given situation.

Improved knowledge of each other's working conditions, an open attitude and a willingness to learn from one another should help to bring about an improvement in the quality of public understanding (see for example Werkö (1982) and Atterstam 1984)).

Some factors to bear in mind

The first ethical and qualitative demands rest with the research workers themselves who, in presenting research theories and results, act as primary informers. Here the self-regulating mechanisms of the national and international scientific community as regards financial support and publication are very important, even though these mechanisms cannot prevent occasional abuse. At the same time the system may sometimes act to inhibit or even repress when it comes to receiving new ideas.

In accordance with research ethics, the scientist should ensure that he or she makes careful interpretations of his or her research results. At the same time, society demands of the scientist that he make available to an increased extent his knowledge and authority in relevant matters, since the process of opinion forming and control must function, even when scientific knowledge is incomplete. The scientist's demand for documentation and certainty in assessments is high compared with what applies, for example, in 'hot news' journalism. The common question in certain situations is, however, *when* is scientific information sufficient for meaningful information to be released about, for example, a cancer risk? Information released too soon with insufficient substantiation can, just like too cautious and delayed information, give rise to legitimate unease among the public. For authorities in risk-control—who must assess whether a decision not to issue warnings or restrictions in some presumed risk situation is less desirable than a decision to do so based on poor quality or incomplete material—it is particularly important in such cases to explain their administrative policy clearly (see Section 7.5).

For journalists working in news media, special conditions of work apply. They must supply news, often with demands for simplification and speed. The journalist's professional role also includes the task of monitoring public bodies and the 'power apparatus' on behalf of the public. This requires a critical attitude with a degree of mistrust. This part of the journalist's professional role can bring complications since, not least when it is a question of cancer, the understanding of risk assessment presumes an awareness of how exceptionally complex and incompletely known the 'cause–effect' relationships are, and where a very long-term perspective is required. As a consequence of the news media's task of watchdog, news supply tends to include items principally of negative value. Where cancer is concerned, this is largely in answer to a widespread fear of cancer, which gives great news value to alarming reports, such as identification of new risks. What may be of great news value from the scientist's point of view is therefore often lacking in news value for the journalist. However, a few of the more sensational results of cancer research have in recent years received good publicity in the mass media.

The specialist press' collaboration in disseminating processed scientific information to certain professional categories and in constituting an information source for news media should also be mentioned. Certainly processed information—the secondary information—can stimulate interest, so that more research results are regarded as sufficiently interesting for further dissemination via the mass media.

In order to take a significant role in disseminating scientific information, such as that relevant to cancer, the mass media ought to demand staff with expertise in, for example, the biomedical field, just as in other specialist fields, such as finance, which must be dealt with in a qualified manner. This could be done by means of a well established network of contacts and/or an adjusted recruitment policy in the larger media, with the employment of persons with research experience. In addition, the question of basic training for journalists should be stressed, since at present little attention is paid in Sweden to the need for staff with some basic knowledge within the relevant fields. The emphasis of the education at the national colleges of journalism lies on training in skills such as journalism, interview technique, style, professional ethics, news evaluation and such like. There is no special training in either natural sciences or the humanities, though some options do exist for certain (limited) study in individual subject areas through a system of extension courses offered to journalists. The Cancer Committee considers that training options for journalists should be improved with a view to making it easier for competence in journalism as such to be combined with a basic training within the medical and natural sciences fields. It is therefore quite reasonable to envisage a shortened training in journalism built into other academic courses.

The same problems affecting basic journalistic training have also been observed in other quarters. There are examples from the larger countries of special arrangements with integrated training in natural sciences and journalism which Sweden might well attempt to make use of, especially if such training were grant aided.

NOTES

1   Most of the resources initially allocated for this service were later transferred to a new control agency, namely the Chemicals Inspectorate. [*Ed. note*.]
2   Further comments on this case and on a coincidental case in the USA (Monsanto as producer of glyphosat) were given in a so-called Special Statement added to the Cancer Committee report by Committee Member Dr Peter Söderbaum, in the Swedish version. From his statement the following may also be quoted: 'The importance that the Cancer Committe attributes to "co-operation and mutual trust" between interested parties in cancer prevention is reflected in the fact that the whole of the present chapter is devoted to the question. It is stressed that Sweden, as part of international co-operation, should promote disclosure of toxicological information to the public. This is relevant in particular for information which is used as the basis for formal approval of drugs, pesticides and similar products. In this matter I would have preferred the Committee to go further in its proposals. The Committee should have stated that all information, e.g., the results of animal tests, that are the basis of approval, without restrictions should be made public and, thereby, available to anyone interested. If this could be achieved under present laws (Secrecy Act) then such a development should be accelerated.' [*Ed. note*.]
3   The investigating group (politicians appointed by the Government, aided by 'experts') has recently (LK, 1987) recommended that current practice in applying the secrecy rules should be geared towards increased openness as regards health risk and safety data for registered pharmaceuticals, obtained, for example, through clinical trials. [*Ed. note*].

13
Health screening for cancer prevention and detection

13.1 Health screening—background

13.1.1 Some general comments

Repeated examination of persons without symptoms—i.e. health or screening controls—in order to prevent or to detect different diseases at an early stage, has been discussed intensively in recent decades. The debate started with considerable optimism which has, however, gradually been replaced by a much more reluctant attitude. The reasons for this are several: some diseases remain undetected despite health controls; through screening some innocent alterations are detected and treated unnecessarily; and the cost–benefit ratio is high, as the yield of detected diseases for which early detection is important is small relative to the costs.

The dominant opinion today is that health controls with a general aim have a very limited value. There may be exceptions for special higher risk groups, for example expectant mothers, children and certain occupational groups.

Greater possibilities for a reasonable yield in relation to efforts and costs may sometimes be obtained by directed health controls or screening: examinations where a specific disease is looked for, and where the prognosis can be improved by early detection. In Sweden, for example, gynaecological health controls for the cytological detection of uterine cervical cancer and its precursor conditions have been established. A committee to examine health screening set up within the Swedish National Board of Health and Welfare in 1978 proposed that directed screening for hypertension, glaucoma and diabetes should also be considered for special age groups. This committee rejected the idea of health controls of a more general type for the reasons mentioned above.

13.1.2 Screening for the detection of cancer and pre-cancerous conditions

Most cases of cancer are at present not detected until symptoms have appeared. As the prognosis of many cancer diseases is dependent upon the extent of the disease at diagnosis, and as the treatment can often be milder and more easily tolerated if given at an early stage, it is natural that screening procedures for cancer have been the object of great interest. Some cancer diseases also have precursor conditions (known as pre-cancerous lesions), and if these lesions can be detected and treated, the cancer can be prevented.

It is not surprising that screening for cancer has created great hopes, and some cancer diseases seem to fulfil the criteria of the Council of Europe Public Health Committee (1974) for diseases suitable for screening:

(a) the disease should be an obvious burden for the individual or for society;
(b) it should have an initial 'silent' stage that can be detected by suitable tests;
c) it should be treatable in such a way that the prognosis is considerably improved.

However, even for cancer, screening has so far had a rather limited application, for several reasons.

The prevalence—the proportion of a population which at a given time has the disease—is very low even for the most frequent cancer diseases. Breast cancer is, for example, the commonest form of cancer in women and about 6 per cent of all women in the West will sooner or later develop the disease. Occasional mammography screening of women above 40 years of age, however, has found only 5–7 cases of breast cancer per 1000 women examined. This means that the screening must be repeated at certain intervals. Many relatively unusual types of cancer cannot be considered at all for screening as the chance of detecting new cases would be extremely small in relation to the costs.

For several common cancer diseases there exist no diagnostic tests suitable for use in screening. Extensive research has been done with the purpose of finding tumour markers, that is, substances produced by the tumours which can be detected in blood or urine. A number of such markers have actually been found (hormones, hormone-like substances, antigens, antibodies, etc.). Some of these markers provide a good way of detecting specific cancer diseases, but these are all so rare that general screening cannot be considered. Also, for some more common cancer types (e.g. breast, colon, stomach and lung cancers), certain tumour markers have been found, but they have too low a sensitivity and specificity to be useful in screening. The diagnostic procedures hitherto used for screening are of a different nature, for example cytological and X-ray examinations, detection of blood in stools and various clinical examinations.

A screening procedure must be harmless or at least entail a very small risk in reaction to the expected benefit. This question has been important in the discussion of mass mammographic screening, in which many women are exposed to a small radiation dose.

Some cancer diseases cannot be radically cured even if they are detected before subjective symptoms have appeared. Examples of this are chronic leukaemia and myeloma (a cancer disease of the bone marrow). Simple tests of sufficient sensitivity exist for the detection of these diseases, but screening for early detection would not be meaningful.

Examples of cancer diseases for which periodic screening has been used or considered are given below.

CANCER OF THE UTERINE CERVIX
By cytological examination of smears from the vagina and cervix, early cervical cancer and pre-cancerous conditions can be detected (known as the Pap smear). This method of gynaecological health control has been used extensively.

BREAST CANCER
By X-ray examination of the breast (mammography), this type of tumour can be detected, often at a very early stage. Periodic screening using mammography is at present being considered in many countries.

CANCER OF THE LARGE INTESTINE
Detection of blood in the stools (e.g. through the Hemoccult test) can disclose cancer in the colon and rectum, as well as some benign tumours which can be precursors of cancer. The specificity of this method is rather low and a rather large proportion of the screened population must be examined further using more complicated methods (X-ray or endoscopy) in order to arrive at a definite diagnosis. The method is at present being tested in several centres but has not yet been introduced as a more general procedure.

LUNG CANCER
Lung cancer can be detected by X-ray examinations and by examination of cells in the saliva and expectorated secretion. Screening with these methods is at present being used on a trial basis for limited high-risk groups (such as heavy cigarette smokers). As lung cancer—even if detected early and treated – usually has a bad prognosis, more general screening for this disease has not been considered.

Cancer of the Urinary Bladder

This can be detected by cytological examination of urine. Screening has been considered and even tested in limited high-risk groups (workers in the rubber and dye industries). However, as cancer of the bladder is rather rare, screening of general populations has not been considered.

Cancer of the Prostate

This type of cancer is the most frequent among males in Sweden. The disease can be detected by palpation via the rectum and cytological examination of secretion from the urethra (after massage of the prostate gland) and of material obtained from a fine-needle biopsy of the prostate gland (via the rectum). As the disease is seldom curable even after early detection, and as many cases have a benign course, general screening is not at present considered.

Oral Cancer

This type of cancer can be detected by simple clinical examination. Mass screening in this form is at present being tested within a WHO project in some parts of India and Sri Lanka, where the disease has a high incidence. It is not being considered in Western countries, where the disease is relatively rare.

Cancer of the Stomach and the Oesophagus

These cancers can sometimes be detected at an early stage by X-ray examination, cytology of gastric fluid, endoscopy and the observation of blood in the stools. In Japan, where both these types of cancer are common, not infrequently affecting young people as well, periodic screening with endoscopy has been tested with some success. In Sweden, screening for stomach cancer has been discussed for particular risk groups, such as persons previously operated on for a gastric ulcer or with pernicious anaemia. More general screening has not been considered.

Primary Liver Cancer

In the commonest form of primary liver cancer (hepatocellular cancer) a sensitive marker has been found (α-fetoprotein). Primary liver cancer is very common in parts of Asia and Africa, probably due to chronic hepatitis B virus infections. Screening with α-fetoprotein has been tested on a large scale in some districts of China, where there is a very high incidence of this cancer. Due to the difficulties of curing this type of cancer and its very low prevalence in the West, screening has not been considered here. A more detailed description and discussion of screening for cancers of the cervix, breast, lung and the large intestine are given in Section 13.2.

13.1.3 Definition of populations suitable for screening

In all screening for cancer, some limitation of those to be screened must be made in order to limit the procedure to parts of the population where the relevant tumour type is common enough for the benefits of detection to balance the efforts and costs involved.

In Sweden, for instance, gynaecological health controls have been concentrated on groups aged 30–49 years, and the randomized trial with mammographic screening to women above 40 years of age.

In special situations it is possible to limit screening to more specific risk groups, for instance smokers, underground miners and workers exposed to asbestos in screening for lung cancer, and persons with pernicious anaemia and those operated on for gastric ulcers when screening for gastric cancer. However the following discussion concentrates mainly on screening of the general population.

13.1.4 Screening problems—theoretical aspects

In a screening, four types of findings can be recognized:

(a) correctly positive tests, i.e. those that give a correct diagnosis of the disease;
(b) correctly negative tests, i.e. those that indicate correctly that the examined persons do not have the disease;
(c) falsely positive tests, i.e. those that indicate the presence of the disease in persons who do not have it;
(d) falsely negative tests, i.e. those that do not give a positive result despite the fact that the examined persons have the disease.

The following measures are often used in order to evaluate the diagnostic ability of a particular screening method.

(a) *Specificity*. The probability that a person with a negative test does not have the disease can be expressed as the number of persons who do not have the disease and have negative tests, divided by the total number of persons without the disease.
(b) *Sensitivity*. The probability that a person with a positive test really has the disease is expressed as the number of persons who actually have the disease and positive tests, divided by the total number of persons with the disease.
(c) *Positive predictive value*. The probability that a positive test is correctly positive is expressed as the proportion of correctly positive tests among all the positive tests.

A test which does not give any false positive findings has maximal specificity (100 per cent) and a test which does not give any false negative findings has maximal sensitivity (100 per cent). The positive predictive value is maximal (100 per cent) if all the positive tests are correctly positive.

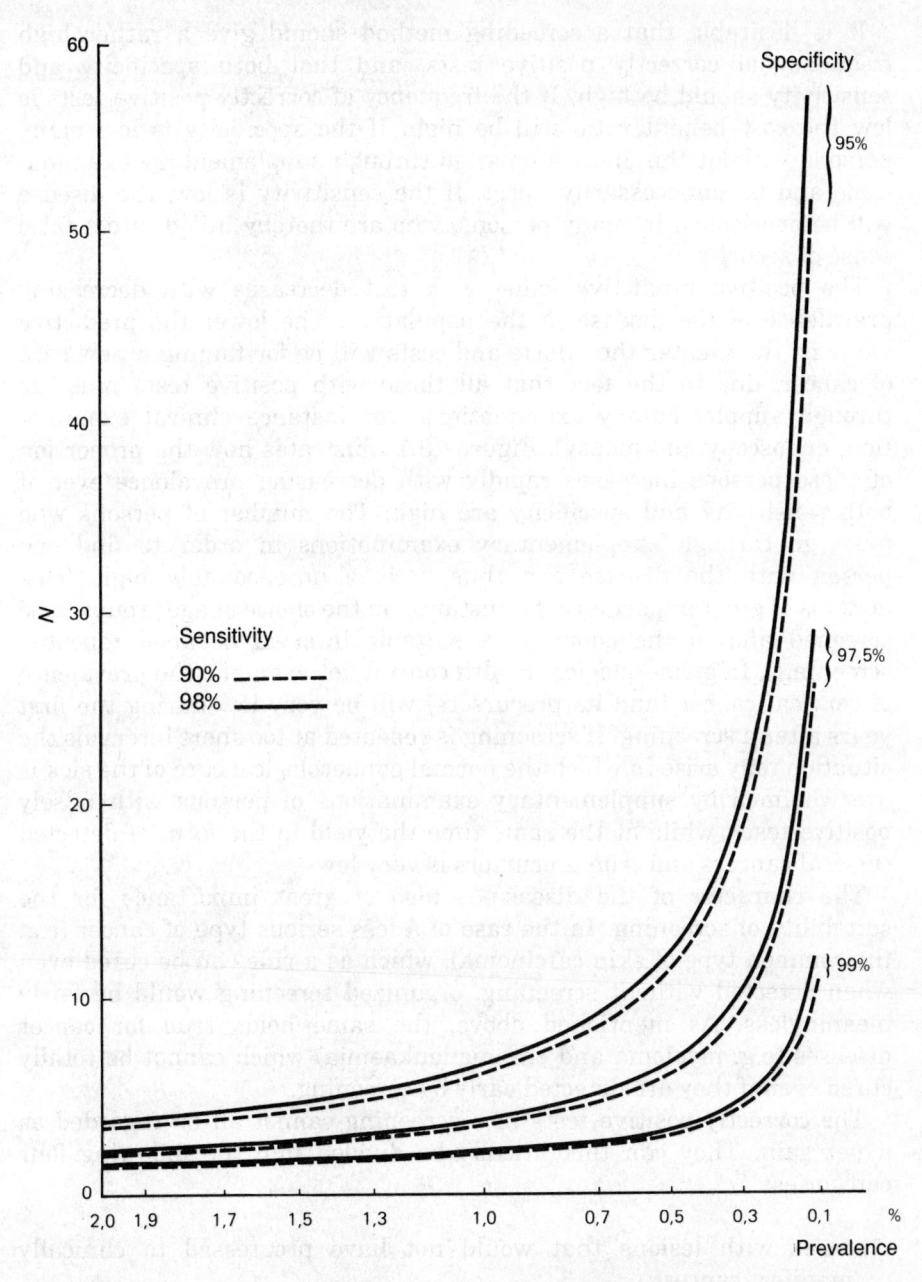

Figure 13.1 The influence of the prevalence on the predictive value. *N* denotes the average number of persons with positive tests who need to be examined further in order to find one person with a correctly positive test (cancer or precursor to cancer). When the prevalence decreases, the number of persons who must undergo supplementary examination in order to detect a true case of cancer (or precursor to cancer) rapidly increases. This is very important, for instance in the choice of age groups to be screened and in determining suitable screening intervals.

It is desirable that a screening method should give a rather high frequency of correctly positive tests, and that both specificity and sensitivity should be high. If the frequency of correctly positive tests is low the cost–benefit ratio will be high. If the specificity is low many persons without the disease must go through supplementary examinations and be unnecessarily upset. If the sensitivity is low, the disease will be overlooked in many persons, who are thereby lulled into a false sense of security.

The positive predictive value of a test decreases with decreasing prevalence of the disease in the population. The lower the predictive value is, the greater the efforts and costs will be for finding a new case of cancer, due to the fact that all those with positive tests must go through supplementary examinations (for instance clinical examination, endoscopy and biopsy). Figure 13.1 illustrates how the proportion of these persons increases rapidly with decreasing prevalence even if both sensitivity and specificity are high. The number of persons who must go through supplementary examinations in order to find one person with the disease can thus become unreasonably high. This factor is of great importance, for instance, in the choice of age groups to be screened and in the choice of a suitable interval between repeated screenings. In gynaecological health control, for example, the prevalence of cervical cancer (and its precursors) will be very low during the first years after a screening. If screening is repeated at too short intervals the situation may arise in which the normal gynaecological care of the sick is overwhelmed by supplementary examinations of persons with falsely positive tests, while at the same time the yield in the form of detected cervical cancers and true precursors is very low.

The character of the disease is also of great importance for the suitability of screening. In the case of a less serious type of cancer (e.g. the common type of skin carcinoma), which as a rule can be cured even when detected without screening, organized screening would be fairly meaningless. As mentioned above, the same holds true for cancer diseases (e.g. myeloma and chronic leukaemia) which cannot be totally cured even if they are detected early by screening.

The correctly positive tests in a screening cannot all be regarded as a net gain. They can theoretically be divided into the following four categories:

(1) cases with lesions that would not have progressed to clinically manifest cancer;
(2) cases which are cured and which would have been cured even without screening;
(3) cases that are cured and which would have been incurable without the screening;
(4) cases which are incurable even when detected by screening.

To which of these categories a person with a correct positive test belongs cannot be decided individually, with the exception of some cases in group (4). This means that people in group (1) must also go through supplementary examinations and treatment. This group can be said to represent an 'artificial' morbidity which is the unavoidable price of the screening process. The size of this group and the character of the treatment are therefore of great importance when the advantages of a screening are weighed against the disadvantages.

In gynaecological health control (screening with Pap smears), group (1) is relatively large as precursor lesions to cervical cancer are the major yield of the screening, and only some of those would have progressed to invasive cancer. The treatment of these precursor lesions (dysplasia and cancer *in situ*) is, however, usually mild and one can therefore accept group (1) being relatively large if the screening has an overall positive effect, in other words if it reduces the incidence and mortality rates of cervical cancer.

In screening for breast cancer by mammography, group (1) is probably smaller, as the main yield of the screening is microscopically invasive breast cancer. However, our knowledge of the natural history of subclinical or minimal breast cancer is incomplete. Some of these lesions would certainly have progressed to clinical cancer. Breast cancer, however, can sometimes grow very slowly, and some of the detected lesions would probably not have proceeded to clinical cancer within the life-span of the patient. Previously, the treatment of early breast cancer detected by mammographic screening was, as a rule, total mastectomy, which many women and doctors regard as mutilating. If group (1) were large and total mastectomy were the only treatment available, then it would be doubtful if screening would be accepted even if it were able to give a certain reduction in the mortality rate from breast cancer. The tendency to accept screening will, of course, be greater if early breast cancer can be treated while preserving the breast (local excision of the tumour) which has been put into practice to an increasing extent in recent years. Screening for cervical and breast cancer illustrates a general and important problem, namely that precursor lesions and early stages of cancer are often detected for which the natural history is incompletely known. Both examples show that the nature of the treatment influences the attitude to screening.

Group (2) above includes cases that would have been detected at a curable stage even without screening. As regards the possibility of cure, the screening is thus unnecessary for this group, but may still be of value if the extent of treatment could be reduced and the treatment thereby made less distressing for the patient.

Group (3), persons who may be treated and cured only as a result of screening, constitute the principal target group. This group can be regarded as the net gain of the procedure, and it is the size of this group that chiefly decides its value.

For group (4), screening can be justified only if earlier treatment could prolong survival and improve the quality of life in patients with incurable but still asymptomatic cancer diseases. This is seldom the case, and the detection of incurable cancer in persons without symptoms often impairs their quality of life.

With some simplification, it could be stated that the value of screening depends not only upon the frequency of correctly positive findings, specificity and sensitivity, but also upon the proportion of the detected cases of cancer (or precursors to cancer) that can be cured due only to the screening. In reality the size of this proportion can be determined only by statistical–epidemiological methods. Over a long observation period the behaviour of the disease is studied in a screened population in order to decide whether screening reduces the mortality of the disease or in other ways reduces its effects in the examined population.

The survival rate, for example 5 or 10 years after diagnosis, is often higher in a group of patients in whom the disease has been detected by screening than it is in a group of patients with symptomatic diseases. This observation is sometimes presented as proof of the benefits of screening, but this is incorrect for two reasons. Firstly, the survival in any group of patients — for example with cancer, diabetes or hypertension—will appear longer if the starting point for the observation is placed at an earlier time (see Figure 13.2, 'lead time bias'). Secondly, screening produces selection of patients with a less malignant and aggressive disease, in which the 'silent' subclinical phase of the disease is generally longer than in patients with more aggressive disease (see Figure 13.3, 'length bias').

Evaluation of a screening procedure requires statistical– epidemiological analyses with comparisons between screened and non-screened populations. Retrospective comparisons of this kind are often of doubtful value, as it may be difficult to find comparable populations from a statistical point of view and biases of different kinds are easily introduced.

The problem can be illustrated by the gynaecological health control programmes for the early detection and prevention of cervical cancer. These health controls started during the 1950s and 1960s in many parts of the world accompanied by great optimism. However, their evaluation involved considerable difficulties, and the value of this type of screening therefore remained controversial for a long time.

For these reasons controlled, prospective studies have definite advantages. In such studies, a screened population is compared with

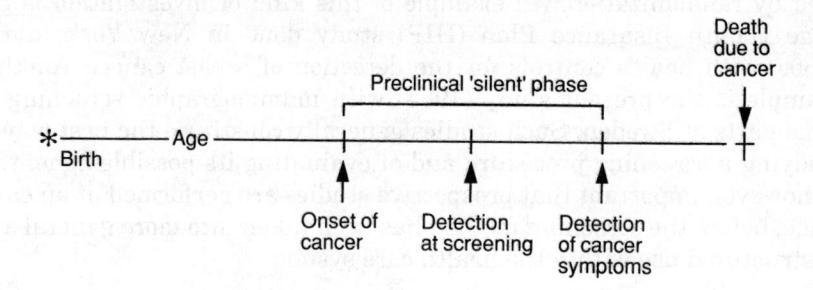

Figure 13.2 Illusory improvement of prognosis by screening ('lead-time bias'). If a cancer disease is detected at screening but not cured, an illusory improvement of the prognosis may occur. The diagram illustrates how the survival time after detection of the disease increases with earlier diagnosis. The survival from birth is, however, the same.

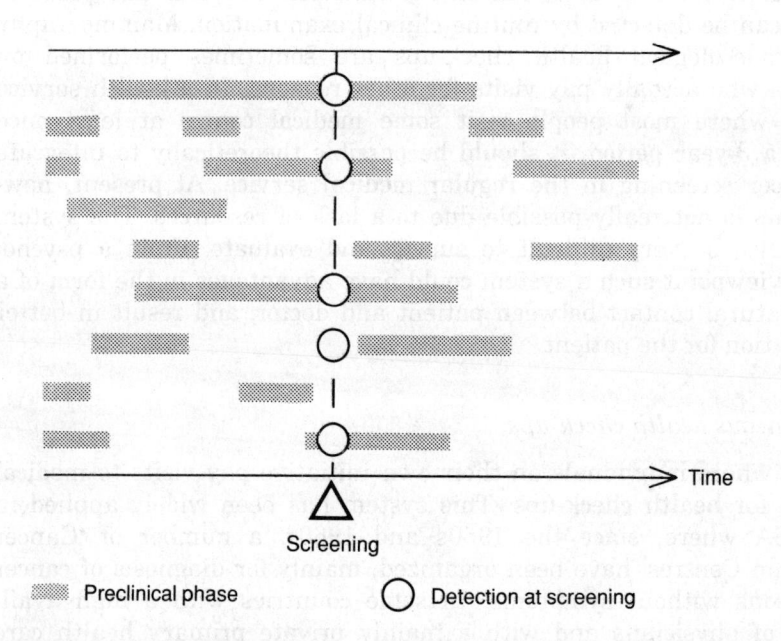

Figure 13.3 The length of the preclinical ('silent') phase influences the probability of detection by screening ('length bias'). The probability of detection is highest for cancers with a long preclinical phase. These are, as a rule, less aggressive and malignant than cancers with a short preclinical phase. The cases detected at screening therefore represent a prognostically more favourable selection.

an adequate control population and statistical comparability is procured by randomization. An example of this kind of investigation is the large Health Insurance Plan (HIP) study done in New York in the 1960s, with health controls for the detection of breast cancer. Another example is the present study (1984) with mammographic screening in some parts of Sweden. Such studies generally constitute the best way of studying a screening procedure and of evaluating its possible benefit. It is, however, important that prospective studies are performed at an early stage, before the screening method has been taken into more general and unstructured use within the health care system.

13.1.5 Organization of health screening

Health control 'en passant' in connection with other visits to medical services

In connection with visits for other reasons to different medical services, screening for cancer can also be done. To certain extent this is already the case for some kinds of cancer. For example skin, oral and prostate cancer can be detected by routine clinical examination. Mammography and gynaecological health check-ups are sometimes performed on patients who actually pay visits for other reasons. In a health service system where most people visit some medical centre at least once during a 3-year period, it should be possible theoretically to integrate all cancer screening in the regular medical service. At present, however, this is not really possible due to a lack of resources. The system would also be very difficult to survey and evaluate. From a psychological viewpoint such a system could have advantages in the form of a more natural contact between patient and doctor, and result in better information for the patient.

Spontaneous health check-ups

This is where individuals on their own initiative pay visits to medical centres for health check-ups. This system has been widely applied in the USA where, since the 1950s and 1960s, a number of 'Cancer Detection Centres' have been organized, mainly for diagnosis of cancer in persons without symptoms. In some countries with a high availability of physicians and with a mainly private primary health care system (for instance the USA and West Germany), it has been rather common for persons without symptoms to go for check-ups, which of course may also cover cancer. In the West German health insurance system, the costs of check-ups for women aged 20 years or more and men aged 45 years or more are reimbursed by insurance, and it is closely specified which examinations for cancer may be included. One advantage of spontaneous check-ups is that this places a greater responsibility on the individuals themselves for their health. Disadvantages can be the fact that factors such as education, money and age may determine who uses the facilities, and that the resources of the medical service will not be used optimally. There is also a risk that health check-ups might be used for too commercial purposes. In Sweden, spontaneous check-ups for the early detection of cancer have been rather limited; some gynaecological examinations and breast examinations, however, can be placed in this category.

Organized health screening

In this case, all persons within a certain population (for instance all women in specified age groups) are invited to be screened. Organized screening with vaginal cytology (gynaecological health control) was introduced in all Swedish counties in the 1950s and 1960s. Since the 1970s, organized mammographic screening has started in some Swedish counties.

In organized screening, the medical authorities bear a great responsibility for the net benefit of the operation. Even if participation is voluntary, those invited have not themselves asked for the examination, and possible negative side-effects must therefore be seriously taken into account. Organized screening is, however, as a rule the most effective and rational method for evaluation of a screening method. Before a screening procedure is introduced in the general population, it should ideally first be evaluated by means of a randomized study, in which a population subjected to organized screening is compared with an adequate control population. If such an evaluation gives a positive result, different organization models for more extensive screening can be discussed. The advantages and disadvantages of screening procedures must be carefully weighed up, including the cost.

13.2 Issues relating to cancer screening in Sweden

13.2.1 Discussion of various cancer types

Four types of cancer have been studied in some depth in relation to the work of the Cancer Committee. These are cancer of the uterine cervix, breast, large intestine and lung. They are all common diseases, for which diagnostic tests suitable for screening exist. Cervical and breast cancer are also rather frequent among relatively young or middle-aged women, and are already the subjects of screening on a regular basis or as trials. Cancer of the lung and large intestine are also common and some trials with screening are currently being conducted in various parts of the world. Official reports on cancer screening have recently been published in two countries—Canada and Norway—having a social structure and a cancer pattern rather similar to Sweden's.

In the Canadian report (Canadian Task Force on the Periodic Health Examination, 1979), the following types of cancer were discussed: cancers of the breast, cervix, large intestine, lung, stomach, prostate, bladder, oral cavity and skin and Hodgkin's disease. According to the report, there were good reasons for considering screening for breast cancer (mammography and clinical examination in women aged 50–59 years) and relatively good reasons for considering screening for cervical cancer (vaginal cytology) in all sexually active women every third year up to the age of 35 years and thereafter every fifth year. Screening for cancer of the large intestine could be considered in selected groups (persons with chronic colitis, familary polyposis or villous adenomas, and persons with a family history of bowel cancer). For none of the other cancers mentioned was sufficient reason found to consider screening.

In the Norwegian report (Siem, 1979), only breast, lung and cervical cancers were discussed. No screening was recommended for breast or lung cancer. Gynaecological health control (vaginal cytology) was recommended for women aged 30–70 years every fifth or, possibly, every third year.

Reports from experts for the Cancer Committee on the screening for the four types of cancer mentioned and on economic aspects of cancer screening have been published separately (Jakobsson, 1984; Petters- sson, 1984a, b; Rudenstam, 1984; Simonsson, 1984; and Håkansson and Jonsson, 1984). Below is a summary, together with judgements made by the Committee.

13.2.2 Gynaecological screening (vaginal cytology)

A little more than 50 years ago, the US physician Papanicolaou described how the examination of cells in secretions from the vagina and cervix could reveal cervical cancer and precursor lesions of such cancer. This test—often called the Pap smear—has high sensitivity and specificity (if precancerous lesions are also included as correctly positive findings). Specimens can be taken and primarily microscopically examined without the presence of a doctor, which makes the test very suitable for screening, from a technical point of view. In the screening of previously unscreened women in Sweden aged 30– 50 years, pathological changes are usually found in 3–6 per cent of those examined. About 25 per cent of these pathological tests represent obvious precancerous lesions or invasive cancer, while the remaining 75 per cent represent less pronounced cytological changes of uncertain

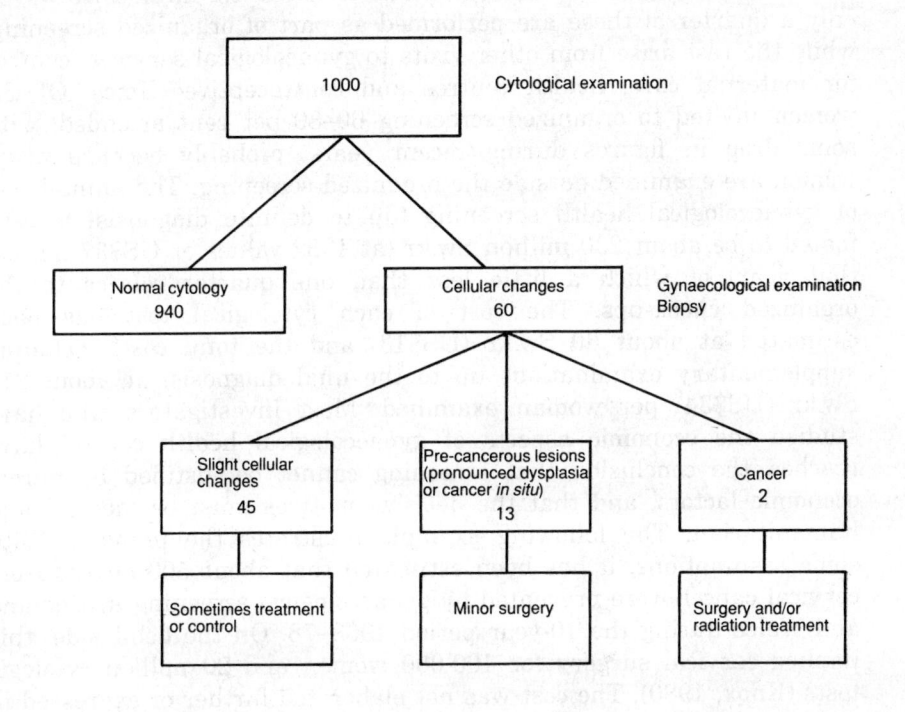

```
                    ┌─────────────────┐
                    │      1000       │  Cytological examination
                    └────────┬────────┘
                   ┌─────────┴─────────┐
        ┌──────────┴──────┐   ┌────────┴────────┐
        │ Normal cytology │   │ Cellular changes│  Gynaecological examination
        │       940       │   │        60       │  Biopsy
        └─────────────────┘   └────────┬────────┘
                    ┌──────────────────┼──────────────────┐
        ┌───────────┴──────┐  ┌────────┴─────────┐  ┌─────┴──────┐
        │ Slight cellular  │  │ Pre-cancerous    │  │            │
        │ changes          │  │ lesions          │  │   Cancer   │
        │                  │  │ (pronounced      │  │     2      │
        │       45         │  │ dysplasia or     │  │            │
        │                  │  │ cancer in situ)  │  │            │
        │                  │  │       13         │  │            │
        └────────┬─────────┘  └────────┬─────────┘  └─────┬──────┘
        ┌───────┴──────────┐  ┌────────┴─────────┐  ┌─────┴──────────┐
        │ Sometimes        │  │                  │  │ Surgery and/or │
        │ treatment        │  │ Minor surgery    │  │ radiation      │
        │ or control       │  │                  │  │ treatment      │
        └──────────────────┘  └──────────────────┘  └────────────────┘
```

Figure 13.4 Schedule for gynaecological health control. The example shows a typical result in the age group 30–50 years. Two cases of invasive cervical cancer were detected among 1000 screened women; 13 cases were detected with obvious precursor lesions (pronounced dysplasia or cancer *in situ*) which could be removed by minor surgery. A large number of slight cellular changes was also found and some of these required treatment and/or control.

significance. A scheme for gynaecological health controls is illustrated in Figure 13.4.

More or less systematic screening with Pap smears was begun in different parts of the world during the 1940s and has since increased progressively. In Sweden, the test was brought into more general use as part of gynaecological examinations during the 1950s. In the mid 1960s, organized screening was started in some counties. In 1967, the Swedish National Board of Health and Welfare recommended organized screening every fourth year between the ages of 30 and 49 years inclusive. In 1973, such screening had begun in all counties with the exception of the municipality of Gothenburg, where it was introduced in 1977.

In the early 1960s, the number of tests in Sweden per year was about 200 000, and this has now risen to about 1.1 million. However, only a quarter of these are performed as part of organized screening, while the rest arise from other visits to gynaecological services, centres for maternal care, health centres and contraceptive clinics. Of the women invited to organized screening 60–80 per cent attended, with some drop in figures during recent years, probably because many women are examined outside the organized screening. The annual cost of gynaecological health screening (up to definite diagnosis) is estimated to be about 230 million Sw.kr (at 1982 values or US$37 million that year) of which a little less than one quarter relates to the organized check-ups. The cost of each cytological test has been estimated at about 80 Sw.kr (US$13) and the total cost, including supplementary examinations up to the final diagnosis, at about 215 Sw.kr (US$34) per woman examined. Most investigators who have studied the economic aspects of gynaecological health control have reached the conclusion that screening cannot be justified by purely economic factors, and that the decisive motives must be medical and humanitarian. The following example illustrates the problem. With some assumptions, it has been estimated that about 500 deaths from cervical cancer were prevented by gynaecological screening in England and Wales during the 10-year period 1968–78. On the debit side, this implied cervical surgery for 100 000 women and 20 million cytologic tests (Knox, 1980). The cost was not elaborated further or expressed in economic terms. Translated to Swedish cost conditions, this would have meant around 7 million Sw.kr at 1982 values or US$1.1 million per death prevented. (This sum is of the same order of magnitude as those examples of actual costs per 'life saved', mentioned in Chapter 7.) An important non-economic cost seen statistically is the fact that 200 women thus had to undergo 'unnecessary' surgery for each death prevented.

Gynaecological health control started in an atmosphere of great optimism and with the belief that it would rapidly reduce incidence and mortality rates of cervical cancer. It is therefore understandable that prospective, randomized studies were not considered. However, the retrospective evaluation of this screening has been more difficult than was originally thought. A decrease in incidence and mortality rates for cervical cancer has certainly been observed in many regions, but there was often a decreasing trend even before the introduction of the screening. Such a trend has also been observed in some countries without screening. It therefore cannot be discounted that factors other than screening may also have played a part in the decreasing rate of cervical cancer (social and hygienic factors, the number of pregnancies, infections, etc.) The value of gynaecological health control is therefore still a somewhat controversial subject. One negative aspect of the screening has been a greatly increased number of minor operations (such as removal of the mucous membrane in the cervix) due to supposed precancerous lesions. In Sweden, this increase has been especially pronounced in younger age groups, in which this type of surgery is 10 times more frequent than the number of detected cancer cases. In Finland, the effect has been considerably less pronounced, and it seems probable that differences in diagnostic judgements and therapeutic routines have played a role here.

Other observations strongly indicate, however, that screening really has reduced the incidence and mortality rates of cervical cancer. In some Canadian districts a striking association has been demonstrated between the rate of gynaecological check-ups and a decrease in the cervical cancer mortality rate. In Finland, Iceland and Sweden, a reduction in the incidence and mortality rates of cervical cancer has also been observed during recent years, especially in the younger age groups, which fits very well with its being an effect of gynaecological health controls.

Figure 13.5 shows trends in the incidence and mortality rates of cervical cancer in Sweden during the period 1960–79 in different age groups. In the age groups 30–39, 40–49 and 50–59 years, an obvious decrease in both incidence and mortality rates occurred while a corresponding change was not observed for the age groups 20–29, 60–69 and 70–79 years. These changes correlate closely with the introduction of organized screening in the age groups 30–49 years over that period. The decreased rates also in the age groups 50–59 years might be due to the fact that many women in this group had been screened earlier during the period.

The experience from Norway, however, is different from that of the other Nordic countries. Organized screening started in 1959 in one Norwegian county. After some years, as no reduced mortality rate in cervical cancer was observed, no general organized gynaecological health control or organized screening was introduced. The frequency of Pap tests has been as high in Norway as in the other Nordic countries, but a reduced mortality rate of cervical cancer has nevertheless not been observed. One explanation for this may be that unstructured health control is less efficient than organized screening.

In 1981, an expert group appointed by the Swedish National Board of Health and Welfare expressed the view that organized health screening was justified and should continue, even if its capacity to reduce the mortality rate in cervical cancer was still not regarded as being fully demonstrated. One essential advantage of health screening was felt to be that many early lesions could be treated with simple and mild methods. To obtain a better survey of the situation, co-ordination of health control within each region was recommended. This could be accomplished with a computerized administrative programme which

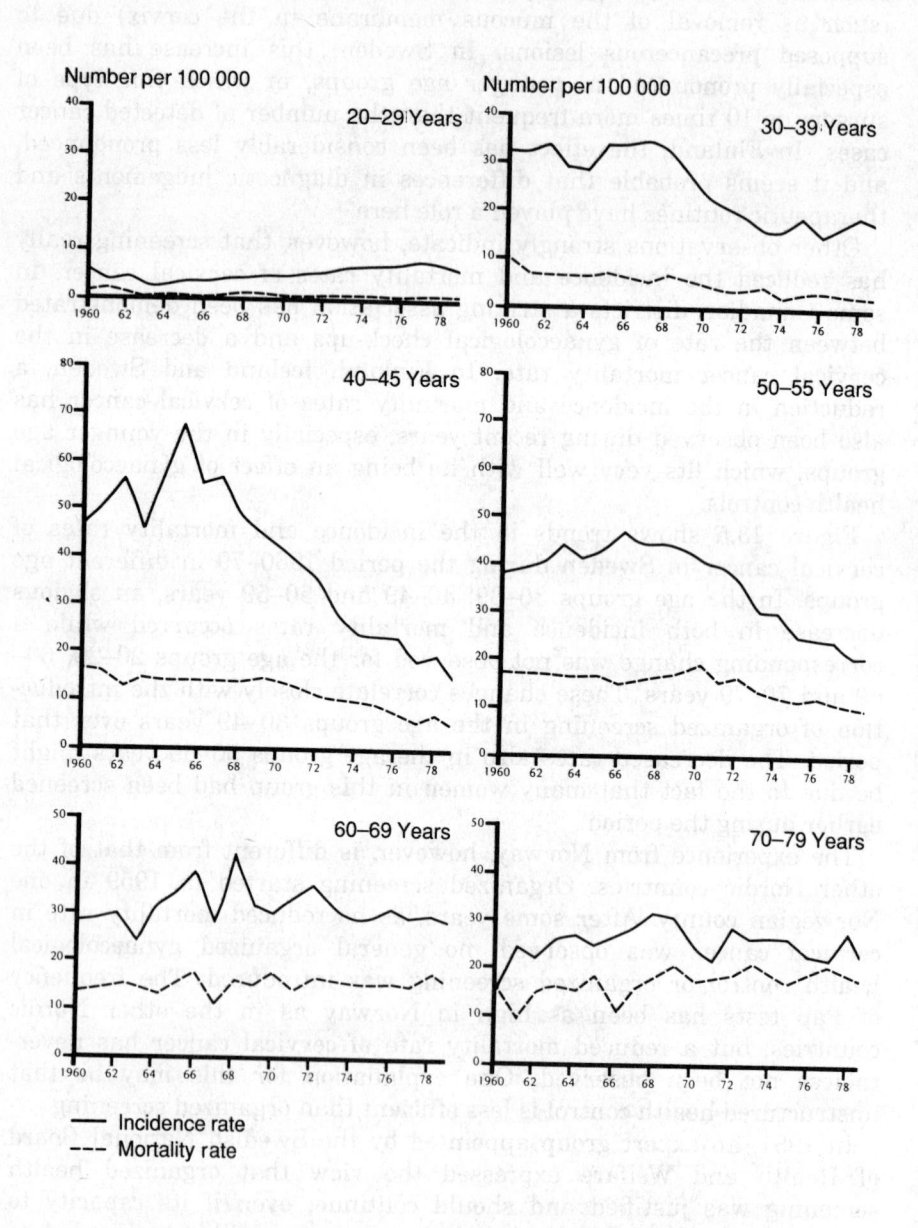

Figure 13.5 Cervical cancer in Sweden. Incidence and mortality rates in different age groups during the period 1960–1979

would also make it possible to avoid unnecessary double tests. The expert group recommended organized screening in the age group 20–59 years of intervals of 3 years. It was estimated that the present number of 1.1 million Pap smears per year should be reduced to 750 000, thanks to the proposed regional administrative programme.

Conclusions

It is unfortunate that a prospective randomized study of gynaecological health screening was not performed at an early stage. Such a study would have made it possible to remove the doubts which have long hung over the effect of this type of screening more quickly. However, retrospective studies from recent years – especially in Finland, Iceland and Sweden – quite clearly indicate that organized gynaecological health control really does reduce the incidence and mortality rates in cervical cancer. Therefore this activity should continue. It should also be pointed out that changes in sexual habits in recent decades may increase the risk of cervical cancer. These changes include earlier intercourse, more sexual partners and a change from mechanical barrier contraceptives (caps and condoms) to birth-control pills and coils.

The Cancer Committee also recommends that the computerized registration system previously proposed by another expert group should be introduced for all Pap tests both within and outside the organized screening programme, in order to rationalize the activity and to avoid duplicated examinations. The expert group referred to had recommended an extension of the screening to women aged 20–59 years (from the present 30–49 years) and a shortening of the intervals from 4 to 3 years. Nevertheless, they assumed that it should be possible to reduce radically the total number of tests due to the proposed data system. It must be stressed, however, that such an effect implies changing not only the organized screening programme, but also the unstructured gynaecological health controls. This problem cannot be solved by an administrative data system alone, but also requires detailed recommendations to all medical units and a high degree of acceptance by these units, otherwise there is a high risk that the number of tests will increase instead of decrease. Some experience of the effects of administrative data programmes should therefore be acquired before a major extension of organized screening is introduced.

From the medical point of view, there seems to be good reason for extending the organized screening to the age group 50–59 years. Incidence and mortality rates in cervical cancer are currently higher in this age group than in the age range 30–49 years (see Figure 13.5). The number of Pap tests performed outside organized screening is also considerably lower in this age group than in younger women. The medical motives for including the age group 20–29 years are much weaker; the incidence of both invasive cervical cancer and positive precursor lesions is very low in this age group. A shortening of the intervals between testing from 4 to 3 years has been suggested, but there are at present no data available indicating that such a shortening would essentially improve the effects of the screening. The effect of gynaecological health control is probably due in essence to the detection and treatment of precursor lesions, which grow very slowly.

Thus the only change now recommended in the present Swedish organized screening programme is an extension to include women aged 50–59 years. Although there are strong indications that screening has reduced incidence and mortality rates in cervical cancer, further analysis of the effects of the present programme would be valuable. In Sweden extensive material has been collected over the past decade. In some counties, for instance, data have been registered which could be of value for the identification of high-risk groups. Certain information has also recently become available at the national level through data recorded from all organized gynaecological screening before 1979. In any case, sufficient time has now passed since the introduction of screening to allow detailed analyses concerning morbidity and mortality to be made. Comparison between the development in counties where screening was introduced early or late, for instance, would be of interest. It is also important to study side-effects, such as the frequency of minor cervical surgery caused by the screening. This frequency may be influenced by routines in the cytological interpretation and may perhaps be reduced without adversely affecting the benefits of screening.

13.2.3 Screening for breast cancer

The possible methods for earlier detection of breast cancer are health check-ups with clinical examination and/or mammography and regular self-examination of the breasts. Different combinations of these measures are possible. Other diagnostic methods which have been tested or considered have too low a specificity or are too complicated for screening. Health controls by clinical examination only have been tried (e.g. in Malmö during the 1960s), but the yield is low in relation to the effort and costs. Mammography, which is a special X-ray examination with low-energy X-rays, was described in the 1920s, but was not brought into general use until the 1960s and 1970s. The method has been progressively developed leading to improved diagnostic information and the reduction of radiation doses, which were originally rather high.

During the 1960s, trials with mammography started, at that time always in combination with clinical examination. The most interesting of these trials was the Health Insurance Plan of Greater New York (HIP) study, which started in 1964. From the insurance register, 62 000 women aged 40–64 years without a previous history of breast cancer were selected. Half of these formed the study group, while the other half served as a control group. All the women in the study group were invited to have breast examinations once yearly for four consecutive years. The examinations included an interview, a clinical examination, mammography and thermography imaging (heat emission from the skin). Only two-thirds of the invited women accepted. A follow-up after 9 years showed that 91 breast cancer deaths had occurred in the study group compared to 128 in the control group, a difference which was statistically significant. This reduction in breast cancer mortality only involved women over 50 years of age.

The study strongly suggested that health screening with close follow-up can reduce breast cancer deaths. Analysis shows that mammography (which in this study seems to have been of rather poor technical quality) can only have contributed to a limited extent to the reduced mortality, and that careful clinical follow-up was the essential factor. Only 33 per cent of the cancers were detected by mammography alone, and in 45 per cent mammography gave a negative result. Also factors such as the standard of health care and degree of self-examination in the control group may have influenced the observed difference. The results of the HIP study therefore need to be verified by further studies before they can be generally accepted, especially if screening systems are used which deviate from the HIP study.

In 1969–79 a screening study using thermography was performed in the Swedish town of Gävle. Thermography turned out to be unsuitable for breast screening due to its very low specificity which produced a large proportion of false positive findings. Women selected by thermography and a control group were subjected to clinical examination and mammography. During this work a radiologist, Bengt Lundgren, introduced mammography with only one film (an oblique projection) as a possible method for screening. This method was used in a neighbouring municipality (Sandviken) where all women aged 35 years or more were invited for mammography. Of those screened, only 4–5 per cent needed to be called back for supplementary mammography and clinical examination. Of the total screened population, somewhat less than 1 per cent had to undergo diagnostic surgery. Breast cancer was found in 5.7 per 1000 screened women and about 50 per cent of these cases were subclinical meaning that they could not be detected by clinical examination (palpation). Similar results were obtained later in several Swedish studies. A schedule for screening with mammography and typical results are demonstrated in Figure 13.6.

The studies in Gävle and Sandviken, like some studies in other countries during recent years (especially the BCDDP study in the USA

Cancer: causes and prevention

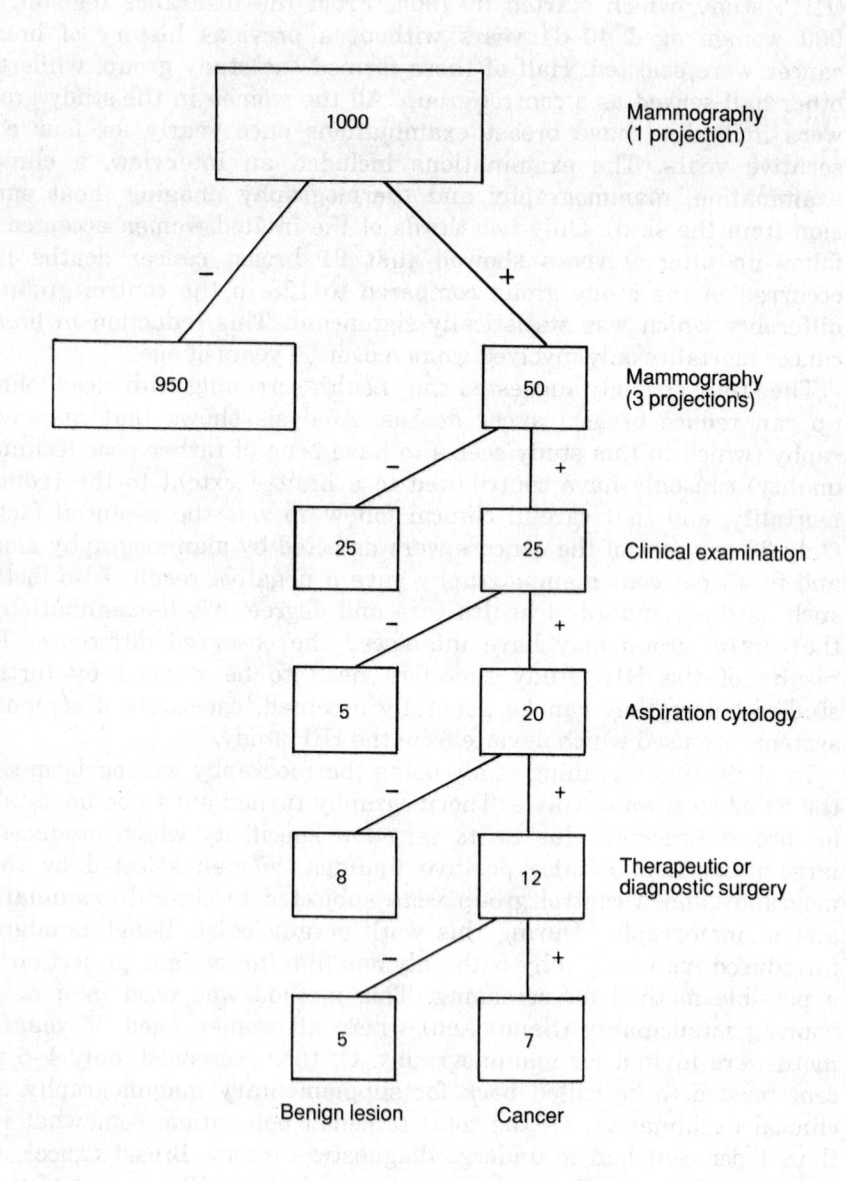

```
                    1000  — Mammography (1 projection)
                   /    \
                  −      +
                 /        \
              950          50  — Mammography (3 projections)
                          /  \
                         −    +
                        /      \
                      25        25  — Clinical examination
                               /  \
                              −    +
                             /      \
                            5        20  — Aspiration cytology
                                    /  \
                                   −    +
                                  /      \
                                 8        12  — Therapeutic or diagnostic surgery
                                         /  \
                                        −    +
                                       /      \
                                      5        7
                                Benign lesion  Cancer
```

Figure 13.6 Schedule for screening with mammography. The example shows a typical result at mammography screening of women aged over 40 years in Sweden: + findings that may imply cancer; − findings that are normal or do not indicate cancer. In the example, seven cases of breast cancer are detected among the 1000 women examined.

and the DOM project in Holland; see Jakobsson, 1984), have shown that mammography using modern techniques has a high specificity and sensitivity. Clinical examination only slightly increases the yield of the primary screening. The debate about breast screening in Sweden has therefore been almost exclusively focused on mammography. An important question has been the possible carcinogenic effect of the radiation doses received. In the present screening trials the radiation dose is about 1 mGy (milligray). No epidemiological evidence exists for a carcinogenic effect at this low dose. In radiological protection, however, it is assumed that the risk is proportional to the dose. With such a linear extrapolation, mammographic screening every third year in women over 40 years of age should induce a few breast cancers per year in Sweden. The annual number of new breast cancers in Sweden is approximately 4000.

Compared with the expected benefits of mammography screening—a reduction in mortality from breast cancer—most people at present regard the theoretical risk of cancer induction as negligible. It is, however, generally recommended that mammography should be avoided for pure health check-ups in women under the age of 40 years. The prevalence of breast cancer in these age groups is very low and, due to the structure of the breasts, mammography is of less diagnostic value than for older groups. The expected benefit to these younger women is not believed to counterbalance the risk of cancer induction by the radiation exposure.

Further developments in Sweden have included more large-scale trials with mammography screening as well as an intense public debate on women's right of access to mammography. Some details are given below.

In 1975, with the Gävle and Sandviken studies in mind, the National Board of Health and Welfare, invited several other county councils to participate in extended trials with mammography. It was agreed that in the counties of Kopparberg and Östergötland, a prospective controlled trial randomized on municipality and parish levels should be performed. The study group—women aged 40 years or more—would undergo mammography screening twice with an interval of 2.5–3 years, before any offer of organized screening of the corresponding control group could be considered. The objective was to see if breast cancer mortality could be reduced.

The screening trial started in Kopparberg in October 1977 and the first screening cycle was completed in May 1980. In Östergötland the corresponding dates were April 1980 and June 1981. A similar trial started in Malmö in January 1977 and a further one in southern Stockholm in 1981. The latter two trials were randomized on an individual basis. In 1982 Gothenburg decided on a mammography screening trial for women aged 40–60 years. The trials in Kopparberg and Östergötland (known as the W–E study) have been co-ordinated by a National Board of Health and Welfare project group.

At a conference in 1982 with participation of experts in mammography, epidemiology and oncology, the Swedish studies were discussed (Andersson et al., 1983). In the Malmö and W–E trials the total study group then comprised about 90 000 women and the total control group about 60 000. The response rate from the women invited was about 75 per cent in the Malmö study and about 90 per cent in the W–E study. The investigation confirmed previous observations, namely, that breast cancer was more frequently detected in the study group and that the tumours in this group were often small and lacked axillary lymph node metastases. It was felt that a significant effect on the breast cancer mortality rate could not be expected until around 1985–6, and some experts regarded even this as too optimistic. The strong shifting of the breast cancer population towards prognostically more favourable stages, however, indicated that a reduction in the mortality rate could be expected in the screened population.

In the age group 40–49 years, the prevalence of breast cancer is quite low, and the National Cancer Institute in the USA recommends that these women should not be subject to mammography screening as the benefit is probably low in relation to the radiation risk. The number of cases in the earliest Swedish studies is probably too few to show whether screening reduces the mortality rate in this group, but when later on the results from the Stockholm and Gothenburg trials became available, it may also be possible to observe screening effects.

Around 1980, screening with mammography became a topic of general debate in Sweden. Large groups of women saw screening with this method as a right for everyone, although there seems to have been some confusion over the significance of the trials in progress. In the Swedish Parliamentary session 1980–1, four motions were put forward concerning mammography screening. Parliament then recommended that all women who suspected they had breast cancer or felt worried about the risk of this disease should, after visiting a doctor and if they themselves wished it, be referred for mammography. At the same time, it stated that there were good reasons to wait for the evaluation of the W–E project before a firm stance was taken on general mammography screening. It was urgent to evaluate the W–E project as soon as was technically possible. Initiatives from county councils towards extended mammography screening on a trial basis should receive active support. The importance of information on self-examination and the adequate education of radiologists and paramedical personnel was underlined.

In Sweden, about 250 000 mammographies were performed in 1980; half of these were the result of the organized trials while the other half were done within the regular medical services. It can be assumed that many of these latter tests were done as check-ups in patients without symptoms.

The cost of general screening in Sweden of all women 40–60 years old with mammography every third year has been estimated as likely to be approximately 40 million Sw.kr in 1982 values (then US$6.7 million) not including the supplementary examination required for definite diagnosis and treatment (Håkansson and Jonsson, 1984). The cost per mammography screening has been assessed at approximately 110 Sw.kr (about US$17). Including the figure for supplementary examinations up to definite diagnosis, the total cost per year has been estimated at 80 million Sw.kr (US$13 million). The additional personnel requirement for such general screening would be about 175 (including around 25 doctors).

The ability of women to notice symptoms themselves is of great importance for the early detection of breast cancer. The diagnosis of clinical breast cancer can certainly be made earlier if women are informed about self-examination. In Sweden information is distributed mainly by out-patient clinics, health centres, company health services, maternity clinics, family planning centres and pharmacies. Some information is also given by the newspapers and television. Women on the mammography trials mentioned above have, as a rule, also been informed about self-examination.

An intensive self-examination programme has been reported from Finland (Gästrin 1977, 1981). However, this programme might seem too obtrusive for many women and in Sweden has only been applied to a limited extent. But how women can be effectively informed about self-examination is an important question and it is possible that the present rather unstructured information eludes many women in the relevant age groups. Even in many Swedish health care regions without screening trials, programmes for the earlier detection of breast cancer through other means are at present being prepared. Among measures of immediate interest are the setting up of special out-patient departments for breast diseases, courses for primary health care staff (general practitioners, company doctors, nurses and midwives) and increased information about self-examination.

Conclusions

Efforts aimed at reducing the effects of breast cancer are extremely important. It is, however, understandable that there remains considerable hesitation concerning the introduction of general mammography screening. At the first screening of women above 40 years about 99.5 per cent of them derive no benefit from the procedure and at repeated screening this percentage is even greater. One disadvantage of screening is that many women must undergo surgery unnecessarily. The evaluation of mammography screening therefore entails considerable problems.

No country has yet (1984) introduced general mammography screening. The Swedish trials carried out should provide unique possibilities for obtaining a scientifically adequate evaluation of the effects of this type of screening. Pending such evaluation, it is not possible to take a stance on general screening. Initial conclusions are likely to relate only to women over 50 years of age. Evaluation of screening in the 40–49 year age group may, however, be possible later on.

The annual number of mammographies performed in Sweden has increased rapidly and further increases can be expected, partly because of the recommendations made by the Swedish Parliament in 1981. This means that within a few years a very large number of mammographies will be performed as check-ups within the regular medical services – besides the mass screening trials – and a computerized administration programme similar to that discussed for gynaecological health control, is likely to be needed. Another requirement will be for adequately trained medical personnel. Few extra staff will be needed, but a knowledge of mammography needs to be included in the basic training of all relevant personnel.

No definite recommendations can be made concerning suitable ages for mammographic health-control but, in general, it does not seem appropriate for women under the age of 40 years without definite symptoms.

Information about self-examination is important for the early detection of breast cancer. At present this is probably not as effective as it could be. It is suggested that the National Board of Health and Welfare, in collaboration with the Swedish Cancer Society, look into the problem (for general aspects of public information see Chapter 9). In this context, some guiding principles would also be of value to Swedish County Councils when developing action programmes for the early detection of breast cancer in their respective areas. Work on an action programme need not be tied to a decision of whether or not to offer general mammographic screening, and it is strongly recommended that preparation of such programmes be undertaken in all areas of the country. A programme should include recommendations concerning referral of patients, indications for mammography, special out-patient departments for breast diseases, information on self-examination and educational programmes for medical staff.

13.2.4 Screening for colo-rectal cancer

Cancer of the large intestine (colon and rectum) is the second most common cancer in Sweden among both men and women. Each year around 3800 new cases are reported and about half of these patients will eventually die from it. People with hereditary polyposis, with ulcerous colitis and with close relatives who have had colo-rectal cancer, run an increased risk. The majority of colo-rectal cancers, however, appear in people without these risk factors. It is generally thought that many of these cancers develop from benign polyps (adenomas), which are considerably more common than cancer.

The prognosis of colo-rectal cancer is dependent upon the size and extent of the tumour at diagnosis. For superficial cancer of the intestinal mucous membrane, 5-year survival rate is almost 100 per cent while, if the cancer has penetrated the mucous membrane and has spread to the lymph nodes, the figure is only 25 per cent. The tumour often grows very slowly and most patients have had their cancer for several years, sometimes 10 or more, by the time it is detected. The scope for detection by screening and for reduction of the mortality rate should therefore be good.

Some cancers can be detected by examination of the rectum with the finger (rectal palpation) and inspection of the lower 25–30 cm of the bowel with a rectoscope. However, rectal palpation discloses only 15 per cent, and rectoscopy only 50 per cent of cancers in the large intestine, and both examinations require a doctor at the initial diagnostic stage. Neither method is therefore suitable for use in screening.

Cancer of the large intestine often causes blood in the stools (as do several types of benign lesions such as haemorrhoids, polyps, and gastric ulcer). The possibility of detecting intestinal cancer early from blood in the stools has been discussed for a long time, but the methods previously had too low a specificity for screening. In 1971, however, a method was reported in which small amounts of faeces could be examined for blood by means of a filter paper impregnated with a chemical reagent (Hemoccult). In order to increase the specificity, meat and fish should not be eaten the day before the test. Usually a sequence of tests is performed, such as one double-test for three days.

The examined person takes the specimen himself. In some countries such as the USA and West Germany, the test has become rather popular. The American Cancer Society, for instance, recommends that all persons over 40 years of age should be examined by rectal palpation, and that those over 50 should be screened annually with a Hemoccult test and examined by rectoscopy every third to fifth year. The West German Federal Health Insurance reimburses the cost of one Hemoccult test per year in persons aged 45 years or over. No medical reports have appeared to show the results of this activity. It represents, in both the USA and West Germany, an unstructured, spontaneous approach to health control rather than a systematic, organized screening.

In more systematic studies of the age groups over 40, usually 1–4 per cent of screened individuals have had a positive test, with an average of about 2 per cent. Among those with positive tests, supplementary examinations have revealed cancer in 2–4 per cent and intestinal polyps in about 25 per cent. The sensitivity is regarded as high. The specificity is low if only cancer is taken into account, but relatively high if polyps (adenomas), which can be precursors to cancer, are also considered. At present two large controlled screening studies are in progress in New York and Minnesota. In Minnesota the participants present a random sample, which makes comparison with a non-screened population possible. Both studies have so far demonstrated that the cancers detected by Hemoccult screening are often in an early stage. A similar experience was recently reported from a randomized study in the Nottingham area in England (Hardcastle et al., 1983).

Statistical evidence of a reduction in the mortality of colo-rectal carcinoma due to screening, however, has not yet been reported. One disadvantage of this method is its low specificity, which means that many persons without cancer must undergo quite complicated supplementary examinations (radiological examinations and endoscopy). In the US and English studies mentioned the participation rate among the invited persons was remarkably low.

At the university hospital in Gothenburg, a randomized study was started in 1982 that included everyone in the municipality born between 1918 and 1922 (about 26 000). Half of these were invited to screening with a Hemoccult test, while the other half served as controls. Of those contacted, 66 per cent participated, which is a much higher rate than in other studies. In a first round of screening, more cases of colo-rectal carcinomas and adenomas were found in the study group and most of these were at an earlier stage than the tumours found in the control group (Kewenter, 1983), but no further details have yet been reported.

Conclusions

Colo-rectal cancer is one of the most frequently occurring malignant tumours. The prognosis is dependent upon the stage at which the cancer is detected and the possibilities of prevention are limited. The potential of screening with the Hemoccult test should therefore be watched closely. According to a crude estimate, a study group of about 40 000 people and a control group at least four times as large are needed in order to demonstrate, within 6–7 years, whether screening reduces the mortality in this cancer. The current (1984) randomized trial in Gothenburg is a pilot study of great value for elucidating the administrative, methodological and medical problems connected with this type of screening. It can also provide important information on the level of interest among the public. Before the Hemoccult test is taken into more general (unstructured) use as a health control method and especially before any general screening programme is considered, a responsibility rests with the appropriate societal bodies to make sure that there has been a scientific evaluation of the method by a more extended controlled trial.

13.2.5 Screening for lung cancer

The morbidity and mortality rates of lung cancer have increased in Sweden during the last 20 years among both men and women. The most important reason for this increase is without any doubt tobacco smoking (see Section 4.2), but other risk factors may also play a certain role, as discussed in Chapters 2 and 6. The treatment results for lung cancer are still poor, and the 5-year survival rate is only a few per cent. In special favourable sub-groups, however, with early, operable cancers a 5-year survival rate of about 25 per cent can be obtained.

Chest radiography and cytology of saliva and expectorated secretion can be used as screening methods for lung cancer. Chest radiography especially can reveal early tumours in the lung parenchyma (often adenocarcinomas) while sputum cytology can disclose early tumours in the central bronchi (often squamous-cell and small-cell carcinomas). Several screening projects using these methods have been performed or are taking place in different parts of the world, including a couple of studies in Sweden. The screening has usually been concentrated on special high-risk groups (cigarette smokers). Certain studies have shown that screening sometimes discloses early cancers with a good prognosis, but there are at present no indications that this health control reduces the mortality rate of lung cancer to any substantial degree. Most cases detected by screening have also had poor prognoses and the slightly increased 5-year survival rate that has sometimes been reported may be misleading and can very likely be explained by the earlier starting point for the observation (see Figure 13.2) and a selection of prognostically more favourable cases.

Conclusions

Present knowledge of the natural history of the disease and screening trials in other countries do not speak in favour of a large-scale screening project in Sweden. It is well known that some sub-groups in society run an increased risk of lung cancer, such as smokers and some persons exposed occupationally to carcinogens (e.g. asbestos, arsenic, nickel, chromium and radon daughters in mines) and probably also persons with a specific hereditary reaction pattern concerning the metabolism of certain carcinogenic substances (polycyclic hydrocarbons). A minority of people with several of these risk factors may run a very high risk of developing lung cancer. It is, however, doubtful if a screening programme in such high-risk groups could substantially improve treatment possibilities and prognoses. Furthermore, definition of an extreme high-risk group would probably create great psychological problems. The main efforts concerning lung cancer should, therefore, be concentrated on prevention, especially a reduction in smoking.

13.3 Psychological aspects of screening for cancer

There are only a few reported studies of the psychological and social aspects of organized screening for cancer. Most of these reports concern the reasons why some persons invited to screening do not participate (Berrino et al., 1979; Fink et al., 1972; Pinotti and Borges, 1977). The most frequent reasons for non-participation seem to be low motivation due to lack of information and fear of cancer, but geographical accessibility also seems to play a role.

In Sweden, participation in gynaecological and mammographic screening has on the whole been satisfactory. Three studies have been reported up to 1981 in Sweden (Blom and Wilhelmsson, 1980; Hansagi et al. 1980, Waldenström, 1981). Two studies concerned breast cancer screening and one gynaecological health control. The studies looked at reactions in women who, after a primary screening, are called back for repeated or supplementary examinations. From the psychological point of view it would be of value to study further the general attitudes of invited persons towards all phases of the procedure, and how much knowledge they have of the aims and the significance of the screening. Such studies should be performed in connection with screenings for cervical cancer, breast cancer and colo-rectal cancer and could help in planning better information for the invited population.

Most people are probably not informed about, or do not understand, the different types of screening results: correctly positive, correctly negative, falsely positive and falsely negative. Authorities, medical staff and scientists lack sufficient knowledge of the psychological and/or social problems that may appear in connection with different findings. It would therefore be of great value to study these problems in connection with current screening programmes.

Women in general seem to have great expectations as regards screening for cervical cancer and breast cancer. This can be seen from discussions in the mass media and from the many political proposals put forward in Sweden, at both the national and the county level.

As breast cancer is the commonest form of cancer in women and as its incidence is increasing, this disease is especially feared. In several county councils efforts have been made to teach women about self-examination of the breasts. Compared to mammography this method may seem crude and old-fashioned. It is therefore important to inform the public about the advantages and limitations of the two methods.

In principle, most women could be taught to palpate their breasts carefully every month. Women who regularly practised self-examination do on average have smaller breast cancers at diagnosis than other women (Greenwald et al., 1978; Foster et al., 1978). Some women, however, seem to be so worried about the possibility of finding a cancer that they do not examine their breasts. Reasons may be that cancer is often associated with death, and also that they fear losing a breast (Gyllensköld, 1976, Rimer, 1976). There seems also to be a tendency among the public to trust experts and modern technology and to underestimate the value of initiative and personal responsibility.

Both information and psychological support in connection with gynaecological and breast screening are often insufficient, especially in relation to repeated or supplementary examinations following suspected positive or inadequate primary screening tests. Studies in various Swedish cities have found that women recalled for supplementary screening for either breast cancer or cancer of the cervix generally suffered severe anxiety (or completely denied such feelings) and felt that they received inadequate information and support from medical staff (Blom and Wilhelmsson, 1980; Waldenström, 1981). Another report showed that women who were invited for mammographic screening, but did not participate, thought that cancer was contagious, always caused pain and was incurable (Hansagi et al. 1980) Nevertheless, a majority of these women considered that organized screening should exist.

Information about cellular alterations found at gynaecological check-ups probably influences the sexual life of these women, a question which, however, has not been studied so far.

It is obvious that information relating to organized screening is important. Screenings have an impersonal character and it is difficult to foresee the psychological reactions of those invited to attend. The invitation letters and letters concerning findings of the screening must therefore be drafted with great care. People called back for repeated or supplementary examinations must have the opportunity to talk to a doctor (or another responsible person on the medical staff without delay).

Furthermore, the responsibility for information, psychological and other support is not limited to the initial stage, that of detecting a cancer. According to one Swedish study (Kagan et al., 1980), about 40 per cent of women with newly diagnosed breast cancer had an obvious need of psychological and social support. Blom and Wilhelmsson

(1980) (see above) also found that women who were operated on considered the contact with medical staff to be insufficient, especially concerning information given before the operation. The resource problems in Sweden in this context are taken up in Chapter 14.

13.4 Overall evaluation

The problems connected with screening for cancer are complicated for many reasons. One is the fact that at screening, precursor stages or very early stages of cancer are often detected, for which the possibility of progression to clinically manifest cancer is incompletely understood. Attitudes towards screening, especially organized screening by contacting selected individuals, are influenced by many factors. Among other things the following questions must be asked. How many people have to be unnecessarily treated and disturbed by the screening? Can the screening result in milder treatment for many patients? Is mortality rate of the cancer disease in question reduced by the screening? Are the costs reasonable in relation to the benefits? One firm belief of the Cancer Committee is that society has a responsibility for a scientific evaluation of a screening method by well-planned prospective trials before it is put to wider use on the general public in organized screening.

Only three screening methods for cancer can at present be considered in Sweden. These are gynaecological check-ups (vaginal cytology), mammography and Hemoccult test for detection of blood in the stools.

Since the 1960s gynaecological screening has been well established in Sweden. There is convincing evidence that this reduces incidence and mortality rates of cervical cancer. The gynaecological check-ups organized by the responsible authorities (the county councils) should, therefore, continue. The remaining controversies concern choice of suitable age groups, screening intervals and coordination between the organized screening programmes and the unstructured screening performed, for instance in connection with maternal care, contraceptive advice and ordinary visits to medical services. Computerized administrative programme for the registration of all Pap smear tests should be used to avoid unnecessary double examinations. The largest amount of statistical material which has already been collected should be subjected to intensive analyses in order better to elucidate the effect of screening on, for instance, the incidence rates of invasive cervical cancer and precancerous lesions, the mortality rate of cervical cancer, and the frequency of operations and other therapeutic measures. In the meantime the present age range for organized screening could be widened to 30–59 years, while retaining the present 4-year screening intervals.

Mammography for early detection of breast cancer has so far not been introduced in any country as a general health control organized by the medical authorities. The current randomized trials in Sweden are therefore very important for evaluating the effects of this type of screening, and they are the object of considerable international interest. These trials should be evaluated before general mammographic screening is considered. More and better information about self-examination, and programmes for early detection of breast cancer should be drawn up. The introduction of an administrative computer programme for the registration of mammographies should also be considered, as a large increase in the number of mammographies can be expected whether or not organized screening is introduced. The medical authorities should be prepared for increased mammographic activity, which may require the education of more radiologists and increased resources for supplementary diagnostic examinations and treatment.

The Hemoccult test for the early detection of adenomas and cancer in the large intestine is the object of increasing interest and is technically well suited for screening purposes. Experience is, however, still limited and so far there is no evidence that this type of screening reduces the mortality rate of colo-rectal cancer. Development should nevertheless be watched closely and it may become desirable for extended randomized trials to be planned in Sweden, similar to the current mammography trials.

The psychological and social problems connected with screening should be studied in more detail than hitherto. Such studies could naturally be co-ordinated with current screening programmes and trials. Even without further studies, it is already quite obvious that the information given to invited and examined persons needs to be improved. A minimum requirement is that all examined persons (even those with negative test results) should get an adequately designed letter giving the result of the examination. Everyone called back for repeated or supplementary examinations should have the opportunity to talk with a doctor or someone else on the medical staff.

The proposed Swedish studies and evaluations should be coordinated by the National Board of Health and Welfare, which should also make recommendations on further activities.

The proposals of the Committee concerning screening for cancer are limited in scope. The reasons for this are partly the uncertainty which is still attached to some types of screening and partly the fact that some continuing randomized screening trials cannot yet be evaluated. However, this important field should be watched carefully. New medical discoveries (such as new screening methods and improved treatment) may in the future increase the possibilities and motivation for screening for cancer. In the foreseeable future, however, the majority of cancers will still not be detected until they have reached a symptomatic stage.

For patients with clinical symptoms, as early a diagnosis as possible is important, as this often increases the probability of successful treatment. It is therefore important that doctors, not least general practitioners, should receive adequate education in cancer diagnostics and that the public should have good access to medical services and be informed about the common symptoms of cancer.

The medical care must be organized in a way that minimizes the timespan from the initial suspicion of cancer to final diagnosis and treatment. This will entail improvement in the education of doctors and the organization of medical services and is partly outside the scope of the Committee (see Chapter 14 on organization of cancer care). These issues seem at present to be more important in the early detection and treatment of cancer than screening is. Special care programmes aimed at specific cancer diseases should make it possible to improve the situation and reduce the delay between first suspicions and treatment.

Addendum

Since 1985 the Swedish National Board of Health and Welfare has made definite recommendations concerning both gynaecological health control (vaginal cytology) and mammographic screening. It recommends organized screening by calling women aged 20–59 to have a Pap smear every third year. As regard mammography screening, analyses of the W-E material (see p. 526) in late 1984 showed a significantly reduced mortality rate from breast cancer in the screened group compared to the unscreened control group (Tabar, et al. 1985). For the whole group of women aged 40–70 years, this reduction was about 30 per cent. The reduction was only observed in women aged 50 years or more, and not in the age group 40–49 years. In the latter age group, however, the number of breast cancer deaths were too few for any definite evaluation. The National Board of Health and Welfare has now recommended general mammographic screening with invitations to all women aged 40–55 years every 18 months, and women aged 55–70 years every 3 years.

14
Review of the organization of cancer care in Sweden

14.1 Current situation

Up to the 1950s there were essentially two approaches to treatment of malignant diseases—surgery and radiotherapy. Parallel with progress in these fields, new methods of treatment have emerged in recent decades, mainly chemotherapy and endocrine therapy. This development, in conjunction with more accurate and earlier diagnosis of cancer, has changed the pattern of cancer care. Curative treatment is increasingly feasible, and effective palliation can be more extensively provided when cure is not achievable. Concomitantly the treatment of cancer has become more complex and resource demanding.

There is every reason to expect these trends to continue, leading to improved and less traumatic methods of treatment, while the numbers of patients presenting for treatment and the time during which treatment is given will increase. Multiplicity of treatment methods and use of combined methods intensify the need for collaboration between various clinical disciplines and sectors of the health services and for special training of doctors and other personnel. It is neither reasonable nor feasible to provide large numbers of hospitals with the specialized resources of personnel and equipment required to meet the rising demands. Some centralization is therefore necessary for provision of appropriate cancer care and for rational utilization of these resources.

For large groups of cancer patients, the treatment required in certain stages of the disease can be achieved only at selected hospitals with access to specialized staff and equipment. Different countries have chosen different ways of organizing special cancer care, in many instances depending on the existing structure of health care and available resources.

Guidelines issued in 1974 by the National Board of Health and Welfare (NBHW) for cancer care in Sweden proposed co-ordination within each of the country's health service regions, each serving a population of 1–1.7 million, by an oncological centre at the regional hospital. The functions of these centres may be summarized as follows:

(a) responsibility for regional cancer registration and some regional cancer statistics, including formulation of guidelines for record keeping within the region;
(b) formulation of cancer management programmes, including routines for follow-up, to be used within the region;
(c) co-ordination, within the framework of accepted management programmes, of the region's resources for cancer care by appropriate distribution of functions between the various units in the health service chain, from primary care centres to the regional hospital and the other way round;
(d) co-ordination of cancer care resources within the regional hospital, by arrangements for interdisciplinary groups;
(e) responsibility for counselling and information on cancer and on management programmes to doctors and health service units within the region;
(f) provision of training in clinical oncology for different categories of health service staff at all educational stages;
(g) promotion of collaboration between basic and clinical oncological research;
(h) surveillance of psychological psychiatric and sociomedical aspects of cancer care;
(i) advice regarding mass screening programmes for cancer and formulation of guidelines for cancer prevention.

The NBHW assumes that the oncological departments at the regional hospitals will have administrative and organizational responsibility for the functioning of the oncological centres. The surgical treatment of cancer will continue to be undertaken within the various, often organ-specialized, departments of surgery.

Although the management of certain cancer forms should be centralized to the regional hospital, the high incidence of other forms necessitates that such cases continue to be the responsibility of the general county health services.

14.2 General guidelines for the future

During the foreseeable future the need for cancer care will increase. This must be emphasized, although quantitative assessment of care requirements cannot be reliably based on existing trends in various cancer forms and age patterns in the population. Nor is it feasible to determine the expected or possible effects of ongoing or projected preventive measures. However, the increasing pressures on resources for cancer care are indicated already by the further evolution of therapeutic methods outlined earlier. At the same time there is a certain gradual shift in policy and resource allocation as regards the Swedish health service, with greater emphasis on preventive measures and primary care (as opposed to hospital treatment). Appropriate progress in cancer care may be impeded if the growing demands on resources in this practical field are not recognized in the ongoing health service reorganization.

Regional cancer centres, including registries covering all cancer cases within the region, are already in operation throughout Sweden.

Co-ordination of existing resources by the oncological centres is essential to satisfy the needs of modern cancer care. Such co-ordination is also the most effective way of utilizing the present limited resources to achieve good cancer management. In practice the development of the oncological centres in Sweden has been uneven, and energetic measures need to be taken rapidly within the six regional health service structures to offer comprehensive cancer care by organizing all oncological centres with regional cancer registries, functioning management programmes and facilities for training all staff categories, for counselling and providing information and for surveillance of the psychological and sociomedical aspects of cancer care. It would be inadvisable, however, to strive for identical organization in all regions of the country. Geographic circumstances, local potentialities, existing organization and customs can warrant differences in organizational solutions.

Centralization is frequently recommended in order to offer cancer patients adequate evaluation of their condition and adequate treatment but it is not advantageous in all respects. A long distance from home, family and friends can be highly distressing to the patient. The constant aim must be, therefore, to strive for a reasonable balance between the need for specialized care, with the requisite equipment and competence of personnel, and patients' desire to be as near to home as possible.

14.3 Co-ordination by interdisciplinary collaboration, cancer management programmes, counselling and information within the health service region

Co-ordination of regional resources for the care of individual cancer patients is currently achieved by interdisciplinary collaboration, management programmes and systems of consultation. It is now widely accepted that assessment of cancer cases in crucial phases of the disease should be made by representatives of various clinical specialities in consultation. A system of this type now exists at all regional hospitals in Sweden. But because many cancer patients are not and will not be treated at the regional hospital, it is essential that there should be facilities for interdisciplinary collaboration also at the county hospitals. In addition, oncological consultation within the framework of other medical services, including long-term, home health and primary care, should be encouraged. This accords with the aim of treating patients at home or as near as possible to home.

Management (or care) programmes are defined as agreed guidelines for care of particular diseases. Each is developed in the light of the organizational conditions and the available resources within the area. Work on management programmes has started in all regions, and several are already in operation for different tumour groups.

Development of management programmes is an important function of an oncological centre. Experience has shown that this work tends to be ineffective unless the administrative duties can be co-ordinated and entrusted to a special secretariat. The extra financial resources thus needed must be provided by the county councils to a greater extent in the future than at present.

Oncological centres have responsibility for advising and informing medical staff and health services regarding cancer diseases. In several countries it is now considered important to extend an information function to include the general public. The view of the Cancer Committee is that this should apply also in Sweden.

14.4 Organization within the county health care framework

Hospitals at county level carry out 'primary' treatment (with a curative intention), supplementary treatment, palliative treatment and follow-up of previously treated patients, often in consultation with an oncological centre at a regional hospital. This pattern of care outside of regional oncological centres will continue in Sweden. The organization of county health services is therefore very important for the quality of cancer care.

Considerable variations exist between counties as regards facilities for cancer care. This may depend on, for example, the size of the county's population, geographic structure, distance from the regional hospital, and the existing organization. So that the quality of care may be acceptable regardless of where the patient lives, however, the existing organization must fulfil certain requirements. One is that important decisions concerning management, even within the county health care framework, should be made by consultation between representatives from different clinical disciplines. Doctors participating in this work should be appropriately trained.

Necessary oncological competence in county hospitals can be achieved in various ways. Permanent posts for trained oncologists at these hospitals provide one possible method. Another possibility is a system for regular consultation from the regional hospital. The approach to this question can differ between counties. All county councils should, however, without undue delay decide upon a strategy for broadening oncological competence within their health services. Without such decisions there is a risk that improvisations necessary to solve acute problems will lead to an organization that will not prove to be rational in the long term. A system of regular consultations from the oncological centre at the regional hospital should guarantee frequent up-dating of oncological knowledge. Permanent posts for specialists in oncology at county hospitals give greater continuity in cancer care.

Progress in radiotherapy necessitates increasingly complicated equipment and, for its proper use, specially trained technical and medical personnel. To establish such an organization in many places throughout the county is neither advisable nor possible. Accurate planning of the resources for radiotherapy at regional hospitals is, therefore, essential. The aim should be to concentrate all curative radiotherapy for cancer at the regional hospital.

14.5 Training

In their daily work nurses instruct and supervise large groups of staff. Oncological training of nurses working in units which care for many cancer patients should, therefore, receive special attention. The increasing use of chemotherapy and radiotherapy demands sound basic and up-to-date knowledge in such nurses. The same applies to training in dealing with emotional reactions connected with cancer and its treatment. In an international perspective, the need for specialization and oncological training of nurses is well recognized. Certain changes in the present training programmes in Sweden should be made in this direction and could lead to appreciable improvements in cancer care.

14.6 Psychological, psychiatric and sociomedical aspects of cancer care

The emotional needs of cancer patients are increasingly recognized. In a number of cancer centres in various countries, teams comprising psychiatrists, psychologists and social workers have been integrated with specialists in somatic cancer care. So far only limited efforts of this kind have been made in Sweden.

Cancer denotes a group of dreaded diseases often associated with physical, emotional and social upheaval to both patients and their relatives. The treatment often has disturbing side-effects and may lead to altered life-style. Much support is given by nursing staff, social workers, psychologists, etc., but, because of lack of suitable training, it is often inadequate. The psychological and sociomedical aspects of cancer care are therefore important responsibilities for oncological centres. Improvements can be achieved by measures aimed directly at patients by education of personnel groups and through research.

Many studies have shown that personnel in oncology departments often suffer from fatigue, irritability and a feeling of inadequacy attributable to the mental strain involved in the work. A prerequisite for more effective emotional support to cancer patients and their families is that personnel, including doctors, should receive some training in psychology and also guidance in difficult situations from professional psychologists or psychiatrists. Such support could, for example, require crisis intervention or provision of resources for social help. For these reasons, posts should be established at all oncological centres for psychiatrists and/or psychologists who should preferably have some psychotherapeutic training.

Patients operated on for breast cancer or laryngeal cancer, or who have some form of stoma, and parents of children with malignant diseases have formed associations to provide support for others in similar situations. The valuable help given by such voluntary organizations includes psychological support. Formation of such associations should be encouraged and they should be recognized as assets in cancer care.

14.7 Prevention of cancer, screening programmes and collaboration between basic and clinical research

The documentation and expertise available in oncological centres must be fully utilized. The regional cancer register can be valuable in epidemiological research and for follow-up of preventive measures. These resources in the oncological centres would also be useful in planning and execution of screening programmes for early diagnosis of cancer.

Many difficulties have been reported from several countries in applying results of experimental cancer research in clinical research and development. The need to improve collaboration between basic and clinical cancer research has been one of the main motives for institution of cancer centres in a number of countries. In Sweden a decisive factor in the achievement of such an integration is that some oncologists have taken up clinical training and research following training in basic research at a university. The facilities for experimental research that are associated with the regional oncological centres have also been shown to encourage integration between basic and applied research.

14.8 Multi-regional collaboration

Treatment of rare tumour forms, or tumours which require highly specialized resources, can be centralized advantageously at a few of the oncological centres. Examples are bone marrow transplantation in acute leukaemia, management of some tumours in children and rare optical malignancies. In Sweden multi-regional collaboration has begun as regards education, formulation of common management programmes, common guidelines for regional cancer registers, etc. This can be valuable in various connections and frequently can help save resources. Such collaboration between oncological centres in different regions should, therefore, be encouraged.

15
Research into cancer and preventive measures

15.1 Starting points

Continued research is necessary in order to be able to reduce the deleterious effects of the cancer diseases. Cancer research today includes not only clinical and epidemiological research into the occurrence, causes, prevention, diagnosis and treatment of different forms of cancer, but also aspects which lead into a number of areas of medicine, natural science and behavioural science. The neoplastic transformation of a normal cell is a disturbance of basic functions of the cell. This fact as well as the reaction of the host organism against cancer-transformed cells makes disciplines such as molecular biology, cell biology, virology, immunology and genetics very significant for cancer research in a wide sense. Research within the behavioural sciences is important e.g. as a means of finding ways for changing people's life-style as an element in the prevention of cancer. Technical research, as well as contributing to methods of diagnosis and treatment, may also indicate new ways to prevent cancer.

Economic and social science are also relevant to a broader perspective: they are essential to analyses, of the decision-making process as such, to cost-benefit analyses in such processes and other analyses of the consequences of one or more possible measures for reducing cancer risks. This research will not be touched upon further in this chapter.

All of the preceding chapters have introduced relevant questions of research and indicated where further research is needed. This is so, among other things, with regard to the present knowledge of the causes and mechanisms of induction of cancer diseases (Chapters 2 and 3), experience from and problems connected with certain types of register or data-base studies with different environmental variables (Chapter 5), information systems for population studies, including early-warning systems (Chapter 8), the relationship between tobacco smoking and cancer (Section 4.2) and between diet and cancer (Section

4.3). Specific projects recommended have included an epidemiological study aiming to provide a quantitative estimate of the risk of radon in homes (Section 10.4), studies of dietary habits and dietary changes and their effects on health (Section 10.2), measurements of exposure, etc., to provide a better basis for evaluating the importance of passive smoking (Sections 4.2 and 10.1), and scientific evaluations of current activities with mass health screening of breast cancer and cervical cancer (Chapter 13). A special programme for research on air pollution in the home and its importance from the point of view of cancer risk as well as factors such as ventilation, etc. (Section 10.5) is connected with conditions in Sweden today. Research into information transmission and influencing of attitudes has been mentioned in connection with the discussion about public health education (Chapter 9).

Toxicological questions and methodological approaches that are important for the understanding of cancer induction through the impact of environmental factors have also been touched upon. The difficulties in quantifying risks have been pointed out in Chapters 7 and 11. Chapter 11 briefly treated the question of toxicological research in connection with a discussion of test methods and test resources for the investigation of mutagenic and carcinogenic effects.

This chapter supplements the previous text by giving examples of more areas of current cancer research in Sweden, by identifying problems which need to be addressed and by discussing certain organizational aspects.

15.2 The organization and financing of Swedish cancer research

15.2.1 Introduction

Besides a basic organization for education and research within the system of higher education and certain permanent resources at some other national organs, financial resources for cancer research in Sweden are mainly obtained from grants. National research councils, official bodies for the financing of mostly 'applied research', within specific spheres (sectors) as opposed to 'basic research' and various funds are among the major sources of these grants. Considerable resources are also provided by the general organization of public health and medical care, and within this, regional oncological centres are likely to play an increasing role in cancer research. Much cancer research in Sweden is financed by funds dependent on collections and donations, but a gradual increase of the support provided by the state is now taking place.

The *Swedish Cancer Society* was instituted in 1951, to support, organize and co-ordinate cancer research and to promote the development of new methods of examination and treatment. In addition, the Society is involved in disseminating information about the aims and conduct of cancer research and about the prevention, symptoms and treatment of cancer diseases. The activities of the Society are financed by collections and gifts and by an annual contribution of 3 million Sw.kr from the state. The total research grants made by the Society during recent years are shown in Table 15.1. Other charitable organizations provide funds for cancer research. These funds support mainly clinical research, and their grants amounted to about 15 million Sw.kr in 1983.

Table 15.1 Grants for cancer research 1976–83 in millions of Swedish kroner from the Swedish Cancer Society, the Medical Research Council and the Natural Science Research Council. In addition, other government agencies contributed about 12 million Sw. kr and local university funds about 15 million Sw. kr to give a total sum of about 90 million Sw. kr in 1983

Year	Swedish Cancer Society Total	State Contribution	Research Councils[a]	Total
1976	20.5	3.0		
1977	23.0	3.0		
1978	26.5	3.0		
1979	28.5	3.0	9.5	38.0
1980	30.0	3.0	14.0	44.0
1981	30.0	3.0	17.8	47.8
1982	31.0	3.0	22.3	53.3
1983	35.5	3.0	27.9	63.4

[a] According to the analyses carried out by the councils themselves of their project grants. For the years 1980–83, included in these sums are grants specifically allocated to cancer research (3.0, 6.0, 9.2 and 12.6 million Sw. kr respectively).

The main support for cancer research by the Swedish Government is through the *Medical Research Council* and the *National Science Research Council*. In addition to this, the Swedish Government makes an annual contribution of 4.8 million Sw.kr to the International Agency for Research on Cancer (IARC), the cancer research organ of the World Health Organization.

The National Council for the Planning and Co-ordination of Research is an organ with certain co-ordinating tasks in relation to other national research councils. It provides grants of its own mainly to areas which appear to be especially important from a societal point of view.

Research on occupational cancer is to a large extent financed by grants from the *Work Environment Fund*, which each year both places certain resources at the disposal of the National Board of Occupational

Safety and Health and supports research directly within institutions and clinics.

Out of a levy on payrolls in Sweden a certain percentage automatically goes to the fund each year, according to law. This is used, among other things, to finance research projects decided by a board of directors. From a budget in 1983 of just over 500 million Sw.kr 130 million went towards research and development (besides the special grants to the control agency mentioned). Direct research grants from the Work Environment Fund for studies of genotoxicity and/or cancer amounted to about 6.5 million Sw.kr in the year 1981 and during its first 10 years of existence amounted to a total of about 30 million Sw.kr. These have been directed mainly towards epidemiological research of occupational and population groups, but also to experimental studies and the development of methods for estimation of genotoxic or carcinogenic risk. An element of special interest from the point of view of disease prevention in the activities of the Work Environment Fund and the National Board of Occupational Safety and Health is their support for technical research with the aim of reducing exposures.

Several other bodies with responsibilities for particular sectors help to finance especially target-oriented cancer research. One is the *Research Council of the National Environmental Protection Board* which is involved in studies of environmental factors and cancer risks in urban environments and the characterization of genotoxic compounds in waste discharges. An average sum for this has been about 1 million Sw.kr during recent years (the early 1980s) for research with a connection to cancer. Also, *the National Products Control Board*, which is linked to the National Environmental Protection Board, has initiated studies concerning genotoxic effects of certain chemical substances and studies of cancer epidemiology. *The National Institute of Radiation Protection*, on average, directs about 2 million Sw.kr of its available research money to relevant projects such as investigations of radiation environments, and certain projects of cancer epidemiology related to radiation risks.

Industrial research and development by individual firms or trade research institutes contributes to the lessening of deleterious effects of cancer diseases through investigating process changes or other techniques for reducing exposures to carcinogenic agents and through development of products for diagnosis and treatment of cancer.

15.2.2 Total resources available to cancer research

In a broad sense, cancer research is the largest area of biomedical research in the world. In the USA, the National Cancer Institute had an annual budget of more than USA$1000 million in 1980, an increase of a factor of 4 over the previous decade. Together with other grants for cancer research in the USA this represents considerably more than half of the total funding for cancer research in the world. The background to these large investments is the hope that cancer can be prevented and treated with much greater success. This led to a special law, The National Cancer Act, through which a specific cancer research programme was initiated in 1971. About 90 fields were identified where considerable gains were expected from an increased investment in research. Progress made in cancer research in the USA during the 1970s as summarized by the National Cancer Advisory Board (1981) and the dramatically improved results of methods of treatments for certain forms of cancer (child leukaemia, Hodgkin's disease and testicular cancer) were emphasized.

A comparison of grants for cancer research in Sweden and in the USA, for example as per capita expenditure, is rendered difficult mainly by two factors. One is that support for biomedical research in the Swedish institutions, over their regular budgets, is proportionally much greater than in the USA. This support has been excluded from the previously mentioned sum of about 90 million Sw.kr annually, in the early 1980s, in grants to cancer research in Sweden (Table 15.1). The second factor concerns the amount of money actually available for research. In the USA, researchers must set aside up to 50 per cent of their grants for the management of their parent institutions and for other costs not directly related to research. The corresponding percentages deducted from project budgets to cover administrative costs in Sweden have long been very low, although they now are tending to increase somewhat. An estimate taking the second but not the first factor into account points at an annual sum of around US$2.5 per person in the USA and about 11 Sw.kr per person in Sweden going directly to research on cancer. The actual value of these sums within each of the two countries seems to be about the same, irrespective of large alterations of the rate of exchange in the first part of the 1980s. Swedish cancer research is, moreover, of a high international standard. In an investigation carried out in the USA (cited in MFR (1983)) it was shown that among the 1000 most cited researchers in the world in the sciences of physics, chemistry and biomedicine during the period 1968–78, 736 were from the USA, 85 from UK, 42 (all of whom were active in the biomedical sciences) from Sweden, 26 from France, 23 from Canada, and 21 from West Germany. Other countries were represented by 13 or fewer researchers.

15.3 Swedish cancer research—types and directions

Basic research regarding the nature and induction mechanisms of cancer takes place within many of the biomedical disciplines at the faculties of medicine and of science. An intensely studied sub-area is *the biochemistry of basic life processes*. Of special interest are studies of the organization of DNA, its transcription product RNA and the translation of RNA to proteins which determine the properties of the cells. Foreign DNA and RNA from viruses are also examined, as well as how the body converts and activates chemicals that may give rise to cancer.

Studies of the basic processes of life are of importance for the understanding of the induction and growth of tumour cells and of how this growth may be influenced by systems of the body or by drugs which interact with the DNA → RNA → protein process.

Within *cell biology*, cell hybridization and chromosome banding has made it possible to analyse the properties of tumour cells and their genetic information in detail. Furthermore, differences between the growth of normal and tumour-transformed cells have been studied. Chromosome banding has shown that the chromosomal aberrations in tumours are not random. As a result of such analyses a Swedish group has been able to localize the genes for a component of antibody molecules. The banding techniques are also tentatively used for tumour diagnosis and for investigations of the effects produced by toxic compounds on the genetic information.

Cytochemical investigations of the DNA pattern in cancer cells (e.g. breast cancer) have, in Swedish studies, been shown to give information about the degree of malignancy of the tumour and can thus probably open the way to improving knowledge of the properties of individual tumours and consequently to a more specific treatment.

Virology and immunology are also areas which are rapidly developing and where Swedish research holds a strong position. Viruses cause certain cancer forms in animals and most probably also in human beings. Proteins produced by the cells both in virus-induced and chemically induced tumours seem to regulate cell growth and appear also to exist in normal cells, although in lower concentration. The discovery made in recent years that certain genes, called *oncogenes*, can exist in the normal DNA of humans as well as in certain tumour viruses has partly blurred the boundary between cell biology and virology. The role of oncogenes during neoplastic transformation is being studied intensively (see Chapter 3). It has previously been possible to show that certain tumour types exhibit recurring chromosomal changes characteristic of each tumour type. In many such cases it has been possible to demonstrate that a 'normal' oncogene has been relocalized from one chromosome to another, and there seems to be a direct link to these cells starting to behave like cancer cells. The products of the oncogenes themselves have in many cases already been isolated and shown to be enzymes with a probable effect on the growth of cells.

In the area of virology, viruses with DNA and RNA as genetic material are being studied. In addition to transmitting its own genetic information to an infected cell, certain RNA viruses may also carry parts of the normal hereditary material of the host cell, thereby bringing the infected cell out of balance and leading to a more rapid transformation than in the case of viruses that do not carry cell information.

Another central area of research deals with changes in the cell surface as a result of virus infection. Since the cell surface is the point of contact of the cell with its surroundings, through which all exterior control is exerted, changes at the surface are potential causes of the aberrant behaviour of tumour cells. Linked to this are the critical questions as to what factors regulate and influence the occurrence of metastases.

Immunology embraces many topical phenomena, e.g. the so-called natural killer cells which may kill tumour cells without previously having learned to recognize them, other mechanisms for cell-mediated killing of tumour cells, how certain cells may impair an immunological response and how interferon may influence immunity. Furthermore, there is intensive work going on to use the monoclonal antibodies for improving diagnostic methods and therapy.

Processes connected with intestinal metabolism are nowadays much in focus with regard to several cancer forms. More attention should be paid to *intestinal bacteria* and their transformation of dietary components (see Section 4.3), as well as metabolic studies of different components of the diet.

The conditions are favourable in Sweden for *clinical oncological research* due to a highly developed health care organization. The study of the *symptomatology and processes of cancer diseases* as well as the *introduction and evaluation of new diagnostic and therapeutic methods* is facilitated by a considerable centralization at the regional level and the co-ordination of the cancer health care through oncological centres and the access to good systems of registration and follow-up. The conditions for clinical cancer research are considerably different from those of basic research because of the close connection with health care, and an important part of the costs are covered, at least indirectly, by the health care budget. A collaboration between basic and clinical research within the cancer area (cf. Section 14.7), which might both be stimulating through the exchange of ideas and make possible a rapid application at the clinical level of findings from basic research, is also important. The existence of oncological centres at the regional hospitals should improve the prospects for such a collaboration, and also for clinical and epidemiological cancer research, which requires cooperation between many institutions and clinics.

Present clinical oncological research includes some large projects which require advanced laboratory techniques and which are usually carried out in collaboration between clinics and academic institutions of medicine. Some of these projects lie in the fields of cell biology (e.g. certain cytogenetic projects), chemistry (projects concerning the biochemistry of certain cancer forms and the metabolism of cancer patients) or immunology and virology (projects concerning, among other things, the Epstein-Barr virus and interferon).

Many projects study hormonal receptors which are molecules in the cell that receive and transmit hormones from the exterior. It has long been known that many types of tumour are inhibited in their growth by the administration of hormones. By measuring the capacity of the tumour cells to bind the hormones, it is possible to make better predictions about which tumours will be susceptible to the action of hormones. Research on receptors in cancer cells from the breast, kidneys, corpus uteri and prostate as well as in leukaemias and malignant lymphomas is also being carried out.

The treatment of tumours with *cytostatics* (cell inhibitors) is a therapeutic method of increasing importance. Many projects are being undertaken concerning the metabolism of different cytostatics in the body. Other projects deal with the possibility of predicting the sensitivity of tumours to different cell inhibitors by studies on tumours growing in tissue culture or in animals.

The testing of cytostatics, in particular for adjuvant treatment (preventive treatment of patients who have been treated with 'radical' surgery or radiation), must often be carried out as controlled prospective multi-centre studies, i.e. with many participating clinics, so that the possible advantages of the treatment can be demonstrated and balanced against the disadvantages. Many such studies are being carried out on a national or regional basis in Sweden and deal with, for example, breast cancer, malignant lymphomas, ovary cancer and stomach cancer.

Controlled studies of the effects of mammographic health control for early detection of breast cancer, and health screening using a method for demonstration of occult blood in faeces for early diagnosis of intestinal tumours (see Chapter 13) are also research projects of great practical interest. There are many projects at present where tumour markers are used in order to follow progress and prognoses in cancer diseases.

Within the areas of *radiotherapy* and *radiobiology* several long-term projects are in progress to examine mechanisms of damage and repair of cells following irradiation. The modification of the effects of radiation, e.g. by different types of dose fractionation, chemical substances and influence on the circulation of the blood, is being investigated. In collaboration with clinical institutions, scientific and technical institutions and industry, development of new apparatus for treatment with highly energetic X-ray and electron irradiation is also under way in Sweden. Treatment of tumours with locally elevated temperatures, known as hyperthermia, has also attracted increasing interest and is the subject of some research projects where the method is combined with cell-inhibiting drugs or radiation therapy.

The development of radiological diagnostics is important for both cancer diagnosis and cancer treatment. Several Swedish research projects have been concerned with *computer tomography*, a technique which has radically improved the possibilities of localizing tumours and planning radiation treatment. NMR (nuclear magnetic resonance) tomography is a totally new technique which, similarly to computer tomography, presents pictures of cross-sections of the body. It is based on the fact that certain atoms (e.g. hydrogen atoms) have magnetic properties which may be analysed with strong magnetic fields and radiowaves. The potential of this technique is being carefully evaluated.

Psychological aspects of tumour diseases are receiving increased attention. Experiences of illness and treatment in breast cancer patients, and family worries in cases of childhood cancer have been studied. Another important question concerns the individual's psychological reactions to attending health check-ups, especially when recalled for further investigation. Special attention needs to be given to providing information in a suitable way in such cases (see Chapter 13).

The introduction of a new method for diagnosis or treatment must be based on the fact that it has been judged to be better than, or equivalent to, existing methods. An important question during the evaluation of different methods is the *ethical aspect*. This concerns particularly the ability of the patients to choose whether to participate in randomized studies where different methods of treatment are compared. This question is not unique to cancer research. Use of randomized clinical investigations must be carefully restricted where the information to the patient can have considerable psychological consequences, as in cancer care (Einhorn, 1983). Ethical committees for the treatment of such questions exist at all educational centres and larger hospitals. and co-operate through a special standing committee under the Medical Research Council. Problems of research and ethics of treatment are also being continuously followed and discussed in other quarters such as the National Board of Health and Welfare.

The significance of *life-style and other environmental factors* for cancer induction is studied partly in projects of a more experimental character, which illuminate the metabolism and effects of different potentially carcinogenic chemical and physical agents, dose–response relationships, etc., and partly in epidemiological projects.

During recent years, much increased interest in *cancer epidemiology* has been noted in Sweden including both descriptive and analytical studies. Swedish epidemiology, however, needs strengthening through research on and development of methodology. This involves the validation of data, sampling methods, statistical models and problems of interpretation of results. Better co-operation with basic research in mathematical statistics should be brought about.

As explained in Chapter 8, Sweden has, like other Nordic countries, very good opportunities of carrying out cancer–epidemiological research due to the access to complete cancer registries and good demographic individual-related data through the personal numbers allocated to all members of the population.

It has been shown earlier (Chapters 5 and 6) that registry data are available already but crude environmental variables usually can be used for analytical as well as descriptive, approaches in cancer epidemiology. Sweden also has good possibilities for proper analytical studies (of cohorts and case-control) since it is relatively easy to follow up populations and obtain data about different environmental variables.

The further development of models for *exposure analysis* of pollutants in occupational and general environments, sampling and quantitative techniques of chemical analysis for the determination of exposures and for biological monitoring of risk groups with regard to specific exposures (see Section 4.4) are tasks of research which are of interest both when it comes to continuous risk management and for future epidemiological investigations. Under the heading 'Epidemiological monitoring' in Chapter 8 the Cancer Committee has, furthermore, discussed the need for development of methods for *early warning* of exposures to agents with a potential cancer risk (genotoxic effect).

Another need is for epidemiological investigations into the effects of preventive measures such as changes in the diet. These are termed *intervention studies* and are particularly important where the causal relationships are not established, which is the case for most human cancers.

Studies of *genetic variation* in personal susceptibility to carcinogenic agents and in the disposition of individuals to develop cancer diseases refer to a central issue in this context.

Experimental investigations of the carcinogenic effects of different agents on animals and mutagenic and other genotoxic effects on cells are also essential from a preventive point of view. When human data are lacking, experimental studies are in many cases the only available way of clarifying potential cancer risks. Current areas of research include the methodology of testing the cancer-initiating effects and promoter effects of agents in experimental animals, clarification of qualitative relations between different genotoxic effects and cancer initiation. In addition, quantitative methods for determination of genotoxic activity in short-term tests (particularly chemical dosimetry by measurement of adducts to DNA or to suitable proteins) for unknown agents, followed by chemical identification should be developed further. The concentration of such adducts is a measure of dose and therefore related to risk, and can be determined both in samples from human beings and in experimental animals and cellular test systems. Adduct determinations should be introduced as widely as possible as a supplement in all laboratory tests so that the use of the results for the quantification of risk is facilitated.

An understanding of dose–response relationships is vital to risk estimation, especially at low levels of chemical and physical environmental factors. These relationships should therefore be examined, primarily in long-term animal tests and in close conjunction with active research into the mechanisms of oncogene activation, promotion, etc.

Adequate resources must be made available for both long-term studies in animals and short-term tests. Facilities for long-term carcinogenicity tests in animals are not widely available in Sweden.

Technical issues are often brought to the fore during cancer preventive measures. In the general environment this applies to, for instance, the elimination of mutagenic and carcinogenic pollutants. In the occupational environment examples are to be found in the introduction of improved techniques of ventilation, of combustion techniques less detrimental to the environment, and in the development of manufacturing processes and products which cause less emission of potentially carcinogenic substances, or lead to either smaller amounts of solid waste or to more easily degradable substances in the waste.

Sweden is well advanced in combustion techniques for heating and other energy purposes including automobiles. This research area is vital if significant long-term improvement in air pollution is to be achieved.

There seems to be a development towards biologically more 'benign' products with regard to both organic and inorganic substances including metals (see also Westermark, 1982) Even in the absence of direct data on cancer risks, it is presumed that such product changes will to some extent imply reduced exposure to carcinogens. Two examples of removal of carcinogens are the replacement of asbestos as an insulator by other inorganic materials, and the substitution of the carcinogenic solvent benzene by other organic liquids in chemical laboratories and industry.

Within manufacturing industry, two major routes are open to cutting down human exposure to carcinogens. One is to improve the degree of containment of processes involving these substances, as in the polymerization of vinyl chloride. The other is to introduce advanced automation, including robots, into processes so that humans do not have to come into immediate contact with hazardous materials.

Swedish research and product development is also called for with regard to foodstuffs (see Section 10.2).

Concluding remarks

Referring to the decisive role of research for improving the situation with regard to cancer diseases, it is obvious that Sweden as a small country has limited resources. It is, therefore, a good strategy to direct research money in particular to areas where a high competence has already been built up, or where the conditions are otherwise judged to be especially favourable. In addition, specific national problems may require special resources.

In this section and in other parts of this report, a number of research issues have been pointed out where Swedish inputs seem natural. The research efforts should be increased, in particular in the areas of epidemiology, toxicology in relation to action mechanisms and genetics, and research into problems associated with the concept of risk and risk management.

15.4 Some organizational issues

To identify cancer research specifically may be possible for research of the type supported by the Swedish Cancer Society and/or carried out at oncological centres or institutions particularly directed towards cancer questions where all the activity is by definition cancer research. In addition there are special programmes or individual projects which have been planned as cancer research within organizations with wider tasks. At the same time, however, it is clear that much of the research which is designated or planned as 'cancer research', in particular basic research, generates knowledge which has a much wider area of application. The question of whether the organization of cancer research, especially in relation to bodies financing research, is suitable, must thus be given a rather general formulation.

The following three requirements apply to funding of research in all areas.

Firstly the *quality* aspect should never be neglected. Quality of research is ensured by two processes. The first is the examination of applications for grants by a team of experts. The second is the refereeing of papers submitted for publication in international scientific journals.

Secondly, the organization of research should function in such a way that it *encourages* the development of *new ideas*. The involvement of several funding bodies with different interests and aims is a positive feature in this respect. Provision should be made for the award of long-term research grants to well-established scientific groups on conditions which do not restrict the researchers from following up new ideas and, if necessary, changing the directions of their work.

Thirdly, a rigid *categorization* of research should *be avoided* since this tends to work against a 'best distribution' of research money. Also, clear boundaries often cannot be drawn between categories such as basic research and applied research. National research councils and other funding bodies should therefore co-operate, as indeed several already do, in, for example, dealing with certain applications.

The bodies funding research in particular sectors in Sweden choose which projects to support not only on the basis of scientific merit, but also on their relevance to the responsibilities of the body involved. A large part of this research is linked to 'programmes', i.e. fairly comprehensive research plans for specific problem areas, often drafted in collaboration with interested researchers. There should be more contacts between sectorial bodies responsible for, among other things, environmental cancer risks. Improved communication between such funding organs and the 'traditional' research councils including, for example, the Swedish Cancer Society is also desirable because of the need to settle borderline matters and to obtain good judgements of the quality and feasibility of proposed projects.

The most important causes of cancer in quantitative terms have been identified as those associated with life-style (see Chapter 6). In Sweden there is no agency with special responsibility for research in these risk areas, in contrast to the risks from occupational exposures, environmental pollutants and so on. It is therefore urgent that the research councils should take up this responsibility.

Particular attention should be directed towards emerging needs for co-ordinated, long-term resource inputs to certain areas of research, for example on the relationship between environmental factors and cancer diseases. Prospective long-term population–based investigations with respect to cancer as well as other chronic diseases and possible causative factors, both of an endogenous and of an exogenous character, have been mentioned previously (Chapter 8). Such projects, perhaps planned to run for several decades, must not be interrupted before time because of lack of continuity in competence or financial resources.

It is not justified to make further proposals for any major changes to the existing organization of cancer research, including measures for cancer prevention, beyond indicating a general need for consultation and co-operation between the diverse bodies involved in supporting the research. In this context, the setting up of an advisory health council to the Government, as proposed in the next chapter, should also be noted. Such a council 'for information and co-ordination within the health sector' could, for example, from time to time discuss and point out areas where cancer research is urgent.

16
Some general conclusions

16.1 Introduction

The Cancer Committee's terms of reference required it to suggest a realistic strategy for prevention of cancer diseases. Economic and other consequences were to be examined and an order of priority indicated for the measures recommended. Problems related to the diagnosis and therapy of these diseases were also to be addressed. In other words, the Committee's brief was to suggest measures to generally reduce the harmful effects of cancer diseases, but with the focus on preventive measures.

In this report, an overall strategy of cancer prevention is discussed in Chapter 7, indicating general conditions for prevention of a cancer disease, and the strategy's major aims and components. Different principles for rank-ordering, in particular of regulatory measures, were treated including cost-benefit analysis in a broad meaning of this concept. In some of the following chapters (Chapters 8–12 and 15), these considerations were developed in more detail, including specific recommendations within certain areas. Thus strategic principles on a number of aspects have been introduced in the contexts where they naturally fit in.

Possibilities for early diagnosis through mass screening programmes have been dealt with in depth in Chapter 13, and the organization of cancer care was reviewed in Chapter 14.

One of the prerequisites for continuing measures to reduce the harmful effects of cancer diseases is good information systems for demographic studies (Chapter 8) and a first-rate national cancer research programme (Chapter 15). This applies to both preventive measures and diagnosis, treatment and other medical care.

The present chapter discusses ways of setting priorities with respect to different types of measures or activities aimed at reducing the harmful effects of cancer diseases, as well as cost aspects in broad outline in connection with a review of the more important recommendations from previous chapters (Sections 16.2 and 16.3).

During the course of the Cancer Committee's work, the clear view emerged that cancer prevention should be integrated into a general approach to measures for risk reduction and health-promotion (see Section 7.3); this then formed a point of departure for the subsequent considerations and proposals with regard to different cancer-preventive measures. In Section 16.4 this concept is developed in a wider perspective. Particularly with the aim of improving the breadth of view at the national level with regard to health-promoting measures, the Committee therefore finally recommends that a health council should be set up as an advisory body to the Government. This would also mean the introduction of a supplementary mechanism in society to channel new knowledge.

16.2 Starting points, preconditions for ordering of priorities, etc.

The importance of cancer diseases

In order to reach a balanced judgement between the need for and the economic possibilities of acting with regard to some specific category of disease, one needs to be able to assess the detrimental effects of this disease or disease category in relation to other diseases or health disturbances at the time a decision is taken. Such comparisons between diseases cannot be specifically addressed here, but some of the principal data on the importance of cancer diseases are summarized in the following (see also Chapter 2).

In Sweden, as in other countries with similar living conditions, cancer is the second largest cause of death after cardiovascular diseases. For a long time the age-standardized cancer mortality has been almost constant in Sweden while there has been some increase in the incidence of cancer diseases as a whole, although the trend is at present not at all clear (see Figure 2.6). Certain cancer forms have shown an increase in frequency while others have gone down. Because the prevalence of a disease—in particular one more common among older people—and the proportion of deaths it causes is dependent on competing causes of death, one obtains a more informative picture of the importance of a disease by looking at its effect on the average life-span. At the present time, the cancer mortality in the total population implies a decrease in the average life-span of 2–3 years, while the average life-span for those afflicted with a cancer disease is shortened, on the average, by about 11 years for men and 16 years for women.

As indicated previously there are great variations between different cancer diseases in their degree of malignancy, curability, age at first appearance, etc. In 1980, the average age at diagnosis of a cancer disease was almost 69 years for men and just over 66 years for women. For specific cancer diseases, the conditions may be different, with an average age at diagnosis of cancer of the cervix and of the breast (women) of 55 and 64 years, respectively, and for cancer of the prostate and malignant melanoma (men) of 73 and 58 years, respectively. About one third of the new cancer cases recorded now refer to persons of working age.

The direct costs of cancer care in Sweden in 1977, expressed in terms of 1980 costs, are believed to have amounted to just over 2000 million Sw.kr (Table 2.11). According to another estimate (quoted in Table 2.12), tumour diseases are responsible for more than 5 per cent of the direct costs of health care and for about 3 per cent of the total morbidity costs in the country. It should be stressed that data on morbidity costs are often difficult to judge since very different bases for the caculation can be used.

Even if the public perception of the nature of cancer diseases, their prevalence and their development over time often seems to have been one-sided or inaccurate—resulting in over-anxiety—it is obvious that this group of diseases does play a very great role, whether viewed from the angle of society as a whole or of people as individuals. *Continued strong action to reduce the harmful effects of cancer diseases is therefore imperative.* Such action must include both disease-preventive measures, early and definite diagnosis, and good treatment and care of those who have developed a cancer disease.

Formulating programmes of measures in this context is often limited by the still imperfect knowledge of the causes of tumour diseases and the induction and development of tumours in the body. Although recent research has made important and sometimes decisive progress, it is not scientifically justified to plan today for extraordinary efforts against cancer diseases or to expect spectacular effects during the foreseeable future from measures that can be taken at the present time. Steadily growing scientific knowledge, improved methods of treatment, and so on, resulting from intensive cancer research programmes all over the world, will gradually improve the possibilities for acting against these diseases. However, this must not be allowed to influence measures that can be taken today to counter living habits or other environmental factors known to be associated with increased cancer risk.

Preventive measures—general principles

In parallel with improving knowledge of how different diseases arise, the matter of disease-preventive measures becomes more and more important. In principle, there is hardly any difference between, on the one hand, efforts to prevent the occurrence of a disease or injury (whether actions are individual related or group related) and, on the other hand, giving medical care to a person who is afflicted with such a disease or injury.

It is often obvious that disease-preventive measures are economically worthwhile, almost irrespective of what basis is used for calculations of morbidity or mortality costs. An expected decrease in the total cost of medical care and/or a reduced loss of production are simple illustrations of how preventive measures are a good economic investment. In other cases this is not so clear; humanitarian aspects should then also be brought into the calculation, as is done for example with regard to the care of elderly people.

Disease-preventive measures as normally perceived within a health care system need to be supplemented by principles applicable to certain situations or health risks, at least where the individual has difficulty in influencing circumstances himself. The basis here is the risk concept. Besides trying to assess the effect on public health in general of different measures to reduce a risk, the decision-maker should also consider individual risks and differences between individuals or population groups in the actual risk situation (see Chapter 7, on the strategy of cancer prevention). Such situations for decision are usually governed by legislation. This also implies that groups outside the traditional health care field will become involved, as decision-makers and cost units, *viz.* a number of control agencies and enterprises (see Chapter 11).

Research activities are an integral part of the strategy to improve possibilities of reducing the occurrence of different cancer diseases. The basic research necessary in this context should be determined mainly by purely scientific considerations. The availability of adequate scientific competence will be one of the governing factors also when priorities of applied research are ordered.

In Sweden, research and development with regard to cancer diseases and cancer risks is financed by certain public bodies and other organizations such as the Cancer Society as well as by the business community. The borderline between these is not drawn up once and for all. According to Swedish statutory risk control, for example, a company should always give priority to research and development activities aimed at identifying and countering risks which are due to that company's own activities. Major public resources also go to research of this kind but the top priority of publicly financed research should be towards problems common to several kinds of industry or towards broader social problems.

Preventive measures—a holistic view of contributions and effects

The overall picture of causes of diseases or health risks should always be considered. Certain known or suspected causes of cancer are also of great importance for the development of other diseases or environmental disturbances, and preventive measures must be looked at in these wider perspectives.

Road traffic in urban areas may be mentioned as an example. The Cancer Committee's estimate (see Section 10.3) is that in Sweden some 100–1000 cancer cases per year may be caused by general air pollution in urban areas (to which road traffic is a dominant contributor, though it cannot be separated from the heating of dwellings, etc.). In 1983 a Swedish governmental committee on car exhausts suggested measures such as the introduction of unleaded petrol and so-called catalytic cleaning of car exhausts in order to reduce air pollution from petrol-driven road traffic. These measures should certainly reduce cancer risks, but a scientific basis is lacking for estimating the magnitude of the effect. The recommendations for the measures were based on all the various negative health and environmental effects involved and there would be little point in discussing what countermeasures regarding car exhausts would be justified by the still uncertain estimates of cancer risks *alone*.

Dietary habits provide another example where over-consumption or a deficiency of certain components of the diet might constitute a common risk factor behind different health effects (see Section 10.2). Thus suspicions have begun to be raised of increased risks of certain types of cancer developing in connection with a high fat intake, a factor which has for a long time been associated with an excess risk of cardiovascular diseases. It is clear, therefore, that reduction of fat intake should be promoted by all possible means even though the effects of such reductions on the total cancer incidence cannot at present be assessed.

It also follows from the two examples mentioned that it would not be meaningful, even theoretically, to try to set priorities on the basis of cancer risks alone, for example between promoting a transition to a less fat-rich diet amongst the Swedish population, on the one hand, and measures to reduce emissions of car exhausts on the other. This is true irrespective of the uncertainty, in both these cases, of the estimates of the size of the cancer risks and of the causal correlations.

Tobacco smoking (Section 10.1) is a rather different example. Here a causal relationship with lung cancer has been clearly demonstrated from a scientific point of view; the influence is great in Sweden as concerns both the total number of lung cancer cases and the (increased) risk for the individual. Aetiological fractions can be calculated with various degrees of certainty also for other forms of cancer (Table 4.6).

The cancer risk alone from tobacco smoking is large enough to warrant drastic countermeasures, and smokers in addition show high excess mortality in certain other diseases.

Although specifically concerned with cancer prevention, the Cancer Committee has pointed out in Section 7.3 that an integrated approach is often necessary with regard to health-promoting actions, risk management, development of new knowledge, etc. For example, health education aiming to influence living habits that might be important for cancer induction should be carried out largely as part of general health-promoting activities (Chapter 9).

Additions to the knowledge-base through research (Chapter 15) and continuous following of trends in cancer diseases, monitoring of risk groups etc., (Chapter 8) are to some extent activities that can be carried out for cancer on its own. This includes functions attached to the central and regional cancer registries. However, it is also necessary to consider cancer-preventive aspects in connection with functions in more general registries or information systems, e.g. the Cause-of-Death Registry or functions related to the different subsystems for epidemiological monitoring now being built (Chapter 8).

Legislation and organization of risk control with regard to chemical and physical agents (Chapter 11) must continue to build on an integrated approach towards all existing risks to humans from, for example, a certain chemical product or a process leading to exposure in the work environment or in the general environment. Furthermore, in some cases it is necessary to consider hazards from such agents to other parts of the environment as well as to humans.

Cancer prevention will in many cases be mainly a question of supplementing existing or planned activities to take account of the specific nature of cancer induction in comparison with other (non-stochastic) health effects, and the risk policy discussed in Section 7.5.

The responsibility for rank ordering of preventive measures, etc., and the organizations concerned

It is presumed that different societal bodies both at the national and at lower administrative levels (in Sweden, especially the county councils) as well as research-financing organizations develop their own strategies as regards cancer prevention including setting priorities. This should apply both to broad risk areas and to specific risk factors. An example of the latter is the risk control of the tens of thousands of existing specific chemical substances, of which some may entail an increased cancer risk to man. The responsibility in Sweden for setting priorities at a detailed level and for judgements of resource needs and the follow-up of costs thus rests in principle with the organizations concerned.

The Cancer Committee has restricted its task to pointing out measures aiming at prevention within a couple of major risk areas either through recommendations of its own or by supporting recommendations made by other official task forces. These are areas where scientifically justified measures are considered realistic at the present time.

What has just been said about the setting of priorities among preventive measures also holds true for other measures to reduce the harmful effects of cancer disease, namely those relating to diagnosis, treatment and other forms of care. According to Swedish law, each county council independently sets the financial budget for its activity and sets priorities between different health care needs (other than for research efforts with national money and contributions from the national budget to certain activities).

A continued adherence or adjustment by the respective responsible organizations to the strategic principles suggested by the Committee could lead to further improved cancer-preventive efforts in the future— in particular in the light of the steadily increasing knowledge of the causes of cancer. This ought to be reflected in the ordering of priorities of available total resources when such decisions are to be taken.

Over and above what is implied by the regional/local self-administration, it rests ultimately with the state authorities (Parliament and Government) to distribute national resources between different societal organizations and to judge possible needs of changes in the legislation. The advisory health council, recommended by the Cancer Committee in the following, the task of which should be directed towards health-promoting measures generally, could facilitate the Government's obligations in this context.

16.3 Survey of more important proposals and overall cost aspects

To a great extent societal mechanisms already exist in Sweden which wholly or partly aim at reducing the damage from cancer diseases, be it research, health care, statutory risk control or other efforts by public authorities, commercial enterprises or voluntary organizations. These mechanisms seem to have usually functioned well with quick reactions (both from politicians and others) to new knowledge or to specific demands for resources. This is not to deny that situations have occurred where people should have acted differently—in particular seen in retrospect. Nor can it be denied that there may exist other deficiencies which should be rectified. However, the major point is that the *present conditions* in Sweden provide a good basis for continued and intensified measures to counteract the harmful effects of cancer diseases.

> A radical improvement of the health status of the Swedish population has taken place during this century, which is reflected in the rapid increase of the average life-span. This has had an impact on both the number of cancer cases and the cancer pattern. A major cause of the increase in absolute numbers of cancer cases has been the increasing proportion of older people in the population.
>
> On the basis of the trend so far, it is difficult to forecast future development of the age-standardized cancer incidence. Certain cancer forms are clearly decreasing in Sweden while others seem to be increasing or remain fairly stable. In all probability, a large proportion of the cancer cases are caused by living habits and other environmental factors. Such factors should be able to be influenced to a considerable extent. The aim of cancer prevention is to reduce the cancer risk; nevertheless, should cancer develop, the aim should be to make it appear later in life than it would have done otherwise.
>
> The need for earlier diagnosis and better treatment and other care of cancer patients remains unchanged alongside increased efforts to prevent these diseases.

Another facet of cancer prevention is that after having long been mainly concerned with reducing involuntary cancer risks from exposure to different agents, attention is increasingly turning to risks in connection with life-style. This should be reflected in the priorities adopted by different bodies for cancer-preventive work—though without neglecting the need for protection of the individual against involuntary risks.

As stated above, the responsibility to transform the Cancer Committee's intentions into detailed plans should very much be the task of each organization concerned. Bearing that in mind, the Committee will just indicate some overall principles which emerge after the previous different proposals have been seen in relation to one another.

These major points are as follows (they should not be taken as being in order of importance):

(a) The general principle of increased commitments to *disease-preventive measures* must be especially promoted. But substantial resources are still needed in the health care system for diagnosis, care and treatment of cancer patients. High priority—also in research—should be attached to achieving *early diagnosis* both through mass health-screenings and through medical examinations carried out for other reasons.

(b) Among known *causal factors*, *tobacco smoking* offers the promise of the best results, on the basis of present scientific knowledge, from attempts to reduce the total cancer incidence. All measures which might conceivably lead to a decrease in smoking ought therefore to be given very high priority. There are also convincing data on the great importance of the *diet* with regard to total cancer incidence, but the scientific data are not so clear for individual dietary components. Research should be intensified, both into the role of individual dietary components for cancer induction, and into possible changes in the population's eating habits.

(c) Today, the most important method of trying to bring down future total cancer incidence seems to be through *health education*. Besides information aiming to influence tobacco use and dietary habits as mentioned above, health education with regard to cancer risks could deal with such matters as alcohol abuse, unwise sunbathing habits and deficient sexual hygiene.

(d) *The statutory risk control* of physical and chemical agents and the efforts that must be made both by industry and by the responsible public authorities remain important. Although the quantitative significance of risk factors covered by such control, in terms of the total cancer incidence, seems to have been fairly limited so far, the importance of the control apparatus must not be underestimated. Its aims are twofold: (*i*) to counteract high individual risks (even if the risk applies to only a few persons) and generally to try to keep any individual's exposure to carcinogenic agents as low as possible (see chapter 7), (*ii*) to counteract previously unknown risk factors with such wide distribution and likelihood of exposure among large population groups that the risk could be of considerable importance to future total cancer incidence even if the individual risk is negligible.

(e) Research and scientific investigations must continue and be further developed in order to add, among other things, the use of efficiently functioning information systems. Cancer research in Sweden has a strong position internationally. Nationwide registries of new cancer cases and cancer death cases are essential for the continuous growth of scientific knowledge and for assessing the effects of measures taken to prevent disease, and the effects of earlier diagnosis or of new methods for treatment of cancer diseases.

Some general conclusions

A conspectus review of the Cancer Committee's proposals by chapter gives the following aspects on costs and cost units. Many Committee recomendations do not carry an exact cost. This is partly because the calculation base is insufficient, partly because it is deliberately left to the implementing bodies to decide on resource allocations in the context of each such body's overall responsibilities.

Chapter 8 deals with health information systems, including early warning of cancer risks, and the prerequisites for epidemiological studies. Good epidemiological monitoring will gradually require a substantial build up of resources, the costs of which will have to be borne both by county councils and the central Government.

Chapter 9 gives strong emphasis to health education, not neglecting the role of the mass media. The county councils will have to carry most of the costs, aided by voluntary organizations.

Chapter 10, Section 1, recommends forceful efforts in particular to drastically reduce tobacco smoking. A programme to deter children from taking up smoking will require a budget of at least 5 million Sw.kr per year for at least 5 years. A joint funding by various interested parties is perceived.

Chapter 10, Section 2, on the diet. In this section, primarily, the dietary habits in Sweden are especially brought into focus, in particular the present high fat intake.

It is difficult to assess the economic consequences of dietary changes to individual households and to the national production and trade, particularly agriculture and the food industry. Moderate changes of dietary habits by the individual, i.e. a reduction of the total fat intake by a few percentage units and a certain increase of intake of other products such as cereals, would not imply cost increases to the Swedish households. After some time the agricultural production would probably change in the direction towards adjustment to the national consumption. Based on the present (1983) national agriculture policy and price regulations, a reduced demand of certain agricultural products as discussed by the Cancer Committee would imply a considerable drop of income in the agricultural sector in a long-term perspective, according to expert judgement obtained by the Committee.

In *Chapter 10, Section 3*, on general air pollution, the Cancer Committee endorsed proposals made by the Car Exhausts Committee that regulations which tighten up the efficiency of car exhausts ought to be issued as soon as possible. The resulting costs should be seen in relation to all health and environmental risks from such emissions; however, they are difficult to elucidate at the moment (1984). The increased production costs for cars with this improved exhaust cleaning has been calculated to about 3000 Sw.kr per vehicle by the Car

Exhausts Committee; the cost will have to be met by the customer. Another proposal working in the opposite direction was a tax reduction (0.2 Sw.kr per litre) of the unleaded petrol required for such cars; also users of a few other car models would benefit if they were to choose the unleaded petrol.

Chapter 10, Section 4, deals with the cancer risks from indoor radon. A proposed study to determine the magnitude of risk in this context will require about 10 million Sw.kr.

The primary target of reducing indoor radon occurrence in existing buildings to a maximum of 400 Bqm^{-3} radon daughters had previously been calculated to cost about 500 million Sw.kr, which will almost totally have to be met by the property owners. One may then add another 20–40 million Sw.kr for locating such dwellings and about 25 million Sw.kr of extra costs per year for producing new dwellings with reasonably low radon concentrations.

Other matters regarding air pollution in the indoor environment and general technical aspects such as ventilation systems (*Chapter 10, Section 5*) will require co-ordinated actions between different public bodies including research-funding organizations.

The Cancer Committee's strategy for cancer prevention presumes the existence of an effective legal control machinery for risks from physical and chemical agents (*Chapter 11*). This machinery should through an increased international co-operation to the extent applicable, be able to meet reasonable demands and expectations from individuals in the general population. In some cases this could mean a need for increased efforts towards the control of cancer risks from chemical agents. As an example the Committee has pointed out that the general knowledge and overview of ongoing exposures is not satisfactory.

Adequate information is not available to the Committee for judging how much of improvement in cancer risk control can be achieved through reallocation of resources from other control sectors by each of the authorities concerned and through measures such as making the control activities more effective by means of increased co-operation with other bodies or through a review of the routines for ordering of priorities on different subject matters within the cancer risk control sector itself. The Committee is disinclined, at least at present, to ask for any particular resource-demanding increases of *the average level* of ambition with regard to the so-called chemical cancer risk control based on current legislation in Sweden. But there could be a need to look more closely at the distribution of tasks and resources between the various responsible authorities in the future.

A more clearly expressed official policy in cancer risk control from the responsible agencies and a tighter control of new chemical substances as an expected result of the work of another governmental group the (Chemical Commission) will no doubt have repercussions also on industry and commerce. However, it is not self-evident that this will always imply increases of net costs for the enterprises concerned, although, for example, the cost of risk reduction in existing plants in some cases have amounted to several million Swedish kroner per cancer case prevented or postponed. In Section 7.5 the Cancer Committee discussed cost–benefit evaluations somewhat more in detail and referred there to some specific case studies undertaken on behalf of the Committee to illuminate economic aspects, an approach considered to be the only feasible way of describing cost consequences of concrete measures taken against specific risk factors. The cost situation of a company might also be affected by what the demands are in other countries for protection against health risks.

Chapter 12 stresses the importance of information for co-operation and as a means for mutual trust in risk management. The role of the mass media calls for well-educated journalists in the fields of medicine/natural sciences. A recommended supplement to education possibilities in Sweden will mean an excess cost for the national higher-education system.

The responsibility for mass health-screening programmes (*Chapter 13*) in Sweden rests with the county councils. A possible introduction of a large-scale mammographic health check-up is one of the main issues discussed by the Committee in this context. A nation-wide programme of this nature has been calculated to cost about 80 million Sw.kr per year. The extra staff needed is around 175 persons.

When addressing the organization of cancer care in Sweden (*Chapter 14*), the Committee stressed, among other things, that there are growing demands on such care which must be recognized in connection with the ongoing restructuring of the health and medical services.

Research plays a decisive role in efforts to limit harmful effects of cancer diseases (*Chapter 15*). According to the Committee at least the same resources as at present (of the order of 100 million Sw.kr per year in the early 1980s), in unchanged real-value terms, should continue to go towards cancer research. Supplementary resources will be needed in the future, especially for long-term, prospective population studies.

According to its terms of reference the Cancer Committee was to 'illuminate to what extent more far-reaching changes in life-style, technology, industrial production, etc., would be needed to considerably reduce the cancer risks' and also look into 'what effects such changes could have on societal economy, employment and material welfare'. As apparent from previous chapters, the investigation has led to the conclusion that scientific information available does not indicate a need for such fundamental changes at the present time or for measures that could have a significant effect on the national economy.

The major resource-consuming research and control activities, the county councils' responsibilities in the health care sector with increased demands on preventive efforts, and specific resource-consuming measures, such as implementation of the proposals of the Car Exhausts Committee, do not in general aim solely at cancer prevention. The same might be said about an implementation of the proposals by the Radon Committee, which could place a heavy financial burden on individual home owners. The dietary changes considered desirable by the Cancer Committee—the long-term economic effects of which are difficult to estimate—are well in line with the main directions of present Swedish dietary recommendations even though these were not drawn up with regard to the association between diet and cancer.

At present the improvement of cancer prevention can therefore hardly be regarded as a new question or as one of a specifically 'cancer-economic' nature. This does not preclude the possibility that future improved understanding of the nature and causes of cancer diseases could warrant changes in society that might have considerable economic consequences.

16.4 Setting up an advisory health council at the national level

Cancer diseases form part of the overall disease panorama and they should therefore be dealt with in this wider context. Stress should also be laid on the fact that many different conditions in society lead to ill health and that the induction of cancer diseases can be related to factors touching different sectors of society. Our living habits influence health a great deal. Obvious health risks are associated with smoking, high alcohol consumption and certain kinds of diet.

In the course of the project Health Services in the 1990s (HS 90) a state-of-the-art report on general health risks in Sweden was published, which illustrates various conditions in the physical environment that can have an influence on human health.

Changes in society have also meant changes in family structure, sexual habits and family planning. In different ways such factors also have an influence on health.

The home environment can produce adverse health effects because of certain chemical substances in building materials and of changes in building techniques. The occurrence of radon in houses (causing exposure to ionizing radiation of a certain type) is another example of a health hazard in the residential environment.

Health risks associated with traffic are well known. Although traffic accidents present the greatest human risk, other risks to health can be related to car exhausts and fuel.

Other factors in our physical environment that can influence health are air and water pollutants, and ionizing and other radiation. The working environment is particularly important. The proportion of employees with long periods of absence because of disease is, for example, considerably higher among manual and factory workers than among office employees. Redundancy generates ill-health, in particular of a psycho-social nature. Shift work is an example of another factor that can have a negative impact on health.

The factors outlined above can cause ill-health of different kinds, with the development of diseases in the circulatory system, respiratory organs and locomotive organs, as well as mental disturbances—and sometimes several adverse health effects simultaneously. As seen from previous chapters, several of the conditions mentioned seem to be related in different ways to the induction and development of malignant tumour diseases; a major part of the cancer in Sweden is probably due to living habits and to some extent to conditions in the work environment and other specific environments. The disease panorama, in general, also shows considerable geographic variation within the country, and this holds true for cancer diseases as well. In order to be able to successfully prevent ill-health in society, one should consider the conditions described here within the framework of an overall health policy. The cancer diseases are then just one part—albeit an important one—of the ill-health that should be prevented as far as possible.

The 1982 Swedish Health Care Act places the responsibility for promoting good health in the whole population on the County Councils. The conditions described above are of importance for this new task of the county councils.

Modern society is complex and measures within one sector of society may lead to unexpected consequences within another sector. At the national level the responsibility for different sectors is compartmentalized. Within the Swedish Government, there are several ministries with responsibility for areas that are of direct significance to the health of the population. This situation led the Cancer Committee to discuss the idea of setting up a special ministry for health and environmental questions, in some ways similar to the arrangements in a number of other European countries. However, it was not possible to obtain a clear enough picture of the likely balance of advantages and disadvantages inherent in such a move to allow any recommendation to be made. Therefore, the ministerial structure has been assumed to remain as at present.

However, information on health risks and co-ordination of measures to promote good health and to prevent health risks are matters of great importance at the national political level, and some improvements—within the system—are called for. The Cancer Committee therefore recommends that a special advisory group for information and co-ordination within the health sector should be set up, affiliated to the Government, preferably to the Ministry of Health and Social Affairs. It could, for example, be called the Advisory Health Council.

This Council would consist of representatives from the scientific community, the county councils, the municipalities, relevant governmental agencies and, of course, of representatives from the ministries mainly concerned. Its main role would be to give advice to the Ministry of Health and Social Affairs, which is responsible for public health, on matters relating to prevention of ill-health and promotion of good health.

Various major themes could be examined by the Council, for example, the effects on health (including cancer when relevant) of residential planning, of dietary habits, of the traffic environment and of redundancy. The Health Council might also discuss more specific issues such as household chemicals and health risks, or a particular group of chemical substances (human exposures in different environments, health effects). Analyses of certain reports, for example the publications from the Swedish Cancer Registry, may be presented to and discussed by the Council. The Government could use the Council as an instrument to continuously follow the general development within the cancer sphere, especially with regard to scientifically based possibilities for preventive work, and to otherwise follow up the intentions of the Cancer Committee presented in this Report.

At the operational level in Sweden, suspected health risks including those causing special public concern are handled by the responsible governmental agencies in co-operation with central laboratories. In Chapter 11 the Cancer Committee has proposed the reinforcement of co-operation between the central agencies so that such matters can be dealt with rapidly and effectively. In some cases it may be necessary also for the Government to be familiar with the cause of a specific alarm and therefore receive fairly comprehensive information. The Advisory Health Council could be an appropriate forum for presentation and discussion of such matters.

Further, it is essential that the distribution of resources and other matters of trade-off can be seen in a general health-policy perspective. This is equally true for establishing a balance between preventive measures and medical treatment. The Council could provide advice to the Government in this respect. The Council should be able to call on special experts to participate in its meetings when this is considered desirable. Experts representing different activities and branches of knowledge should likewise be able to aid in preparing different matters before meetings and to aid in the reporting of research results.

In contrast to permanent agencies, the Council as a body would not have any formal responsibilities or executive functions. The actual costs incurred directly by the Council should be minimal.

The Advisory Health Council ought to pay particular attention to health risks that may appear in a long-term perspective through human activities today. This applies especially to assessment of possible health risks to future generations through the influence of genotoxic substances or ionizing radiation on the genetic material of the parent generation, or through human activities in the physical environment which could later give rise to health risks (mainly by delayed exposure, for example through toxic waste).

The proposed Advisory Health Council, to advise and inform the Government and to propose and co-ordinate new action, is well in line with recommendations issued by the World Health Organization (WHO) in 1981, in the document 'Managerial process for national health development'. In this document, the WHO recommended the setting up of 'National Health Councils', adapted to the specific conditions in each country, in order to ensure that health matters are dealt with across borders of different kinds.

Appendix 1
Summary

The following text is from the original summary (in English—with some minor additional changes) of the Cancer Committee's recommendations in its report Cancer—orsaker, förebyggande m.m. (SOU 1984:67), chapters 1–6 giving the scientific background having been deleted.

Part II

In Part II of this report, which covers Chapters 7–16, systematic treatment is given to various prerequisites and measures for reducing the harmful effects of cancer diseases. This includes (*a*) ways and means of preventing cancer, with reference to the data and viewpoints given in Chapters 2–6 and (*b*) certain questions of diagnosis and therapy, as well as the organization of cancer care. Emphasis is put on certain areas of special importance for cancer research.

Chapter 7

Chapter 7 discusses a strategy of cancer prevention: it specifies the general prerequisites for stopping the induction of cancer, the main aims of the strategy and its components. Taking as basic the importance of a philosophy for the assessment of risks and the adoption of remedial measures, the chapter considers various principles for rank-ordering, especially of regulatory measures, including cost--benefit analysis in the broad sense of this term. In some of the subsequent chapters these assessments are elaborated, together with concrete proposals in certain areas. Here the Committee has defined the strategic principles as a number of points in contexts where discussion of this kind fit in naturally.

The Cancer Committee makes the following observations, among others:

Summary

(a) It should be possible to influence the causal factors in living habits and in the rest of the environment which contribute to the induction of cancer.
(b) Inasmuch as total prevention is impossible, preventive measures should seek to reduce the cancer risk; should cancer develop nevertheless, the aim should be to make it appear later in life than it would have done otherwise.
(c) The concept of risk is central in cancer prevention, as well as within areas where all chains of events are not foreseeable, and where the trauma (disease), seen biologically, is a random effect.
(d) The strategy should have two main aims:(i) the total incidence of cancer shall be brought down; (ii) 'unacceptable' individual risks shall be remedied; further, attention should be paid to the possibility that coming generations may be harmed.
(e) Cancer forms one part of the overall disease pattern; hence measures to prevent cancer must be seen in this larger picture.
(f) The cancer prevention strategy should encompass both known risks or risk areas and unknown or insufficiently known risks; it involves not only concrete measures that seek to prevent cancer directly or indirectly, but also continued accretions to the corpus of knowledge on the basis of researches and investigations.
(g) Follow-up studies of health effects and other consequences of taken measures are important, especially if the measures are farther reaching.
(h) Questions of cancer prevention affect many interested parties, and it must be assumed that public bodies with responsibility for preventive measures, as well as business firms, voluntary organizations, scientists and research-financing institutions will each devise their strategy to promote an effective system of cancer prevention.
(i) The following risk areas/causal factors concerning cancer should form components of the strategy even if the requisite measures may greatly differ in their nature and scope: consumption of tobacco and alcohol, eating habits including specific dietary factors, sexual habits, infections, general air pollution, factors in the work environment, consumer articles, ionizing radiation and ultraviolet radiation, and iatrogenic factors.
(j) The central authorities responsible for the statutory risk control of physical and chemical agents should formulate and document a risk policy relating to cancer.
(k) Medical/scientific assessments relating to identification and estimation of risks, with critical examination of available scientific data, should be segregable from the social and political assessments that lie in risk evaluation and decisions on direct control measures; it follows that risk evaluations cover such matters as risk acceptance and 'how much proof' is necessary to justify taking action in a

particular situation, as well as questions of technical and economic prerequisites for reduction of risk.
(l) A rank ordering of regulatory measures will depend on such things as how the value of cost and benefit is measured: a process in which monetary and non-monetary magnitudes (e.g. experience of risk and uneven distribution of risks and benefits in the population) are to be determined, after which they should be presented in a way that makes it easier for the decision-makers to see where the conflicts lie.
(m) With respect to comparable, controllable risks in the environment (primarily ionizing radiation and chemical substances with cancer-initiating properties), efforts should be made to devise identical principles of safety; the principles developed in the field of radiation protection would then be guiding.
(n) The assumption of a linear dose–response relation in the low-dose range should also underlie the regulation of chemical substances, unless available data clearly indicate the existence of a 'threshold dose' for effect.
(o) Carcinogenic causal factors greatly vary in strength (carcinogenic potency), which in combination with actual exposure indicates the magnitude of risk. However, there are often palpable difficulties of determining, with good scientific accuracy, the carcinogenic potency of chemical substances; including determination of whether or not a factor lacks importance from the risk aspect.
(p) At the same time as reduced exposure to chemical carcinogens should be aspired to as a general rule, allowance should be made for the feasibility of grading risks and of fixing threshold doses in certain instances for substances which do not bind to DNA.

Chapter 8

Discussed in Chapter 8 are information systems including early warning of cancer risks. Most of the discussion pertains to population-based information systems and the prerequisites for epidemiological studies.

In order to learn about the presence, causes and effects of a disease in a population, it is necessary to have information systems containing data both about the victims (e.g. incidence and mortality registers) and about other individuals in the population (e.g. demographic basic data).

The Committee briefly describes different epidemiological methods of working, after which it goes at greater length into information systems for the health and medical services, especially the Cancer Registry, an incidence register that was set up in 1958, and a Causes-of-Death Registry that has been giving specifics about different cancer diseases since 1951. These files contain individual-related data (via civic registration numbers), which greatly enhance the feasibility of undertaking epidemiological studies, e.g. on statistical correlations between a cancer disease and living conditions or other more specific environmental factors.

A more or less explicit monitoring function attaches to certain registers of the kind referred to in the present context. A separate subsection is devoted to a general discussion of epidemiologic monitoring, which may involve not only surveillance of known risks but also indications of previously unknown risks.

Some light is shed on matters of international co-operation, with particular reference to epidemiological cancer research.

The Cancer Committee makes the following observations:

(a) Because of its population-based information systems and other nation-specific conditions, Sweden is very well positioned to engage in studies of cancer diseases as well as of other, especially chronic diseases, and in that way undertake a commitment to do epidemiological work that adds to the international corpus of knowledge about different diseases and their causes. Towards that end every advantage should be taken of opportunities to work together with other countries, especially the Nordic countries. Particular emphasis should be put on the importance of population-based, secular research programmes in the form of prospective studies.
(b) It will be necessary to have the Swedish university system develop better opportunities for education in epidemiology, with emphasis on postgraduate studies.
(c) Requirements can be formulated saying that certain general population data should always be easily available for epidemiological research activities; the reference here is to official data that already enter into the present system of civil registration. Here it is desirable to improve accessibility to already ADP-recorded data on kinships (parents) and on earlier addresses.
(d) Essential data about patients undergoing treatment, therapy or examinations should be recorded in a comparable manner both on a day-to-day basis and in special research projects.
(e) It is assumed that epidemiological monitoring programmes, or subsystems of such programmes seen generally, will be further developed in the course of the next few years.

Over and above the foregoing, the Committee makes certain observations that especially stem from the cancer diseases:

(a) Systematic collection and analysis of data on incidence of cancer and causes of death should be seen as parts of a larger system for epidemiologic monitoring.

(b) High-quality, nation-wide data about cases of cancer that have occurred (the Cancer Registry) and about deaths related to cancer (in the Cause-of-Death Registry) are of fundamental importance for cancer epidemiology.

(c) The division of labour that has evolved in practice between the central Cancer Registry at the National Board of Health and Welfare and the regional registry of neoplasms at oncological centres has major advantages.

(d) Some performance demands defined by the Committee should be imposed on cancer registrations in order to minimize time lags and to promote analytical functions.

(e) The basis for registration of death causes should be improved and, among other things, the routines for returning reports on deaths and causes of death should be reviewed to permit separation into legal-administrative and medical processing, respectively.

(f) Responsibility for the medical part of cause-of-death registration should be transferred from the Central Bureau of Statistics to the National Board of Health and Welfare.

(g) Apart from the health variables that are followed in a general epidemiological monitoring process, efforts should also be made as part of this process to improve documentation on exposure to conceivable risk factors in the environment, including living habits; further, consideration should be given to the feasibility of setting up sample banks with specimens of human cells and tissues.

(h) Epidemiological studies of cancer incidence—having regard to such things as the long latency period for most cancer diseases—should be supplemented by monitoring of other clinical parameters that could be related to initial phases of the cancer- induction process. Active efforts should be made to pursue further research and development for this purpose.

(i) Responsibility for expansion of an epidemiological monitoring service rests primarily with the health authorities (County Councils), in partnership with other interested parties. Further, the pivotal force, at least for parts of activities such as cancer epidemiology, should lie at regional level with the assistance of oncological centres.

(j) It is the responsibility of the National Board of Health and Welfare to co-ordinate and plan epidemiological monitoring at national level, and the National Institute of Environmental Medicine should answer in all essential respects for the operative part of this activity.

(k) Good epidemiological monitoring will gradually require a substantial build up of resources, the costs of which will have to be borne both by county councils and the Government.

Chapter 9

The subject of Chapter 9 is health education of the kind which seeks to change living habits as one way of preventing diseases such as cancer, even if such education is seen here as part of a broader programme of prevention.

An account is given of some of the main health education ideas contained in the project called 'Health Services in the 1990s' (Hälso- ochsjukvård inför 90-talet, HS 90), which assigns health education a key role for the offensive thrust of the new health care policy. Since health education is an activity that depends in no small measure on broad collaboration, the chapter presents an account of (a) the formal division of responsibilities between public agencies with regard to health education and (b) the other major parties having an interest at the local and regional plane which can work together on health education in varying degrees. Since the county councils bear the overall responsibility for health education, a separate account is given of what the councils are currently doing in this field. County council health education is described as an activity in the process of evolving, with councillors pressing ahead by trial and error as regards goals, methods, target groups, etc. Against this background, the chapter then discusses a number of strategic issues, where factors which limit the information effect as well as factors which can apparently enhance the effect of health education are illuminated. Next, the Committee discusses certain ethical issues which must be highlighted in all public affairs information of the kind that seeks to influence attitudes, norms and living habits. The Committee also takes up the question of mass-media participation in the health information process.

The Cancer Committee observes that:

(a) Under the Health Care Act, the county councils bear the overall reponsibility for health education, an activity that chiefly forms a natural part of the duties of primary care.
(b) By decision of Parliament and Cabinet, the National Board of Health and Welfare is required to lend support and service to the authorities in charge of the medical services to enable them to develop their health education programmes. Such assistance will be especially important during the build-up phase.

The Cancer Committee makes the following points among others:

(a) Health education which seeks to change living habits is a central instrument of prevention where the total incidence of cancer is concerned.
(b) Health education whose goal is to prevent cancer should be regarded as an integral part of general health education.
(c) Since health education which seeks to change living habits can

never be seen as an isolated medical issue unrelated to social and cultural patterns and to other living conditions, integrated approaches at different levels of society and co-operation between different parties will be needed.
(d) The county councils should develop effective forms of collaboration between the different fields of their own activities, other professional carers, public agencies and various voluntary organizations.
(e) Educational authorities, county councils and other public agencies should consider the need to train people in the conduct of health education.
(f) The design, execution and evaluation of health education concerning cancer risks must be tackled on an interdisciplinary basis, and the National Board of Health and Welfare should take the initiative to mount a comprehensive discussion of these matters.
(g) Society, acting through its designate agencies, should be entitled to make greater use of public service announcements about health education via the broadcasting media (radio and television). Further, it will be desirable to have the mass media take greater part in dissemination of health information on the basis of their own programming.

Chapter 10

Under the heading, 'Special measures in certain risk areas', the Cancer Committee takes up five such areas for more detailed discussion in Chapter 10.

Section 10.1 is concerned with tobacco use and tobacco products. Proceeding from the summary and conclusions drawn in earlier chapters about the significance of tobacco use for cancer incidence and how the risks associated with exposure to tobacco smoke in the environment should be judged at the present time, the Cancer Committee considers the feasibility of cutting back sharply on tobacco use generally and smoking in particular. Today's formal possibilities for product control are also examined. Considered briefly is the question of how to follow up the effects of future measures. An added reminder made in the present context is this: we still lack data on specifically Swedish conditions of exposure to carcinogenic substances in the environment which are due to smoking tobacco.

The Cancer Committee makes the following points, among other:

(a) Tobacco smoking is the largest single, statistically significant cause of cancer in Sweden. Each year approximately one in every six cancer cases, or about 5500 cases in all, are induced by smoking. Moreover, smokers account for higher-than-average death rates from certain other diseases.

(b) The smoker runs risks so great that imports and sales of tobacco products in Sweden would not be allowed if medical considerations alone were to govern.
(c) Exposure to tobacco smoke in the environment, so-called passive smoking, entails a certain risk of cancer. Naturally, the individual risk will vary with exposure conditions and is probably low as a rule, but there is no precluding the possibility that such risk is substantial in extreme cases, as in premises where many persons smoke for long periods.
(d) In all circumstances a great many passively exposed persons will be involved, where certain groups in particular, such as children, stand little chance of avoiding exposure through actions of their own.
(e) A goal should be that no one shall be exposed to tobacco smoke in the environment against his or her will.

To gauge the effect of measures taken against smoking tobacco, the following points may be laid down:

(a) The development of lung-cancer incidence, in particular, correlates directly with the development of smoking habits; the lung cancer risk will increase especially if smoking has started early in life.
(b) The incidence of lung cancer among men in Sweden is high and still nearly four times the women's rate, which is certainly due to earlier differences of smoking habits.
(c) Smoking has gone up sharply among women, and lung cancer incidence is consequently on the rise and may be expected to continue increasing considerably unless the pattern of smoking habits is changed.
(d) The risk of developing lung cancer will drop off sharply even within a few years if one stops smoking; this will also hold for anyone who has been smoking heavily for a long time.

When it comes to taking concrete measures, the Cancer Committee submits the following viewpoints and proposals:

(a) Several investigating groups in recent years have pointed out the health hazards associated with smoking. But since the measures subsequently taken have proved to be inadequate, vigorous exertions must continue to be made and their special emphasis put on drastic curtailment of tobacco consumption.
(b) Towards that end, health education and other measures which can stimulate and help people stop smoking should be intensified.
(c) It will be especially important to take measures which discourage people from starting to smoke. Further, over and above existing activities, more resources will have to be deployed to sustain special efforts aimed at deterring children and young people from

starting to smoke in the first place; wherever possible, such new efforts should be co-ordinated in a special programme which should be accorded the status of a national cause.
(d) The price of tobacco products should be used to damp consumption, with the movement of prices in each case not to be slower than that of the consumer price index; all tobacco products should be subject to the same policy of taxation.
(e) Legislative possibilities for product control similar to those which apply to other biologically active chemical substances should be available for all tobacco products; such control should be financed by charges levied on manufacturers and importers.
(f) Trends in smoking habits should be continuously followed by the designated governmental agency; any health changes of the kind that can be related to tobacco consumption should be especially followed by means of epidemiological monitoring.

Section 10.2 is concerned with diet and eating habits. It observes that food and drink (in addition to the air we breathe) constitute the greatest 'potential for exposure' to environmental factors seen generally, yet at the same time intake of nutrients and fluids is essential to life.

In addition to questions of possible cancer risks from such chemical substances as pollutants for instance through micro-organisms or food additives, more and more research has come to focus on the importance of dietary composition (food components which contribute, to or perhaps counteract, the induction of cancer), in other words our eating habits. Here, the Cancer Committee takes up: the likely importance of individual dietary components (also touched upon are cancer risks associated with use of alcohol; the bounds of statutory risk control (see Chapter 11) and the responsibility of central governmental agencies for health education and other information addressed to the general public; the possibility of issuing dietary recommendations aimed at cancer prevention, and the means available to change people's eating habits. Conceivable effects of dietary changes are especially discussed.

Under this heading the Cancer Committee makes the following observations:

(a) Taken together, epidemiological experimental research findings convincingly show that diet matters a great deal for total cancer incidence; as yet, however, the detailed knowledge available is not such as to permit precise quantification.
(b) Intensified research into this field should also be started in Sweden.
(c) The cautious conclusions that can now be drawn about the significance of individual components for cancer and that can be translated into dietary recommendations, compare well with the advice already given by Swedish experts and with the nutritional recom-

mendations of the National Food Administration. It is assumed that these make due allowance not only for dietetic needs but also for the opportunity to let choice of diet promote health and combat known diet-related diseases (other than cancer).
(d) A lowering of fat intake stands out as most urgent at the present time. In that connection a probable favourable effect on the incidence of at least some cancer diseases can be added to other expected positive effects, not least as regards cardiovascular diseases.
(e) The long-term goal for society's measures should be to bring down the total fat intake in stages to an average of less than 30 per cent of the energy intake. Here a first sub-goal to aim at in the next decade could be a reduction to 35 per cent from the present nearly 40 per cent.
(f) As a rule, the planning of diets, adjusted for individual needs in accordance with the Swedish nutritional recommendations now in force, should move towards the lower value in the specified interval for total fat intake (25–35 per cent of the energy requirement): in particular, persons whose fat intake is extremely high should lower it.
(g) Other aspects of the diet are that it should be varied, which is in accordance with the present nutritional recommendations. In this context the importance of fruit and vegetables, as well as wholegrain cereal products, should be especially pointed out.
(h) Health education and other targeted information should be the primary method of promoting what science now considers the most nutritious diet possible in homes and institutional kitchens (school catering services, company canteens, etc.). However, attention should also be paid to questions such as product supply, pricing and the like.
(i) The effects of measures taken should be studied in order to illuminate how altered eating habits affect people's health, and in so doing determine such matters as the extent to which the incidence of different cancer diseases changes.

Section 10.3 deals with general air pollution. Many factors bear upon the quality of air in a locality, among them automotive exhausts, the heating of homes and houses, other generation of energy, industrial processes, incineration of waste, etc. In this section the Cancer Committee has chiefly dwelt on the dominant problem of urban settlements, namely road traffic (but where the pollutants as a rule cannot be distinguished from, say, residential heating).

The air inhaled in the urban environment contains a great many different pollutants, as a rule in very low concentrations. Here the Cancer Committee has made certain assessments of the extent of cancer risks. For the rest it has mainly taken up the proposals, put forth earlier by the Car Exhausts Committee, for measures to reduce exhaust emissions and ambient pollutant concentrations caused by road traffic.

The Cancer Committee makes the following observations, among others:

(a) According to reasonable assumptions, the number of cancer cases per annum which are due to general air pollution (in urban areas) should fall within the range of some 100–1000 cases.
(b) The Car Exhausts Committee has identified several known or feared negative health and environmental effects of automotive exhausts as a basis for its proposals to limit ambient pollutant concentrations.
(c) In principle, the committee has endorsed the proposals made by the Car Exhausts Committee (report No. 1983:27 in the *SOU* series, later made more stringent in a communication to the Government dated 7 December 1983, with reference to its concerted statement of reasons.
(d) Preventive measures against general air pollution, particularly from road traffic, should be taken where this is technically and economically feasible, also having special regard to involuntary exposure and to cancer risks.
(e) Among other things, requirements for an effective catalytic cleaning of exhaust from petrol-driven passenger cars should be introduced at the earliest opportunity, and unleaded petrol should be available and be used where this is technically possible.
(f) Continued research is desirable, especially into the mutagenic/carcinogenic effects of different exhaust gas components. Greater attention should be paid to the role of diesel operation for health hazards and to the development of diesel technology with a view to reducing emissions.

In Section 10.4 the Cancer Committee deals with the risks of cancer associated with decay products of the radioactive gas radon in houses. Radon, an element that occurs in nature, is capable of contaminating indoor air by way of unsuitable building materials and through leakage into houses from the ground. A cardinal question is to gauge the dimensions of the cancer risk. The Committee also endorses the measures proposed by the Radon Committee to reduce the potential for exposure to radon both in existing and future buildings.

The Cancer Committee makes the following points, among others:

(a) As a first reminder, the Swedish Institute of Radiation Protection (SSI) has estimated that present concentrations of radon daughters in Swedish dwelling units may in future cause about 1100 cases of

lung cancer per annum, with a factor of uncertainty that gives the interval about 300—3000 cases.
(b) The scientific basis for estimation of risk is as yet greatly defective.
(c) On the basis of its own deliberations, the Cancer Committee concludes that a figure in the region of the lower limit in SSI's risk interval looks most probable.
(d) The only way to ascertain the extent of this potentially grave health problem is to do a well-planned radon-epidemiological study which specifically relates to Swedish conditions.
(e) Such an investigation will presumably have to be very comprehensive and take anything from four to seven years to complete. Moreover, the research design of this project should be interdisciplinary and integrated, with formal ties to some appropriate public body such as the National Institute of Environmental Medicine.
(f) In all circumstances the proposals made by the Radon Committee in report No. 1983:6 in the *SOU* series should be implemented now as a minimum measure. Additionally, the feasibility should be explored of making it easier for homeowners who so wish to lower the concentration of radon daughters below the level proposed by the Committee.

In addition to discussing general air pollution with special reference to urban settlements (in Section 10.3), the Cancer Committee summarizes in Section 10.5 the question of air pollution in the indoor environment as a general phenomenon. Included are not only such things as tobacco smoke with its potential concomitant of passive smoking (see Section 10.1) and indoor radon (see Section 10.4), but also the presence of the same general air pollutants as in outdoor air. Substances from building materials or formed from micro-organisms or in the course of food preparation may affect the quality of indoor air.

Occupational exposures stemming from processes or product handling in the working environment are treated elsewhere in this report.

The Cancer Committee points out the following:

(a) Certain cancer risks that have been partly considered from other aspects in the foregoing can be associated with air pollution in the indoor environment.
(b) The incidence and concentration of different air pollutants indoors is due in part to technical solutions of problems posed by for example, building materials and ventilation. Hence concerted efforts in the form of a programme to deal with cancer risks in the indoor environment generally, and the residential environment in particular, should be made as an adjunct to research and control measures which focus on specific agents.
(c) The initiatives taken to date and the activities now going on with this aim in mind are deserving of continued support.

Given its overall responsibilities for health, the National Board of Health and Welfare should aspire to co-ordinate its efforts more in consultation with various bodies, among them the National Institute of Environmental Medicine and the Swedish Council for Building Research.

(d) It is desirable, not only from the scientific but also from the administrative viewpoint, to make concerted and integrated approaches to air pollution as a phenomenon; where appropriate, guidelines (hygienic threshold limits) for pollutants in the outdoor environment should allow for possible concentrations indoors.

(e) Threshold limit values for agents in public places and other communal premises and in the residential environment may in certain cases supplement other measures aimed at reducing health hazards.

Chapter 11

The subject of Chapter 11 is the statutory control of risks. Various points of view and proposals are set forth by way of supplementing the strategy for cancer prevention described in Chapter 7.

The Cancer Committee has not aspired to analyse, in any greater depth, the legislation that is relevant in order to counteract cancer risks. Besides, some of the legislation is now being reviewed by other bodies, among them the Chemicals Commission, with a view to future revision. A brief presentation is made of the most important legislative areas, from which it appears that certain basic principles remain the same, even though the legislative products involved have different vesting dates and bear reference in parts to different risk conditions. More than one law or Act of Parliament may well become applicable to specific risk factors, all according to how prevalent they are.

The chapter discusses some issues which refer (a) to the basis for making risk estimates, especially with regard to chemical agents and (b) the evaluation of risks and measures of direct control. Certain conclusions are drawn from the foregoing as regards the organizational structure of governmental agencies and other bodies.

Various points are made by the Cancer Committee, among them:

(a) The medical/scientific analysis of cancer risks for humans associated with exposure to specific substances or with mixed exposures is usually a troublesome procedure. It assumes a capability for making sophisticated scientific assessments of all available data on the properties of chemical agents and their effects.

(b) Identical or similar scientific data should be assessed in the same way by different governmental agencies in the Swedish system of risk control. Among other things, there should be common criteria

on which to base evaluation of substances which should be considered carcinogens within the meaning of the law.
(c) The basis for assigning orders of priority to risk estimates should focus on exposure analysis of already known agents, or agents that are suspected on good grounds of being carcinogenic (including products, handling methods, processes, emissions, etc.), rather than on large-scale measures to bring forth new data on the properties and effects of other agents.
(d) In addition, priorities should be ordered for certain resources to permit risks to be identified in situations where exposure is presumably high in individual cases and/or where a great many persons are being exposed.
(e) Regulating agencies' overview of exposures to chemical agents is partly insufficient. Seen generally, information about and access to exposure data should be improved.
(f) The question of resources for the testing of cancer risks is closely associated with the general build-up of toxicological competence and toxicological research and development facilities in Sweden.
(g) Decisions on risk control taken by a governmental agency should, to a greater extent than is now the case, be documented in a readily accessible manner, with summaries of risk estimates, cost–benefit analyses and other data of material importance for the decisions.
(h) The results of measures taken should be clarified by means of special efforts in connection with inspection, supervision and the like. Over and above the foregoing, continuing adequate surveillance to ensure compliance with regulations is of great importance—and so it is, too, for the trust that the individual puts in society's control apparatus.
(i) International co-operation aimed at facilitating statutory risk control is vital, both as regards the work of research and investigation, including the performance of tests, the formulation of policy and, where applicable, the taking of administrative measures.
(j) There should be more domestic collaboration among authorities, especially the regulatory agencies. Such co-operation should be institutionalized in particular for the medical/scientific analysis of risks. For this purpose it will have to be assumed that extramural scientific experts are brought into committees, joint working parties or similar bodies on an *ad hoc* basis or for longer periods.

Chapter 12

In Chapter 12 the Cancer Committee dwells on the role that information plays for interaction and mutual trust in the process of risk control. The candour and confidentiality of information are discussed, as are the possibilities for hearings and the like. The chapter dicusses the output of scientific information, its transmission and quality, and notes tendencies to belittle the importance of research.

In the opinion of the Cancer Committee:

(a) The trust that not least the general public puts in the statutory process of risk control will very much depend on its access to information.
(b) For this reason and in the interests of free research, there must be laid down the principle of unimpeded access to scientific and other information on file with a governmental agency which deals with the assessment of health hazards, if any. Although no direct change in existing secrecy legislation is proposed, efforts should be made to promote an international accord, which lets such information be communicated more openly.
(c) The vast output of data on risks, risk factors and ways and means of combatting risks is to be found in the international scientific literature. More often than not, however, the transmission of information, especially to laymen, is bound up with difficulties.
(d) Apart from the information services that certain scientific libraries render in response to inquiries, governmental agencies in risk control, and not least the mass media, play an important role in the active dissemination of information.
(e) The quality of information merits particular consideration. Towards that end great emphasis must be put on the mass-media employment of journalists who have a thorough grounding in the natural sciences, which means that improved facilities should be offered for their education and training.

Chapter 13

The subject of Chapter 13 is health examinations (screening programmes) which try to detect cancer or pre-cancerous lesions. Considered against the background of various criteria and requirements to permit making judgement of which diseases lend themselves to diagnosis by means of mass health examinations, the Committee elects to discuss four diseases in greater detail: cancers of the cervix, breast, intestine and lungs. The Committee considers each of these diseases separately, and also illuminates the information that is available to pass judgement on the preconditions for 'invitational' health check-ups and their value.

In this connection the Cancer Committee takes up the complex of problems bound up with diagnoses based on mass health examinations, as exemplified by questions such as the following: How many persons must be treated and unnecessarily worried because of the health check-up? Will it follow from the health check-up that treatment can be mitigated for many patients? Can mortality from this particular form of cancer be reduced? Are the costs reasonably proportionate to the benefits?

The Committee also deals with the psychosocial aspects of mass health examinations.

With respect to mass health examinations for cancer, the Committee observes:

(a) The complex of problems bound up with mass health examinations are complicated, partly because the spontaneous course of pre-cancerous lesions or cases of very early cancer that are often detected is incompletely known.
(b) Since retrospective evaluation of a health check-up's effects often entails considerable difficulties and uncertainty, a well-controlled pilot scheme is usually preferable.
(c) Society is reponsible for evaluation of a health check-up method on the basis of an adequate pilot scheme, before the method is accepted for a general, invitational health check-up.
(d) At present only three forms of mass health examinations for cancer are being considered in Sweden: a gynaecological health check-up (cervical cancer), a mammographic health check-up (breast cancer) and a health check-up which seeks to detect blood in the stool (intestinal cancer).
(e) Improved diagnosis of symptomatic cancer is now probably of greater importance for reducing the effects of cancer diseases compared with invitational health examinations.

The Cancer Committee proposes the following:

(a) Invitational gynaecological health check-ups under the auspices of the medical service authorities are to continue and extend from their present scope (covering the age group 30–49 years to include the age group 30–59 years with specimens to be taken every 4 years as at present.
(b) Data management programmes are to be introduced, by region or county, for the registration of all vaginal smear tests with the aim of better co-ordinating the organized invitational health check-up with other gynaecological health check-ups.
(c) A more accurate information base is to be produced to permit the passing of judgement on various matters, for instance determining the adequate extent of, and suitable examination interval for, the invitational gynaecological health check-up through (i) in-depth analysis of the statistical on gynaecological health check-ups that has been gathered in conjunction with the National Board of Health and Welfare Cancer Registry and by some county councils

and (ii) study of the medical activity that has been generated by health check-ups.
(d) Trials with invitational, mammographic health check-ups in the Malmö municipality and by the county councils in the counties of Kopparberg and Östergötland should be continuously evaluated in statistical–medical terms. As soon as a sufficient information base is in hand, a position is to be taken towards general, invitational health check-ups.
(e) Mammography for the sole purpose of health screening is to be avoided for women under the age of 40 yeaars.
(f) Both an ongoing study in the Gothenburg municipality and similar studies abroad concerning early diagnosis of intestinal neoplasm. through demonstrating the presence of blood in the stool (Hemoccult test), should be carefully followed and possibly be made to underpin an expanded pilot scheme of controlled trials with invitational health check-ups.
(g) The psychosocial aspects of mass health examinations for cancer are to be studied to a greater extent then in the past.
(h) Proposed studies and evaluations are to be co-ordinated by the National Board of Health and Welfare.

Chapter 14

The organization of cancer care in Sweden is the subject of Chapter 14. Here the exposition proceeds from a summary of the 1974 guidelines put out by the National Board of Health and Welfare (NBHW), concerned with the planning of clinical oncology, wherein are stated the principles governing the allocation of resources and competencies as between different levels of health care. Against this background the Committee then describes the development of oncological care in Sweden after 1974. Here are illuminated various matters concerning the trade-off to be struck between the need to centralize resources and the need of patients for nearness to home. This exposition leads over to a section which deals with the development of cancer care at the regional level, where oncological centres are strategically placed to co-ordinate the resources of the health-care region, and to another section concerned with cancer care at county level. Here the text goes at length into how the need for oncological competence among physicians is going to be met within the county care framework. With the same aim in mind, which is to raise the quality of cancer care, the Committee discusses various ways of bringing about improved training of nurses and improved psychological care.

In the opinion of the Cancer Committee:

(a) The build-up of regional oncological centres should be pursued in

line with proposals contained in the NBHW Guidelines: Planning of Clinical Oncology (32/1974).
(b) The practical and necessary development of cancer care, having regard to the growing demands that are put on such care, are to be borne in mind in connection with the current restructuring of the health and medical services.
(c) If the intentions spelled out in the NBHW guidelines are to be realized, the regional oncological clinics must have adequate capacity.
(d) Patients should also be assured of access to oncological competence within the county care framework on the strength of measures to be taken by the individual county councils, and the need for such expertise should be borne in mind for planning the further education and in-service training of physicians.
(e) The resources available to radiation therapy, which require sophisticated technical equipment, specially trained personnel and a sizeable population of patients for their efficient utilization, should be concentrated on the oncological regional clinics and not be further expanded within the county care framework.
(f) The training of nurses in cancer care is vital matter into which UHÄ (the Office of the Chancellor of Swedish Universities and Colleges) should inquire more closely, and in so doing should consider the potentials for improvement identified by the Cancer Committee.
(g) The psychological care of cancer patients should be improved, first and foremost through the establishment of special posts for physicians and psychologists at oncological centres, not least for purposes such as personnel guidance.
(h) The information service provided by oncological centres should be made to include the transmission of information to the general public.
(i) The authorities in charge of the medical services should aspire to more effective collaboration between the oncological centres of different health care regions, especially so that resources can be jointly utilized for the functions of diagnosis, care therapy and training.

Chapter 15

Research into cancer and measures to prevent cancer are taken up in Chapter 15, and one is reminded that the Cancer Committee has directly or indirectly dealt with research matters in all the previous chapters in those contexts where they naturally belong.

The total funds that go towards cancer research in Sweden are great compared with the funding of other research in this country. In 1983 awards of project grants to pay for cancer research amounted to about

90 million Sw.kr, of which the Swedish Cancer Society accounted for just over one-third.

The Committee identifies a number of research issues and areas where Swedish contribution would appear to be highly motivated: for instance, in basic biomedical research, research into clinical oncology, major epidemiological and experimental studies of living habits and other environmental factors of importance for the induction of cancer, technical problem formulations aimed at the implementation of measures to prevent cancer, etc. The chapter goes on to discuss the overall organization of cancer research, and takes up such matters as quality and efficiency, contacts between research-financing bodies and co-operation on major programmes, as well as the overall need for resources. The foregoing does not include activities or projects of the kind which should be financed through the health authorities or by way of the governmental budget (through responsible agencies) or where the Committee has previously recommended special financing channels.

The Cancer Committee makes the following points, among others:

(a) Research plays a crucial role in efforts to limit the harmful effects of cancer diseases.
(b) The cancer research conducted in Sweden, albeit a small country whose resources are accordingly limited, is of great importance and in some areas Swedish researchers might be regarded as international leaders.
(c) It primarily devolves upon the research community and the research-financing bodies to order their own priorities within the constraints set by available resources; no organizational changes are proposed.
(d) Stepped-up research efforts are desirable, especially in the areas of epidemiology, toxicology in relation to action mechanisms and genetics, and research into the problems associated with risks and remedial measures.
(e) It is up to the research councils and the sectorial research bodies themselves to assess the resources they require, having regard to the carrying-out of the intentions that the Cancer Committee has expressed.

Chapter 16

Chapter 16 lists some general priorities to order for activities intended to counteract the harmful effects of cancer diseases. After which the Cancer Committee does a conspectus review of its proposals to allow for certain cost aspects as well as cost carriers. The need for overview at the national level is discussed, partly to keep a very general hold on measures to promote health, partly to follow up new knowledge and the intentions of the Cancer Committee.

The Cancer Committee makes these observations, among others:

(a) Cancer diseases constitute an important part of the country's health problems. Effective and vigorous steps must continue to be taken to mitigate the harmful effects of cancer, which means putting particular emphasis on prevention, diagnosis, and the treatment and care of cancer patients.
(b) In principle, responsibility for the ordering of priorities at detailed level and for assessments of resources required and follow-ups of costs, in accordance with the proposals that the Committee has made above, should directly rest with the respective official bodies concerned, with particular consideration to be paid to that strategy for cancer prevention which the Committee has outlined.
(c) Moreover, the costs of implementing the Committee's proposals can seldom be seen as a matter that involves cancer alone.

With regard to the ordering of general priorities, the Cancer Committee submits the following:

(a) The general principle of increased commitments to preventive measures must be especially upheld.
(b) Substantial resources are still needed in the health care system for diagnosis, care and treatment of cancer patients, with high priority attaching not least to questions of early diagnosis.
(c) Tobacco smoking offers promise of the best results, based on the present state of scientific knowledge, from attempts to reduce the total cancer incidence; further, the great importance of diet justifies intensified research, as into the role of individual dietary components for cancer induction, and changes in the population's eating habits within the framework of present Swedish dietary recommendations.
(d) Today, the most important method of trying to bring down the future total cancer incidence seems to be through health education.
(e) In addition, societal control of physical and chemical agents is needed for various purposes, notably to help and protect the individual.
(f) The build-up of knowledge through research and development work must continue and be further developed.

Lastly, the Committee proposes that an advisory body to the Government should be set up in order to follow developments and to initiate proposals for, and to facilitate co-ordination of, nation-wide efforts to prevent ill health and to promote good health.

Editorial comments on later events

What has happened in Sweden since 1984 with a bearing on the recommendations made by the Cancer Committee?

First to be noted is that the Committee report, with few exceptions, was very well received by Swedish society, as shown in the traditional rround of comments from a great number of agencies and organisations. Howeer, it is often difficult to pinpoint measures taken thereafter as being results of this Committee report in particular; cancer prevention issues as such or as part of a more general health policy or risk management policy have been raised in several other contexts as well.

Secondly, no comprehensive analysis or follow-up has been made (as yet) of how the Committee's way of thinking has influenced priority setting, decision making and attitudes in Sweden.

Generally speaking, measures towards prevention of cancer diseases have been further developed and intensified during the latter half of the 1980s. Among other things it may be mentioned that:

(a) The Cancer Committee report formed part of the base for a Government bill on the future directions of health and medical care in Sweden, during the Parliamentary session 1984–5. The strategy implies more stress on health promotion and more health policy considerations in all sectors of societal planning.

(b) Under an existing high-level group for co-operation between the Government and the county councils regarding health and medical care in Sweden, chaired by the Prime Minister, a sub-group has been set up for 'public health' especially. This group is to give advice in health policy matters and to prepare for such matters to be taken up for discussion by the high-level group. The need to address public health issues in a practical and concrete way as well as to increase co-operation across administrative sector borders have governed the choice of members to the public health group. Special task forces under the public health group are now working on more detailed recommendations to reduce the risks of cancer (and or coronary diseases) and on improving epidemiological monitoring of health risks.

(c) Cancer-epidemiological research has been given increased support through new chairs for professors and better financial resources.

(d) Mass screening with mammography is gradually being introduced by the county councils in their respective areas. However, the analysis and evaluation work continues in special projects, simultaneously.

(e) During the 3-year period 1986–9 extra resources from the national budget were allocated to health education in order to prevent smoking debut.

In 1988 a special adviser was assigned by the Government to look into the existing public anti-tobacco policy with the view of reducing tobacco consumption, for example through a legally instituted right for people to a smoke-free environment, advertising bans and better use of the price instrument. In 1989 Parliament underlined that smoking is a major public health problem and that Parliamentary representatives ought to be asked to participate in the work being done by the governmental adviser.

A slow decrease or stagnation has been noted in smoking habits in Sweden and in 1988 and the snuff consumption went down for the first time since 1969.

(f) A group of experts affiliated to the National Board of Health and Welfare and the National Food Administration has produced (new) guidelines for health promotion work, with respect to diet and physical exercise. The goal is to reduce fat intake to 35 percent over a longer period. So far, a reduction in the total population from 40 to 38 percent has been observed during the last decade.

A special health project in the county of Stockholm, starting in 1987, may be mentioned as an example of regional activities. This project is unique in so far as it aims at better cancer prevention by turning to the *total* population in the area, in order to improve dietary habits in a number of specified ways. Another means is to make healthy food more easily available in shops and restaurants.

(g) The National Board of Health and Welfare together with the National Radiation Protection Institute has issued recemmendations on avoidance of excessive sunbathing, especially by children, in order to limit development of malignant melanoma.

(h) The rules concerning motor vehicle exhausts have tightened in several ways; for example, catalytic cleaning is required for petrol-operated cars from the 1989 models. Unleaded fuel is now widely available. Vapour recovery nozzles are being introduced at petrol stations according to local decisions.

(i) A recommendation by the responsible agency to reduce the limit value for radon daughters from 400 to 200 Bq m^{-3} in the existing residential environment has been given in to the Government for consideration.

A large epidemiological study of radon with respect to cancer risks has been started, the results of which are expected some time during 1991–2.

(j) A Toxicology Advisory Council has been set up as a common resource to governmental agencies working with statutory risk control. The aim is to increase the agency capability to make scientifically sound risk assessments and to harmonize assessment policies between agencies.

(k) Safety policies in radiation protection are gaining acceptance also within other risk areas in Sweden as officially expressed, by for example, the National Environmental Protection Board with regard to the release of chemicals and cancer risks.

Appendix 2
References

All references marked * are background documents that have been used as a source of information, but have not always been cited within the text. A full list of these documents can be found within Appendix 3.

Chapter 2

Bolander, A.-M. and Lindgren, G., 1981, Material to the Swedish Cancer Committee 1981 and later supplements with elaborations of data from the Swedish Cause-of-Death Registry and the Cancer Registry, *Committee Records 46/81*. In Swedish.

Bridbord, K., Decoufle, P,, Fraumeni, J.F., Hoel, D.G., Hoover, R.N., Rall, D.P., Saffiotti, U., Schneiderman, M.A. and Upton, A.C., 1978, *Estimates of the Fraction of Cancer in the United States Related to Occupational Factors*, 15 September, Bethesda: National Cancer Institute, National Institutes of Health.

Cairns, J., Lyon, J.L. and Skolnick, M. (Eds), 1980, Cancer incidence in defined populations, in *Banbury Report 4*, Cold Spring Harbor, NY: Cold Spring Harbor Laboratory. See also Lyon, J.L., Gardner, J.W. and West, D.W., Cancer risk and lifestyle: cancer among mormons from 1967–1975, pp. 3–28, and Phillips, R.L., Kuzma, J.W. and Lotz, T.M., Cancer mortality among comparable members versus non-members of the seventh-day adventist church, pp. 93–102.

Cancer Incidence in Sweden 1959–1980, Socialstyrelsen. [Swedish National Board of Health and Welfare].

International Union Against Cancer, 1970, *Cancer Incidence in Five Continents*, Vol. II.

Carlsson, G., Arvidsson, O., Bygren, L.O. and Werkö, L., 1979, Liv och hälsa [Life and health], *Allmänna Förlaget*. In Swedish.

Dödsorsaker 1959–1980 [Cause of Death 1959–1980], Statistiska centralbyrån (SCB) [Statistics Sweden]. In Swedish with table captions in English.

Doll, R. and Peto, R., 1981, The causes of cancer: quantitative estimates of avoidable risks of cancer in the United States today, *JNCI*, **66**, 1191–1308.

Epstein, S., 1979, *The Politics of Cancer*, San Francisco: Sierra Club Books.

Fraumeni, J.F. Jr et al., 1975, *Atlas of Cancer Mortality for US Counties 1950–1969*, Bethesda: National Institutes of Health, 1975.

Herzman, P. and Lindgren, B., 1980, Sjukdomarnas samhällsekonomiska kostnader 1964–75 [The costs of diseases from a socio-economic point of view 1964–75], *IHE-meddelande 2 [Institute of Health Economics, Communication 2]*, Lund.

Higginson, J. and Muir, C.S., 1979, Environmental carcinogenesis: misconceptions and limitations to cancer control, *JNCI* **63**, 1291–8.

Hofsten, E. and Lundström H., 1976, *Swedish Population History 1750–1970*, Section 8, Stockholm: Statistics Sweden.

Larsson, L-G., Sandström, A., Damber, L., 1982, *Cancer in the counties of Västernorrland, Västerboffen and Norrboffen, Sweden*, 1959–1978, University Hospital, Umeå.
Magnus, K., 1981, Cancerepidemiologi, in Romanus, R., Larsson, L.-G., Rosengren, B. and Rudenstam, C.M. (Eds) *Klinisk Onkologi*, pp. 12–26. In Swedish.
SPRI [Planning and Rationalization Institute for the Health and Social Services], 1981, Project 3102/December 1981. Håkansson, S., and Marké, L.-Å., *Kostnader för Cancervården i Sverige 1980* [*Costs of Cancer Care in Sweden 1980*]. In Swedish.
Weisburger, J.H., Cohen, L.A. and Wynder, E.L., 1977, on the etiology and metabolic epidemiology of the main human cancers, in Hiatt, H., Watson, J.D. and Winsten, J.A. (Eds) *Origins of Human Cancer, Cold Spring Harbor Conferences*, Vol. 4, pp. 567–602, Cold Spring Harbor, NY: Cold Spring Harbor Laboratory.
Wynder, E.L. and Gori, G.B., 1977, Contribution of the environment to cancer incidence: an epidemiologic exercise, *JNCI*, **58**, 825–32.

Chapter 3

Bridges, B.A., Clemmensen, J. and Sugimura, T., 1979, Cigarette smoking–does it carry a genetic risk? *Mutat. Res.*, **65**, 71–81.
*Ehrenberg, L., 1984b, Radiation risks and radiation protection: a generally useful model, *Swedish Departmental Series Ds S 1984:6*, Ministry of Health and Social Affairs. In Swedish.
Ehrenberg, L. and Osterman-Golkar, S., 1980, Alkylation of macromolecules for detecting mutagenic agents, *Teratogen. Carcinogr. Mutagen.*, **1**, 105–27.
Ehrenberg, L. and Osterman-Golkar, S., 1983, in Castellani, A. (Ed.) *The Use of Human Cells for the Evaluation of Risk from Physical and Chemical Agents, NATO ASI-Series A: Life Sciences*, Vol. 60, p. 295, New York: Plenum Press.
Ehrenberg, L., Moustacchi, E. and Osterman-Golkar, S., 1983, International commission for protection against environmental mutagens and carcinogens, Dosimetry of genotoxic agents and dose–response relationships of their effects, *Mutat. Res.*, **123**, 121–82.
Holm, L.-E., Eklund, G. and Lundell, G., 1980, Incidence of malignant thyroid tumours in humans after exposure to diagnostic doses of iodine-131. II. Estimation of thyroid gland size, thyroid radiation dose, and predicted versus observed number of malignant thyroid tumours, *JNCI*, **65**, 1221–4.
*Holmberg, B. and Ehrenberg, L., 1984, Origin of cancer: basic phenomena and theories, *Swedish Departmental Series Ds S 1984:5*, Ministry of Health and Social Affairs. In Swedish.
Klein, G., 1982, Epstein Barr virus, malaria and Burkitt's Lymphoma, *Scand. J. Infect. Dis. Suppl.*, **36**, 15–23.
Knudson, A.G., 1971, *Proc. Natl. Acad. Sci. USA*, **678**, 820.
Littlefield, N.A., Farmer, J.H., Gaylor, D.W. and Sheldon, W.G., 1979, Effects of dose and time in a long-term, low-dose carcinogenic study, in Staffa, J.A. and Mehlman, M.A. (Eds) *Innovations in Cancer Risk Assessment* (ED_{01} Study), Special issue *J. Env. Pathol. Toxicol.*, **3**(3), 17–34.
Murphree, A.L. and Benedict, W.F., 1984, *Science*, **223**, 1028.
*Nilsson, R. and Ehrenberg, L., 1984, Which conclusions can be drawn on cancer risks from epidemiologic and experimental data? *Swedish Departmental Series Ds S 1984:6*, Ministry of Health and Social Affairs.
OECD, 1981, *Guidelines for Testing of Chemicals*, Paris:OECD. Office of Technology Assessment (OTA), 1981, *Assessment of Technologies for Determining Cancer Risks from the Environment*. Washington, DC: GPO.
Osterman-Golkar, S. and Ehrenberg, L., 1983, Dosimetry of electrophilic compounds by means of hemoglobin alkylation, *Ann. Rev. Public Health*, **4**, 397–402.
*Säfwenberg, J.-O., 1980 Notes on promoters, cocarcinogens and inhibitors (used by the Cancer Committee as a basis for an inventory of exposure data). (Unpublished.)
Staffa, J.A. and Mehlman, M.A. (Eds), 1979, *Innovations in Cancer Risk Assessment (ED_{01} Study)*, special issue *J. Env. Pathol. Toxicol.*, **3**(3).
*Tornqvist, M., 1984. Genotoxicity of NO_x in air pollution and of its reaction products

including nitrite, *Swedish Departmental Series Ds S 1984:5*, Ministry of Health and Social Affairs. In Swedish.
UNSCEAR, 1977, *United Nation's Scientific Committee on the Effects of Atomic Radiation, Sources and Effects of Ionizing Radiation,* New York: United Nations.
* von Bahr, B., Ehrenberg, L., Scalia-Tomba, G.-P. and Säfwenberg, J.-O., 1984b, Study of different models for dose-response relationships, *Swedish Departmental Series Ds S 1984:5.*
Weisburger, J.H. and Williams, G.M., 1982, Metabolism of chemical carcinogens, in Becker, F.F. (Ed.), *Cancer,* New York: Plenum Press, pp. 241–333.

Section 4.2

BEIR (Committee on the Biological Effects of Ionizing Radiations), 1980, *The Effects on Populations of Exposure to Low Levels of Ionizing Radiation,* Washington, DC: National Academy of Sciences.
Bergman, H. and Axelson, O., 1983, Passive smoking and indoor radon daughter concentration. *Lancet,* **ii**, 1308. See also Bergman, H. et al., 1984, *Third International Conference on Indoor Air Quality and Climate,* Stockholm, Vol. 2, p. 79.
Best, E.W., Walker, C.B., Baker, P.M. et al., 1967, Summary of a Canadian study of smoking and health, *Can. Med. Assoc. J.*, **96**, 1104–8.
Brunnemann, K.D. and Hoffmann, D., 1978, in *Environmental Aspects of N-Nitroso Compounds, IARC Sci. Publ. 19,* p.343.
Buckley, J.D., Doll, R., Harris, R.W., Vessey, M.P. and Williams, P.T., 1981, Case–control study of the husbands of women with dysplasia or carcinoma of the cervix uteri, *Lancet,* **ii**, 1010–15.
Cameron, P., Kostin, J.S., Zaks, J.M. et al., 1969, The health of smokers' and nonsmokers' children, *J. Allergy,* **43**, 336–41.
Cederlöf R, Friberg, L., Hrubec, Z. and Lorich, U., 1975, *The Relationship of Smoking and Some Social Covariables to Mortality and Cancer Morbidity,* Parts 1 and 2, Stockholm: The Department of Environmental Hygiene, Karolinska Institute.
Chan, W.C. and Fung, S.C., 1982, *Cancer campaign*, in Grundmann, E. (Ed.) *Cancer Epidemiology*, Vol. 6, p.199, Stuttgart: Gustav Fischer.
Colley, J.R., 1974, Respiratory symptoms in children and parental smoking and phlegm production, *Br. Med. J.*, **2**, 201–4.
Correa, P., Pickle, L.W., Fontham, E., Lin, Y. and Haenszel, W., 1983, Passive smoking and lung cancer, *Lancet,* **ii**, 595–7.
Damber, L. and Larsson, L.-G., 1983, University Hospital, Umeå, Personal communication.
Doll, R., 1978, Atmospheric pollution and lung cancer, *Environ. Health Perspect.*, **22**, 23-31.
Doll, R. and Hill, A.B., 1964, Mortality in relation to smoking: ten years' observations of British doctors, *Br. Med. J.* **1**, 1460–67.
Doll, R. and Peto, R., 1976, Mortality in relation to smoking: 20 years' observations on male British doctors, *Br. Med. J.*, **2**, 1525–36.
Doll, R. and Peto, R., 1981, The causes of cancer: quantitative estimates of avoidable risks of cancer in the United States today, *JNCI,* **66**, 1191–1308.
Druckrey, H., Preussmann, R., Ivankovic, '. and Schmähl, D., 1967, Organotrope carcinogene Wirkungen bei 65 versch, denen *N*-Nitroso-Verbindungen an BD-Ratten, *Z. Krebsforsch.*, **69**, 103–201.
*Ehrenberg, L., 1984a, An attempt to estimate cancer risks due to passive smoking, *Swedish Departmental Series Ds 1984:5,* Ministry of Health and Social Affairs. In Swedish.
Emanuel, W.,1931, Uber das Vorkommen von Nicotin in der Frauenmilch nach Zigarettengenuss, *Z. Kinderheilkunde,* **52**, 41–6.
Engholm, G., Englund, A., Hallin, N. and von Schmalensee, G., 1982, *Rapport över Undersökningar Rörande Eventeull Förekomst av Biologiska Effekter inom Andningsorganen av Exposition för Glasfiber/Mineralull (MMMF) inom Byggnadsindustrin i Sverige [Report on Studies Concerning Possible Biological Effects in the Respiratory Tract from Exposure to Glass Fibre/Mineral Wool (MMMF) in the*

Building Trade in Sweden], Bygghälsan och Arbetarskyddsfonden [The Construction Industry Foundation for Industrial Safety and Health and the Swedish Work Environment Fund], 78/130. In Swedish.

Everson, R.B., 1980, Individuals transplacentally exposed to maternal smoking may be at increased cancer risk in adult life, *Lancet*, **ii**, 123–7.

Fagerström, K.-O., 1981, Tobacco smoking, nicotine dependence and smoking cessation (Doctorial thesis), *Acta Universita Upsaliensis*.

Garfinkel, L., 1980, Cancer mortality in nonsmokers: prospective study by the American Cancer Society, *JNCI* **65**, 1169–73.

Garfinkel, L., 1981, Time trends in lung cancer mortality among nonsmokers and a note on passive smoking, *JNC1*, **66**, 1061–6.

Greenberg, L.A., Lester, D. and Haggard, H.W., 1952, Absorption of nicotine in tobacco smoking, *J. Pharmacol. Exp. Therap.*, **104**, 162–7.

Haenszel, W. and Taeuber, K.E., 1964, Lung-cancer mortality as related to residence and smoking histories. II. White females, *JNCI*, **32**, 803–38.

Haenszel, W., Loveland, D.B. and Sirken, M.G., 1962, Lung-cancer mortality as related to residence and smoking histories. I. White males, *JNCI*, **28**, 947–1001.

Hammond, E.C., 1966, *Natl Cancer Inst. Monogr.*, **19**, 127.

Hammond, E.C. and Horn, D., 1958, Smoking and death rates; report on forty-four months of follow-up of 187 783 men. In total mortality, *JAMA*, **166**(10), 1159–72.

Hammond, E.C. and Selikoff, I.J. 1981, Passive smoking and lung cancer with comments on two new papers, *Environ. Res.*, **24**, 444–52.

Hardee, G.E., Stewart, T. and Capomacchia, A.C., 1983, Tobacco smoke xenobiotic compound appearance in mothers' milk after involuntary smoke exposures. I. Nicotine and cotinine, *Toxicol. Lett.*, **15**, 109–12.

Harlap, S. and Davies, A.M., 1974, Infant admissions to hospital and maternal smoking, *Lancet*, **i**, 529–32.

Hemminki, K., Saloniemi, I., Salonen, T., Partanen, T. and Vainio, H., 1981, Childhood cancer and parental occupation in Finland, *J. Epidemiol. Community Health*, **35**, 11–15.

Higgins, I.T.T., 1976, Epidemiological evidence on the carcinogenic risk of air pollution, in *Environmental Pollution and Carcinogenic Risks*, IARC Sci. Publ. 13.

Hiller, F.C., *et al.*, 1982, *Am. Rev. Respir. Dis.*, **125**, 406.

Hinds, M.W. and Kolonel, L.N., 1980, Maternal smoking and cancer risk to off-spring, *Lancet*, **ii**, 703.

Hirayama, T., 1975, Cancer epidemiology in Japan (meeting abstract), *J. Jpn. Soc. Cancer Ther.*, **12**, 2.

Hirayama, T., 1981a, Non-smoking wives of heavy smokers have a higher risk of lung cancer: a study from Japan, *Br. Med. J.*, **282**, 183–5.

Hirayama, T., 1981b, *Br. Med. J.*, **283**, 916.

Hirayama, T., 1983, Passive smoking and lung cancer: consistency of association, *Lancet*, **ii**, 1425.

Holma, B., Kjaer, G. and Stokholm, J., 1979, Air pollution, hygiene and health of Danish schoolchildren, *Sci. Total Environ.*, **12**, 251–86.

*Holmberg, B. and Ehrenberg, L., 1984, Origin of cancer: basic phenomena and theories, *Swedish Departmental Series Ds S 1984:5*, Ministry of Health and Social Affairs. In Swedish.

Hrubec, Z., 1983, Statens Miljömedicinska Laboratorium [Swedish National Institute of Environmental Medicine], Personal communication.

Kahn, H.A., 1966, The Dorn study of smoking and mortality among U.S. veterans: report on eight and one-half years of observation, *Natl Cancer Inst. Monogr.*, **19**, 1–125.

Knoth, A. Bohn, H. and Smidt, F., 1983, Passivrauchen als Lungenkrebsursache bei Nichtraucherinnen, *Med. Klin.*, **78**, 66.

Larsson, L.-G., Sandstrom, A. and Damber, L., 1982, *Cancer in the Counties of Vasternorrland, Vasterbotten and Norrbotton, Sweden, 1959–1978*, Umeå: University Hospital, Centre of Oncology.

Löfroth, G., Nilsson, I. and Alfheim, I., 1983, in Walters, M.D. (Ed.) *Short Term Bioassays in the Analysis of Complex Environmental Mixtures III*, New York: Plenum Press.

Lund, E. and Zeiner-Henriksen, T., 1981, Smoking as risk factor for different forms of cancer among 26,000 men and women in Norway. Matching of the group of smokers with the cancer registry over a 12-year period, *Tidsskr. Nor. Laegeforen*, **101**, 1937–40.

Miller, G.H., 1978, *J. Breathing*, **41**, 5. See also Miller, G.H., 1981, Non-smoking wives of heavy smokers have higher risk of lung cancer, *Br. Med. J.*, **282**, 985.

Miller, G.H., 1983, Personal communication.

Mörck, H.J., Linde, J. Agner, E., Heim, H.O., Gyntelberg, F. and Neilson, P.E., 1982, Tobaksforbrug og rygevaner i Norden 1920–1980, [Tobacco consumption and smoking habits in the Scandinavian countries 1920–1980], *Nordisk Medicin* **97**, 134–46.

NBHW, 1980 *Cancer Incidence in Sweden*.

Nicolov, I.G. and Chernozemsky, I.N. 1979, Tumours and hyperplastic lesions in Syrian hamsters following transplacental and neonatal treatment with cigarette smoke condensate, *J. Cancer Res. Clin. Oncol.*, **94**, 249–56.

NTG, 1975, Nordiska tobaksarbetsgruppens betänkande [Report by a Nordic Tobacco Working Group]. In Swedish.

NTS, 1982, *Tobaken och Vi [Tobacco and Us]*. In Swedish.

Österdahl, B.-G. and Slorach, S., 1983, Volatile *N*-nitrosamines in snuff and chewing tobacco on the Swedish market, *Food Chem. Toxicol.*, **21**, 759–62.

Pelkonen, O., Kärki, N.T., Koivisto, M., Tuimala, R. and Kauppila, A., 1979, Maternal cigarette smoking, placental aryl hydrocarbon hydroxylase and neonatal size, *Toxicol. Lett.*, **3**, 331–5.

Perlman, H.H., Dannenberg, A.M. and Sokoloff, N., 1942, The excretion of nicotine in breast milk and urine from cigarette smoking, *J. Am. Med. Assoc.*, **120**, 1003–9.

Petrakis, N.L., Dupuy, M.E., Lee, R.E., Lyon, M., Maack, C.A., Gruenke, L.D. and Craig, J.C., 1982, in Bridges *et al.* (Eds) *Banbury Report 13*, p. 67, Cold Spring Harbor, NY: Cold Spring Harbor Laboratory.

Pike, M.C. and Henderson., B.E., 1981, in Gelboin, H.V. and Tsó, P.O.P. (Eds) *Polycyclic Hydrocarbons and Cancer*, Vol. 3, p. 317, New York: Academic Press.

Pirani, B.B., 1978, Smoking during pregnancy, *Obstet. Gynecol. Survey*, **33**, 1–13.

Preston-Martin, S., Yu M. C., Benton, B. and Henderson, B.E., 1982, *N*-nitroso compounds and childhood brain tumors: a case-control study, *Cancer Res.*, 42, 5240–5.

Reif, A.E., 1981, Effect of cigarette smoking on susceptibility to lung cancer, *Oncology*, **38**, 76–85.

Repace, J.L. and Lowrey, A.H., 1980, Indoor air pollution, tobacco smoke, and public health, *Science*, **208**, 464–72.

Rogot, E. and Murray, J.L., 1980, Smoking and causes of death among U.S. veterans: 16 years of observation, *Public Health Report 95*, pp. 213–22.

Rylander, R., Peterson, Y. and Snella, M.-C., 1984, ETS - environmental tobacco smoke, *Euro. J. Resp. Dis.*, 65, (133).

SCB (Statistics Sweden), 1965, *Rökvanor i Sverige, en Postenkätundersökning Våren 1963 [Smoking Habits in Sweden, A Mail Survey–Spring 1963]*, Stockholm: SCB. In Swedish but with table captions in English.

SCB (Statistics Sweden), 1977, Levnadsförhållanden. Social rapport om ojämlikheten i Sverige [Living conditions. Social report on the 'inequality' in Sweden], *Report 22*, p. 117–23. In Swedish.

Schmeltz, J. *et al.*, 1975, *Prev. Med.*, **4**, 66.

Smoking or Health., 1977, Third Report from the Royal College of Physicians of London, London: Pitman Medical.

Stepney, R., 1980, *Br. J. Addict.*, **75**, 81–8.

Svenska Tobaks AB [Swedish Tobacco Ltd], 1980, 1983, Brochures, annual reports, personal communications.

Tager, I.B., Weiss, S.T., Rosner, B. and Speizer, F.E., 1979, Effect of parental cigarette smoking on the pulmonary function of children, *Am. J. Epidemiol.*, **110**, 15–26.

TC (Swedish Tobacco Committee), 1981, Report on reduced tobacco use, *Swedish Official National Investigation Series 18*. In Swedish.

*Törnqvist, M., 1984, Genotoxicity of NO_x in air pollution and of its reaction products including nitrite, *Swedish Departmental Series Ds S 1984:5*, Ministry of Health and Social Affairs. In Swedish.

Trichopoulos, D., Kalandidi, A. and Sparros, L., 1983, Lung cancer and passive smoking: conclusion of Greek study, *Lancet*, **ii**, 677–8. See also answer to criticism by Trichopoulos, D., 1984, *Lancet*, **i**, 684.
Trichopoulos, D., Kalandidi, A., Sparros, L. and MacMohon, B., 1981, Lung cancer and passive smoking, *Int. J. Cancer*, **27**, 1–4.
UICC (Union Internationale Centre le Cancer), 1976, *Lung Cancer, Technical Report Series*, Vol. 25, Geneva: UICC.
UNSCEAR (United Nations Scientific Committee on the Effects of Atomic Radiation), 1972, *Effects*, Report to the General Assembly, with annexes, Vol. 2, New York: United Nations.
UNSCEAR (United Nations Scientific Committee on the Effects of Atomic Radiation), 1977, *Sources and Effects of Ionizing Radiation*, New York: United Nations.
US Department of Health, Education and Welfare, Public Health Service, 1964, *Smoking and Health*, Report of the Advisory Committee to the Surgeon General of the Public Health Service, *Public Health Service Publication 1103*.
US Surgeon General, 1979, *Smoking and Health*, US Department of Health, Education and Welfare.
US Surgeon General, 1980, *The Health Consequences of Smoking for Women*, US Department of Health and Human Services.
US Surgeon General, 1981, *The Health Consequences of Smoking: The Changing Cigarette*, US Department of Health and Human Services.
US Surgeon General, 1982, *The Health Consequences of Smoking Cancer*, US Department of Health and Human Services.
Vaught, J.B., Gurtoo, H.L., Parker, N.B., LeBoeuf, R. and Doctor, G., 1979, Effects of smoking on benzo[a]pyrene metabolism by human placental microsomes. *Cancer Res.*, **39**, 3177–83
Vineis, P., Frea, B., Uberti, E., Ghisetti, V. and Terracini, B., 1983, Bladder cancer and cigarette smoking in males: a case-control study, *Tumori*, **69**, 17–22.
von Schmalensee, G., 1983, Personal communication.
Weber, A., Fischer, T. and Grandjean, E., 1979, Passive smoking in experimental and field conditions, *Environ Res.*, **20**, 205–16.

Section 4.3

Alcantara, E.N. and Speckmann, E.W., 1976, Diet, nutrition, and cancer, *Am. J. Clin. Nutr.*, **29**, 1035–47.
Alpert, M.E., Hutt M.S.R, Wogan G.N., and Davidson C.S., 1971, Association between aflatoxin content of food and hepatoma frequency in Uganda, *Cancer*, **28**, 253–60.
Armstrong, B.K., 1977, in Hiatt E.H.H., Watson, J.D. and Winsten, J.A. (Eds), *Origins of Human Cancer*, p. 557–65, Cold Spring Harbor, NY: Cold Spring Harbor Laboratory.
Armstrong, B.K. and Doll, R., 1975, Environmental factors and cancer incidence and mortality in different counties with special reference to dietary practices. *Int. J. Cancer*, **15**, 617.
Baumann, C.A. and Rush, H.P., 1939, *Am. J. Cancer*, **35**, 213.
Bjelke, R., 1978, Dietary factors and the epidemiology of cancer of the stomach and large bowel, *Aktuel Ernaehrungsmed Klin Prax*, Suppl. 2, 10–17.
Bull, R.J., Robinson, M., Meier, J.R. and Stober, J., 1982, Use of biological assay systems to assess the relative carcinogenic hazards of disinfection by-products, *Environ. Health Perspec.*, **46**, 215–27.
Buncher, C.R., Kuzama, R.J. and Forcade, C.M., 1977, Drinking water as an epidemiologic risk factor for cancer, *Origins of Human Cancer*, pp. 347–56, Cold Spring Harbor, NY: Cold Spring Harbor Laboratory).
Callen, D.F., Wolf, C.R. and Philpot, R.M., 1980, Cytochrome P-450 mediated genetic activity and cytoxicity of seven halogenated aliphatic hydrocarbons in Saccharomyces cervisiae, *Mutat. Res.*, **77**, 55–63.
Carroll, K.K., 1975, Experimental evidence of dietry factors and hormone-dependent cancers, *Cancer Res.*, **35**, 3374.

Carroll, K.K. 1977, in Winnick, M. (Ed.) *Nutrition and Cancer*, New York: John Wiley and Sons.
Carroll, K.K. and Khor, H.T., 1975, Dietary fat in relation to tumorigensis, *Progr. Biochem. Pharmacol.*, **10**, 308–53.
Chan P.-C. and Cohen, L.A., 1975, Dietary fat and growth promotion of rat mammary tumors, *Cancer Res.* **35**, 3384–6.
Clemens, T.L., Hill, R.N., Bullock, L.P., Johnson, W.D., SuHatos, L.G. and Vesell, E.S., 1979, Chloroform toxicity in the mouse: role of genetic factors and steroids, *Toxicol. Appl. Pharmacol.*, **48**, 117–30.
Cohen, S.M., Wittenberg, J.F. and Bryan, G.T., 1976, *Cancer Res.*, **36**, 2334.
Crump, K.S. and Guess, H.A., 1980, *Drinking Water and Cancer: Review of Recent Findings and Assessment of Risks*, Report prepared by Science Research Systems Inc. for the Council on Environmental Quality, USA.
Cummings, J., 1981a, Fibres. Symposium on 'dietary factors influencing the risk of cancer', Stockholm. *Vår Föda*, **33**, suppl. 1.
Cummings, J.H., 1981b, Proc. Nut. Soc., **40**, 7.
DeRouen, T.A. and Diem, J.E., 1977, Relationships between cancer mortality in Louisiana drinking-water source and other possible causative agents, in Hiatt, E.H.H., Watson, J.D., Armstrong, B.K. and Winsten, J.A. (Eds), *Origins of Human Cancer*, pp. 331–45, Cold Spring Harbor, NY: Cold Spring Harbor Laboratory.
Dich, J., Åkerstrand, K., Andersson, A., Lönberg, E., Josefsson, E. and Jansson, E., 1979, Konserveringsmedels förekomst och inverkan på mögel- och mykotoxinbildning i matbröd. [Presence of preservatives and their effects on growth of mould and formation of mycotoxins in bread], *Vår Föda*, **31**, 385–403. In Swedish.
Doll, R. and Peto, R., 1981, The causes of cancer: quantitative estimates of avoidable risks of cancer in the United States today, *JNCI*, **66**, 1191–1308.
Dungal, N.J., 1961, *Am. Med. Assoc.*, **178**, 789.
*Ehrenberg, L., 1984c, Early warning systems (for detection of risk factors in populations/individuals), *Swedish Departmental Series Ds S 1984:5*, Ministry of Health and Social Affairs. In Swedish.
Engst, R. and Fritz, W., 1977, Food–hygienic toxicological evaluation of the occurrence of cancerogenic hydrocarbons in smoked products, *Acta Alim. Pol. III*, **(XXVII)3**, 255–67.
Feron, V.J., Kruysse, A. and Woutersen, R.A., 1982, *Eur. J. Cancer Clin. Oncol.*, **18**, 13–31.
Gori, G.B., 1979, Dietary and nutritional implications in the multifactorial etiology of certain prevalent human cancers, *Cancer*, **43**, 2151–61.
Gottlieb, M.S. and Carr, J.K., 1982, Case–control cancer mortality study and chlorination of drinking water in Louisiana, *Environ. Health Perspect*, **46**, 169–77.
Gray, G.E., Pike, M.C. and Henderson, B.E., 1979, Breast-cancer incidence and mortality rates in different countries in relation to known risk factors and dietary practices, *Br. J. Cancer*, **39**, 1–7.
Guzikowski, G., 1980, *Asbestifibrer i Dricksvatten. Litteratursammanställning och Pilotundersökning av Svenska Dricksvatten. [Asbestos Fibres in Drinking-water. Literature Review and Pilot Study of Swedish Drinking-waters]*. In Swedish.
Haenszel, W., Kurihara, M., Locke, F.B., Shimuzu, K. and Segi, M., 1976. Stomach cancer in Japan, *J. Natl. Cancer Inst.*, **56**, 265–74.
Harvey, R.F., Pomara, E.W. and Heaton, K.W., 1973, *Lancet*, **1**, 1278.
Hogan, B., 1979, *Nature*, **277**, 261.
*Holmberg, B. and Ehrenberg, L., 1984, Origin of cancer: basic phenomena and theories, *Swedish Departmental Series Ds S 1984:5*, Ministry of Health and Social Affairs. In Swedish.
Hopkins, G.J. and Carroll, K.K., 1979, Dietary polyunsaturated fat versus saturated fat in relation to mammary carcinogenesis, *Lipids*, **14**, 155–158.
Jansson, B., 1983, Intracellular potassium and sodium ions and their relations to cancer, Paper presented at the International Symposium on the Health Effects and Interactions of Essential and Toxic Elements, Lund, 13–18 June. See also Jansson, B., 1981, in Malt, R.A. and Williamson, R.N.C. (Eds), *Colonic Carcinogenesis*, Proceedings of the 31st Falk Symposium, p. 109, Lancaster: M T P Press.

Joossens, J.V., Kesteloot, H. and Amery, A., 1979, Salt intake and mortality from stroke, *N. Engl. J. Med.*, **300**, 1396.

Josefsson, E. and Nygren, S., 1981, Volatile N-nitrosocompounds in foods in Sweden, *Vår Föda*, Suppl. 2/81.

Kanarek, M.S. and Young, T.B., 1982, Drinking water treatment and risk of cancer death in Wisconsin, *Environ. Health Perspect.*, **46**, 179–86.

Kritchevsky, D., 1977, *Federal Proceedings*, **36**, 1692.

Kuhnlein, U., Bergström, D. and Kuhnlein, H., 1981, Mutagens in feces from vegetarians and non-vegetarians, *Mutat. Res.* **85**, 1–12.

Lavik, P.S. and Baumann, C.A., 1943, Further studies on tumorpromoting action of fat, *Cancer Res.* **3**, 749–56.

Lijinsky, W. and Shubik, P., 1964, Benzo(a)pyrene and other polynuclear hydrocarbons in charcoal-broiled meat, *Science*, **145**, 53–5.

MacMahon, B., 1979, Dietry hypotheses concerning the etiology of human breast cancer, *Nutr. Cancer*, **1**, 38–41.

Matsukura, N., Kawacki, T., Morino, K., Ohgaki, H., Sugimura, T. and Takayama, S., 1981, *Science*, **218**, 346.

Miller, A.B., 1983, Nutrition and cancer–an overview, in Wynder, E.L., Leveille, G.A., Weisburger, J.H. and Livingston, G.E. (Eds) *Environmental Aspects of Cancer: The Role of Macro and Micro Components of Foods*, pp. 10–44, Westport, CT: Food and Nutrition Press

Mirvish, S.S., Wallcave, L., Eagen, M. and Shubik, P., 1972, Ascorbate–nitrite reaction: possible means of blocking the formation of carcinogenic N-nitroso compounds, *Science*, **177**, 65–8.

Modan, B., Barell, V., Lubin, F. and Modan, M., 1975, Dietary factors and cancer in Israel, *Cancer Res.* **35**, 3503–6.

Natarajan, A.T., 1980, Personal communication. See also Obe, G. *et al.*, 1980, *Mutat. Res.*, **73**, 377; Obe, G., Karzinogene und mutagene Wirkung von Alkohol, in Zang, K., (Ed.) *Genetik des Alkoholismus*, Stuttgart: Kohlhammer-Verlag.

National Cancer Institute, 1976. *Report on Carcinogenesis Bioassay of Chloroform*, US Department of Health, Education and Welfare.

NBHW, 1981, Nitrogen compounds in ground water. In the series Socialstyrelsen redovisar 1981:9. Stockholm. In Swedish.

NEPB, 1984, J. Nilsson, personal communication.

*Nilsson, R. and Ehrenberg, L., 1984, Which conclusions can be drawn on cancer risks from epidemiologic and experimental data?, *Swedish Departmental Series, Ds S 1984:6*, Ministry of Health and Social Affairs. In Swedish.

Norin, H., Gottling, L. and Linnman, L., 1981, Trihalometaner i svenska dricksvatten [Trihalomethanes in Swedish drinking-waters], *Swedish National Institute of Environmental Medicine Report 1/1981*. In Swedish.

Pereira, M.A., Lin, L.-H., Lin, C., Luppitt, H.M. and Herren, S.L., 1982, *Environ. Health Perspect.*, **46**, 151–62.

Peto, R., Doll, R., Buckley, J.D. and Sporn, M.B., 1981, Can dietary beta-carotene materially reduce human cancer rates? *Nature*, **290**, 201–8.

Rannug, U., 1980, Mutagenicity of effluents from chlorine bleachings in the pulp and paper industry, in Jolley *et al.* (Eds) *Water Chlorination: Environmental Impact and Health Effects*, Vol. 3, (Ann Arbor: Ann Arbor Science Publishers.

Reddy, B.S., Hedges, A.R., Laakso, K. and Wynder, E.L., 1978, *Cancer*, **42**, 2832.

Reitz, R.H., Fox, T.R. and Quast, J.F., 1982, *Environ. Health Perspect.* **46**: 163–8.

Rieger, R. and Michaelis, A., 1960, *Abh. Deut. Akad. Wiss.*, *Berlin KI Med.*, **1**, 54–5.

Rothman, K. and Keller, R.J., 1972, The effect of joint exposure to alcohol and tobacco on risk of cancer of the mouth and pharynx, *Chronic Dis.*, **25**, 711–16.

Schrauzer, G.N., 1976, Selenium and cancer: a review, *Bioinorg. Chem.*, **5**, 275–81.

Selikoff, I.J., Hammond, E.C.and Seidman, H., 1973, Cancer risk of insulation workers in the United States, in Bogovski, P., Gibson, J.C., Timbrell, V. and Wagoner, J.C. (Eds) *Biological Effects of Asbestos*, Lyons:IARC.

Shils, M.E., 1979, Diet and nutrition as modifying factors in tumor development, *Med. Clin. North Am.* **63**, 1027–41.

Simon, V.E. and Tardiff, R.G.I., 1978, Water chlorination, in Jolley, R.L. (Ed.) *Environmental Impact and Health Effect*, Vol. 2 (Belford: Ann Arbor).

Spingarn, N.E., Slocum, L.A. and Weisburger, J.H., 1980, Formation of mutagens in cooked foods. II. Foods with high starch content, *Cancer Lett.*, **9**, 7–12.
Sugimura, T. and Nagao, M., 1979, Mutagenic factors in cooked foods, *CRC Crit. Rev. Toxicol.*, **6**, 189–209.
Sugimura, T., Nagao, M., Kawachi, T., *et al.*, 1977, Mutagens–carcinogens in food, with special reference to highly mutagenic pyrolytic products in broiled foods, in Hiatt, H.H., Watson, J.D. and Winsten, J.A. (Eds) *Origins of Human Cancer*, Vol. 1, pp. 561–1577, Cold Spring Harbor: Cold Spring Harbor Laboratory.
Swedish Ministry of Agriculture, 1982, *Acidification Today and Tomorrow*, Stockholm: Environment '82 Committee.
Tannenbaum, A., 1942, The genesis and growth of tumors. III. Effects of a high fat diet, *Cancer Res.*, **2**, 468.
Thoms, Chr. and Joelsson, A., 1982, Nitrat i grundvattentäkter i Sverige [Nitrate in Swedish ground waters], *Memorandum Series 1598*, Swedish National Environmental Protection Board. - In Swedish.
*Törnqvist, M., 1984, Genotoxicity of No_x in air pollution and of its reaction products including nitrite, *Swedish Departmental Series Ds S 1984:5*, Ministry of Health and Social Affairs. In Swedish.
Tulinius, H., 1981, *Nutr. Cancer*, **2**(4), 200, see also (1979) *Nutr. Cancer*, **1**(2), 61.
Tuyns, A.J., 1978, Alcohol, *Health Res. World*, **2**, 20–31.
Tuyns, A.J., Péquignot, G. and Jensen, O.M., 1977, *Bull. Cancer (Paris)*, **64**, 45–60.
US National Research Council, 1982, Committee on diet, nutrition and cancer, Assembly of Life Sciences, Washington: National Academy Press.
Victorin, K., 1980, Trihalometaner i dricksvatten. Litteraturgenomgådering [Trihalomethane in drinking-water. Literature review and toxicologic evaluation], *Swedish National Laboratory of Environmental Medicine Report 1*. In Swedish.
Victorin, K. and Stenström, T., 1975. Nitratbildning i vattenledingsvatten, [Formation of nitrate in water supply systems], *Memorandum Series 650*, Swedish National Environmental Protection Board. In Swedish.
*von Bahr, B., Ehrenberg, L., Scalia-Tomba, G.-P. and Säfwenberg. J.-O., 1984b, Study of different models for dose-response relationships, *Swedish Departmental Series Ds S 1984:5*, Ministry of Health and Social Affairs. In Swedish.
Watson, A.F. and Mellanby, E., 1930, Tar cancer in mice; condition of skin when modified by external treatment or diet, as factors in influencing cancerous reaction, *Br. J. Exp. Pathol.*, **11**, 311–22.
Wattenberg, L.W. and Loub, W.D., 1978, Inhibition of polycyclic aromatic hydrocarbon-induced neoplasia by naturally occurring indoles, *Cancer Res.*, **38**, 1410–13.
*Westermark, T., 1984a, Models for the formation of mutagenic substances in food preparation and preservation. Possible formation of mutagenic substances in biological tissue through high effect pulses and contact with hot objects, *Swedish Departmental Series Ds S 1984:5*, Ministry of Health and Social Affairs. In Swedish.
Willett, W.C., Polkm, B.F. and Morris, J.S. *et al.*, 1983, Prediagnostic serum selenium and risk of cancer, *Lancet*, **ii**, 130–4.
Wynder, E.L., 1975, The epidemiology of large bowel cancer, *Cancer Res.* **35**, 3388–94.
Wynder, E.L. and Hirayama, T., 1977, Comparative epidemiology of cancers of the United States and Japan, *Prev. Med.*, **6**, 567–94.
Wynder, E.L. and Reddy, B.S., 1977, in Winnick, M. (Ed.) *Nutrition and Cancer*, p.55, New York: John Wiley.
Zaridze, D., 1983, *Epidemiology of prostatic cancer*, Lecture given at 3rd Congress of the European Society of Urological Oncology and Endocrinology, 24–26 November, Rome.
Zoeteman, B.C., Hrubec, J., deGreef, E. and Kool, H.J., 1982, Mutagenic activity associated with by-products of drinking water disinfection by chlorine, chlorine dioxide, ozone and UV irradiation, *Environ. Health Perspect.*, **46**, 197–205.

Section 4.4

*A literature survey on the presence of carcinogenic substances in the environment, IVL, 1980 (Institute for Water and Air Pollution Research, summary). (Unpublished.)

Albert, R.E., et al., 1983, Risk Anal. **3**, 101
Åkerstrand, K. and Josefsson, E., 1979, Mögel och mykotoxiner i böor och ärter [Moulds and mycotoxins in beans and peas], Vår Föda, **31**, 405–14. In Swedish.
Berlin, M. et al., 1977, Biologiskt index för och kromosomförändringar vid bensenexposition [Biological index of and chromosome changes due to benzene exposure], Report 771018, Institutions for Hygiene and Genetics, University of Lund. In Swedish.
Brandt, L., Nilsson, P.G. and Mitelman, F., 1978, Br. Med. J., March 4, 553.
Byrén, D. and Holmberg, B., 1974, Two possible cases of angiosarcoma of the liver in a group of Swedish vinyl chloride–polyvinyl chloride workers. Ann. NY Acad. Sci., **246**, 249–50.
Cederlöf R., Doll, R., Fowler, B., Friberg, L., Nelson, N. and Vouk, V. (eds), 1978, Air pollution and cancer: risk assessment methodology and epidemiological evidence. Report of a task group, Environ. Health. Perspect., **22**, 1–12.
Crouch, E. and Wilson, R. 1981, Regulation of carcinogens, Risk Analysis, **1**, 47.
Dich, J., Åkerstrand, K., Andersson, A., Lönberg, E., Josefsson, E. and Jansson, E., 1979, Konserveringsmedels förekomst och inverkan på mögel- och mykotoxinbildning i matbröd [Presence of preservatives and their effects on growth of mould and formation of mycotoxins in bread], Vår Föda, **31**, 385–403. In Swedish.
Doll, R. and Peto, R., 1981, The causes of cancer: quantitative estimates of avoidable risks of cancer in the United States today, JNCI, **66**, 1191–1308.
Dunkelberg, H., 1982, Carcinogenicity of ethylene oxide and 1,2-propylene oxide upon intragastric administration to rats, Br. J. Cancer, **46**, 924–33.
EEC, 1979, Council Directive 79/831.
*Ehrenberg, L., 1984c, Early warning systems (for detection of risk factors in populations/individuals), Swedish Departmental Series Ds S 1984:5, Ministry of Health and Social Affairs. In Swedish.
Ehrenberg, L., 1980, Methods of comparing risks of radiation and chemicals. The rad equivalence of stochastic effects of chemicals, in Radiobiological Equivalents of Chemical Pollutants, p. 23, Wien: International Atomic Energy Agency (IAEA).
*Ehrenberg, L., 1984a, An attempt to estimate cancer risks due to passive smoking, Swedish Departmental Series Ds 1984:5, Ministry of Health and Social Affairs. In Swedish.
Ehrenberg, L. and Törnqvist, M., 1984, Cancer risks due to pollutants in ambient air of urban areas, Swedish Departmental Series Ds S 1984:5, Ministry of Health and Social Affairs. In Swedish.
Ehrenberg, L., Moustacchi, E. and Osterman-Golkar, S. 1983. International commission for protection against environmental mutagens and carcinogens. Dosimetry of genotoxic agents and dose–response relationships of their effects, Mutat. Res., **123**, 121–82.
Ehrenberg, L., Osterman-Golkar, S., Segerbäck, D., Svensson, K. and Calleman, C.J., 1977, Evaluation of genetic risks of alkylating agents. III. Alkylation of haemoglobin after metabolic cnversion of ethene to ethene oxide in vivo, Mutat. Res., **45**, 175–84.
Englund, A.J., 1980, Toxicol. Environ. Health, **6**(516), 1267–73.
*Ericsson, S.-O., 1984, Case study—the presence of asbestos in relation to brake linings, clutches, thermal insulation, fire protection, etc., Swedish Departmental Series Ds 1984:1, Ministry of Health and Social Affairs. In Swedish.
*Excerpt from IARC'S 1982 summary (vol. 1–29) on the carcinogenic risks of chemicals to humans. (Unpublished.)
*Exposure data from the National Board of Occupational Safety and Health. (Unpublished.)
Forsberg-Karlsson, J., Ehrenberg, L., Osterman-Golkar, S. and Hussein, S., 1983, Quantitative risk estimate of genotoxic effects of benzo(a)pyrene (BaP), Report 1982 for the Swedish project Coal–Health–Environment, Technical Report Series 80, Statens Vatten Fallsverk [Swedish National Power Administration]. In Swedish.
Griesemer, R.A. and Cueto Jr, C., 1980, Toward a classification scheme for degrees of experimental evidence for the carcinogenicity of chemicals for animals, in IARC Sci. Publ. 27.
Gustafsson, K.H., 1981, Rester av etylenklorhydrin i vissa importerade industrikryddor

[Residues of ethylene chlorolydrin in certain imported spices], *Vår Föda*, **33**, 15–21. In Swedish.

Hammond, E.C. *et al.*, 1979, *Ann. NY Acad. Sci.*, **330**, 473–90.

Hardell, L., 1981, Epidemiological studies on soft-tissue sarcoma and malignant lymphoma and their relation to phenoxyacid or chlorophenol exposure, *Umeå University Medical Dissertations*, New Series, **65**.

Hogstedt, C., Malmqvist, N. and Wadman, B., 1979a, *J. Am. Med. Assoc.*, **241**, 1132–3.

Hogstedt, C., Rohlén, O., Berndtsson, B.S., Axelson, O. and Ehrenberg, L., 1979b, A cohort study on mortality and cancer incidence among employees exposed to chemicals in the production of ethylene oxide, *Br. J. Ind. Med.*, **36**, 276–80.

Holmberg, B. and Ahlborg, V., 1983, *Environ. Health Perspect.*, **47**, 1–30.

*Holmberg, B. and Säfwenberg, J.-O., 1984, Occupational cancer—a survey, *Swedish Departmental Series Ds S 1984:5*, Ministry of Health and Social Affairs. In Swedish.

Holmberg, B., Elofsson, S., Holmlund, L., Maasing, R., Molina, G. and Westerholm, P., 1979, Dödlighet och cancersjuklighet hos arbetare i svensk PVC-bearbetande industri [Mortality and cancer incidence of workers in the Swedish PVC-processing industry], in *Arbete och Hälsa 4*, Swedish National Board of Occupational Safety and Health. In Swedish.

Holmberg, B., Englund, A., Gumaelius, K., Holmlund, L., Kestrup, L., Maasing, R. and Westerholm, P., 1982, Retrospektiv kohortstudie över två svenska gummiindustrier [A retrospective cohort study of two Swedish industrial rubber plants], in *Arbete och Hälsa 34*, Swedish National Board of Occupational Safety and Health. In Swedish.

IARC, 1979, *IARC Monographs*, Vols 1–20 amd Suppl. 1.

IARC, 1982, Monographs on the evaluation of the carcinogenic risk of chemicals to humans; chemicals, industrial processes and industries associated with cancer in humans, *IARC Monographs*, Vols 1–29 and Suppl. 4.

Ishinishi, N. *et al.*, 1980, Carcinogenicity of beryllium oxide and arsenic trioxide to the lung of rat by an intratracheal instillation, *Fukuoka Iqaku Zasshi*, **71**(1), 19–26.

Johnsson, A. and Berg, A., 1978, Analys av 1,2-dibrometan, 1,2-dikloretan och bensen i omgivande luft [Analysis of 1,2-dibromethane, 1,2-dichloroethane and benzene in ambient air], *Memorandum Series 1122*, Swedish National Environmental Protection Board. In Swedish.

Josefsson, E. and Nygren, S., 1981, Volatile N-nitroso compounds in foods in Sweden, *Vår Föda*, **33**, suppl. 2, 147.

Joyner, R.E., 1964, *Arch. Environ. Health.*, **8**, 700–10.

Jung, Z., 1971, *Haupt. Geschlechskr.*, **46**, 35–6.

Lundberg, P., Svensson, E., Holmberg, B. and Hogstedt, C. 1983. Kriteriedokument för gränsvärden–polyaromatiska kolväten [Criteria documents of hygienic limit values–polyaromatic hydrocarbons], in *Arbete och Hälsa*, Swedish National Board of Occupational Safety and Health. In Swedish.

Löfroth, G. and Ames, B.N., 1978, Mutagencicity of inorganic coupounds in Salmonella typhimurium: arsenic, chromium and selenium (Abstr.), *Mutat. Res.* 53(1), 65–6.

Lynch, D.W., Lewis, T.R. and Moorman, W.J., 1982, Chronic inhalation toxicity of ethylene oxide and propylene oxide in rats and monkeys—a preliminary report, *The Toxicologist*, **2**, 11–12.

Mackay, D., 1979, Finding fugacity feasible, *Environ. Sci. Technol.*, **13**, 1218–23.

Mackay, D. and Paterson, S., 1981, Calculating fugacity, *Environ. Sci. Technol.*, **15**, 1006–14.

McPherson, K., Neil, A., Vessey, M.P. and Doll, R. 1983, Oral contraceptives and breast cancer (Letter), *Lancet*, **ii**, 1414–15.

*Memorandum, 1980 with certain information based on data from IARC and NCI (used by the Cancer Committee as a basis for an inventory of exposure data). (Unpublished.)

Morgan, R.W., Claxton, K.W., Divine, B.J., Kaplan, S.D. and Harris, V.B., 1981, *J. Occup. Med.*, **23**, 767–70.

NBOSH (National Board of Occupational Safety and Health), 1981, Exposure data submitted to the Cancer Committee. Unpublished document. In Swedish.

NBHW (National Board of Health and Welfare), 1981, Exposure data from the Department of Drugs. Unpublished. In Swedish.

NBHW (National Board of Health and Welfare), 1983, Department of Drugs official statement on carcinogen and mutagen effects plus toxic effects on reproduction of

metromidazole, tinidazole and ornidazole, in *Cirkulärskrivelse 1983:4*. In Swedish.
NEPB (National Environmental Protection Board (Naturvårdsverket)) 1981, Exposure data submitted to the Cancer Committee. Unpublished document. In Swedish.
NEPB (National Environmental Protection Board), 1982, Kadmium, förekomst, användning, bestämmelser. [Cadmium–occurrence, use, regulations], *Memorandum Series 1602*. In Swedish.
NFA (National Food Administration), 1981, Exposure data submitted to the Cancer Committee. Unpublished document. In Swedish.
NFA (National Food Adminstration), 1982, Pesticide residues in fruits and vegetables on the Swedish market 1976–1980, *Vår Föda*, **34** (Suppl. 3).
Nicholson, W.J. et al., 1981, Quantification of occupational cancer; Meeting March 29–April 2, 1981, *Banbury Report 9*, Cold Spring Harbor: Cold Spring Harbor Laboratory.
Nilsson, R. and Ehrenberg, L., 1984, Which conclusions can be drawn on cancer risks from epidemiologic and experimental data? *Swedish Departmental Series Ds S 1984:6*, Ministry of Health and Social Affairs.
NPCB (National Products Control Board), 1982, Exposure data submitted to the Cancer Committee. Unpublished document. In Swedish.
OECD, 1981/2, *Hazard Assessment Project OECD Working Party on Exposure Analysis, Final Report*, Berlin: Umweltbundesamt.
OECD, 1983, Provisional data interpretation guides (DIGs) for initial hazard assessment of chemicals, *ENV/CHEM/CM/83.3*, May, Paris.
Olin, G.R. and Ahlbom, A., 1980, *Environ. Res.*, **22**, 154–61.
Osborne, J.S., Adamek, S. and Hobbs, M.E., 1956, Some components of gas phase of cigarette smoke, *Anal. Chem.*, **28**, 211–15.
(OTA) (Office of Technology Assessment), 1981, *Assessment of Technologies for Determining Cancer Risks from the Environment*, June, Washington DC.
Pershagen, G. and Vahter, M., 1979, Arsenic. A toxicological and epidemiological appraisal, *Memorandum Series 1128*, Swedish National Environmental Protection Board.
Pershagen, G., Nordberg, G. and Björklund, N.-E., 1983, Carcinomas of the respiratory tract in hamsters given arsenic trioxide and/or benzo(a)pyrene by the pulmonary route, *Environ. Res.*, in press.
Pershagen, G., Wall, S., Taube, A. and Linnman, L. 1981, On the interaction between occupational arsenic exposure and smoking and its relationship to lung cancer, *Scand. J. Work. Environ. Health*, **7**, 302–9.
Persson, I. et al., 1983, Practice and patterns of estrogen treatments in climacteric women in a Swedish population. A descriptive epidemiological study. Part I, *Acta Obstet. Gynecol. Scand.*, **62**, 289–302.
Pike, M.C., Henderson, B.E., Krailo, M.D., Duke, A. and Roy, S., 1983, Breast cancer in young women and use of oral contraceptives: possible modifying effect of formulation and age at use, *Lancet*, **ii**, 926–30.
Pike, M.C., Robert, D., Gordon, J., Brian, D., Henderson, B.E., Herman, M.D., Menck, R. and SooHoo, J., 1975, Air pollution, in Fraumeni, J. (Ed.) *Persons at High Risk of Cancer*, New York: Academic Press. See also Pike, M.C. and Henderson, B.E., 1981, in Gelboin, H. and Tsó, P.O.P. (Eds) *Policyclic Hydrocarbons and Cancer*, Vol. 3, p. 317, New York: Academic Press.
Rossman, T.G., Meyn, M.S. and Troll, W., 1977, Effects of arsenite on DNA repair in *Escherichia coli.*, *Environ. Health Perspect.*, **19**, 229–33.
Rossman, T.G., Stone, D., Molina, M. and Troll, W., 1980, Absence of arsenite mutagenicity in *E. coli* and Chinese Hamster cells, *Environ. Mutagen.*, **2**, 371–9.
Rudnay, P. and Borzongi, M., 1981, The tumorigenic effect of treatment with arsenic trioxide, *Magyar Oncologia*, **25**, 73–7.
*Säfwenberg, J.-O., 1980, Notes on promoters, cocarcinogens and inhibitors (used by the Cancer Committee as a basis for an inventory of exposure data). (Unpublished.)
Sandberg, E., Vaz, R., Albanus, L., Mattsson, P. and Nilsson, K., 1982, Förorening i livsmedel av mjukgörande ämnen i plastfilm [Contamination of foods by plasticizers in plastic foil], *Vår Föda*, **34**(9–10), 470–82. In Swedish.
Simons, T.J., 1983, Development of three-dimensional numerical models of the Great Lakes, *Sci Ser. 12*, Ontario: Canada Center of Inland Water.

Simons, T.J., 1980, Circulation models of lakes and inland seas, *Can. Bull. Fish. Aquat. Sci.*, **203**.
Slorach, S. Gustafisson, J.-B., Jorhem, L. and Mattsson, F., 1983, Intake of lead, cadmium and certain other metals via a typical Swedish weekly diet. *Vår Föda*, Suppl. 1/83.
Snellings, W.M., Weill, C.S. and Maronpot, R.R., 1981, Final report on ethylene oxide two-year inhalation study in rats, *Project Report 44–20*, Bushy Run Research Center, PA.
Streisinger, G., 1983, Extrapolations from species to species and from various cell typoes in assessing risks from chemical mutagens, *Mut. Res.*, **114**, 93.
Swedish Special Panel, 1982, Risk assessments of certain pesticides. Background report to an *ad hoc* governmental committee on the use of chemicals in agriculture and forestry. *Library of Ministry of Agriculture, Stockholm.* In Swedish.
Swenberg., J.A. *et al.*, 1983, *Carcinogenesis* **4**, 945–52.
Takanaka, S. *et al.*, 1983, Carcinogenicity of cadmium chloride aerosols in rats, *JNCI*, **70**, 367.
Thiess, A.M., Schwegler, H., Fleig, I. and Stocker, W.G., 1981, *J. Occup. Med.*, **23**, 343–7.
Tomatis, L., 1979, *Ann. Rev. Pharmacol. Toxicol.*, **19**, 511–30.
*Törnqvist, M., 1984, Genotoxicity of NO_x in air pollution and of its reaction products including nitrite, *Swedish Departmental Series Ds S 1984:5*, Ministry of Health and Social Affairs. In Swedish.
US EPA (US Environmental Protection Agency), 1978, *Carcinogen Assessment Group's Report on Population Risk to Arsenic Exposures*. See also Anderson, E.L., 1982, in *Workshop on Quantitative Estimation of Risk to Human Health from Chemicals*, July 12, Rome, and WHO, 1981, Arsenic, *Environmental Health Criteria 18*, Geneva:WHO.
US EPA, 1979a, *Carcinogen Assessment Group's Final Report on Population Risk to Ambient Benzene Exposures*, 10 January.
US EPA, 1979b, Methodology for estimating direct exposure to new chemical substances, *EPA 560/13–79–008*, July, Washington, DC: Office of Toxic Substances.
US FDA (Food and Drug Administration) Bureau of Foods, 1982, *Toxicological Principles for the Safety Assessment of Direct /Food Additives and Color Additives Used in Food*, Washington, DC: Food and Drug Administration.
US National Research Council (Committee on diet, nutrition and cancer, Assembly of life sciences), 1982, *Diet, Nutrition and Cancer*, Washington, DC: National Academy Press.
*von Bahr, B., Ehrenberg, L., Scalia-Tomba, G.-P. and Säfwenberg, J.-O., 1984b, Study of different models for dose-response relationships, Swedish Departmental Series Ds S 1984:5, Ministry of Health and Social Affairs. In Swedish.
*Wall, S. and Taube, A., 1983, The Rönnskär case—an epidemiologic study of lifespan and mortality patterns among workers in a smelter industry, *Swedish Departmental Health Series Ds S 1983:5*, Ministry of Health and Social Affairs. In Swedish.
WHO, 1979. Mycotoxins, *Environmental health criteria 11*, Geneva: WHO.
Wilmot, W.A., 1976, A numerical model of the effects of reactor cooling water on fjord circulation I and II. Swedish Meteorological and Hydrological Institute Reports, *Hydrology and Oceanography, RHO 6*.
Wood, W.P., 1981, Comparison of environmental compartmentalization approaches. OECD Chemicals Group, Working Party of Exposure Analysis (EXPO), *Room Doc. 80.21*.

Section 4.5

Ambio, 1982, Nuclear war: the aftermath, pp. 112–13.
Anderstam, B., Hamnerius, Y., Hussain, S. and Ehrenberg, L., 1983, Studies of possible genetic effects in bacteria of high frequency electromagnetic fields, *Hereditas*, **98**, 11–32.
Åsard, P. E., 1982, *Strålskydd inom Sjukvården, Expertrapport, Röntgenverksamheten inom Stockholms Läns Landsting, Dimensionering och Organization [Radiation Protection in the Public Health Service. Expert Report on X-ray Use in Stockholm County]*, Stockholm County Council. In Swedish.

References

Astrup Jensen, A., 1982, Melanoma, flourescent lights, and polychlorinated biphenyls, (Letter), *Lancet*, **ii**, 935.
BEIR III, (Committee on the Biological Effects of Ionizing Radiations), 1980, *The Effects on Populations of Exposure to Low Levels of Ionizing Radiation*, Washington, DC: National Academy of Sciences.
Berâl, V., Evans, S., Shaw, H. and Milton, G., 1982, Malignant melanoma and exposure to fluorescent lighting at work, *Lancet*, **ii**, 290–3.
Cohen, B.L., 1982, Failures and critique of the BEIR III lung cancer risk estimates, *Health Phys.*, **42**, 267–84.
Crutzen, P.J., 1971, *J. Geophys. Res.*, **76**, 7311.
Crutzen, P.J., 1974, *Ambio*, **I**, 201.
Crutzen, P.J. and Birks, J.W., 1982, *Ambio*, **II**, 114.
Damber, L. and Larsson, L.G., 1982, Combined effects of mining and smoking in the causation of lung carcinoma, *Acta Radiol. Oncol.*, **21**, 305–13.
Edling, C., 1983, Doctorial thesis, Linköping. See also Axelson, O. *et al.*, *Scand. J. Work Environ. Health*, **5**, 10.
*Ehrenberg, L., 1974, Genetic toxicology of environmental chemicals, *Acta Biol, Yugosl. Ser. F. Genetika*, **6**, 367–98.
Ehrenberg, L., 1978, Dos–responssamband för biologiska effekter av joniserande strålning; tillämpning vid riskuppskattning[Dose–response relationships for biological effects of ionizing radiation; application in risk estimation], Report to the Swedish Energy Commission, *Swedish Departmental Series Ds I 1978:24*, 1:1–1:177. In Swedish.
Ehrenberg, L., 1984a, An attempt to estimate cancer risks due to passive smoking, *Swedish Departmental Series Ds S 1984:5*, Ministry of Health and Social Affairs. In Swedish.
*Ehrenberg, L., 1984b, Radiation risks and radiation protection A generally useful model, *Swedish Departmental Series Ds S 1984:6*, Ministry of Health and Social Affairs. In Swedish.
*Eklund, G., 1984, The Cancer Registry: trends in age—specific incidence, *Swedish Departmental Series Ds S 1984:4*, Ministry of Health and Social Affairs. In Swedish.
Elwood, J.H. and Lee, J.A.H., 1975, Recent data on the epidemiology of malignant melanoma, *Semin. Oncol.*, **2**, 149–54.
Farber, E. and Cameron, R. 1980, The sequential analysis of cancer development, *Adv. Cancer Res.*, **31**, 125–226.
Gellin, G.A., Kopf, A.W. and Garfinkel, L., 1969, Malignant melanoma. A controlled study of possibly associated factors, *Arch. Dermatol.*, **99**, 43–8.
Ham, W.T.Jr, Mueller, H.A. and Sliney, D.H., 1976, Retinal sensitivity to damage from short wavelength light, *Nature (London)*, **260**, 153–5.
Hersey, P., Bradley, M., Hasic, E., Haran, G., Edwards, A. and McCarthy, W.H., 1983, Immunological effects of solarium exposure, *Lancet*, **i**, 545–8.
Holman, C.D., Mulroney, C.D. and Armstrong, B.K., 1980, Epidemiology of preinvasive and invasive malignant melanoma in Western Australia, *Int. J. Cancer*, **25**, 317–23.
*Holmberg, B. and Ehrenberg, L., 1984, Origin of cancer: basic phenomana and theories, *Swedish Departmental Series Ds S 1984:5*, Ministry of Health and Social Affairs. In Swedish.
Hultqvist, B., 1956, Studies of naturally occurring radiations, *Kungl. Svenska Vetenskapsakademiens Handlingar* [Royal Swedish Academy Archives], 4th series, Vol. 6, No. 3.
ICRP, 1977, Publication 26, Recommendations of the International Commission on Radiological Protection, *Ann. ICRP*, **1**,(3).
IVA/BEEF, 1983, Biologiska effekter av hogspänningsledningars elektromagnetiska fält. [Biological effects of the electromagnetic fields of high voltage lines], Swedish Academy of Engineering Sciences (IVA), *IVA Report 240*. In Swedish.
Kvåle G., 1982, in Magnus, K. (Ed.) *Trends in Cancer Incidence*, p. 185, Washington, DC: Hemisphere.
Lancaster, H.O. and Nelson, J., 1957, *Med. J. Aus.*, April 6, 452.
Larsson, L.G. and Damber, L., 1982, Interaction between underground mining and smoking in the causation of lung cancer: A study of non-uranium miners in northern Sweden, *Cancer Detect. Prev.*, **5**, 385–89.

Lerman, S., 1980, *Ophthal. Res.*, **12**, 303. See also Lerman, S., 1980, *Radiant Energy and the Eye*, New York: MacMillan.
Lindell, B., 1978, Source-related detriment and the commitment concept: applying the principles of radiation to non-radioactive pollutants, *Ambio*, **7**, 250–9.
*Lindell, B., 1984, How large is a reasonably acceptable risk? *Swedish Departmental Series Ds S 1984:6*, Ministry of Health and Social Affairs. In Swedish.
Magnus, I.A. and Young, A.R., 1981, Modification of photocarcinogenesis by 5-methoxypsoralene and sunscreens, *Proc Int. Psoralene SIR, Paris*, pp. 371–81, Oxford: Pergaman Press.
Magnus, K., 1977a, *Cancer*, **40**, 389.
Magnus, K., 1977b, Incidence of malignant melanoma of the skin in the five Nordic countries: significance of solar radiation, *Int. J. Cancer*, **20**, 477–85.
Magnus, K., 1981, Habits of sun exposure and risk of malignant melanoma: an analysis of incidence rates in Norway 1955–1977 by cohort, sex, age, and primary tumor site, *Cancer*, **48**, 2329–35.
Magnus, K., (Ed.), 1982, *Trends in Cancer Incidence: Causes and Practical Implications*, Proceedings of a Symposium held in Oslo, Norway, 6–7 August 1980, Washington, DC: Hemisphere. See in particular papers by Muir, C.S. (p. 363), Muir, C.S. and Nectoux, J. (p. 365), Teppo, L. (p., 393), Armstrong B.K., Holman, C.D.J., Ford, J.M. and Woodings, T.L. (p. 399).
NBHW (Swedish National Board of Health and Welfare), 1976, Patientsäkerhet vid röntgenundersökningar. [Patient safety during X-ray examination], in *Socialstyrelsen Anser. 4*. In Swedish.
*NIRP, 1984, [Survey of Swedish collective radiation doses. Data from the National Institute of Radiation Protection] (presented by S. Grapergiesser), *Swedish Departmental Series Ds S 1984:2*, Ministry of Health and Social Affairs. In Swedish.
Radford, E.P., 1980, Human health effects of low doses of ionizing radiation: the BEIR III controversy, *Radiat. Res.*, **84**, 369–94.
Saxén et al., 1977, Epidemiology of lung cancer in Scandinavia, *IARC Sci. Publ. 16*, p. 217.
SEC, 1978, Energy, Report by the Swedish Energy Commission, *SOU 1978:49*, Stockholm: Liber Förlog. In Swedish.
Snihs, J.-O. et al., 1981, Radiation protection in Swedish mines, *Swedish National Institute of Radiation Protection Report 81-20*.
Sober, A.J., Lew, R.A., Fitzpatrick, T.B. and Marvell, R., 1979, Solar exposure patterns in patients with cutaneous melanoma–a case control series (meeting abstract), *Clin. Res.*, **27**, 536A.
Swanbeck, G. and Larkö O., 1982, Solljus och UV-strålning som orsak till hudcancer [Solar light and UV-radiation as a cause of skin cancers], *Nord Med.*, **97**, 277–9. In Swedish.
UNSCEAR (United Nations Scientific Committee on the Effects of Atomic Radiation), 1977, Report to the General Assembly, United Nations, New York.
UNSCEAR (United Nations Scientific Committee on the Effects of Atomic Radiation), 1982, *Ionizing Radiation: Sources and Biological Effects*, New York: United Nations.
US National Research Council, 1982, *The Committee on Chemistry and Physics of Ozone Depletion and the Committee on Biological Effects of Increased Solar Ultraviolet Radiation, Report*, Washington, DC: National Academy Press.
WHO (World Health Organization), 1984, *Effects of Nuclear War on Health and Health Services*, Report (1983) by an international expert group, Geneva: WHO.

Section 4.6

Archer, V.E., Gillam, J.D. and Wagoner, J.K. 1976, Respiratory disease mortality among uranium miners, *Ann. NY Acad. Sci.*, **271**, 280–93.
Archer, V.E. et al., 1973, *J. Occup. Med.*, **15**(3), 204–11.
Bingham, E. and Falk, H., 1969, The modifying effect of cocarcinogens on the threshold response. *Arch. Environ. Health*, **19**, 779–83.
Bohrman, J.S., 1983, Identification and assessment of tumor-promoting and cocar-

cinogenic agents: state-of-the-art in vitro methods, *CRC Crit. Rev. Toxicol.*, **11**(2).
Curtis, H.J. and Tilley, J., 1972, The role of mutations in liver tumor induction in mice, *Radiat Res.*, **50**, 539–42.
Curtis, H.J., Czernik, C. and Tilley, J., 1968, Tumor induction as a measure of genetic damage and repair in somatic cells of mice, *Radiat. Res.*, **34**, 315.
Hammond, E.C. et al., 1979, Asbestos exposure, cigarette smoking and death rates, *Ann. NY Acad. Sci.*, **330**, 473–90.
Hopkins, G.K. and Carroll, K.K., 1979, Relationship between amount and type of dietary fat in promotion of mammary carcinogenesis induced by 7,12-dimethylbenz(a)anthracene, *JNCI*, **62**, 1009–12.
Larsson, L.-G. and Damber, L., 1982, Interaction between underground mining and smoking causation of lung cancer: a study of nonuranium miners in Northern Sweden, *Cancer Detect. Prevent.*, **5**, 385–9.
Miettinen, O.S., 1982, Causal and preventive interdependence. Elementary principles, *Scand. J. Work Environ. Health*, **8**, 159–68.
Office of Technology Assessment (OTA), 1981, *Assessment of Technologies for Determining Cancer Risks from the Environment*, Washington, DC: GPO.
Pershagen, G., Wall, S., Taube, A. and Linnman, L., 1981, On the interaction between occupational arsenic exposure and smoking and its relationship to lung cancer, *Scand. J. Work Environ. Health*, **7**, 302–9.
Reddy, B.S., Narisawa, T. and Weisburger, J.H., 1976, Effect of a diet with high levels of protein and fat on colon carcinogensis in F344 rats treated with 1,2-dimethylhydrazine, *JNCI*, **57**, 567–9.
Reddy, B.S., Watanabe, K. and Weisburger, J.H., 1977, Effect of high-fat diet on colon carcinogenesis in F344 rats treated with 1,2-dimethylhydrazine, methylazoxymethanol acetate, or methylintrosourea, *Cancer Res.*, **37**, 4156.
Saffiotti, U., 1980, The problem of extrapolating from observed carcinogenic effects to estimates of risk for exposed populations, *J. Toxicol. Environ. Health*, **6**, 1309–26.
Saracci, R., 1981, in McDonald, J.C. (Ed.) *Recent Advances in Occupational Health*, Vol. 1, p. 119, Edinburgh: Churchill Livingstone.
*Wall, S. and Taube, A., 1983, The Rönnskär case—an epidemiologic study of lifespan and mortality patterns among workers in a smelter industry, *Swedish Departmental Health Series Ds S 1983:5*, Ministry of Health and Social Affairs. In Swedish.
Warwick, G.P., 1971, Metabolism of liver carcinogens and other factors influencing liver cancer induction, in *Liver Cancer, IARC Sci. Publ. 1*, pp. 121–57.
Wattenberg, L.W., 1977, Inhibitors of chemical carcinogenesis, *Adv. Cancer Res.*, **26**, 197–226.
Weisburger, J.H. and Weisburger, E.K., 1963, Pharmacodynamics of carcinogenic analyses of aromatic amines, and nitrosamines, *Clin. Pharmacol. Therap.*, **4**, 110.
Witschi, H., Williamson, D. and Lock, S., 1977, Enhancement of urethan tumorigenesis in mouse lung by butylated hydroxytoluence, *JNCI*, 58, 301.
Witschi, H.P., Hakkinen, P.J. and Kehrer, J.P., 1981, Modification of lung tumor development in A/J mice, *Toxicology*, **21**, 37–45.

Chapter 5.

*Berglund, K., Ekman, G. and Dzieciaszek, D., 1984, Influence of socio-economic variables on cancer incidence in the Swedish municipalities, *Swedish Departmental Series Ds S 1984:4*, Ministry of Health and Social Affairs. In Swedish.
Bolander, A.-M. and Lindgren, G., 1981, Material for the Swedish Cancer Committee 1981 (and later supplements) with elaborations of data from the Cause of Death Registry and the Cancer Registry, *Committee Records 46/81*. In Swedish.
Cairns, J., 1975, *Sci. Am.*, **233**, 64.
Cederlöf, R., Friberg, L., Hrubec, Z. and Lorich, U., 1975, *The Relationship of Smoking and Some Social Covariables to Mortality and Cancer Morbidity*, Parts 1 and 2, Stockholm: The Department of Environmental Hygiene, Karolinska Institute.
Doll, R., 1978, An epidemiological perspective of the biology of cancer, *Cancer Res.*, **38**, 3573–83.
Doll, R. and Peto, R., 1981, The causes of cancer: quantitative estimates of avoidable

risks of cancer in the United States today, *JNCI*, **66**, 1191–1308.
*Ehrenberg, L. and Ekman, G., 1984, Cancer diseases in Sweden: studies on variations in mortality and incidence, *Swedish Departmental Series Ds S 1984:4*, Ministry of Health and Social Affairs. In Swedish.
Einhorn, J., Rapaport, E., Wennström, G. and Wiklund, K., 1978, Cancer--miljöregistret tillgängligt för forskning [The Cancer–Environment Registry now available for research], *Läkartidningen*, **75**, 3415–17. In Swedish.
Einhorn, J. et al., 1980, *Cancer Risks and Environmental Factors, an Investigation Based on the New Cancer–Environment Registry*, Report to Arbetarskyddsfonden (the Swedish Work Environment Fund). In Swedish.
*Eklund, G., 1984., The Cancer Registry: Trends in age-specific incidence, *Swedish Departmental Series Ds S 1984:4*, Ministry of Health and Social Affairs. In Swedish.
*Ekman, G., Ehrenberg, L. and von Bahr, B., 1984, Diagnostic intensity, a confounding factor in epidemiologic analysis of the *CMR*, *Swedish Departmental Series Ds S 1984:4*, Ministry of Health and Social Affairs. In Swedish.
Hakulinen, T. and Pukkala, E., 1981, Future incidence of lung cancer: forecasts based on hypothetical changes in the smoking habits of males, *Int. J. Epidemiol.*, **10**, 233–40.
Hakulinen, T. and Pukkala, E., 1982, in Magnus, K. (Ed.) *Trends in Cancer Incidence*, p. III, Washington, DC: Hemisphere.
Hammond, E.C., 1966, *Natl Cancer Inst. Monogr.*, **19**, 127.
Johansson, L. and Ekman, G., 1983, Stockholm: Statistics Sweden. In press.
Kvåle, G., 1982, in Magnus, K. (Ed.) *Trends in Cancer Incidence*, p. 185, Washington, DC: Hemisphere.
Lynge, E., 1982, The Danish occupational cancer study, in *Prevention of Occupational Cancer–International Symposium, ILO Occupational Safety and Health Series 46*, Geneva:ILO.
Malker, H. and Weiner, J., 1984, Cancer–miljöregistret. Exempel På utnyttjande av registerepidemiologi inom arbetsmiljöområdet [The Cancer–Environment Register. Examples of the use of register epidemiology in the work environment field], Swedish National Board of Occupational Safety and Health, in *Arbete och häsa* 9. In Swedish.
Mellström, D., 1981, 'Life style, ageing and health among the elderly', Doctorial thesis, Göteborg.
NBHW (Swedish National Board of Health and Welfare, 1982, *Cancer Incidence in Sweden 1979*.
*Nilsson, R. and Ehrenberg, L., 1984, Which conclusions can be drawn on cancer risks from epidemiologic and experimental data? *Swedish Departmental series Ds S 1984:6*, Ministry of Health and Social Affairs.
Pettersson, F., Björkholm, E. and Karnström, L. 1982, in Magnus, K. (Ed.) *Trends in Cancer Incidence*, p. 293, Washington, DC: Hemisphere.
Sandstad, B., 1982, in Magnus, K. (Ed.) *Trends in Cancer Incidence*, p. 103, Washington, DC: Hemisphere.
Saxén, E.A., 1982, in Magnus, K. (Ed.) *Trends in Cancer Incidence*, p. 5, Washington, DC: Hemisphere.
*Swenson, D., 1984, A description of certain central registers of importance to cancer registration in the future, *Swedish Departmental Series Ds S 1984:4*, Ministry of Health and Social Affairs. In Swedish.
SCB (Statistics Sweden), 1965, *Smoking habits in Sweden. A Mail Survey–Spring 1963*, Stockholm. In Swedish but with table captions in English.
SCB (Statistics Sweden), 1981a, Mortality Environment Registry 1961–1970, *Memorandum series* **5**. In Swedish.
SCB (Statistics Sweden), 1981b, Dödstal efter kön, ålder och dödsorsak [Death rates by sex, age and cause of death], in *Statistiska meddelanden, HS 1981: 10.1–10.3*. In Swedish.
Teppo, L., Pukkala, E., Hakama, M., Hakulinen, T., Herva, A. and Saxén, E., 1980, Way of life and cancer incidence in Finland, *Scand. J. Soc. Med. Suppl.*, **19**, 1–84.
*von Bahr, B., Bolander, A.-M. and Ehrenberg, L., 1984. Cancer mortality as a function of age, marital status and region, studied by a weighted multiplicative Poisson model, *Swedish Departmental Series Ds S 1984:4*, Ministry of Health and Social Affairs. In Swedish.

*Wall, S. and Taube, A., 1983, The Rönnskär case—an epidemiologic study of lifespan and mortality patterns among workers in a smelter industry, *Swedish Departmental Health Series Ds S 1983:5*, Ministry of Health and Social Affairs. In Swedish.

Wiman, L.-G. and Jansson, O., 1980, in *Records from the Annual Meeting of the Swedish Medical Society, 1980*. Stockholm. In Swedish.

Chapter 6.

Adami, H.-O., 1977, Epidemiology and endocrinology in breast cancer. Results of a case control study, (Thesis) *Acta Universita Upsaliensis*, **286**.

Buckley, J.D., Doll, R., Harris, R.W., Vessey, M.P. and Williams, P.T., 1981, Case-control study of the husbands of women with dysplasia or carcinoma of the cervix uteri, *Lancet*, **ii**, 1010–15.

Cederlöf, R., Doll, R. Fowler, B., Friberg, L., Nelson, N. and Vouk, V. (Eds), 1978, Air pollution and cancer: risk assessment methodology and epidemiological evidence. Report of a task group, *Environ. Health Perspect.*, **22**, 1–12.

Doll, R. and Peto R., 1981, The causes of cancer: quantitative estimates of avoidable risks of cancer in the United States today, *JNCI*, **66**, 119–1308.

EHE, 1977, Energi–Hälsa–Miljöverkningar vid användning av fossila bränslen, [Energy-Health-Environment. Health and environmental effects from the use of fossil fuels], Report by a committee, *SOU 1977:68*, Stockholm: Liber Förlag. In Swedish.

*Ehrenberg, L. and Ekman, G., 1984, Cancer diseases in Sweden: studies on variations in mortality and incidence, *Swedish Departmental series Ds S 1984:4*, Ministry of Health and Social Affairs. In Swedish.

*Ehrenberg, L. and Törnqvist, M., 1984, Cancer risks due to pollutants in ambient air of urban areas, *Swedish Departmental Series Ds S 1984:5*, Ministry of Health and Social Affairs. In Swedish.

Einhorn J. et al. 1980, *Cancer Risks and Environmental Factors, an Investigation Based on the New Cancer-Environment Register*, Report to Arbetarskyddsfonden [the Swedish Work Environment Fund]. In Swedish.

Ekman, G., 1983, *Mutat. Res.*, 123, 180 (Appendix to Ehrenberg et al., *ibid.*, p. 121).

Fox, A.J. and Adelstein, A.M., 1978, Occupational mortality: work or way of life? *J. Epidemiol. Community Health*, **32**, 73–8.

Hammond, E.C., 1966, *Natl. Cancer Inst. Monogr.*, **19**, 127.

Higginson, J. and Muir, C.S., 1979, Environmental carcinogenesis: misconceptions and limitations to cancer control, *JNCI*, 63, 1291–8.

Hogstedt, C., Gustavsson, A. and Frenning, B., 1983, *Mortality and Exposure among Swedish Chimney Sweeps*, Report to Arbetarskyddsfonden (the Swedish Work Environment Fund) Project 80/67. In Swedish.

Holmberg, B. and Ahlborg, U. (eds), 1983, Proceedings of a symposium on Biological tests in the evaluation of mutagenicity and carcinogenicity of air pollutions with special reference to motor exhausts and coal combustion products, *Environ. Health Persp.*, **47**.

*Holmberg, B. and Ehrenberg, L., 1984, Origin of Cancer: basic phenomena and theories, *Swedish Departmental Series Ds S 1984:5*, Ministry of Health and Social Affairs. In Swedish.

Jenkins, C.D., 1983, Social environment and cancer mortality in men. *New Engl. J. Med.* 308, 395–8. See also Jenkins, C.D., 1984, *New Engl. J. Med.*, **310**, 130.

Kasl, S.V., 1984, Stress and health, *Ann. Rev. Publ. Health*, **5**, 319–41.

Lund, E., Zeiner-Henriksen, T., 1981, Smoking as risk factor for different forms of cancer among 26,000 men and women in Norway. Matching of the group of smokers with the cancer registry over a 12-year period, *Tidsskr. Nor. Laegeforen*, **101**, 1937–40.

MacMahon, B., Cole, P. and Brown, J., 1973, Etiology of human breast cancer: a review, *JNCI*, **50**, 21–42.

Malker, H., 1982, Swedish National Board of Occupational Safety and Health, Personal communication.

Malker, H. and Weiner, J. 1984, The Cancer–Environment Registry, Examples of the use of register epidemiology in the work environment field, Swedish National Board of Occupational Safety and Health, in *Arbete och hälsa 9*. In Swedish.

Möller, G. and Möller, E., 1975, Considerations of some current concepts in cancer research, *JNCI*, **55**, 755–9. See also Möller, E. and Möller G., 1976, Relevance of the immune system to the incidence of cancer, *Läkartidningen*, **73**, 3105–7.

Rogot, E. and Murray, J.L., 1980, Smoking and causes of death among U.S. veterans: 16 years of observation, *Publ. Health Rep.*, **95**, 213–22.

Skegg, D.C., Corwin, P.A., Paul, C. and Doll, R., 1982, Importance of the male factor in cancer of the cervix, *Lancet*, **ii**, 581–3.

*Törnqvist, M., 1984, Genotoxicity of NO_x in air pollution and of its reaction products including nitrite, *Swedish Departmental Series Ds S 1984:5*, Ministry of Health and Social Affairs. In Swedish.

US National Research Council, 1982, *Diet, Nutrition, and Cancer*, Report by a committee, Assembly of Life Sciences, Washington, DC: National Academy Press.

*Wall, S. and Taube, A., 1983, The Rönnskär case—an epidemiologic study of lifespan and mortality patterns among workers in a smelter industry, *Swedish Departmental Series Ds S 1983:5*, Ministry of Health and Social Affairs. In Swedish.

Wynder, E.L. and Gori, G.B., 1977, Contribution of the environment to cancer incidence: an epidemiologic exercise, *JNCI*, **58**, 825–32.

Chapter 7

*Ehrenberg, L., 1984b, Radiation risks and radiation protection: a generally useful model, in *Swedish Departmental Series Ds S 1984:6*, Ministry of Health and Social Affairs. In Swedish.

*Ericsson, S.-O., 1984, Case study—the presence of asbestos in relation to brake linings, clutches, thermal insulation, fire protection, etc., in *Swedish Departmental Series Ds S 1984:1*, Ministry of Health and Social Affairs. In Swedish.

ILO, 1974, *Convention on occupational cancer*, no. 139, article 2, Geneva.

ILO, 1977, *Occupational safety and health series* no. 39, Geneva.

*Lindell, B., 1984, How large is a reasonably acceptable risk?, *Departmental Series Ds S 1984:6*, Ministry of Health and Social Affairs. In Swedish.

*Nilsson, R. and Ehrenberg, L., 1984, Which conclusions can be drawn on cancer risks from epidemiological and experimental data? *Departmental Series Ds S 1984:6*, Ministry of Health and Social Affairs. In Swedish.

O'Riordan, T., 1979, Environmental impact analyses and risk assessment in a management perspective, in *Energy Risk Management*, G.T. Goodman and W.D. Rowe (eds), London: Academic Press, pp. 21–36.

Rall, D.P., 1978, Thresholds? *Environ. Health Perspect.*, **22**, 163–5.

*Soderbaum, P., 1984a, Actors' perspectives in health and environment protection, *Departmental Series Ds S 1984:6*, Ministry of Health and Social Affairs. In Swedish.

*Soderbaum, P., 1984b, Strategies for documentary basis of decision making, *Departmental Series Ds S 1984:6*, Ministry of Health and Social Affairs. In Swedish.

*Westermark, T., 1984b, Four case studies—cancer disease in industrial employees, environmental risks, counter - measures, costs, *Departmental Series Ds S 1984:1*, Ministry of Health and Social Affairs. In Swedish.

Chapter 8

*Ehrenberg, L., 1984c, Early-warning systems (for detection of risk factors in populations/individuals), *Departmental Series Ds S 1984:5*, Ministry of Health and Social Affairs. In Swedish.

Foster, F., 1980, Chief Health Statistician, Department of Health, New Zealand, Personal communication, *Swedish Cancer Committee Archives 6/79*.

*Swenson, D., 1984, A description of certain central registers of importance to cancer registration in the future, in *Swedish Departmental Series Ds S 1984:4*, Ministry of Health and Social Affairs. In Swedish.

*Wall, S. and Taube, A., 1983, The Rönnskär case—an epidemiological study of life span and mortality patterns among workers in a smelter industry, *Swedish Departmental Series Ds S 1983:5*, Ministry of Health and Social Affairs. In Swedish.

Chapter 9

Abortion Committee, 1983, Family planning and abortion, *SOU 1983:31*, Stockholm: Liber Förlag. In Swedish.
HS '90 Group, 1981a, Health risks. Report from the project 'Health Services in the 1990s', *SOU 1981:1*, Stockholm: Liber Förlag. In Swedish.
HS '90 Group, 1981b, Bases and guidelines for further work. Report from the project 'Health Services in the 1990s', *SOU 1981:4*, Stockholm: Liber Förlag. In Swedish.
NTS (Swedish National Smoking and Health Association), 1970, Smoking decreases in the USA. Interview with Dr D. Horn, *Tobaken och Vi*, **15**, 23–5. In Swedish.
Puska, P., 1983, Effectiveness of nutrition education strategies, Paper given at the plenary session of the 4th European Nutrition Conference, Amsterdam, 24-27.5.
Puska, P., McAlister, A., Pekkola, J. and Koskela, K., 1981, Television in health promotion: evaluation of a national programme in Finland, *Int. J. Health Educ.*, **24**(4).
Puska, P., Salonen, J.T., Nissinen, A., Tuomilehto, J., Vartiainen, E., Korhonen, H., Tanskanen, A., Rönqvist, P., Koskela, K. and Huttunen, J., 1983, Change in risk factors for coronary heart disease during ten years of a community intervention programme (North Karelia project), Br. Med. J., 287, 1840.
Qvarnström, U., Riis, U. and Svensson, P.-G., 1980, Care, education, information. Ideas of changes within the medical care system, *The Tema Series*, University of Linkoping. In Swedish.
Salonen, J. T., Puska, P., Kottke, T.E., Tuomilcheto, J. and Nissinen, A., 1983, Decline in mortality from coronary heart disease in Finland from 1969 to 1979, *Br. Med. J.*, **286**, 1857–60.

Chapter 10

Bruce, A., 1981, Swedish nutritional recommendations, *Vår Föda*, **33**, 354–72. In Swedish.
C Ex Committee, 1983, Cars and better air quality. Report of the Car Exhausts Committee, *SOU 1983:27*, Stockholm: Liber Förlag. In Swedish.
DHG (Diet and Health Group under the '1983 Food Committee'), 1984, Report. *Swedish Departmental Series J 1984:9*, Ministry of Agriculture. In Swedish.
Ehrenberg, L. and Ekman, G., 1983, Notes on aggregated analyses in an epidemiological study. (Unpublished.) *Cancer Committee Archives 37/83*. In Swedish.
*Ehrenberg, L. and Törnqvist, M., 1984, Cancer risks due to pollutants in ambient air, In *Swedish Departmental Series Ds S 1984:5*, Ministry of Health and Social Affairs. In Swedish.
Fagerström, K.-O., 1981, Tobacco smoking, nicotine dependence and smoking cessation (Doctorial thesis), *Acta Universita Upsaliensis*.
Hunt, W. A., Barnett, W. and Branch, L. G., 1971, Relapse rates in addiction programs, *J. Clin. Psych.*, **27**, 455–6.
*Lindvall, C., 1984, Food products and meals - different ways to reduce fat consumption, in *Swedish Departmental Series Ds nS 1984:6*, Ministry of Health and Social Affairs. In Swedish.
NACNE (National Advisory Committee on Nutritional Education), 1983, *Proposals for nutritional guidelines for health education in Britain*, London: The Health Education Council.
*NAMB (Swedish National Agricultural Market Board, Research and Analysis Division), 1984, The possibilities of reducing total fat intake through food pricing, in *Swedish Departmental Series Ds S 1984:6*, Ministry of Health and Social Affairs. In Swedish.
NEPB, 1981,. Decree regarding control of air pollution, etc., from gasoline fuelled automobiles, The Swedish National Environmental Protection Board, *Statue-code SNFS 1981:3, MS:2*, Stockholm: Liber Förlag. In Swedish.
NFA (Swedish National Food Administration), 1981, Dietary factors influencing the risk of cancer, *Vår Föda*, **33**, Suppl. 1.
NIEM, 1983, Cars and better air quality. Health risks from car exhausts, Report by the

National Institute of Environmental Medicine, SOU 1983:28, Stockholm: Liber Förlag. In Swedish.
*NIRP, 1984, Survey of Swedish collective radiation doses. Data from the National Institute of Radiation Protection (presented by S. Grapergiesse), *Swedish Departmental Series DSS 1984:2*, Ministry of Health and Social Affairs. In Swedish.
NPA (Swedish National Power Administration), 1983, Effects on health and the environment from the use of coal. Main report and two major background documents: No. 1 on techniques for the use of coal and No. 2 with detailed descriptions and analyses of health/environment effects. ISBN 91-7186-191-2 (189-0 and 190-4 respectively). In Swedish.
Radon Committee, 1983, Radon in houses, *SOU 1983:6*, Stockholm: Liber Förlag. In Swedish.
Rasmussen, S. et al., 1981, The relationship between indoor radon and lung cancer: a study of feasability of an epidemiological study, *MIT Technical Report EPA-1*.
SCB (Statistics Sweden), 1965, *Smoking Habits in Sweden. A Mail-Survey, Spring 1963*. In Swedish, but with table captions in English.
Slorach, S.A., 1981, Nitrate, nitrate and nitrosoamines consumption and health risks, *Vår Föda*, **33**, 324–34. In Swedish.
Spengler, J.D. and Sexton, K., 1983, Indoor air pollution: a public health perspective, *Science*, **221**, 9–23.
TC (Swedish Tobacco Committee), 1981, Report on reduced tobacco use, *SOU 1981:18*. In Swedish.
*Törnquist, M., 1984, Genotoxicity of NO in air pollution and of its reaction products including nitrite, in *Swedish Departmental Series Ds S 1984:5*, Ministry of Health and Social Affairs. In Swedish.
US National Research Council, 1982, Committee on diet, nutrition and cancer. Assembly of Life sciences, National Research Council, *Diet, Nutrition and Cancer*, Washington, DC: National Academy Press.
US Surgeon General, 1979, *Smoking and Health*, US Department of Health, Education and Welfare.
US Surgeon General, 1981, *The Health Consequences of Smoking: The Changing Cigarette*, US Department of Health and Human Services.

Chapter 11

Chemicals Commission, 1984, Report on the control of chemicals, *SOU 1984:77*, Stockholm: Liber Förlag. In Swedish.
*Holmberg, B. and Säfwenberg, J.-O., 1984b, Chemically induced cancer: Policy and scientific risk philosophy—an international outlook, in *Swedish Departmental Series Ds S 1984:6*, Ministry of Health and Social Affairs. In Swedish.
ILO, 1974, *Convention on Occupational Cancer 139*, Article 2, Geneva:ILO.
*Nilsson, R. and Ehrenberg, L., 1984, Which conclusions can be drawn on cancer risks from epidemiological and experimental data?, in *Swedish Departmental Series Ds S 1984:6*, Ministry of Health and Social Affairs. In Swedish.
OECD, 1982, Decision of the Council concerning the minimum pre-marketing set of data in the assessment of chemicals, *Document C(82)196*, Paris.
UHÄ, 1982, Toxicology: education, research, testing, Report by the Swedish National Board of Universities and Colleges, in *UHÄ Reports 26*. In Swedish.
US National Research Council, 1983, *Risk Assessment in the Federal Government: Managing the Process*, Washington,DC: National Academy Press.

Chapter 12

Atterstam, I., 1984, Doctor meets journalist: a collision between cultures? *Läkartidningen*, **81**, 2419–20. In Swedish.
EEC, 1979, Council Directive 79/831.
INRA, 1982, Report on information about risks in the working environment, *SOU 1982:30*, Stockholm: Liber Förlag. In Swedish.

LK, 1987, Report on drug legislation, *SOU 1987:20*, Stockholm: Liber Förlag. In Swedish.
MDN, 1982, Report on environmental information, *SOU 1980:24*, Stockholm: Liber Förlag. In Swedish.
OECD, 1983a, Recommendation of the Council concerning the OECD list of non-confidential data on chemicals, *Document C(83)98*.
OECD, 1983b, Recommendation of the Council concerning the protection of proprietary rights to data submitted in notifications of new chemicals, *Document C(83)96*.
Werkö, L., 1982, Scientists and mass media: how can they see eye-to-eye? *Làkartidningen*, **79**, 3041–2.

Chapter 13

From the specially prepared background documents, marked *, some key references have been extracted and included here, marked +. [*Ed. note.*]

+Ackerman, L.V. and Katzenstein, A.L., 1977, The concept of minimal breast cancer and the pathologist's role in the diagnosis of 'early carcinoma', *Cancer*, **39**, 2755–63.
+Andersson, I., 1980, Mammographic screening for breast carcinoma, Dissertation, Malmö.
Andersson, I., Bjurstam, H., Fagerberg, G., Hellström, L., Lundgren, B. and Tabâr, L., 1983, Breast cancer screening using mammography in Sweden, *Läkartidningen*, **80**, 2559–62. In Swedish.
+Beahrs, O.H., Shapiro, S. and Smart, C., 1979, Report of the working group to review the National Cancer Institute—American Cancer Society Breast Cancer Detection Demonstration Projects, *J. Natl. Cancer Inst.*, **62**, 641–709.
+Berlin, N., 1981, Breast cancer screening. The case for screening women younger than 50 years, *JAMA*, **245**, 1060.
Berrino, F., Chiappa, L., Olivero, S., Todeschin, P., Turolla, E. and Vegetti, P., 1979, Study of women who did not respond to screening for cervical cancer, *Tumori*, **65**, 143–55.
Blom, H. and Wilhelmsson, M., 1980, Having a breast tumour: reactions at health examination and diagnosis, in *Early Detection of Breast Cancer*, Scientific symposium, Swedish Cancer Society. In Swedish.
+Boyes, D.A., *et al.*, 1980, The foundations of cervical cancer screening: a cohort study of cervical cancer screening in British Columbia, *J. Epidemiol. Community Health*.
+Breslow, L., Thomas, L.B. and Upton, A. C., 1977, The National Cancer Institute *ad hoc* working groups on mammography in screening for breast cancer and a summary report of their joint findings and recommendations, *J. Natl. Cancer Inst.*, **59**, 468–541.
+British Breast Group, 1978, Screening for breast cancer. Statement by British Breast Group, *Br. Med. J.*, **2**, 178–80.
Canadian Task Force on the Periodic Health Examination, 1979, *Can. Med. J.*, **121**, 1–45.
+Clarke, E.A. and Anderson, T.W., 1979, Does screening by 'Pap' smears help prevent cervical cancer? A case control study, *Lancet*, **ii**, 1–4.
+Christopherson, W.H. and Scott, M.A., 1977, Trends in mortality from uterine cancer in relation to mass screening, *Acta Cytol.*, **21**, 5–9.
+Consensus Development Conference Statement, 1980, *Cervical cancer screening, 25 July 1980*, Bethesda: National Institutes of Health.
Council of Europe Public Health Committee, 1974, Screening as a tool of preventive medicine: a critical assessment of the organisational and economic aspects of screening, Report by a working party 1972–4, Strasbourg.
+de Waard, F., Rombach, J.J. and Colette, H.J.A., 1978, The DOM project for the early detection of breast cancer in the city of Utrecht, The Netherlands, in Miller, A.B. (Ed.) *Screening in Cancer*, Geneva: International Union Against Cancer.
+Eddy, D.M., 1980, *Screening for Cancer: Theory, Analysis and Design*, New York: Prentice-Hall.
+Ericsson, J., Mattson, B. and Petterson, F., 1975, Gynaecological Screening in Sweden—follow-up of woman examined 1967–70, *Läkartidningen*, **74**, 1047–9. In Swedish.
+Farrands, P.A., Griffiths, R.L. and Britton, D.C., 1981, The Frome Experiment—value

of screening colorectal cancer, *Lancet*, 6 June, 1231–2.
Fink, R., Shapiro, S. and Roester, R., 1972, Impact of efforts to increase participation in repetitive screenings for early breast cancer detection, *Am. J. Publ. Health*, **62**, 328–36.
Foster, R.S., Lang, S.P. Constanza, M.C., Worden, J.J., Haines, C.R. and Yates, J.W., 1978, Breast self-examination practices and breast cancer stage, *New Engl. J. Med.*, **299**, 265–70.
+Frumorgen, P. and Demling, L., 1979, Early detection of colorectal cancer with a modified Guiac test, in Winawer, S.J. (Ed.) *Colorectal Cancer: Prevention, Epidemiology and Screening*, New York.
+Gardner, J.W. and Lyon, J.L., 1977, Efficacy of cervical cytologic screening in the control of cervical cancer, *Preventive Medicine*, **6**, 487–99.
Gästrin, G., 1977, Self-examination for detection of breast cancer, *Lardsfingens Tidshrift*, **8**. In Swedish.
Gästrin, G., 1981, *Breast Cancer Control*, Stockholm: Almquist and Wiksell.
Gilbertsen V.A., McHugh, R., Schuman, L. and Williams, S.E., 1980, The earlier detection of colorectal cancers, *Cancer*, **45**, 2899–2901.
+Greegor, D.H., 1971, Occult blood testing for detection of asymptomatic colon cancer, *Cancer*, **28**, 131–4.
+Green, G.H., 1978, Cervical cancer and cytologic screening in New Zealand, *Br. J. Obstet. Gynaecol.*, **85**, 881–6.
Greenwald, P., Nasca, P.C., Lawrence, C.E., Horton, J., McGarrah, R.P., Gabriele, T. and Carlton K., 1978, Estimated effect of breast self-examination and routine physician examinations on breast cancer mortality, *New Engl. J. Med.*, **299**, 271–3.
Gyllensköld, K., 1976, *Of Course One Takes Fright. Talks With Women Treated for Breast Cancer*, Stockholm: Forum. In Swedish.
+Hakama, M., 1980, Mass screening for cervical cancer in Finland, in *Screening in Canada, A Report of the UICC International Workshop Toronto, Canada, 24–27 April, 1978, UICC Technical Report Series 40*, pp. 73–92.
*+Håkansson, S. and Jonsson, E., 1984, Costs of screening activities, in *Swedish Departmental Series Ds S 1984:3*. In Swedish.
Hansagi, H., Jakobsson, S. and Lundgren, B., 1980, Attitudes to screening for breast cancer—a population study, in *Early Detection of Breast Cancer*, Scientific symposium, Swedish Cancer Society. In Swedish.
+Hardcastle, J.D., Balfour, T.W. and Amar, S.S., 1980, Screening for symptomless colorectal cancer by testing for occult blood in general practice, *Lancet*, 791–3.
Hardcastle, J.D., Farrands, P.A., Balfour, T.W., Chamberlain, J., Amar, S.S. and Sheldon, M.G., 1983, Controlled trial of faecal occult blood testing in the detection of colorectal cancer, *Lancet*, **ii**, 1–4.
+Hastings, J.B., 1974, Mass screening for colorectal cancer, *Am. J. Surg.*, **127**, 228–33.
+Haugen, A., 1976, Mass screening for cancer of the uterine cervix in the county of Ostfold, Norway, *De PCa Symposium*, New York.
+Helfrich, G.B., Petrucci, P. and Webb, A., 1981, Mass screening for colorectal cancer planning, implementation, results, *International Symposium on Colorectal Cancer*, New York.
+Helm, G., Johnsson, J.-E. and Lindberg, L.-G., 1980, The impact of cytological screening on the incidence of invasive cervical cancer, *Acta Obstet. Gynecol. Scand.*, **59**, 271–3.
*Jakobsson, S., 1984, Mass-screening for breast cancer, in *Swedish Departmental Series Ds S 1984:3*, Ministry of Health and Social Affairs. In Swedish.
Kagan, A., Olsson, A., Shalit, B. and Levi, L., 1980. Identity of needs for psycho-social support in post-mastectomy (carcinoma of the breast) patients, *Internal Report 124*, Stress research laboratory, Karolinska Institute.
Kewenter, J., 1983, Personal communication.
Knox, E.G., 1980, Cancer of the uterine cervix. Information for planning control measures and for measuring their effectiveness, *UICC Symposium on Trends in Cancer Incidence*, Oslo, 5–8 August, 1980.
+Knox, E.G., 1982, Cancer of the uterine cervix, in Magnus, K. (Ed.) *Trends in Cancer Incidence. Causes and Practical Implications*, Washington, DC: Hemisphere.
+Kristein, M.M., 1980. The economics of screening for colorectal cancer, *Social Sci. Med.*, **14C**, 275–84.

+Land, C.E., 1980, Estimating cancer risks from low doses of ionizing radiation, *Science*, **209**, 1197–1203.
+Langeland, P., 1970, Population screening for female breast tumours. A clinical investigation, *Acta Radiol.*, Suppl., 297.
+La Salle, D. and Leffall Jr, 1981, Colorectal cancer—prevention and detection, *Cancer*, **47**, 1 March, Suppl.
+Lundgren, B., 1979, Population screening for breast cancer by single view mammography in a geographic region in Sweden, *JNCI*, **62**, 1373–9.
Lundgren, B. and Jakobsson, S., 1979, Single view mammography screening. Three year follow up of interval cancer cases, *Radiology*, **130**, 109–12.
+Melamed, M.R., Flehinger, B.J., Zaman, M.B., Heelan, R.B., Hallerman, E.T. and Martini, N., 1981, Detection of true pathological stage I lung cancer in a screening program and the effect on survival, *Cancer*, **47**, 1182–7.
+Miller, A.B., Lindsay, J. and Hill, G.B., 1976, Mortality from cancer of the uterus in Canada and its relationship to screening for cancer of the cervix, *Int. J. Cancer*, **17**, 602–12.
+National Board of Health and Welfare, 1976, Gynaecological mass screening in Sweden 1968–73, *Statistics HS 1976:1*
+National Cancer Institute Consensus Development Panel on Breast Cancer Screening, 1978, Statement on Recommendations, *J. Natl. Cancer Inst.*, **60**, 1523–4.
+Nou, E., Stenkvist, B. and Grafman, S., 1979, Bronchial carcinoma. A prospective 5 year study of unselected carcinoma population in a Swedish county, *Scand. J. Resp. Dis.*, Suppl. 104, 43–82.
*Pettersson, F., 1984a, Mass-screening according to Paparicolamos method, in *Swedish Departmental Series Ds S 1984:3*, Ministry of Health and Social Affairs. In Swedish.
*Pettersson, F., 1984b, Literature survey—Gynaecological health control, in *Swedish Departmental Series Ds S 1984:3*, Ministry of Health and Social Affairs. In Swedish.
Pinotti, J.A. and Borges, S.R., 1977, Effective follow-up of detected cases of cancer of the cervix uteri, *Bol. Off. Sanit. Panam.*, **82**, 223–36.
+Prescott, N. et al., 1980, Cost effectiveness of screening for occult blood in the stool: another look, *New Engl. J. Med.*, **303**.
Rimer, J. J., 1976, The impact of mass media on cancer control programs, in Cullen, J.W., Fox, B.H. and Isom, R.N. (Eds) *The Behavioural Dimensions*, New York: Raven Press.
Rudenstan, C.-M., 1984, Mass-screening for detection of tumours in the colon and rectum, in *Swedish Departmental Series Ds S 1984:3*, Ministry of Health and Social Affairs. In Swedish.
+Schneider, I. and Twiggs, L.B., 1972, The costs of carcinoma of the cervix, *Obstet. Gynecol.*, **40**, 851–9.
+Schwartz, M., 1978, A mathematical model used to analyse breast cancer screening strategies, *Operations Res.*, **26**(6).
+Schweitzer, S.O. and Luce, B.R., 1979, A cost-effective approach to cancer detection, *US DHEW, Publ. (PHS) 79–3237*, Washington, DC: National Center for Health Services Research.
+Shapiro, S., 1978, Efficacy of breast cancer screening, in Miller, A.B. (Ed.) *Screening in Cancer*, Geneva:International Union Against Cancer.
Siem, H., 1979, Mass screening and health controls, Groups on health services research under the Norwegian General Sciences Council, *Report 2*, Oslo. In Norwegian.
*Simonsson, B.G., 1984, Screening for early detection of lung cancer, in *Swedish Departmental Series Ds S 1984:3*, Ministry of Health and Social Affairs. In Swedish.
+Strax, P., 1977, The role of thermography as compared with mammography, *Int. J. Radiation Oncol. Bio. Phys.*, **2**, 751–2.
+Tabár, L. and Gad, A., 1981, Screening for breast cancer: the Swedish trial, *Radiology*, **138**, 219–22.
Tabár, L, et al., 1985, The first results from a randomized study in the count of Kopparberg and Östergötland (the W-E project). Reduced breast cancer mortality through health screening with mammography, *Läkartidningen*, **82**, 1551. In Swedish.
+Taylor, W.F., Fontata,R. S., Uhlenhopp, M.A. and Davis, C.S., 1981, Some results of screening for early lung cancer, *Cancer*, **47**, 1114–20.
Waldenström, U., 1981, *Do I have cancer? A Survey of Women's Experiences of Cervix*

Uteri Cell Changes, Report from Women's clinic, Falcon Hospital. In Swedish.
+Weiss, W., Samec, H.J., Gulz, W., Ruizer, E. and Neymahr, A., 1980, Erfahrungen mit dem Haemocculttest bei 8, 784 Patienten, *Wiener Klim Wschr I*.
+Widow, W. *et al.*, 1978, Roentgenographic chest screening in the detection and survival of patients with lung cancer, *Annals thoracic surgery*, **26**, 406–12.
+Winawer, S.J., Andrews, M., Flehinger, B., Sherlock, P., Schottenfield, D. and Miller, D.G., 1980, Progress report on controlled trial of fecal occult blood testing for the detection of colorectal neoplasia, *Cancer*, **45**, 2959–64.
+Winchester, P., Shull, H.J., Scanlon, E.F., Murrell, J.V., Smeltzer, C., Vrba, P., Iden, M., Sheelman, D.H., Magpayo, P., Dow, J.W. and Sylvester, J., 1980, A mass screening program for colorectal cancer using chemical testing for occult blood in the stool, *Cancer*, **45**, 2955–8.

Chapter 15

Einhorn, J., 1983, Patient information from random clinical studies, *Läkartidningen*, **80**, 4767. In Swedish.
MFR, 1983, Information from the Swedish Medical Research Council, 4, No. 3. In Swedish.
National Cancer Advisory Board, 1981, Decade of discovery—advances in cancer research 1971–81, *US Department of Health and Human Sciences NIH Publication 81-2323*.
Westermark, T., 1982, Chemical threats to the environment; a systematics of evaluation, *Bull. Sci. Tech. Soc.*, **2**, 171–8.

Appendix 3
Background documents

Background documents to the report	Published in
Cancer diseases in Sweden: Studies on variations in mortality and incidence L. Ehrenberg and G. Ekman	Ds S 1984:4
Cancer mortality as a function of age, civil status and region, studied by a weighted multiplicative Poisson model B. von Bahr, A.-M. Bolander and L. Ehrenberg	Ds S 1984a:4
Diagnostic intensity, a confounding factor in epidemiologic analysis of the CMR[*] G. Ekman, L. Ehrenberg and B. von Bahr	Ds S 1984:4
Influence of socio-economic variables on cancer incidence in the Swedish Municipalities K. Berglund, G. Ekman and D. Dzieciaszek	Ds S 1984:4
The Cancer Registry: Trends in age-specific incidence G. Eklund	Ds S 1984:4
A description of certain central registers of importance to cancer registration in the future D. Swenson	Ds S 1984:4
The Rönnskär-case—an epidemiologic study of lifespan and mortality patterns among workers in a smelter industry S. Wall and A. Taube	Ds S 1983:5

Origin of cancer: basic phenomena and theories B. Holmberg and L. Ehrenberg	Ds S 1984:5
Study of different models for dose-response relationships B. von Bahr, L. Ehrenberg, G.-P. Scalia-Tomba and J.-O. Säfwenberg	Ds S 1984b:5
Notes on promoters, cocarcinogens and inhibitors (used by the Cancer Committee as a basis for an inventory of exposure data) J.-O. Säfwenberg	Unpublished document (1980)
Genotoxicity of NO_2 in air pollution and of its reaction products including nitrite M. Törnqvist	Ds S 1984:5
An attempt to estimate cancer risks due to passive smoking L. Ehrenberg	Ds S 1984a:5
Models for the formation of mutagenic substances in food preparation and preservation. - Possible formation of mutagenic substances in biological tissue through high effect pulses and contact with hot objects T. Westermark	Ds S 1984a:5
Radiation risks and radiation protection: A generally useful model L. Ehrenberg	Ds S 1984b:6
How large is a reasonably acceptable risk? B. Lindell	Ds S 1984:6
Early warning systems (for detection of risk factors in populations/individuals) L. Ehrenberg	Ds S 1984:c
Memorandum with certain information based on data from IARC and NCI (used by the Cancer Committee as a basis for an inventory of exposure data)	Unpublished document (1980)
Exposure data from the National Board of Occupational Safety and Health	Unpublished document (1980)

Exposure data from the National Environment Protection Board	Unpublished document (1981)
A literature survey on the presence of carcinogenic substances in the environment (the Institute for Water and Air Pollution Research. Summary)	Unpublished document (1980)
Exposure data from the National Food Administration	Unpublished document (1981)
Exposure data from the Department of Drugs of the National Board of Health and Welfare	Unpublished document (1981)
Mass-screening for breast cancer S. Jakobsson	Ds S 1984:3
Mass-screening according to Papanicolauos method F. Pettersson	Ds S 1984a:3
Literature survey—gynaecological health control F. Pettersson	Ds S 1984b:3
Mass-screening for detection of tumours in the colon and rectum C.-M. Rudenstam	Ds S 1984:3
Screening for early detection of lung-cancer Bo G. Simonsson	Ds S 1984: 3
Costs of screening activities S. Håkansson and E. Jonsson	Ds S 1984:3
Exposure data from the National Products Control Board	Unpublished document (1982)
Survey of Swedish collective radiation doses. Data from the National Institute of Radiation Protection	Ds S 1984:2

Case study—the presence of asbestos in relation to brake linings, clutches, thermal insulation, fire protection, etc. S.-O. Ericsson, Consulting Engineer	Ds S 1984:1
Occupational cancer—a survey B- Holmberg and J.-O. Säfwenberg	Ds S 1984a:5
Cancer risks due to pollutants in ambient air of urban areas L. Ehrenberg and M. Törnqvist	Ds S 1984:5
Actors' perspectives in health and environment protection P. Söderbaum	Ds S 1984a:6
Excerpt from IARC's 1982 summary (vol. 1–29) on the carcinogenic risks of chemicals to humans	Unpublished document
Strategies for documentary basis of decision making P. Söderbaum	Ds S 1984b:6
The possibilities of reducing total fat intake through food pricing The National Agricultural Market Board, Research and Analysis Division	Ds S 1984:6
Food products and meals—different ways to reduce fat consumption C. Lindvall	Ds S 1984:6
Which conclusions can be drawn on cancer risks from epidemiologic and experimental data? R. Nilsson and L. Ehrenberg	Ds S 1984:6
Chemically induced cancer: Policy and scientific risk philosophy—an international out-look B. Holmberg and J.-O. Säfwenberg	Ds S 1984b:6
The Rönnskär case—an epidemiologic study of lifespan and mortality patterns among workers in a smelter industry	Ds S 1983:5
Some case-studies on measures to reduce cancer risks	Ds S 1984:1
Survey of Swedish collective radiation doses	Ds S 1984:2
Mass-screening for early diagnosis of cancer	Ds S 1984:3
Cancer diseases in Sweden, variations in incidence and mortality, etc.	Ds S 1984:4
Certain medical/scientific aspects on cancer risks	Ds S 1984:5

*Accronym for a data-file obtained from the Swedish Cancer Registry and the 1960 population census, containing i.a. information on an individual basis.

Appendix 4
Committee members and experts

The Swedish Cancer Committee was set up by the Government in the middle of 1979 and finished its task by the end of 1984. The following information pertains to this period, with some up-dating.

Full members

K. Sune D. Bergström
MD; Nobel laureate; Professor of Chemistry, the Karolinska Institute; Emeritus 1981; Chairman of the Cancer Committee.

Engelsbrektsgatan 21
S-114 32 Stockholm

Lars G. Ehrenberg
PhD; Professor of Radiobiology, Stockholm University; Emeritus 1987.

Institutionen för radiobiologi
Stockholms universitet
S-106 91 Stockholm

Jerzy Einhorn
MD; Professor of Radiotherapy, the Karolinka Institute; Head of the Oncological Centre at the Karolinska Hospital.

Karolinska sjukhuset
Radiumhemmet
Box 60500
S-104 01 Stockholm

Lars T. Friberg
MD; Professor of Public Health Sciences, the Karolinska Institute; Director, National Institute of Environmental Medicine; Emeritus 1986.

Institutet för miljömedecin
Box 60208
S-104 01 Stockholm

Bengt E. Gustafsson
MD; OD; Professor of Medical
Symbiology, the Karolinska
Institute.

(Deceased)

Karin Gyllensköld
PhD; Associate Professor in
Educational Psychology, Stockholm
University.

Karolina Institutet
Department of Psychotherapy
Stadshagsgården
Sit Göransgatan 126, vån 13
S-112 45 Stockholm

Bo E.G. Holmberg
PhD; Professor and Head of
Division, National Institute of
Occupational Medicine.

Arbetsmiljöinstitutet
Ekelundsvägen 16
S-171 84 Solna

Lars-Gunnar Larsson
MD; Professor and Head of the
Oncological Centre at Umeå
Regional Hospital; Emeritus 1985.

Östra Kyrkogatan 21
S-902 45 Umeå

Lars H. Lindau
MEng; Head of Technical
Department, National
Environmental Protection Board.

Statens Naturvårdsverk
S-171 85 Solna

Curt Mileikowsky
DEng; Associate Professor in
Physics, Royal Institute of
Technology; Industrialist.

Ulla M. Swarén
Pharm.L; Head of Chancery,
Swedish Council of Environmental
Information; from 1982 Chief
Secretary, Cancer Committee; from
1985 Senior Adviser, National
Environmental Protection Board.

Statens Naturvårdsverk
S-171 85 Solna

O. Peter W. Söderbaum
PhD; Asociate Professor in Natural
Resources Economy, Swedish
University of Agricultural Sciences.

Institutionen för ekonomi
Sveriges Lantbruksuniversitet
Box 7013
S-750 07 Uppsala

Thorsten K.L. Thor
Head of Planning and
Rationalization Institute of the
swedish Health and Social Services
(SPRI); from 1988 Manager,
County Council of Kristianstad.

Landstinget
Box 522
S-291 25 Kristianstad

E.G. Torbjörn Westermark
DEng; Professor of Nuclear
Chemistry, Royal Institute of
Technology; Emeritus 1988.

Lalugaardsvägen 5
S-183 38 Täby

Associated experts

Sven Alsén
MD; Assistant Director General,
National Board of Health and
Welfare; Retired 1982.

Trollvägen 26
S-133 34 Saltsjöbaden

Anders B. Englund
MD; Chief Secretary, Cancer
Committee; from 1982 Executive
Director, Union International
Contre le Cancer; from 1985
Medical Director, Swedish
Construction Industry Foundation
for Industrial Safety and Health.

Bygghälsan
Box 706
S-182 17 Danderyd

E. Birgitta Liliewall
BL; Ministry of Health and Social
Affairs; from 1986 another
Government organization within
the health care area.

Hälso- och sjukvårdens
ansvarsnåmnd
Box 3539
S-103 69 Stockholm

Besides the associated experts above, appointed by the Government, the Cancer Committee received assistance from several other experts most of whom are found among the authors of background documents according to Appendix 3.

With particular reference to matters regarding 'diet and cancer' there was a contribution from:

Jan-Åke Gustafsson
MD; Professor of Medical
Nutrition, the Karolinska Institute.

Center for Nutrition and
Toxicology
Novum
S-141 57 Huddinge